Laryngology

A Case-Based Approach

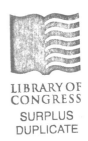

Laryngology

A Case–Based Approach

Jacqueline Allen, MBChB, FRACS, ORL-HNS
S. A. Reza Nouraei, MBBChir, PhD, FRCS, FRCS (ORL-HNS)
Guri S. Sandhu, MBBS, MD, FRCS, FRCS (ORL-HNS), hon FRAM

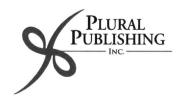

PLURAL
PUBLISHING
INC.

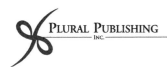

5521 Ruffin Road
San Diego, CA 92123

e-mail: information@pluralpublishing.com
Web site: https://www.pluralpublishing.com

Typeset in 10/12 Palatino by Achorn International
Printed in the United States of America by Integrated Books International

NOTICE TO THE READER
Care has been taken to confirm the accuracy of the indications, procedures, drug dosages, and diagnosis and remediation protocols presented in this book and to ensure that they conform to the practices of the general medical and health services communities. However, the authors, editors, and publisher are not responsible for errors or omissions or for any consequences from application of the information in this book and make no warranty, expressed or implied, with respect to the currency, completeness, or accuracy of the contents of the publication. The diagnostic and remediation protocols and the medications described do not necessarily have specific approval by the Food and Drug administration for use in the disorders and/or diseases and dosages for which they are recommended. Application of this information in a particular situation remains the professional responsibility of the practitioner. Because standards of practice and usage change, it is the responsibility of the practitioner to keep abreast of revised recommendations, dosages, and procedures.

Library of Congress Cataloging-in-Publication Data

Names: Allen, Jacqueline, author. | Nouraei, S. A. Reza (Seyed Ahmad Reza), author. |
    Sandhu, Guri S. (Guri Singh), author.
Title: Laryngology : a case-based approach / Jacqueline Allen, S. A. Reza Nouraei, Guri Sandhu.
Description: San Diego, CA : Plural Publishing, Inc., [2020] |
    Includes bibliographical references and index.
Identifiers: LCCN 2019022602 | ISBN 9781944883591 (paperback) |
    ISBN 1944883592 (paperback) | ISBN 9781944883621 (ebook)
Subjects: MESH: Otorhinolaryngologic Diseases | Child | Adult | Case Reports
Classification: LCC RF46 | NLM WV 140 | DDC 617.5/1—dc23
LC record available at https://lccn.loc.gov/2019022602

Contents

Foreword

When I was an otolaryngology resident, every textbook that I owned was organized by topics. They were all similar structure—they started with anatomy and physiology and then went into detailed descriptions of individual conditions/procedures. Most of the lectures we received were similarly ordered. This is how I learned. This is how most of us learned.

When I started as a junior Attending and was asked to give lectures to the residents, I followed what I knew—I started with anatomy/physiology and then expounded on the individual condition or surgical procedure. Although informative, I often found it difficult to engage the residents. Many would nod off in that dark room. I was also not convinced that the material helped them much when they came across a patient with complex issues that didn't "fit" the textbook descriptions. After a few years, I switched to a case-based approach, with positive results. The residents seemed more alert and attentive and I felt that they were really able to apply that knowledge to actual cases that they saw in clinic.

Over the years, education theory has shifted away from the "classic curriculum" that has relied on facts and figures to more progressive education styles. Case-based learning (CBL) is popular in many fields, including business, law, and now, medicine. CBL is learner centered and relies on real work scenarios to teach concepts. Cases often offer a wealth of information and the instructor has the freedom to explore many topics, as guided by the discussion. Learners tend to relate to the content and therefore are typically more engaged. Overall, I have found CBL a great tool and have incorporated it in my educational endeavors.

This book brings the concept of CBL to print form. While similar texts do exist, this one is quite comprehensive, covering almost every topic in modern laryngology. The book is also unique in that it includes contributions from renowned laryngeal specialists from many parts of the world, giving it a unique multinational flavor not found in competing texts. Given all this, this text stands to become a "must read" for the serious student of laryngology. I am excited to be a part of it.

Milan R. Amin, MD

Preface

Communication and social interaction are characteristics that define human culture and enrich our social fabric. The ability to speak and engage in discourse has been admired since civilization began. For the third of the population who make their living using their voice, any disturbance or perturbation in vocal ability may have devastating consequences. Even now most social gatherings revolve around good food, good wine, and good company. The social stigmatization of not being able to participate in a family meal or order and eat food from a menu, or wearing a tracheostomy or feeding tube impacts patients of all ages, ethnicities, and genders. This is what makes laryngology a critical and relevant specialty.

In the age of celebrity chefs and pop music stars, laryngologists play a key role in managing the problems and expectations of both professionals and the general public. It is hugely satisfying to help return phonation to the voiceless and diet to the dysphagic. It is what drives us and pushes us to explore novel pathways.

This book examines cases that appear in laryngology clinics every day. Some are common and others rare; however, each one requires thoughtful assessment and management. We have had the good fortune of collaborating with some of the leading experts in global laryngology who have given their knowledge, expertise, and experience to provide the cases for this book and to discuss the varied management options as they see it. While every surgeon has her/his own personal approach, these illustrative cases demonstrate the breadth of options and critical thinking needed to give your patients the best care. We are most grateful to the many contributors who have given their time and effort unstintingly and have helped us create a book that we feel is practical, current, and comprehensive. We hope that you will enjoy and find useful the case discussions, and recognize among these cases patients with whom you have dealt or will see in the future.

Jacqueline Allen, MBChB, FRACS ORL-HNS
S. A. Reza Nouraei, MBBChir, PhD, FRCS, FRCS (ORL-HNS)
Guri S. Sandhu, MBBS, MD, FRCS, FRCS (ORL-HNS), hon FRAM

Contributors

Lacey Adkins, MD
Assistant Professor
Department of Otolaryngology–Head and Neck Surgery
Louisiana State University Health Sciences Center
    New Orleans
Baton Rouge, Louisiana
Chapter 53

Jahangir Ahmed, MA(CANTAS), FRCS-ORL-HNS, PhD
Consultant Head and Neck Surgeon
Barts Health NHS Trust
The Royal London Hospital
London, United Kingdom
Chapters 29 and 41

Jacqueline Allen, MBChB, FRACS ORL-HNS
Laryngologist
University of Auckland
Auckland, New Zealand
Chapters 7, 43, 51, and 55

Theodore Athanasiadis, PhD, FRACS ORL-HNS
Flinders University
Adelaide, South Australia
Chapter 46

Michael S. Benninger, MD
Chairman, Head and Neck Institute
The Cleveland Clinic
Professor and Chair
Department of Otolaryngology–Head and Neck Surgery
Cleveland Clinic Lerner College of Medicine
Cleveland, Ohio
Chapter 26

Jane Bickford, BAppSc (SpPath), PhD, CPSP
Senior Lecturer, Speech Pathology
College of Nursing and Health Sciences
Flinders University
Adelaide, Australia
Chapter 49

Sarah N. Bowe, MD
Pediatric Otolaryngology Fellow
Department of Otolaryngology
Massachusetts Eye and Ear Infirmary
Boston, Massachusetts
Chapter 5

Matthew Broadhurst, MD, FRACS
Director, Queensland Voice Centre
Director, Queensland Centre for Otolaryngology
Queensland, Australia
Chapter 23

Raymond Brown, MD
Department of Otolaryngology-Head and Neck Surgery
UT Health San Antonio
San Antonio, Texas
Chapter 12

Paul C. Bryson, MD, FACS
Associate Professor of Otolaryngology-Head and
    Neck Surgery
Director, Voice Center
Head, Section of Laryngology
Cleveland Clinic
Cleveland, Ohio
Chapter 21

Hannah Burns, MBBS, BSc, FRACS
Visiting Medical Officer
Department of Otolaryngology
Queensland Children's Hospital
Senior Lecturer
University of Queensland
Brisbane, Australia
Chapter 4

Colin R. Butler, PhD, FRCS (ORL-HNS)
Pediatric ENT Fellow
Great Ormond Street Hospital
London, United Kingdom
Chapter 30

Dinesh Chhetri, MD
Professor of Head and Neck Surgery
UCLA Voice Center for Medicine and the Arts
University of California, Los Angeles
Los Angeles, California
Chapter 3

Lesley F. Childs, MD
Assistant Professor of Otolaryngology–Head and
    Neck Surgery
Associate Medical Director
Clinical Center for Voice Care
University of Texas Southwestern Medical Center
Dallas, Texas
Chapter 15

Declan Costello, MA, MBBS, FRCS (ORL-HNS)
Consultant
Ear, Nose, and Throat Surgeon
Laryngologist
Queen Elizabeth Hospital
Birmingham, United Kingdom
Chapter 22

Anna Pamela C. Dela Cruz, MD
Department of Otorhinolaryngology
University of the Philippines
Philippine General Hospital
Manila, Philippines
Chapter 44

Sebastian Doeltgen, PhD, MSP(Dist)
Associate Professor
Head of Teaching Section, Speech Pathology
College of Nursing and Health Sciences
Flinders University
Adelaide, Australia
Chapter 49

Lisa A. D'Oyley, MS, CCC-SLP
Supervisor, Speech Language Pathology
Department of Otolaryngology–Head and Neck Surgery
University of Washington Medical Center
Chapter 24

Kranthi Earasi, MD
Doctor of Medicine
Drexel University College of Medicine
Philadelphia, Pennsylvania
Chapter 19

Alexandar Gelbard, MD
Associate Professor
Co-Director, Vanderbilt Center for Complex Airway
    Reconstruction
Department of Otolaryngology, Vanderbilt University
    School of Medicine
Nashville, Tennessee
Chapter 38

Nick Gibbons, FRCS (ORL-HNS), MD
Consultant Otolaryngologist and Voice Surgeon
University Hospital Lewisham
London, United Kingdom
Chapter 20

Christopher J. Hartnick, MD
Professor
Department of Otology and Laryngology
Harvard Medical School
Division Director, Pediatric Otolaryngology
Director, Pediatric Airway, Voice, and Swallowing
    Center
Chief Quality Officer for Otolaryngology
Boston, Massachusetts
Chapter 5

Georgina Harris, BSc, MBBS, FRACS
ENT Consultant
St. Vincent's Hospital
Laryngologist
Voice Assessment Centre
St. Vincent's Clinic
Sydney, Australia
Chapter 9

Kate J. Heathcote, FRCS (ORL-HNS)
Consultant and ENT Surgeon
The Robert White Centre for Airway Voice and
    Swallowing
Pool Hospital NHS Foundation Trust
Poole, United Kingdom
Chapter 31

Mandy Henderson, MSc
Speech-Language Pathologist
Starship Children's Hospital
Auckland, New Zealand
Chapter 10

Matthew R. Hoffman, MD, PhD
Division of Otolaryngology
Department of Surgery
University of Wisconsin School of Medicine and
    Public Health
Madison, Wisconsin
Chapter 28

Maggie-Lee Huckabee, PhD
Director
UC Rose Centre for Stroke Recovery and Research
Professor
Department of Communication Disorders
The University of Canterbury
Christchurch, New Zealand
Chapter 484

James H. Hull, PhD, FRCP
Consultant Repertory Physician
Royal Brompton Hospital
London, United Kingdom
Chapters 36, 37, and 47

Aphrodite Iacovidou, MBChB, MSc, MRCS (ENT)
ENT Department
Imperial College Healthcare NHS Trust
London, United Kingdom
Chapter 40

Aaron J. Jaworek, MD
Clinical Assistant Professor
Department of Otolaryngology–Head and Neck
  Surgery
Drexel University College of Medicine
Philadelphia, Pennsylvania
Specialty Physician Associates
Bethlehem, Pennsylvania
Chapter 19

Michael M. Johns III, MD
Director
USC Voice Center
Professor
Otolaryngology Head and Neck Surgery
University of Southern California
Los Angeles, California
Chapter 33

James J. Johnston, MBChB, PhD
University of Auckland
Auckland, New Zealand
Chapter 7

Andrew J. Kinshuck, DOHNS, MD, FRCS (ORL-HNS)
Consultant Otolaryngology and Head and Neck Surgery
Aintree University Hospital
Liverpool, United Kingdom
Chapters 36 and 47

Maggie Kuhn, MD, MAS
Assistant Professor
Otolaryngology–Head and Neck Surgery
University of California, Davis
Sacramento, California
Chapter 50

Melda Kunduk, PhD, CCC-SLP
Associate Professor
Department of Communication Sciences and Disorders
Louisiana State University
Baton Rouge, Louisiana
Chapter 53

Andrée-Anne Leclerc, MSc, MD, FRCS
Division of Otolaryngology
University of Montréal
Montréal, Quebec, Canada
Chapters 16 and 35

Rebecca Leonard, PhD
Professor Emeritus
Department of Otolaryngology–Head and Neck Surgery
University of California, Davis
Sacramento, California
Chapter 34

Wendy Liu, MD, MBBS
Resident Medical Officer
Royal North Shore Hospital
Sydney, Australia
Chapter 52

Peter Loizou, BSc (Hons), BM, DOHNS, MRCS (Eng), MEd, DIC FRCS (ORL-HNS)
Postgraduate Fellow
Head and Neck Surgery
Westmead Hospital
Sydney, Australia
Chapter 52

Albert L. Merati, MD, FACS
Professor, Chief, Division of Laryngology
Department of Otolaryngology–Head and Neck Surgery
University of Washington
Chapter 24

Alasdair D. Mace, MB, BS, DLO, FRCS (ORL-MNS)
Consultant Otolaryngologist, Head and Neck
Clinical Lead for Head and Neck Cancer
Imperial College Healthcare NHS Trust
London, United Kingdom
Chapter 41

Ken MacKenzie, MBChB, FRCS(Ed)
Visitor Professor, School of Psychological Sciences
 and Health
University of Strathclyde, Glasgow
Consultant Otorhinolaryngologist Head and Neck
 Surgery
Queen Elizabeth University Hospital
Glasgow, United Kingdom
Chapter 17

Phoebe Macrae, PhD
Senior Lecturer
University of Canterbury
Deputy Director
Rose Centre for Stroke Recovery and Research
Christchurch, New Zealand
Chapter 48

Murali Mahadevan, MBChB, FRACS
Adjunct Associate Professor
University of Auckland
ORL Surgeon, Starship, ADHB
Auckland, New Zealand
Chapter 8

Silvia G. Marinone-Lares, MD
Department of Otolaryngology–Head and Neck
 Surgery
Auckland District Health Board
Auckland, New Zealand
Chapters 8 and 55

Ted Mau, MD, PhD
Professor
Director, Clinical Center for Voice Care
Department of Otolaryngology–Head and Neck Surgery
University of Texas Southwestern Medical Center
Dallas, Texas
Chapter 15

Timothy M. McCulloch, MD, FACS
Chair, Division of Otolaryngology
Department of Surgery
University of Wisconsin School of Medicine and
 Public Health
Madison, Wisconsin
Chapter 28

Andrew J. McWhorter, MD
Director
Our Lady of the Lake/Louisiana State University
 Voice Center
Professor
Department of Otolaryngology–Head and Neck
 Surgery
Louisiana State University Health Sciences Center
 New Orleans
Baton Rouge, Louisiana
Chapter 53

Valeria Silva Merea, MD
Assistant Attending
Head and Neck Service, Department of Surgery
Memorial Sloan Kettering Cancer Center
New York, New York
Chapter 26

Anna Miles, PhD
Senior Lecturer
Speech Science
University of Auckland
Auckland, New Zealand
Chapters 10 and 51

Robert J. Morrison, MD
Assistant Professor
Department of Otolaryngology–Head & Neck
 Surgery
University of Michigan
Ann Arbor, Michigan
Chapter 38

Omar Mulla, MBBS, MRCS, DOHNA, FRCS (ORL-HNS)
Specialist Trainee in Otolaryngology
Yorkshire Deanery
Leeds, United Kingdom
Chapter 25

Rebecca C. Nelson, MD
Head & Neck Institute
Cleveland Clinic Foundation
Cleveland, Ohio
Chapter 26

Lluís Nisa, MD, PhD
Department of Otorhinolaryngology–Head and Neck
 Surgery
Inselspital, Bern
University Hospital, and University of Bern
Bern, Switzerland
Chapter 2

S. A. Reza Nouraei, MBBChir, PhD, FRCS, FRCS (ORL-HNS)
Robert White Professor of Laryngology
  University of Southampton
Consultant Laryngologist & Tracheal Surgeon
The Robert White Centre for Airway Voice and
  Swallowing
Poole Hospital NHS Foundation Trust
Poole, United Kingdom
Chapters 18 and 39

Daniel Novakovic, FRACS, MBBS, MPH, BSc
Otolaryngologist, Head and Neck Surgeon
Associate Professor
University of Sydney Medical School
Medical Director, Dr. Liang Voice Program
University of Sydney
Sydney, Australia
Chapter 32

Ashli O'Rourke, MD
Associate Professor
Evelyn Trammell Institute of Voice and
  Swallowing
Medical University of South Carolina
Charleston, South Carolina
Chapter 54

Michael Petrou
Lecturer in Medical Microbiology
Faculty of Medicine
European University of Cyprus
London, United Kingdom
Chapter 27

Kristina Piastro, MD
Laryngology Fellow
NYU Voice Center
Brooklyn, New York
Chapter 14

Natasha Quraishi, MA (Cantab), MBBS
Foundation Year One Doctor
Department of Otolaryngology
Charing Cross Hospital
Imperial College Healthcare NHS Trust
London, United Kingdom
Chapters 18 and 27

Marc Remacle, MD, PhD
Professor
Department of Otolaryngology–Head and Neck Surgery
Voice and Swallowing Disorders Unit
Center Hospitalier de Luxembourg
Luxembourg City, Luxembourg
Chapter 44

Faruque Riffat, BSc, MBBS, MS, FACS, FRACS
Department of Surgery
Westmead Hospital
Sydney, Australia
Chapter 52

Clark A. Rosen, MD
Francis Lewis Morrison, MD Endowed Chair in
  Laryngology
Department of Otolaryngology–Head and Neck
  Surgery
Chief, Division of Laryngology
Co-Director, UCSF Voice & Swallowing Center
University of California, San Francisco
Chapters 16 and 35

David E. Rosow, MD, FACS
Director, Division of Laryngology and Voice
Associate Professor of Otolaryngology
University of Miami Miller School of Medicine
Assistant Professor of Clinical Voice Performance
University of Miami Frost School of Music
Miami, Florida
Chapter 45

Jason Rudman, MD
Otolaryngology–Head and Neck Surgery Resident
University of Miami/Jackson Memorial Hospital
Miami, Florida
Chapter 45

Michael J. Rutter, BHB, MBChB, FRACS
Professor
Division of Pediatric Otolaryngology
Cincinnati Children's Hospital Medical Center
Cincinnati, Ohio
Chapter 6

Kishore Sandu, MD
Department of Otolaryngology–Head and Neck
    Surgery
CHUV Lausanne University Hospital
Lausanne, Switzerland
Chapter 2

Robert T. Sataloff, MD, DMA
Professor and Chairman
Department of Otolaryngology–Head and Neck
    Surgery
Senior Associate Dean for Clinical Academic
    Specialties
Drexel University College of Medicine
Philadelphia, Pennsylvania
Chapter 19

Claudia Schweiger, MD, PhD
Research Fellow
Cincinnati Children's Hospital
Cincinnati, Ohio
Hospital de Clinicas de Porto Alegre and
    Universidade
Federal of Rio Grande do Sul
Porto Elegre-RS, Brazil
Chapter 6

Julia Selby, PhD, MMedSci, MSc, MA
Consultant Speech and Language Therapist
Upper Airway Service
Royal Brompton Hospital
London, United Kingdom
Chapter 37

Sophie G. Shay, MD
Department of Head and Neck Surgery
University of California, Los Angeles
Los Angeles, California
Chapter 3

Hagit Shoffel-Havakuk, MD
Assistant Professor
USC Voice Center
University of Southern California
Los Angeles, California
Chapter 33

Douglas Sidell, MD, FAAP
Assistant Professor of Otolaryngology
Director, Pediatric Aerodigestive Program
Director, Pediatric Voice and Swallowing
    Clinics
Department of Otolaryngology–Head and Neck
    Surgery
Division of Pediatric Otolaryngology
Stanford University
Palo Alto, California
Chapter 3

Blake Simpson, MD
Professor, Director of the UT Voice Center
University of Texas Health Science Center at San
    Antonio
San Antonio, Texas
Chapter 12

**Taranjit Singh Tatla, BSc (Hon), MBBS, DLO, FRCS
    (ORL-HNS), PhD**
Consultant, ENT-Head & Neck Surgeon
London Northwest University Healthcare NHS Trust
London, United Kingdom
Chapter 40

Faez H. Syed
Case Western Reserve School of Medicine
Cleveland, Ohio
Chapter 21

Kimon Toumazos, MBChB
Otolaryngology Trainee
Adelaide, South Australia
Chapter 46

Ibrahim Uygun, MD
Pediatric Surgeon
Associate Professor
Dicle University
Diyarbakır, Turkey
Chapter 11

Anne E. Vertigan, PhD
Director, Speech Pathology
John Hunter Hospital
University of Newcastle–Centre for Asthma and
    Respiratory Disease
Hunter Medical Research Institute
New Lambton Heights, Australia
Chapter 42

Emma Wallace
Post-doctoral Research Associate
Adelaide Institute for Sleep Health
Flinders University
Adelaide, South Australia
Chapter 48

Emil Schwarz Walsted, MD, PhD
Department of Respiratory Medicine
Bispebjerg Hospital
Copenhagen, Denmark
Hon. Clinical Researcher
Department of Respiratory Medicine
Royal Brompton Hospital
London, United Kingdom
Chapter 36

Mark G. Watson, FRCS
Consultant Laryngologist, Head & Neck Surgeon
Doncaster Royal Infirmary
Doncaster, United Kingdom
Chapter 25

Emily Wilson, MS, CCC-SLP
Lecturer, Department of Speech and Hearing Sciences
Speech Language Pathologist, Department of
    Otolaryngology–Head and Neck Surgery
University of Washington Medical Center
Chapter 24

Christopher T. Wootten, MD, MMHC
Associate Professor, Department of Otolaryngology
Vanderbilt University Medical Center
Pediatric Otolaryngology Service Chief Clinical Officer
Director, Pediatric Otolaryngology Fellowship
Nashville, Tennessee
Chapter 1

Chadwin Al Yaghchi, MD, PhD, FRCS, DOHNS
Consultant Laryngologist, Ear Nose and Throat
    Surgeon
National Centre for Airway Reconstruction
Imperial College Healthcare NHS Trust
London, United Kingdom
Chapter 29

VyVy N. Young, MD
Associate Professor
Department of Otolaryngology–Head and Neck
    Surgery
University of California, San Francisco
San Francisco, California
Chapter 13

Angela Zhu, MPhil
Medical Student
University of Miami Miller School of Medicine
Miami, Florida
Chapter 45

SECTION I

PEDIATRIC

CHAPTER 1

Congenital Stridor

Christopher T. Wootten

CASE

Case Vignette

The patient is a 17-day-old female with stridor from birth. She was born at 33 weeks gestation, weighing 2.23 kilograms, to a G1P1 18-year-old mother via spontaneous vaginal delivery. The umbilical cord was not wrapped around the neck, and no forceps were required to assist delivery. Apgar scores were 8 at 1 minute and 9 at 5 minutes. While mild inspiratory stridor was noted shortly after birth, by 2 weeks of life, stridor had become severe and associated with substernal retractions and intermittent desaturations—particularly with feeding. She is currently comfortable and active on 0.5 L nasal cannula oxygen with mild inspiratory stridor that worsens with agitation. She has no dysmorphic features; however, she is jaundiced. Flexible nasopharyngoscopy and laryngoscopy demonstrate patent choanae bilaterally. There are no pooled secretions in the vallecula or pyriform sinuses. The epiglottis is slightly omega-shaped, and the supra-arytenoid tissues are prominent. However, a view of the vocal folds is afforded, and the vocal folds fail to abduct bilaterally.

Brain MRI without contrast demonstrates normal brain with age-appropriate myelination and no evidence of cerebellar tonsillar herniation. Laboratory evaluation found total bilirubin to be in the high-normal range.

Discussion Points

1. Describe the necessary and efficient steps to initially stage dysfunction in this infant with stridor.

2. Differentiate between congenital bilateral abductor paralysis and congenital bilateral adductor paralysis in terms of disease presentation, workup, and management.
3. Describe the role of laryngeal reinnervation surgery in the management of congenital bilateral vocal fold movement impairment (BVFMI).

CASE RESOLUTION

Initial Evaluations

Stridor that is initially noted a few weeks after birth and that is escalating in magnitude is a fairly common reason for otolaryngology consultation in infancy. Statistically, the most common cause of inspiratory stridor in infancy is laryngomalacia. Indeed, >80% of infantile stridor is attributable to laryngomalacia,[1] with unilateral vocal fold immobility being the second most common cause of stridor within the first year of life. Bedside flexible endoscopy demonstrated some features of laryngomalacia (slightly omega-shaped epiglottis and prominent supra-arytenoid tissues), but the inability to abduct the vocal folds seemed to be responsible for this infant's noisy breathing. Due to infants' intrinsically high respiratory rate and dependence on a liquid diet, respiratory distress manifested as stridor commonly disrupts the suck-swallow-breathe sequence.[2]

Indeed, most congenital laryngeal anomalies make it difficult for infants to feed normally. Besides suck-swallow-breathe sequence disruption seen with significant laryngomalacia or bilateral vocal fold paralysis, unilateral vocal fold paralysis adds the dimension of glottic incompetence. Infants aspirate when they cannot fully close the laryngeal inlet. Repetitive aspiration may predispose an infant to continuous oxygen use. However, supplemental oxygen is not a long-term treatment for vocal cord paralysis or laryngomalacia in the absence of concomitant pulmonary dysfunction (such as bronchopulmonary dysplasia). This patient is receiving 0.5 L/min oxygen by nasal cannula—a considerable flow rate for a 17-day-old infant.

Of the diagnostic modalities employed in the workup of neonatal stridor, flexible nasopharyngoscopy and laryngoscopy is the highest yield.[3,4] In this patient, bedside flexible laryngoscopy showed failure to abduct the glottis bilaterally. While congenital bilateral vocal cord paralysis is rare, bilateral abductor paralysis is far more common than congenital bilateral adductor paralysis.[5] Failure to adduct the vocal cords results in glottis incompetence instead of the biphasic stridor that typifies abductor paralysis.[5] Motor findings aside, the bedside flexible laryngoscopy is also important as a means to evaluate laryngopharyngeal sensation and the safety of the patient's swallow. Patients with pooled secretions in the vallecula and/or pyriform sinuses or, worse, in the endolarynx demonstrate an increased aspiration risk.[6]

While flexible laryngoscopy identified bilateral paramedian positioning of the vocal cords in this patient, some diagnostic questions remain. Namely, these diagnostic questions are: (1) is the inability to abduct the glottis due to congenital paralysis (a neurological phenomenon) or cricoarytenoid (CA) joint fixation (a mechanical phenomenon)? and (2) what is the etiology of the bilateral congenital vocal cord paralysis? Rigid microlaryngoscopy with palpation of the cricoarytenoid joints is necessary to distinguish paralysis from fixation. Some authors advocate for laryngeal electromyography (LEMG) of the thyroarytenoid and posterior cricoarytenoid muscles under a light plane of anesthesia to further characterize the paralysis.[7] However, early work by Berkowitz found normal LEMG signals.[8,9] If rigid microlaryngoscopy with palpation of the CA joints demonstrates normal joint mobility and the absence of posterior glottic or subglottic scar, the diagnosis is presumed to be neurological. At this point, the etiology of the bilateral true vocal cord paralysis is best assessed with MRI of the brain, head, and neck in an attempt to discover a central or peripheral nervous system dysfunction.[4]

Even with the introduction of high-resolution imaging, most cases of congenital bilateral vocal cord paralysis (BVCP) are idiopathic.[10] The most common abnormality associated with BVCP found on MRI is an Arnold–Chiari malformation (ACM). There are four types of hindbrain herniation that characterize ACM, with type 2 ACM being the subtype most associated with congenital BVCP.[11] With type II ACM, the cerebellar tonsils and the vermis herniate through the foramen magnum. Up to one-third of infants and children with ACM type II, myelomeningocele, and associated hydrocephalus will have brainstem dysfunction.[11] In one series by Choi, 50% of these patients had BVCP, and Holinger described a series of BVCP where 16% of cases were attributable to ACM type II.[11,12] The surgical management of ACM type II is controversial, but patients with severe respiratory symptoms should be considered for decompression. Six percent to 21% of patients fail to improve or have an ephemeral benefit from surgical decompression.[11] Aside from ACM, MRI may demonstrate a cerebral vascular accident. When imaging fails to demonstrate a central or peripheral nervous system lesion, genetic etiologies of BVCP have been reported in case reports and small series.[5,13–16]

Comorbidities

The patient has jaundice of unknown significance. Laboratory testing confirmed the total bilirubin to be in the high-normal range.

Support System

The patient was born to a young, first-time mother with limited resources. The father of the baby was never present at the hospital and appears to no longer be involved with the patient's mother. By day-of-life 19, the neonatal intensive care team became increasingly concerned with the mother's state of mind—seemingly overwhelmed and displaying a flattened affect. She began to speak of putting the child up for adoption.

Patient Preferences and Expectations

Given the primary team's concerns about whether Mom could care for this child at home in her current emotionally detached state, any therapeutic stance came with some risk. Breathing comfortably, swallowing safely, and voicing loudly are the outcomes families hope for when therapeutic options for congenital BVCP are considered. Ideally, no treatment is necessary beyond careful observation and a hope for spontaneous recovery of vocal cord movement (65% recover spontaneously in the report by Lesnik et al).[3] Because the patient remained symptomatic and with an oxygen requirement, tracheotomy represented a "safe" and standard therapy, while endoscopic options, such as unilateral cordotomy, vocal cord lateralization, and posterior cricoid augmentation, seemed to have less certain gains and altered the larynx in the process.[3,10] Ultimately, the patient's mother opted for tracheotomy.

PROCEDURAL STRATEGIES

Indications

While the ability to feed on a thin liquid diet seems instinctive and effortless for infants, the reflexes necessary for feeding are easily derailed by interruption of the suck-swallow-breathe sequence. As such, early correction of significant dyspnea through tracheotomy may prevent oral aversion. Waiting weeks or months to make the decision to perform tracheotomy likely corresponds to weeks or months of inadequate or impossible oral intake. By the time the tracheostomy tube is inserted, a gastric tube may be required as well.

Miyamoto et al in a series of 22 patients reported a 68% tracheotomy rate.[10] Similarly, Lesnik in a series of 19 patients intubated shortly after birth for stridor associated with BVCP noted 74% required tracheotomy due to failure to extubate.[3] Earlier reports favored tracheotomy more heavily.[10] Certainly, among the options for surgical management of BVCP, tracheotomy is the most studied. Rates of spontaneous recovery of vocal cord function range from 33% to 65%,[3,17] and tracheotomy has the theoretical advantage of restoring an airway without altering laryngeal anatomy. Given Mom's uncertainty about keeping her child or putting her up for adoption, it would be imprudent to enter into a treatment pathway that might take some time to heal fully (such as posterior cricoid split and graft placement) or produce an outcome that leaves both breathing and swallowing functions partially impaired (such as cordotomy or vocal cord lateralization operations).

Contraindications

There are important psychosocial limitations of neonatal tracheotomy. For a first-time parent contemplating bringing home a "sick child," the presence of a tracheostomy may seem to heighten the complexity and fragility of the child. This can interfere with mother–child

bonding, adversely affecting the overall health of the baby. Further, the standard safety requirements in place for discharging a child to home with a tracheostomy include: (1) the requirement that at least two competent adults intimately involved in the child's care be fully trained and certified in the care of a child with a tracheostomy prior to discharge and (2) the requirement that the child be discharged to a "stable" home environment with functional utilities, climate control, and a clean and safe environment. Thus, while placement of a tracheostomy may be a common and surgically conservative option, psychosocial factors among the child's caregivers may complicate discharge.

Beyond these important psychosocial factors, there are medical contraindications to surgical interventions, including tracheotomy. Between 32% and 54% of infants with congenital BVCP may be managed with observation alone or at least respond favorably to an intervention that obviates tracheotomy. Favoring observation are reliable, observant parents, a stable home environment (preferably close to a medical center), and a clear mandate to the family to present the child for medical evaluation in the event of escalating stridor and respiratory distress.[3,10] Because spontaneous recovery of vocal cord movement is reported to be between 50% and 68%, children who are compensating well for their BVCP should be considered for simple observation to obviate the long-term morbidities of early surgical interventions.[17]

Expected Results

Tracheotomy provides a definitive surgical airway to children suffering from a variety of upper airway obstructions.[18] Tracheostomy tubes of different diameters and lengths, with and without a cuff to support mechanical positive-pressure ventilation, are available. Between 32% and 68% of children will eventually resolve their BVCP. The timing of spontaneous resolution is highly variable. One-third regained glottis movement by 6 months in one study; yet, spontaneous resolution has been noted as late as 11 years of age.[19]

Team Experience

Pediatric airway surgery should only be undertaken in a pediatric hospital equipped with the appropriate complement of pediatric anesthesia specialists, operating room technicians, nurses, and equipment.

Similarly, the hospital must contain a pediatric intensive care unit or dedicated airway step-down unit that is comfortable managing neonates following tracheotomy or other airway interventions. In particular, postoperative tracheostomy care is best accomplished with a multidisciplinary team approach that directs hospital caregivers and family members to adhere to a standardized clinical pathway.[20]

Risk–Benefit Analysis

While tracheotomy is seen as a conservative operation in the spectrum of pediatric airway surgery, tracheotomy carries some risks in the neonate. In the short term (the first week following tracheotomy), accidental decannulation is a concern, alongside mucus plugging. Under both circumstances, the patient may suffer from acute airway obstruction. While infants are sedated following tracheotomy to allow maturation of the stomal tract, they are particularly vulnerable to plugging due to an inadequately humidified ventilator circuit. Following the first safe tracheostomy tube change, the infant is usually assessed for the ability to feed by mouth. The presence of tracheostomy impairs the infant's ability to safely swallow due to elimination of the subglottic air cushion and the mechanical resistance to laryngotracheal elevation during the swallow imparted by the tracheostomy tube. In the long term, tracheotomy carries the risk of airway scarring, including suprastomal airway collapse, or "A-frame" or lambdoid deformity at the stoma site. In contrast to other surgical interventions in BVCP, however, the scarring incurred by tracheotomy is at least distributed within the trachea, instead of at the level of the glottis.

Before considering any operation to improve the ease of airflow in an infant with BVCP, recall that around 30% may not require tracheotomy,[17] and >60% of these will go on to demonstrate spontaneous recovery of true vocal cord (TVC) motion.[3] Thus, in the treatment of congenital BVCP any surgical therapy must be weighed against simple observation.

Therapeutic Alternatives

- *Non-invasive positive pressure ventilation.* Humidified high-flow nasal cannula (HHFNC) and nasal continuous positive airway

pressure (NCPAP) ventilation are two airway augmentative technologies commonly employed in neonates with respiratory distress. There is evidence to support HHFNC and NCPAP over conventional mechanical ventilation delivered via an endotracheal tube in this population. By avoiding instrumentation of the larynx, laryngeal function is preserved, and there is no risk of laryngotracheal scarring. The net result is a diminished rate of bronchopulmonary dysplasia, nosocomial pneumonia, and sepsis.[21] The risks of non-invasive positive pressure ventilation pertains mostly to the secondary effects their mode of delivery may have on the delicate, largely non-ossified craniofacial skeleton of the neonate (eg, flattened midface, columellar damage). If non-invasive positive pressure ventilation fails, patients often require some surgical intervention.

- *Vocal cord lateralization.* Vocal cord lateralization depends on a mobile cricoarytenoid joint. A suture is passed on either side of the vocal process of the ipsilateral arytenoid (or through it). Placing tension on the suture by tying it externally to the straps muscles or laryngotracheal framework lateralizes the posterior aspect of the vocal cord. There are a handful of techniques described to accomplish this—either by passing the sutures transcervically ("outside in") or using an endoscopic needle driver ("inside out").[22,23] One advantage of vocal cord lateralization compared with other posterior glottic operations is its reversibility. Given the challenging, confined space of the neonatal larynx, vocal cord lateralization is usually described as a means to achieve decannulation after tracheotomy for BVCP in individuals with insufficient recovery of movement. Based on published series, single-operation success rates with vocal cord lateralization are <50% as judged by ensuing rates of decannulation.[10,17,24] Most children require some additional procedure, such as a contralateral lateralization, cordotomy, or partial or complete arytenoidectomy) to ultimately achieve decannulation.

- *Cordotomy.* Because the posterior glottis is disproportionally responsible for airflow compared with the anterior glottis, a simple transverse incision into the posterior vocal fold can noticeably improve airflow across a paralyzed larynx. The natural tension of the thyroarytenoid muscle tends to further pull open the vocal cord incision, enhancing its effects. Cordotomy is simple to perform with a CO_2 laser affixed to a micromanipulator. Other methods of cordotomy using a CO_2 fiber wave guide are reported in adults. However, cordotomy has certain drawbacks as a therapy for BVCP in infants. First, it is destructive, and the resulting scarring along the vocal fold may leave the child with long-lasting dysphonia related to an enlarged posterior glottic chink or an evolution of scar into the cricoarytenoid joint. Like vocal cord lateralization, single-operation success (as measured by subsequent decannulation) is low in congenital bilateral TVC paralysis (TVCP).

- *Arytenoidectomy.* When endoscopic cordotomy alone is insufficient to achieve decannulation in infantile bilateral TVCP, several authors report the addition of a partial or complete arytenoidectomy. In fact, "arytenoidectomy," as reported in the literature, is a diverse category of operations designed to remove some portion of the arytenoid cartilage to increase posterior glottis airflow. In adults suffering from bilateral TVCP, there are descriptions of cartilage excision and defect closure through the endoscopic suture-advancement of adjacent mucosa. A partial arytenoidectomy resects the vocal process (and its associated vocal cord epithelium) and the anterior body of the arytenoid. The posterior arytenoid, with its muscular process, is left in vivo. In a total arytenoidectomy, an incision is carried endoscopically from the medial surface of the arytenoid onto the aryepiglottic fold, and microlaryngeal instrumentation is used to excise cartilage (with subsequent defect closure). Through an open laryngofissure, a J-shaped incision on the arytenoid mucosa can allow the surgeon to gain access to the entire body of the arytenoid, allowing total excision. Again, the mucosal defect is closed, and either endoscopic or open arytenoidectomy can be combined with suture lateralization of the posterior vocal fold remnant. This combination was noted to be the most efficacious in a 2003 review of several techniques used to manage BVCP in children.[25]

In contrast, many authors favor simple ablative arytenoidectomy procedures that do not incorporate preservation of mucosa or mucosal flap advancement. Frequently, microscissors or a CO_2 laser are used to remove the anterolateral arytenoid (including the vocal process and posterior true vocal cord).[26] This operation is fairly simple to perform. However, the raw, possibly charred surfaces of cartilage stimulate granulation tissue formation. The resulting scar fibrosis tends to fill in the posterior glottic defect, degrading the benefit to posterior airflow over time. Single-operation success with arytenoidectomy in infants with BVCP is <50%. However, most large series report spontaneous recovery of vocal cord movement at some delay after tracheotomy as the most common mechanism of decannulation.

- *Posterior augmentation grafting (laryngoplasty).* Theoretically, posterior glottic augmentation with autologous cartilage offers several advantages over the above-listed procedures. Cartilage expansion of the posterior glottis is: (1) not destructive to the vocal folds, (2) effective for paralyzed vocal cords or fixed cricoarytenoid joints, and (3) highly customizable to achieve the amount of desired posterior glottic distraction. However, cartilage expansion of the posterior glottis requires exposure to completely divide the posterior plate of the cricoid. This may be accomplished endoscopically with monopolar cautery, scissors, an ultrasonic aspirator, and/or a CO_2 laser.[27,28] More traditionally, cartilage expansion of the posterior plate of the cricoid is performed via a vertical anterior incision through the first tracheal ring, the cricoid, and into the lower portion of the thyroid cartilage. From this exposure, the posterior plate of the cricoid is split and augmented with cartilage graft insertion. The extent to which the operation is employed is limited by its difficulty—an endoscopic cordotomy or partial arytenoidectomy using a CO_2 laser is much simpler than an endoscopic posterior cartilage graft laryngoplasty. Further, the open approach posterior cricoid augmentation carries the stigma of a visible scar on the neck and the inherent risks of open operation. Regardless of the approach to posterior cricoid cartilage augmentation, an endotracheal tube is maintained as a stent for several days while the child recovers from this single-stage operation in an intensive care unit.

- *Tracheotomy.* Tracheotomy remains the most common intervention to correct the burden of disease associated with bilateral TVCP. In recent series, approximately 2/3 of children with BVCP of any etiology undergo tracheotomy,[10,17] and approximately 2/3 achieve decannulation. Children with idiopathic BVCP seem to have the highest likelihood of disease resolution. Overall, tracheotomy is a safe and effective therapy for upper airway obstruction of any etiology. However, a minimal tracheostomy-related mortality in young children is 1.4%.[17] Tracheostomy plugging is the most common cause of pediatric tracheostomy-related death, emphasizing the need for proper humidification of these small cannulas at all times.

  The execution of a pediatric tracheotomy is beyond the scope of discussion, but there are a few common themes that distinguish infant tracheotomies from those performed in older individuals. Specifically, in infants, a vertical tracheotomy is preferred to a transverse incision or a Bjork-flap. Typically, left and right stay sutures of non-absorbable material are placed on either side of the midline tracheotomy. During the early phase prior to the first tube change, the tracheostomy device is secured around the neck with ties rather than having the faceplate sewn to the skin of the neck. Given the high growth velocity across childhood, the variety of standard tracheostomy sizes available for use in children far exceeds those employed in adults.

Cost-Effectiveness

Infants affected with BVCP often have a prolonged stay in a neonatal intensive care unit prior to making the decision to perform tracheotomy. However, regardless of the indication for pediatric tracheotomy, Lewis et al[29] studied the postoperative course and the average hospital charges associated with that stay. The average stay in their population in 1997 was 50 days *after* undergoing tracheotomy, and the average charge was US$200,000. That sum is equivalent to over US$304,000 in 2017.[29] The actual cost of pediatric tracheostomy care is high because it is labor intensive, and many

institutions are turning to multidisciplinary care teams to achieve desirable outcomes.

Informed Consent

The child's mother was counseled as to the risks, benefits, and alternatives to tracheotomy. Among the risks listed were long-term damage to the laryngotracheal framework, altered voicing, altered swallowing, hemorrhage, and accidental decannulation or mucus plugging, leading to respiratory arrest. The in-patient pediatric otolaryngology nurse practitioner circled back with the mother to confirm her understanding of the principles of tracheotomy, why the operation was being proposed, and how the child would be cared for after tracheotomy. The child's mother was introduced to another mother whose child had recently undergone tracheotomy.

TECHNIQUES AND PERIOPERATIVE CARE

Anesthesia and Perioperative Care

Prior to retrieving the patient from the neonatal intensive care unit, we discussed the operative and anesthetic plans with the anesthesiology team. Specifically, we would require the patient to be "asleep but spontaneous"—that is, anesthetized to the point of relaxation, but not so deep that shallow spontaneous respiration is suppressed. We would start the case with a microlaryngoscopy and tracheobronchoscopy to, once again, confirm BVCP. For this portion of the operation, 100% FiO_2 would be acceptable, and it would be delivered via an endotracheal tube held in the pharynx (recall the patient is spontaneously ventilating). Following the endoscopy, we planned to intubate the trachea with an appropriately sized tube and proceed with tracheotomy. At this point, FiO_2 should be lowered to below 40%.

After the discussion of the general operative and anesthetic plan, the patient was transported directly from the neonatal intensive care unit on a Jackson–Reese ventilator. Once in the operating room, a single dose of cephazolin was administered as appropriate prophylaxis for a clean-contaminated case involving a skin incision. Because the child already had intravenous (IV) access, sevofluorane induction was not required. Instead, general anesthesia was induced and maintained with a totally intravenous anesthesia (TIVA) technique, which obviates surgical team exposure to inhalational agents while operating on and within the airway.

The airway framework was palpated along the anterior surface of the neck, and the planned transverse incision was marked in a pre-existing neck crease around the level of the cricoid cartilage. Lidocaine 0.5% with epinephrine 1:200,000 was infiltrated into the incision site. The anesthesia team was alerted to the concentration of epinephrine and the anticipated spike in heart rate. Following microlaryngoscopy and tracheobronchoscopy, the child was positioned on a gel shoulder roll to extend the neck. After all rearrangement of cardiac monitoring leads and after placement of the monopolar grounding pad, a strip of 1-inch silk tape was taped from the right superior corner of the bed, across the mentum, and back up to the left superior corner of the bed. This maneuver maintained the neck in extension and maximized the relatively limited anterior cervical access afforded by the neonate.

Instrumentation

For the initial microlaryngoscopy and tracheobronchoscopy, we used a gauze pad across the maxillary gingiva, and laryngeal exposure was provided by a battery-powered #1 Phillips intubation laryngoscope. With an endotracheal tube being held in the pharynx with the same left hand that was holding the laryngoscope, a 4 mm 0-degree Storz (Karl Storz, Tuttlingen, Germany) Hopkins rod telescope was used to perform microlaryngoscopy and tracheobronchoscopy. The author prefers to size the airway with uncuffed endotracheal tubes, but to secure the airway for tracheotomy using a cuffed endotracheal tube one half-size smaller than the optimally sized uncuffed tube. If the appropriately sized uncuffed endotracheal tube is a 2.0, 2.5, or 3.0 mm inner diameter, then there are no cuffed tubes available in a half-size smaller, so uncuffed tubes are used to secure the airway during tracheotomy. Once the trachea is incised and the stay suture and stomal maturation sutures have been placed, the trachea is cannulated with a Bivona TTS (Smiths Medical, Minneapolis, MN, USA) cuffed tracheostomy tube. The length of the tube selected (neonatal vs pediatric) is chosen based on the perceived distance from the tracheotomy to the carina and the amount of residual soft tissue between the surface of the neck and the tracheotomy site. Typically, for infants in the first 6 to 9 months of life, a neonatal length tube is placed at tracheotomy. Regardless, a thin flexible fiberoptic bronchoscope is always passed down the tube to confirm its position within the airway prior to case completion.

Anatomic Dangers and Other Risks

There are several anatomic dangers pertaining to infantile tracheotomy. First, the neck is short, and intraoperatively the surgeon must clearly delineate the cartilage framework to ensure that the level of entry into the airway is indeed somewhere between the second and fourth tracheal rings. Likewise, it is essential that some rigid endotracheal tube or ventilating bronchoscope is securing the airway. In infants, the trachea is similar in rigidity to the carotid arteries that flank it. To reduce the risk of malpositioning of the tracheostomy tube within the airway and to mitigate accidental decannulation, subcutaneous fat must be removed from the neck skin surrounding the stoma.

Surgical Technique

The neck was incised transversely to access the airway. The subcutaneous fat underlying the incision was debulked with monopolar cautery. Next, the straps muscles were divided in the midline, from the thyroid notch superiorly to below the thyroid gland's isthmus inferiorly. Senn retractors were used to retract the muscles away from the laryngotracheal framework. A fine hemostat was used to dissect beneath the thyroid isthmus, which was, in turn, divided using monopolar cautery without suture ligature. Pause was given to inspect the laryngotracheal framework and to identify the midline of the third and fourth tracheal rings. A marker was used to denote the site of a vertical tracheotomy incision. Prior to making the incision, however, 4-0 Prolene stay sutures were placed on either side of midline for use in an airway emergency in the event of accidental decannulation in the early postoperative period. After the stay sutures were placed, 4-0 chromic gut suture was used to coapt the skin of the neck to the anterior surface of the trachea, just lateral to the stay sutures. Only after these maturation sutures were placed and tied down was the midline tracheotomy incision made. This minimized the time spent with a ventilator leak and helped keep the lungs maximally recruited. A Bivona (Smiths Medical, Minneapolis, MN, USA) 3.0 mm

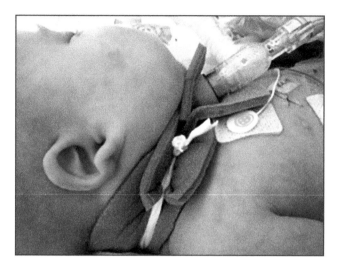

Figure 1–1. A silver-impregnated barrier dressing is placed around the neck to prevent irritation and ulceration by the twill ties during the early post-tracheostomy phase.

inner diameter TTS neonatal tracheostomy tube was placed. After confirming a return of carbon dioxide, the cuff was minimally inflated to maintain a seal. A small flexible bronchoscope confirmed the position of the tube within the airway. A silver-impregnated barrier sponge dressing was placed around the neck (Figure 1–1), and the tracheostomy tube was tightly secured around the neck with a cotton twill tie.

LONG-TERM MANAGEMENT

Referral

Upon discharge, the infant was breathing comfortably via the tracheostomy, and more than half of her nutrition was provided by gastric tube feedings. Follow-up was scheduled with the Complex Aerodigestive Evaluation Team (CADET), a multispecialty group that includes otolaryngology, pulmonology, gastroenterology, speech pathology, and nutrition.

Follow-Up Tests and Procedures

Going forward, the patient needs to be periodically evaluated for return of vocal cord movement and the adequacy of the glottic airway. Regardless of whether she recovers movement, we believe a young child with

a tracheostomy requires surveillance every 6 months in the operating room to assess and treat suprastomal granulation tissue and to monitor for other tracheostomy-related complications, such as anterior tracheal erosion by the cannula. Additionally, operative assessment allows the surgeon to determine whether the tracheostomy tube is appropriately sized, and to recommend specific size adjustments to the tube as the child grows. Finally, operative assessment allows the surgeon to palpate the cricoarytenoid joints to determine whether BVCP is becoming complicated by joint immobility and/or posterior glottic stenosis.

Having achieved partial recovery of glottic movement, the patient was eventually decannulated around 18 months of age. However, she continued to have airway issues. By 24 months, she had accumulated several emergency room visits for recurrent croup-like symptoms. A repeat microlaryngoscopy/tracheobronchoscopy was performed, noting immobility of the left cricoarytenoid joint, and reduced abduction of the right true vocal fold (Figure 1–2). After a comprehensive aerodigestive workup, including a 23-hour esophageal impedance evaluation, videofluoroscopic swallow study, and flexible bronchoscopy, she was deemed a candidate for endoscopic posterior costal cartilage graft laryngoplasty.[27] Because there was no frank scar between the vocal cords posteriorly, we performed an endoscopic split of the cricoid submucosally using heavy endoscopic scissors. Autologous rib

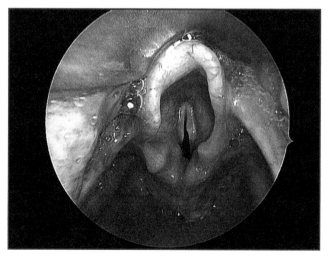

Figure 1–2. Supraglottic view of the patient's airway following decannulation. The patient began to have recurrent croup-like illnesses, and an inadequate glottic airway is suggested.

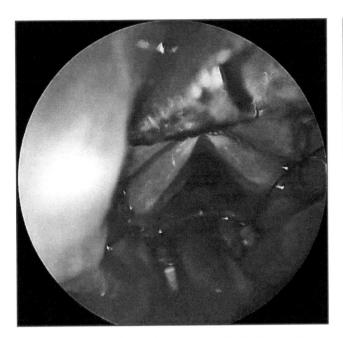

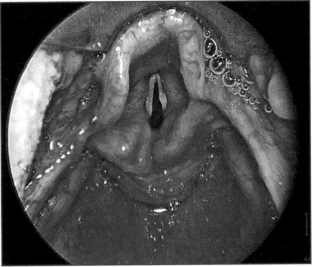

Figure 1–4. The same patient approximately 5 months postoperatively. Note improved glottic airway after costal cartilage graft augmentation of the posterior larynx.

Figure 1–3. Supraglottic view of the patient's airway midway through an endoscopic, submucosal cricoid split and posterior cricoid augmentation with autologous rib. A heavy alligator is seating the graft between the split halves of the posterior cricoid plate. A vocal cord spreader enhances glottic distraction.

was carved into an I-beam shape, and slid into a submucosal pocket between the arytenoids to expand the cricoid plate (Figure 1–3). The overlying posterior glottic and subglottic mucosa provided immediate coverage to the graft. The single stage operation was supported with 7 days of transnasal intubation, where the endotracheal tube functioned as a stent. After a period of healing, the obstructive airway symptoms abated (Figure 1–4).

Quality Improvement

Outcomes assessment in pediatric laryngotracheal stenosis usually centers on whether or not the child is tracheostomy dependent—ie, did the child achieve a cannula-free airway? Our patient achieved decannulation, but it was not durable secondary to the accumulated effects of airway manipulation and time. The left cricoarytenoid joint became fixed, and the mobility achieved on the right was inadequate to avoid recurrent croup-like illness and frequent visits to the emergency department. Thus, she was recommended for augmentation laryngoplasty. While a Myer–Cotton

grade[30] may be assigned to the airway of a child with BVCP, the absence of luminal scar and the triangular shape of the airway at this location tend to allow an air leak around relatively large tubes. The McCaffrey staging system is better suited for staging glottic stenosis or other slit-like lesions,[31] as it does not depend on a leak around an endotracheal tube to correlate with disease severity.

In adults and older children, physiologic staging using spirometry and pulmonary function testing can complement these anatomic staging systems. Likewise, domains of breathing, swallowing, and voicing can be inventoried using patient-reported outcomes. The Clinical COPD Questionnaire is a 10-item adoption of a chronic obstructive pulmonary disorder (COPD) questionnaire that has been shown to correlate with airway disease burden from airway stenosis in adults. The feeding and swallowing impact survey has been used successfully in laryngeal cleft repair functional assessment in children.[32] Likewise, Pullens[33] recently commented on the Pediatric Voice Handicap Index and the Dysphonia Severity Index in laryngotracheal reconstruction patients. Significant voice disturbance was noted in this population.

Gustafson[34] reviewed a Cincinnati experience of 200 single-stage laryngotracheoplasty operations, finding an overall decannulation rate of 96%. However, 36% of the patients in this single-stage operation series were not tracheostomy dependent preoperatively.

Hartnick[35] analyzed an overlapping population of 199 laryngotracheal reconstructions (both double- and single-staged) for subglottic stenosis for operation-specific decannulation rates (for double-staged operations) and operation-specific extubation rates (for single-staged operations). This "operation-specific" designation substantiates that not all large reconstructive efforts are successful in the larynx in one operation.

Discussion Points

1. Describe the necessary and efficient steps to initially stage dysfunction in this infant with stridor.

   - Flexible nasopharyngoscopy and laryngoscopy is an essential first step in the workup of an infant with stridor. Visualization of the glottis in a neonate presents unique challenges. The respiratory rate is rapid, and with airway distress, the patient may be heaving. This results in a great deal of motion in the laryngopharyngeal airway. It is a good idea to record the endoscopic exam so that the movement of the larynx can be reviewed to ascertain the nature and extent of BVFMI.
   - Rigid microlaryngoscopy and bronchoscopy are necessary once BVFMI is confirmed on flexible laryngoscopy. Rigid evaluation allows for palpation of the cricoarytenoid joints and aids in the differentiation between poor motor input (Video 1–2) to the larynx and joint fixation (with or without adequate motor input). Certainly, overt posterior glottic stenosis secondary to fibrosis may be seen in older infants and young children, and posterior glottic stenosis contributes to BVFMI as well.
   - For patients with soft, mobile cricoarytenoid joints and no evidence of interarytenoid scar, MRI of the brain, brainstem, and upper chest allows for comprehensive evaluation of salient neurological tracts responsible for glottic movement. Special attention must be paid to the posterior fossa, where an ACM may be discovered. Type II ACM is most commonly associated with BVCP.
   - Flexible nasopharyngoscopy and laryngoscopy are required as they offer an assessment of glottic movement and pooling of secretions in the oropharynx

and hypopharynx, which suggests laryngopharyngeal sensory deficits, and should raise concerns for feeding safety. In a fiberoptic endoscopic evaluation of swallowing (FEES), oral secretions can be dyed with food coloring. Likewise, formula/expressed breast milk can be dyed. With a flexible nasopharyngoscope in place just below the margin of the soft palate, dye can be traced through the pharynx to assess the safety and the efficacy of the swallow. FEES allows the endoscopist to see specifically how the supraglottic and glottic laryngeal structures protect the airway from aspiration. A video fluoroscopic swallow study (VFSS) (also commonly known as a "modified barium swallow") is a complementary instrumental evaluation of swallowing. Here, images are typically acquired in a sagittal plane while the infant feeds on a liquid meal to which barium has been added. While VFSS in a sagittal plane will miss nuances of anatomy such as laryngeal penetration occurring over the left aryepiglottic fold, instead of the right aryepiglottic fold, VFSS is particularly useful in all the anatomy related to a swallow at the same time. In contrast, the view afforded by FEES "whites out" when the pharynx constricts around the scope.

2. Differentiate between congenital bilateral abductor paralysis and congenital bilateral adductor paralysis in terms of disease presentation, workup, and management.

   - Congenital abductor bilateral vocal cord paralysis presents with airway obstruction due to a failure of the vocal cords to abduct during inspiration. In neonates, inspiratory or biphasic stridor results from narrowing of the glottic inlet. Retractions, cyanosis, and feeding difficulties are commonly associated with congenital abductor bilateral vocal cord paralysis.
   - Congenital adductor bilateral vocal cord paralysis presents with glottic incompetence, weak cry, and aspiration. Flexible endoscopy demonstrates an open glottis during exhalation, cough, cry, and feeding. Congenital adductor bilateral vocal cord paralysis is more rare than abductor paralysis.

The few series in the literature characterizing this population notes a common association with chromosomal anomalies.[5] Spontaneous recovery of vocal cord function is variable and incomplete.

3. Describe the role of laryngeal reinnervation surgery in the management of BVFMI.

- Infants lacking in cricoarytenoid joint fixation or posterior glottic stenosis who fail to resolve abductor bilateral vocal cord paralysis and remain tracheotomy dependent beyond infancy may be considered for a variety of operations to achieve decannulation. The most intuitive operation to restore neurological function to a paralyzed larynx would be a laryngeal reinnervation. In children with acquired paralysis, for example, following a patent ductus arteriosus ligation, the recurrent laryngeal nerve is known to be normal, but dennervated "upstream" of the larynx. In congenital BVCP, movement has not been demonstrated. In a large series by Miyamoto,[10] bilateral laryngeal reinnervation was performed, but the patient remained tracheostomy dependent at the end of the study period. To date, the efficacy of laryngeal reinnervation in this population with congenital BVCP remains unknown.

REFERENCES

1. Zoumalan R, Maddalozzo J, Holinger LD. Etiology of stridor in infants. *Ann Otol Rhinol Laryngol.* 2007; 116(5):329–334.
2. Thorne MC, Garetz SL. Laryngomalacia: review and summary of current clinical practice in 2015. *Paediatr Respir Rev.* 2016;17:3–8. doi:10.1016/j.prrv.2015.02.002.
3. Lesnik M, Thierry B, Blanchard M, Glynn F, Leboulanger N. Idiopathic bilateral vocal cord paralysis in infants: case series and literature review. *Laryngoscope.* 2015;July:1724–1728. doi:10.1002/lary.25076.
4. Hasniah AL, Asiah K, Mariana D, Anida AR, Norzila MZ, Sahrir S. Congenital bilateral vocal cord paralysis. *Med J Malaysia.* 2006;61(5):626–629. http://www.ncbi.nlm.nih.gov/pubmed/17623966.
5. Berkowitz RG. Congenital bilateral adductor vocal cord paralysis. *Ann Otol Rhinol Laryngol.* 2003:764–767.
6. Willging JP, Thompson DM. Pediatric FEESST: fiberoptic endoscopic evaluation of swallowing with sensory testing. *Curr Gastroenterol Rep.* 2005;7(3):240–243. doi:10.1007/s11894-005-0041-x.
7. Maturo SC, Braun N, Brown DJ, Chong PS, Kerschner JE, Hartnick CJ. Intraoperative laryngeal electromyography in children with vocal fold immobility. *Arch Otolaryngol Head Neck Surg.* 2011;137(12):1251–1257.
8. Berkowitz RG, Sun Q, Pilowsky PM. Congenital bilateral vocal cord paralysis and the role of glycine. *Ann Otol Rhinol Laryngol,* 2005;114(6):494–498.
9. Berkowitz RG. Laryngeal electromyography findings in idiopathic congenital bilateral vocal cord paralysis. *Ann Otol Rhinol Laryngol,* 1996:105:207–212.
10. Miyamoto RC, Parikh SR, Gellad W, Licameli GR, York N. Bilateral congenital vocal cord paralysis: a 16-year institutional review. *Otolaryngol Head Neck Surg,* 2005:241–245. doi:10.1016/j.otohns.2005.02.019.
11. Choi SS, Tran LP, Zalzal GH. Airway abnormalities in patients with Arnold-Chiari malformation. *Otolaryngol Head Neck Surg.* 1999;121(6):720–724. doi:10.1053/hn.1999.v121.a98013.
12. Holinger PC, Holinger LD, Reichert TJ, Holinger PH. Respiratory obstruction and apnea in infants with bilateral abductor vocal cord paralysis, meningomyelocele, hydrocephalus, and Arnold-Chiari malformation. *J Pediatr.* 1978;92(3):368–373. doi:10.1016/S0022-3476(78)80421-1.
13. Hoeve HLJ, Brooks AS, Smit LS. JS-X syndrome: a multiple congenital malformation with vocal cord paralysis, ear deformity, hearing loss, shoulder musculature underdevelopment, and X-linked recessive inheritance. *Int J Pediatr Otorhinolaryngol.* 2015;79(7):1164–1170. doi:10.1016/j.ijporl.2015.05.001.
14. Hsu AK, Rosow DE, Wallerstein RJ, April MM. Familial congenital bilateral vocal fold paralysis: a novel gene. *Int J Pediatr Otorhinolaryngol.* 2015;79(3):323–327. doi:10.1016/j.ijporl.2014.12.009.
15. Omland T, Brøndbo K. Paradoxical vocal cord movement in newborn and congenital idiopathic vocal cord paralysis: two of a kind? *Eur Arch Otorhinolaryngol,* 2008;(265):803–807. doi:10.1007/s00405-008-0668-y.
16. Berkowitz RG, Bankier A, Moxham JP, Frcs C, Gardner RJM. Chromosomal abnormalities in idiopathic congenital bilateral vocal cord paralysis. *Ann Otol Rhinol Laryngol,* 2001:624–626.
17. Funk RT, Jabbour J, Robey T. Factors associated with tracheotomy and decannulation in pediatric bilateral vocal fold immobility. *Int J Pediatr Otorhinolaryngol.* 2015;79(6):895–899. doi:10.1016/j.ijporl.2015.03.026.
18. Wootten CT, French LC, Thomas RG, Iii WWN, Werkhaven JA, Cofer SA. Tracheotomy in the first year of life: outcomes in term infants, the Vanderbilt experience. *Otolaryngol Head Neck Surg,* 2006:365–369. doi:10.1016/j.otohns.2005.11.020.
19. Jomah M, Jeffery C, Campbell S, Krajacic A. Spontaneous recovery of bilateral congenital idiopathic laryngeal

paralysis: systematic non-meta-analytical review. *Int J Pediatr Otorhinolaryngol.* 2015;79(2):202–209. doi:10.1016/j.ijporl.2014.12.007.

20. Abode KA, Drake AF, Zdanski CJ. A Multidisciplinary children's airway center: impact on the care of patients with tracheostomy. *Pediatrics,* 2016137(2). doi:10.1542/peds.2015-0455.

21. Alexiou S, Panitch HB. Seminars in fetal & neonatal medicine physiology of non-invasive respiratory support. *Semin Fetal Neonatal Med.* 2016;21(3):174–180. doi:10.1016/j.siny.2016.02.007.

22. Lichtenberger G. Reversible immediate and definitive lateralization of paralyzed vocal cords. *Eur Arch Oto-Rhino-Laryngology.* 1999;256(8):407–411. doi:10.1007/s004050050176.

23. Lichtenberger G. Reversible lateralization of the paralyzed vocal cord without tracheostomy. *Ann Otol Rhinol Laryngol.* 2002;111(1):21–26.

24. Lidia Z, Magdalena F, Mieczyslaw C. Endoscopic laterofixation in bilateral vocal cords paralysis in children. *Int J Pediatr Otorhinolaryngol.* 2010;74(6):601–603. doi:10.1016/j.ijporl.2010.02.025.

25. Hartnick CJ, Brigger MT, Willging JP, Cotton RT, Myer CM. Surgery for pediatric vocal cord paralysis: a retrospective review. *Ann Otol Rhinol Laryngol.* 2003;112(1):1–6.

26. Yilmaz T, Süslü N, Atay G, Özer S, Günaydin RÖ, Bajin MD. Comparison of voice and swallowing parameters after endoscopic total and partial arytenoidectomy for bilateral abductor vocal fold paralysis: a randomized trial. *JAMA Otolaryngol Head Neck Surg,* 2013;139(7):712–718. doi:10.1001/jamaoto.2013.3395.

27. Inglis AF, Perkins J a, Manning SC, Mouzakes J. Endoscopic posterior cricoid split and rib grafting in 10 children. *Laryngoscope.* 2003;113(11):2004–2009. doi:10.1097/00005537-200311000-00028.

28. Yawn RJ, Daniero JJ, Gelbard A, Wootten CT. Novel application of the Sonopet for endoscopic posterior split and cartilage graft laryngoplasty. *Laryngoscope.* 2016;126(4):941–944. doi:10.1002/lary.25596.

29. Lewis CW, Carron JD, Perkins JA, Sie KC, Feudtner C. Tracheotomy in pediatric patients: a national perspective. *Arch Otolaryngol Head Neck Surg.* 2003;129(5):523–529. doi:10.1001/archotol.129.5.523\r129/5/523 [pii].

30. Myer CM, O'Connor DM, Cotton RT. Proposed grading system for subglottic stenosis based on endotracheal tube sizes. *Ann Otol Rhinol Laryngol.* 1994;103(4 pt 1):319–323. doi:10.1177/000348949410300410.

31. McCaffrey T V. Classification of laryngotracheal stenosis. *Laryngoscope.* 1992;102(12 pt 1):1335–1340. doi:10.1288/00005537-199212000-00004.

32. Fracchia MS, Diercks G, Yamasaki A, et al. Assessment of the feeding Swallowing Impact Survey as a quality of life measure in children with laryngeal cleft before and after repair. *Int J Pediatr Otorhinolaryngol.* 2017;99:73–77. doi:10.1016/j.ijporl.2017.05.016.

33. Pullens B, Hakkesteegt M, Hoeve H, Timmerman M, Joosten K. Voice outcome and voice-related quality of life after surgery for pediatric laryngotracheal stenosis. *Laryngoscope.* 2017;127(7):1707–1711. doi:10.1002/lary.26374.

34. Gustafson LM, Hartley BE, Liu JH, et al. Single-stage laryngotracheal reconstruction in children: a review of 200 cases. *Otolaryngol Head Neck Surg.* 2000;123:430–434. doi:10.1067/mhn.2000.109007.

35. Hartnick CJ, Hartley BEJ, Willging JP, et al. Surgery for pediatric subglottic stenosis: Disease-specific outcomes. *Ann Otol Rhinol Laryngol.* 2001;110(12):1109–1113. doi:10.1177/000348940111001204.

CHAPTER 2

Laryngomalacia

Lluís Nisa and Kishore Sandu

Laryngomalacia (LM) is the leading cause of stridor in newborns, diagnosed in up to 75% of infants with congenital stridor.[1] LM was originally described in the early nineteenth century as "congenital stridor." In the 1940s Jackson and Jackson coined the term LM (derived from Greek, literally meaning *soft larynx*).

Symptom onset usually occurs within the first 2–4 weeks of life, with a high-pitched inspiratory stridor. Stridor tends to increase within the next few months and symptom exacerbations are usually observed during exertion (feeding, crying, agitation and supine position). LM has a self-limiting course in approximately 80% of the cases with complete resolution of symptoms at age 12 to 24 months.[2–4] In the remaining cases, clinical course can be complicated by chronic symptoms of upper airway obstruction, disordered swallowing, failure to thrive, dyspnea at rest, or cardiopulmonary complications (cor pulmonale, cardiac failure). In such cases, a full workup including endoscopic assessment of the upper airway in anesthesia and surgical management needs to be considered. Exceptionally and especially in contexts of polymorbidity severe airway compromise may require tracheotomy.[5,6]

DEFINITION

LM describes a dynamic narrowing of the supraglottic larynx during inspiration. The classical form of LM is a

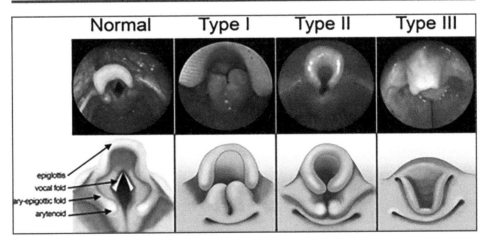

Figure 2–1. Types of laryngomalacia. Type I showing inward collapse of the aryepiglottic (AE) folds and redundant cuneiform cartilages; type II has short AE folds and tubular epiglottis; and type III shows backward tilt of the epiglottis completely obstructing the airway.

congenital anomaly. The epiglottis, the arytenoids, and aryepiglottic folds all tend to collapse during inspiration, resulting in the typical, high-pitched, inspiratory stridor seen in children with LM. While many classifications exist, they are not necessarily easy to apply in clinical routine and do not carry significant prognostic value. Most commonly, from an endoscopic perspective, three main types (Figure 2–1) of obstruction can be distinguished[7,8]:

- Type I: inward collapse of the aryepiglottic folds
- Type II: long and tubular (omega-shaped) epiglottis with short aryepiglottic folds
- Type III: posterior collapsing epiglottis

Late-onset or state-dependent LM features the same endoscopic findings of classical LM but presents in older children. So far, three forms have been described (altered-feeding, altered-sleep, and exercise-induced LM).[5,6]

CASE PRESENTATION

Case 1: Non-Complicated Mild Laryngomalacia

A 2-month-old girl presented with a 6-week history of stridor exacerbated during meals and cry, with intermittent cough episodes. Growth and neurological development were both age appropriate. The parents denied choking or cough attacks. No apneic episodes were observed during sleep.

Social: no passive smoking. No relevant family history.

Initial Assessment

History. Red flag symptoms include failure to thrive, dyspnea with permanent or severe intercostal or xiphoidal retraction, impossible breathing-swallowing coordination with choking episodes, cyanosis with feeding, or possible signs of obstructive sleep apnea. These symptoms would warrant urgent endoscopic assessment by means of flexible nasolaryngotracheal endoscopy in spontaneous breathing as well as direct laryngoscopy in the operating room.

Examination. Head and neck examination with emphasis on in-office flexible laryngoscopy. Red flag findings include episodes of apnea and cyanosis. In case of a positive anamnesis for swallow disorders an in-office fiberoptic endoscopic evaluation of swallowing (FEES) should be performed. Red flag findings include significant aspiration and impossible breathing- swallowing coordination with apnea and/or cyanosis.

Investigations. As mentioned above, the gold standard for the diagnosis of LM is in-office flexible laryngoscopy. A videofluoroscopic swallow study (VFSS) is in general not needed for patients with LM.

Diagnosis

Office flexible laryngoscopy reveals an excessive mucosal redundancy at the level of the arytenoids and interarytenoid space with inward collapse during inspiration (ie, type I LM).

Management

- Milk thickener
- Non-pharmacological anti-reflux management: avoid decubitus after meals, head at 30° during sleep, avoiding prone decubitus
- Reflux suppressing medication is not prescribed in absence of red flags or findings evoking laryngopharyngeal reflux (LPR)

At Review

In case of symptomatic relief (or at least lack of symptom progression), adequate food intake, and normal development, follow-up is performed until complete symptom regression. In case of moderate symptom progression anti-reflux therapy is to be considered and continued equally until complete symptom regression. In case of alarm signs or disease manifestations beyond age 18 months of age a full diagnostic workup, including endoscopic evaluation under anesthesia, ought to be carried out to confirm diagnosis of LM and in search of a second synchronous aerodigestive lesion. Medical comorbidities must be looked for, especially gastroesophageal reflux (GERD)/LPR and neurological and cardiopulmonary disease.

CASE 2: FAILED SUPRAGLOTTOPLASTY AND ITS SURGICAL SALVAGE

Initial Assessment

A male infant born at 38 weeks of gestation via cesarean delivery presented an uneventful perinatal story. Three weeks after birth he developed a permanent inspiratory stridor. Within the next 2 weeks feeding difficulties and intermittent choking with cyanosis and aspiration episodes during breast-feeding complicated the clinical picture. Endoscopic examination revealed a type II LM. Conservative management with thickened milk and anti-reflux medications did not result in significant improvement and the parents sought reevaluation 3 weeks later.

At this point the child underwent laser supraglottoplasty (SGP) at age 2 months at another institution with a good immediate postoperative course.

At Evaluation

After a symptom-free interval of 4 weeks the stridor recurred, and oral feeding quickly became impossible.

Reassessment

Given the feeding difficulty, the child was admitted and immediate endoscopy under anesthesia was performed. Dynamic fiberoptic examination of the larynx revealed a marked fibrosis of the aryepiglottic folds resulting in permanent posterior collapse of the epiglottis with subtotal obstruction of the supraglottic airway (morphologically resembling type III LM). Vocal fold abduction was preserved and complete examination of the upper aerodigestive tract was otherwise irrelevant.

Diagnosis

Cicatricial supraglottic stenosis after SGP.

Management

Revision SGP was undertaken (Figures 2–2 and 2–3). Suspension laryngoscopy was installed. General

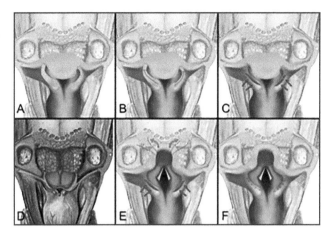

Figure 2–2. Schema showing correction of supraglottic stenosis. (A) Supraglottic stenosis with retroverted epiglottis. (B) T-shape incision on the fibrosed and shortened aryepiglottic (AE) folds. (C) Mobilization of bilateral piriform sinus mucosae. (D) Scarification of the vallecular, lingual surface of epiglottis and base of tongue mucosae using CO_2 laser. (E) Epiglottopexy sutures fixing the epiglottis to base of tongue. (F) Endoscopic mucosal suturing to reestablish the AE folds.

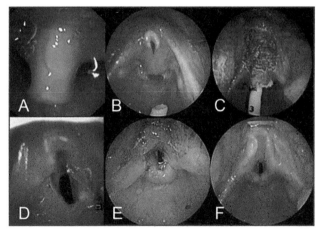

Figure 2–3. Intraoperative images. (A) Severe retroversion of the epiglottis (photograph taken with a videobronchoscope with the patient breathing spontaneously). (B) Supraglottic stenosis (photograph taken with 0° endoscope under suspension laryngoscopy). (C) Scarification of the vallecular, lingual surface of epiglottis and base of tongue mucosae using CO_2 laser. (D) Mobilization of bilateral piriform sinus mucosae. (E) Supraglottic correction by endoscopic suturing and reestablishing the AE folds and epiglottopexy. Please note the fully mucosalized supraglottis. (F) Postoperative result at 3 months.

anesthesia was given using total intravenous anesthesia (TIVA) with the child breathing spontaneously and intermittent passing of a translaryngeal tube when required. The supraglottis, vocal cords, and trachea were intermittently anesthetized with 0.5% Novesine spray. The aberrant scar tissue at the level of the aryepiglottic folds was incised with the ultra-pulse CO_2 laser. Submucosal dissection was performed in order to advance a mucosal flap from the medial aspect of the piriform sinus. The flap was used to cover the mucosal defect of the aryepiglottic folds and was endoscopically sutured with Vicryl 5.0. An epiglottopexy was performed by scarifying the mucosae at the level of the lingual surface of the epiglottis, the valleculae, and the base of the tongue with the CO_2 laser. The epiglottis was subsequently sutured to the base of the tongue with a Lichtenberger needle carrier.

This needle carrying 3.0 Vicryl suture was passed from the inside and emerged on the outside. The Vicryl sutures were knotted and buried in the subcutaneous tissue. Two or three such sutures fixed the epiglottis to the base of tongue. The full mucosal resurfacing of the supraglottis along with an epiglottopexy allowed good healing and prevented recurrence of the stenosis. The epiglottopexy prevented backward tilt of the supraglottis during this healing process.

Evolution

Respiratory support by means of non-invasive ventilation was needed for 2 days after surgery. Feeding via nasogastric tube took place for 4 days following surgery and oral intake was progressively resumed after 5 days. Initial bronchoaspiration improved over the next few days with assistance of swallowing therapy and stridor disappeared within 2 weeks. No further complications were observed after a follow-up period of 9 months.

CASE 3: LATE-ONSET LARYNGOMALACIA

A 34-month-old boy presented with a history of night snoring, common nighttime arousals, constant mouth breathing, and frequent aggressive behavior. The personal story was marked by a diagnosis of congenital LM, but the symptoms had completely regressed with acid suppressive therapy by age 12 months. Voice and swallowing were normal according to the parents.

Initial Assessment

Head and neck examination showed a child in good general condition, with almost constant buccal breathing as well as adenoid hypertrophy with subtotal obstruction of the choanae and a tonsillar hypertrophy with 75% obstruction of the oropharyngeal lumen. Stertor without stridor was heard even when the child was awake. Fiberoptic evaluation of the larynx showed an omega-shaped (tubular) epiglottis with an otherwise normal supraglottic tone and no inspiratory collapse.

An in-patient polysomnography was carried out showing a severe obstructive sleep-apnea syndrome (OSAS) with an apnea-hypopnea index (AHI) of 19.7.

Diagnosis

OSAS within accompanying adenotonsillar hypertrophy.

Management and Evolution

The child underwent adenotonsillotomy at another institution without immediate postoperative complications. Three months after surgery the parents reported that, in spite of a short-lived period of symptom improvement after surgery, the sleep was still disordered and the child continued to snore. A new polysomnography was obtained 3 months after the surgery and showed a persistent OSAS (AHI = 15.2). Careful examination of video recording during polysomnography demonstrated presence of stridor during the REM phases of sleep.

Assessment and Management

Sleep endoscopy under spontaneous breathing was performed by introducing a pediatric bronchoscope through the nose. Laryngoscopy revealed an omega-shaped epiglottis with posterior collapse as well as inward collapse of the supraglottic mucosa during inspiration. The final diagnosis was that of late-onset LM. Having discussed the therapeutic strategy with the parents prior to surgery, CO_2 laser SGP as well as revision tonsillectomy were performed during the same anesthesia. Proton pump inhibitor (PPI) therapy was started postoperatively.

At Review

The immediate postoperative course was uncomplicated. Patient review 3 months after SGP revealed a complete remission of sleep-related symptoms. The polysomnography at that time showed an AHI of 6.1.

DISCUSSION

Etiology

LM is characterized by an insufficient tone of the supraglottis. Its exact etiology remains elusive and is thought to be largely multifactorial. Firstly, the newborn larynx has specific anatomical features which are thought to facilitate the development of LM. The newborn epiglottis and indeed the entire supraglottis are proportionally longer than in adults. The arytenoid cartilages are prominent and the interarytenoid space is proportionally larger and deeper than in adults. Furthermore, the aryepiglottic folds are shorter and have a lower basal tonus than in adults, hence conferring a tendency of the posterior supraglottic structures to an inward collapse. Secondly, it is suggested that laryngeal cartilages in the newborn are more flaccid and tend to more easily collapse during inspiration.[9–11]

Toward 18 to 24 months of age the proportions of the supraglottis gain a shape more similar to that of the adult larynx, hence usually resulting in full remission of symptoms.[12] Moreover it has been equally shown that the mucosa in children with LM tends to be edematous.[11] This edema is thought to be the consequence of both LPR and sustained mucosal trauma due to the increased inspiratory effort in these children.[13,14] While the anatomical configuration of the larynx may partially contribute to the clinical manifestations of LM, a neurological component of LM was postulated over a century ago. In this respect, Thomson and Turner demonstrated that alterations of the peripheral vagal nervous system may result in supraglottic collapse.[15] Further empirical observation shows that sedation in infants and seizures, strokes, or hypoxic brain insults potentially result in typical findings of LM. Symptoms of acquired LM in this context of neurological alterations tend to regress when the underlying neurological cause resolves.[16,17] More recently, Munson et al[18] provided histological evidence of nerve hypertrophy in the submucosal branches of the superior laryngeal nerve in patients with severe LM in comparison with age-matched healthy autopsy specimens.

The ensemble of these observations constitutes the foundation of the sensorimotor integrative etiologic theory of LM, most comprehensively exposed by Dana Thompson.[19] Thompson demonstrated an alteration of the laryngeal adductor reflex, which in turn is responsible for the tone and function of the supraglottis. The afferent pathway of the laryngeal adductor reflex is triggered at the level of mechanoreceptors and the chemoreceptors situated in the supraglottic mucosa. The peripheral stimuli are forwarded via the superior laryngeal nerve to the brainstem. After processing the afferent information, an efferent motor response is elicited via the vagus nerve.[19] Thompson indeed demonstrated that the baseline laryngopharyngeal sensory testing thresholds to trigger the laryngeal adductor reflex are higher in patients with LM and GERD than in those with LM, GERD, and neurological disease, but not in those with LM and neurological disease only when compared with patients with LM and no medical comorbidities.[19] Reported rates of GERD/LPR (defined as the penetration of liquid or gaseous acid/non-acid reflux into the pharyngolarynx) in children with LM are variable and situated somewhere between 65% and 100%, with approximately two-thirds of these patients displaying severe GERD.[20,21] LPR and GERD do not necessarily co-occur and in spite of efforts to identify clear diagnostic criteria based on laryngoscopy features and pH monitoring, due to the fact that both LPR symptoms and findings are variable and non-specific, a consensual clinical definition of LPR remains elusive.[21–23] In spite of such difficulties for the definition of LPR, empirical data show that laryngeal reflux penetration is more likely in children with an increased laryngopharyngeal sensory threshold.[24,25] In light of the high prevalence of GERD/LPR in children with LM, it has been suggested that GERD/LPR may alter the peripheral afferent sensory innervation of the larynx. The specific anatomical and perhaps histological features of the newborn and infant's larynx, combined with some degree of immaturity at the central nervous system level, may lead to the clinical manifestations of LM.[19]

DIAGNOSTIC ASPECTS

The diagnostic approach in the infant with LM needs to address three essential points:

1. Confirming the diagnosis of LM
2. Identifying associated comorbidities
3. Establishing disease severity degree

Confirming the Diagnosis of LM

Most diseases involving the larynx affect one or several of its functions, namely, breathing, airway protection/breathing-swallowing coordination (through its sphincter-like function), and speech. Since LM affects the supraglottis, two of these functions (breathing and breathing-swallowing coordination) can be affected.

With this in mind, accurate history-taking is an essential component in the diagnostic approach of the child with congenital stridor. About the leading symptom of LM, stridor, a detailed inquiry on its onset, evolution, and exacerbating factors (eg, crying, feeding, decubitus) should be obtained. While stridor intensity does not correlate to disease severity, its onset within the first 2 to 4 weeks of life is typical, although not

exclusive of LM.[19] Stridor which presents immediately after birth of beyond 3–4 months of age should evoke other diagnoses of congenital stridor (subglottic stenosis, posterior laryngeal clefts, vocal fold paralysis, etc).

Special attention should be paid to evaluation of swallowing. Anamnesis should include feeding modality (bottle vs. breast-feeding, or combination) and swallowing-related symptoms such as coughing, choking, regurgitations, and cyanosis during feeding.

With respect to clinical examination, the mainstay for the positive diagnosis of LM is in-office flexible fiberoptic laryngoscopy (FFL) in an awake patient. FFL allows dynamic evaluation of the larynx during breathing and has a very high diagnostic accuracy (approximately 90%).[26,27] In-office FFL should not go beyond the vocal cords and is sufficient for the diagnosis of LM in

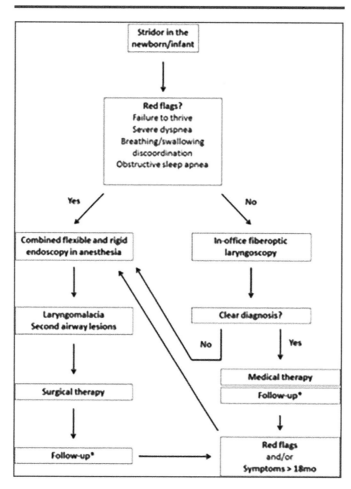

Figure 2–4. Workflow for the diagnostic and therapeutic approach in children with laryngomalacia. *Follow-up is to be regularly performed as long as symptoms persist.

the absence of the red flags (Figure 2–4). Furthermore, FFL can be combined with FEES in children with swallowing dysfunction (choking with cyanosis, cough, regurgitations/emesis). FEES allows dynamic assessment of swallowing and diagnosis of penetration/aspiration.

Infants with LM should be inspected in search of retractions (supraclavicular, subcostal, intercostal, or thoracoabdominal swing).

In case of red flags or unclear diagnosis, combined flexible and rigid endoscopy under anesthesia should be undertaken (see Figure 2–4). The intervention begins with a flexible endoscopic examination of airway from nares to carina and mainstem bronchi by using a flexible bronchoscope in a child in spontaneous breathing. Achieving spontaneous respiration requires an optimal level of anesthesia depth which would allow performing the procedure while avoiding an excessive depth which would preclude spontaneous breathing.[28] Constant collaboration and communication between surgeon and anesthetist is key for success.

The flexible bronchoscope is introduced into the nose, and permeability of the nasal cavities and the choanae is evaluated. The presence of an adenoid and/or tonsillar hypertrophy must be equally noted. Dynamic evaluation of the pharynx and specifically the presence of retrolingual or lateral pharyngeal obstruction are to be carefully assessed. In case of LM, its exact characteristics and sites of collapse must be very precisely observed in order to perform surgical correction (flaccid and posterior collapse of the epiglottis, short aryepiglottic folds, or collapsing arytenoids). A classical pitfall when endoscopically evaluating LM includes inadequate evaluation and/or documentation of vocal cord mobility. A normal vocal cord movement means optimal and symmetric abduction of the arytenoid cartilage and vocal ligament with each inspiration. Before the vocal cords are passed with the bronchoscope, the larynx is sprayed with Novesine and the entire tracheobronchial tree is examined. Direct laryngoscopy and suspension laryngoscopy with the use of a rigid telescope of different angulations are equally performed.

While discussing diagnosis with the parents, the anamnesis and the findings of FFL ought to prompt the surgeon to establish the odds of a surgical indication, which could eventually be carried out at the same time as diagnostic endoscopy. In contrast, however, in case of unclear diagnosis or unexpected findings in the course of diagnostic endoscopy, the therapeutic strategy should be established at a later time to avoid pitfalls. The note on pre-anesthesia evaluation is of utmost importance, as FFL has been shown to provide a better assessment of disease severity than direct laryngoscopy under total intravenous anesthesia.[26]

Identifying Associated Comorbidities

Even though LM is by far the most common cause of congenital stridor, differential diagnosis includes other conditions such as vocal cord paralysis (15–20%), subglottic stenosis (10–15%), laryngeal webs and atresia (5%), saccular cysts and laryngoceles (2%), subglottic hemangiomas (1.5–3%), and laryngotracheal clefts (0.5–1.5%).[29] It must be kept in mind that presence of synchronous airway lesions (SALs) in children with LM is equally possible and may have an impact on management approaches and outcomes. Rates of SALs in children with LM are variable and range from 7.5% to 64%.[13,30–33] The discrepancy of SAL reported rates is most likely due to the diagnostic technique used, included population, and physician's experience. The most common SALs diagnosed in patients with LM are subglottic stenosis and tracheomalacia.[13,30]

Diagnostic assessment should equally allow identifying relevant medical comorbidities. The most common medical comorbidity in children with LM is GERD/LPR, with an estimated prevalence as high as 70–100%.[20,34–36] The variable incidence rates are most likely due to the different diagnostic studies performed as well as variable diagnostic criteria used.

Severity of GERD seems to correlate with severity of LM symptoms.[19,34] FFL may show indirect signs of GERD/LPR, mainly mucosal edema or erythema (especially affecting the posterior glottis), but such findings are not specific or sensitive enough to establish the diagnosis.[37] It is therefore important to keep in mind that in case of severe LM with life-threatening manifestations, if severe GERD/LPR is suspected, or in case of symptom progression under acid suppression therapy, a formal diagnostic test (ie, 24-hour dual-probe pH manometry or monitoring) is essential.[37–39]

Other medical comorbidities, primarily neurological, cardiac, and multisystem syndromes, are diagnosed in a considerable proportion of children with severe disease.[40] More specifically, these comorbidities include Down syndrome (especially children with congenital heart disease), Pierre Robin sequence, CHARGE association (*c*oloboma, *h*eart defects, choanal *a*tresia, *g*rowth *r*etardation, *g*enital abnormalities, and *e*ar abnormalities), unspecific psychomotor retardardation, and Arnold–Chiari malformation.[13,30,40–42] In this sense, close collaboration between otolaryngologists and pediatricians is essential. This is especially true in entities like Arnold–Chiari malformation and hydrocephalus, which are amenable to posterior fossa decompression with possible resolution of airway manifestations without need of laryngeal surgery. In case of severe disease or if stridor first appears after 4 months of age, a high suspicion index is essential in order not to miss such entities. A brain MRI should be obtained in such cases.

Finally, the role of polysomnography in the assessment of children with congenital LM is controversial. A recent prospective study with a small population of children with LM showed that polysomnography was not a useful tool to determine disease severity.[43] Indeed, average AHIs in children who underwent SGP and those who did not were not significantly different. While probably not useful for severity stratification, available data seem to suggest a role of polysomnography for the assessment of surgical outcomes in patients with preoperative OSAS.[44,45]

Establishing Disease Severity Degree

Assessing degree of severity requires a comprehensive anamnesis and physical examination. Thompson[41] suggested a classification of LM based on the symptom severity:

- Mild LM (40% of patients): children present with inspiratory stridor without or only occasionally with mild symptoms of swallowing disorder, especially cough and choking/regurgitation
- Moderate LM (40% of patients): characterized by inspiratory stridor as well as frequent feeding-related difficulties and eventually failure to thrive
- Severe LM (20% of patients): features severe respiratory symptoms with cyanosis or even apnea and severe feeding difficulties with aspiration and failure to thrive

The difference between mild and moderate LM is the frequency of feeding-related symptoms as well as resting average oxygen saturation (SaO_2) (99% vs 96%).[41] Simons et al[46] demonstrated that swallowing dysfunction is common in children with LM regardless of disease severity or comorbidities; hence, suggesting that failure to thrive and presence of complications such as aspiration pneumonia are probably more meaningful criteria to define degrees of severity.

Shah and Wetmore proposed the SWAN mnemonic technique to assess the severity of LM: S = severity of stridor, W = weight gain, A = age at presentation, and N = neurologic status.[47]

MANAGEMENT

Therapeutic strategies in infants with LM are very much dependent on disease severity. Since 80% of patients with LM present with mild to moderate disease, most patients can be managed either symptomatically or medically.

It is essential to advise parents on the importance of non-pharmacological anti-reflux measures. These include use of thickened milk, avoiding decubitus position after meals, raising the head of the bed ensuring a stable 30° elevation of the children's upper body, and avoiding prone decubitus at all times.

Given the prominent association between LM and GERD/LPR, acid suppression therapy is most commonly advocated in cases of moderate LM. An H_2-receptor blocker (eg, ranitidine 3 mg/kg/day) or proton pump inhibitors (eg, omeprazole 1–2 mg/kg/day) can be used in the management of LM. Nevertheless, due to lack of evidence, optimal dosage and length of therapy are not established and largely depend on institutional experience.[20] While it is obvious that data derived from randomized clinical trials comparing placebo versus anti-reflux therapy would be extremely useful, it would be difficult to justify such a trial in a population which generally shows improvement under this treatment. Furthermore, endpoints would be difficult to evaluate, as the most commonly used criteria to define improvement are based on subjective evaluation of symptoms and thus are subject to observer bias.

It is unclear how long acid-suppressing therapy must be pursued in case of SGP, but some authors suggest prolonged postoperative administration to avoid aberrant scar formation.[19,20,41]

In case of symptom progression in spite of optimal acid suppression therapy, of failed SGP, of severe life-threatening symptoms, or in a context of comorbidities, diagnostic testing with impedance pH should be carried out. Fundoplication may be indicated in severe cases of LM, especially in children with relevant medical comorbidities or life-threatening manifestations.[1]

It is worth noting that while acid suppressant therapy is commonly prescribed and considered safe, emerging evidence suggests that long-term PPI therapy given to children younger than 6 months of age may be associated with an increased risk of bone fractures by age 6 years.[48]

Concerning surgery, the classical approach in the past for relief of airway obstruction in children with severe LM was tracheotomy. However, with the introduction of endoscopic laryngeal surgery, SGP under suspension laryngoscopy progressively became the mainstay of treatment for children with LM.[7,49,50]

The exact surgical procedure depends on the type of LM, and the surgical strategy should be established according to the findings in the awake patient. For cases with excessive supraglottic mucosa, the latter can be excised above the arytenoid cartilage, making sure to leave the interarytenoid space intact. Short aryepiglottic folds can be incised keeping close to the epiglottis or even including the borders of the epiglottis in case of tubular or omega- shaped variants. Finally, a posteriorly collapsing epiglottis can be fixed to the base of the tongue by means of epiglottopexy. Here we describe our experience for the surgical salvage of supraglottic stenosis following failed SGP (see Figures 2–2 and 2–3). Our team has recently described another technical variant of SGP that consists of saving 2 to 3

mm of mucosal island at the junction of the ary- and pharyngo-epiglottic folds with excision of the supra-arytenoid tissue in order to minimize aberrant scarring, which could result in supraglottic stenosis (Figure 2–5). The advantage of leaving this mucosal island is to buffer the backward tilt of the epiglottis during scarring of the aryepiglottic folds.

SGP is carried out under suspension microlaryngoscopy and may be performed with laser (especially CO2 laser), cold-steel instruments, or microdebriders used to remove redundant mucosa.[1,7,50–52] Each instrument has advantages and disadvantages. Modern-day ultrapulse CO_2 lasers are very precise and allow adequate hemostasis. A complication like supraglottic stenosis (SPGS) is dreaded after SGP. No association has been found between development of SPGS and the technique of SGP using either cold steel or laser.[5]

Logically, the larger the mucosal resection during SGP, the higher the chances of getting SPGS. An important aspect to consider is the type of anesthesia, as parallel access to the airway must allow oxygenation and surgical access to the larynx. Intermittent apnea/oxygenation has been classically used in the setting of endoscopic laryngeal surgery. Nevertheless, newborns and small infants have a rather limited apnea tolerance and the intervention times are too short to properly carry out SGP. SGP can often be performed under spontaneous breathing or with a small endotracheal tube in situ, always keeping in mind basic safety rules when using the CO_2 laser.[53] High-flow nasal oxygen therapy (HFNOT) exploits the phenomenon of a ventilatory mass flow, also known as *apneic oxygenation*, which is widely used for the respiratory support of children without the need for endotracheal intubation.[54] Early reports suggest that HFNOT could be a precious tool for tubeless endoscopic laryngeal surgery, including SGP.[55]

It is important to keep in mind that in some scenarios, endotracheal intubation is going to be required due to patient-specific features, especially in cases of pulmonary and cardiac comorbidities or difficult larynx exposure. Pierre Robin sequence and syndromes such as CHARGE, Noonan, and Down are systematically associated with difficult or impossible laryngeal suspension exposure. In such cases, a two-surgeon approach is a useful alternative: While one surgeon exposes the larynx with a rigid laryngoscope or a Macintosh laryngoscope blade, the other performs the procedure with the possibility to work with both hands.

Postoperative care depends on institutions and patient-related features. In our institution, routine

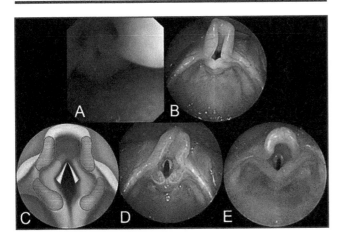

Figure 2–5. Mucosal-island saving supraglottoplasty. (A) Type II LM with severe supraglottic collapse. (B) Severe LM with short AE folds and tubular epiglottis. (C) Schematic representation: excision of the lateral epiglottic rims and saving 2 to 3-mm mucosal island at the junction of the ary- and pharyngo-epiglottic folds. Additional excision of the supraglottic tissue and lengthening of bilateral AE folds. (D) Intraoperative photograph. (E) Postoperative result at 4 months.

cases without intraoperative complications are extubated at the end of SGP with an overnight surveillance in the pediatric intensive care unit with non-invasive ventilation BiPAP (bilevel positive airway pressure). Feeding after surgery is initiated immediately, though this depends on each individual situation. Feeding after epiglottopexy is started after 5 days to allow sufficient time for the epiglottis to cicatrize and adhere to the base of tongue.

PROGNOSIS AND OUTCOMES

As mentioned above, approximately 80% of children have self-limited disease with only mild breathing- and swallowing-related manifestations.[2] Association of GERD/LPR is common, and medical comorbidities (especially neurologic and cardiac disease) complicate the overall management.[34,56] Approximately 10% of children with congenital LM require SGP. Of these, it is estimated that some 20–50% are going to require revision SGP or in extreme cases tracheostomy. The major determinant for SGP failure or need for ultimate tracheostomy seems to be once more related to the presence of GERD/LPR and other medical comorbidities, but also age at the time of surgery (<2 months).[40,41,56] SALs and particularly subglottic stenosis and craniofacial malformations all have adverse effects on surgical outcomes after SGP.[30,57]

It is estimated that children with two medical comorbidities in addition to GERD/LPR carry 5 times higher risk of revision SGP, and those with three comorbidities 10 times more risk to require tracheostomy.[41] Prematurity, in the absence of other comorbidities, does not seem to impact the outcome after SGP. Nevertheless, a gestation age of less than 32 weeks may be associated with higher rates of dysphagia. Swallowing therapy should be especially considered in this group of children.[58]

Children and especially younger infants tend to be smaller in weight and stature than healthy children of the same age at the time of SGP. However, most of these children tend to display a significant weight and stature gain in the few months following SGP.[59] Follow-up of children conservatively managed is essential, as it is estimated that approximately 30% of children with moderate disease will eventually progress to severe disease within 2 months. Risk factors for disease progression include presence of SALs, aspiration, comorbidities, a resting SAO2 <92%, and cyanosis.[19]

LATE-ONSET OR STATE-DEPENDENT LARYNGOMALACIA

Amin and Isaacson[60] coined the term *state-dependent LM* to describe children with normal breathing while awake who featured disordered breathing and LM endoscopic features during sleep.

Adenotonsillectomy is the mainstay of treatment for children with OSAS. Nevertheless, surgery results in full remission of OSAS only in a small proportion of children, hence indicating a multifactorial origin.[61–63] Careful evaluation of a video recording either at home or in the course of a polysomnography ought to allow distinguishing between simple snoring and stridor.

Subsequent observations have identified two additional groups of patients with such forms of late-onset LM: exercise-induced LM and feeding-disorder LM.[64] Feeding-disordered LM features redundant posterior glottic tissue with supra-arytenoid prolapse at rest and exacerbated during swallowing. PPI therapy tends to yield improvement of symptoms, but persistent symptoms may warrant SGP. Exercise-induced LM features characteristics of asthma or allergy without improvement under bronchodilator or anti-allergic therapy. Although these patients tend to have GERD, PPI rarely leads to improvement and SGP is most often needed.[64]

SUMMARY

Laryngomalacia is the leading cause of congenital stridor, with symptom onset within 2 weeks after birth. LM may associate respiratory distress of variable severity, disordered feeding due to impossible breathing/swallowing coordination eventually leading to failure to thrive, and in severe cases complications such as cor pulmonale and cardiac failure. Approximately 80% of children with congenital LM present with mild or moderate disease with full symptom resolution without any management or under acid suppressing medication and life style modifications by age 12–18 months. Those with severe disease or suspected comorbidities should undergo endoscopic evaluation in total anesthesia and eventually surgical management with supraglottoplasty. Prognosis of congenital LM is most often excellent in the absence of comorbidities.

Late-onset or state-dependent LM represents a different disease in older children with clinical and endoscopic features of LM. Most patients with late-onset LM require surgical management.

REFERENCES

1. Richter GT, Thompson DM. The surgical management of laryngomalacia. *Otolaryngolog Clin North Am.* 2008;41: 837–864, vii.
2. Dobbie AM, White DR. Laryngomalacia. *Pediatr Clin North Am.* 2013;60:893–902.
3. Belmont JR, Grundfast K. Congenital laryngeal stridor (laryngomalacia): etiologic factors and associated disorders. *Ann Otol Rhinol Laryngol.* 1984;93:430–437.
4. Apley J. The infant with stridor; a follow-up survey of 80 cases. *Arch Dis Child.* 1953;28:423–435.
5. Denoyelle F, Mondain M, Gresillon N, Roger G, Chaudre F, Garabedian EN. Failures and complications of supraglottoplasty in children. *Arch Otolaryngol Head Neck Surg.* 2003;129:1077–1080; discussion 80.
6. Roger G, Denoyelle F, Triglia JM, Garabedian EN. Severe laryngomalacia: surgical indications and results in 115 patients. *Laryngoscope.* 1995;105:1111–1117.
7. Holinger LD, Konior RJ. Surgical management of severe laryngomalacia. *Laryngoscope.* 1989;99:136–142.
8. Kay DJ, Goldsmith AJ. Laryngomalacia: a classification system and surgical treatment strategy. *Ear Nose & Throat J.* 2006;85:328–331, 336.
9. Sutherland GA, Lamber Lack, H. Congenital laryngeal obstruction. *Lancet.* 1897;150:653–656.
10. Manning SC, Inglis AF, Mouzakes J, Carron J, Perkins JA. Laryngeal anatomic differences in pediatric patients with severe laryngomalacia. *Arch Otolaryngol Head Neck Surg.* 2005;131:340–343.
11. Chandra RK, Gerber ME, Holinger LD. Histological insight into the pathogenesis of severe laryngomalacia. *Intl J Pediatr Otorhinolaryngol.* 2001;61:31–38.
12. Ayari S, Aubertin G, Girschig H, Van Den Abbeele T, Mondain M. Pathophysiology and diagnostic approach to laryngomalacia in infants. *Eur Ann Otorhinolaryngol Head Neck Dis.* 2012;129:257–263.
13. Dickson JM, Richter GT, Meinzen-Derr J, Rutter MJ, Thompson DM. Secondary airway lesions in infants with laryngomalacia. *Ann Otol Rhinol Laryngol.* 2009;118: 37–43.
14. Zoumalan R, Maddalozzo J, Holinger LD. Etiology of stridor in infants. *Ann Otol Rhinol Laryngol.* 2007;116: 329–334.
15. Thomson JTA. On the causation of congenital laryngeal stridor of infants. *BMJ.* 1900:1561–1563.
16. Wiggs WJ, Jr., DiNardo LJ. Acquired laryngomalacia: resolution after neurologic recovery. *Otolaryngol Head Neck Surg.* 1995;112:773–776.
17. Rowe-Jones J, Moore-Gillon V, Hamilton P. Acquired laryngomalacia: epiglottis prolapse as a cause of airway obstruction. *Ann Otol Rhinol Laryngol.* 1993;102:485–486.
18. Munson PD, Saad AG, El-Jamal SM, Dai Y, Bower CM, Richter GT. Submucosal nerve hypertrophy in congenital laryngomalacia. *Laryngoscope.* 2011;121:627–629.
19. Thompson DM. Abnormal sensorimotor integrative function of the larynx in congenital laryngomalacia: a new theory of etiology. *Laryngoscope.* 2007;117:1–33.
20. Hartl TT, Chadha NK. A systematic review of laryngomalacia and acid reflux. *Otolaryngol Head Neck Surg.* 2012;147:619–626.
21. Campagnolo AM, Priston J, Thoen RH, Medeiros T, Assuncao AR. Laryngopharyngeal reflux: diagnosis, treatment, and latest research. *Int Arch Otorhinolaryngol.* 2014; 18:184–191.
22. Belafsky PC, Postma GN, Koufman JA. The validity and reliability of the reflux finding score (RFS). *The Laryngoscope.* 2001;111:1313–1317.
23. Abou-Ismail A, Vaezi MF. Evaluation of patients with suspected laryngopharyngeal reflux: a practical approach. *Curr Gastroenterol Rep.* 2011;13:213–218.
24. Thompson DM. Laryngopharyngeal sensory testing and assessment of airway protection in pediatric patients. *American J Med.* 2003;115 (suppl 3A)166S–168S.
25. Aviv JE, Liu H, Parides M, Kaplan ST, Close LG. Laryngopharyngeal sensory deficits in patients with laryngopharyngeal reflux and dysphagia. *Ann Otol Rhinol Laryngol.* 2000;109:1000–1006.
26. Hartzell LD, Richter GT, Glade RS, Bower CM. Accuracy and safety of tracheoscopy for infants in a tertiary care clinic. *Arch Otolaryngol Head Neck Surg.* 2010;136:66–69.
27. Lima TM, Goncalves DU, Goncalves LV, Reis PA, Lana AB, Guimaraes FF. Flexible nasolaryngoscopy accuracy in laryngomalacia diagnosis. *Braz J Otorhinolaryngol.* 2008; 74:29–32.
28. Best C. Anesthesia for laser surgery of the airway in children. *Paediatric Anaesthesia.* 2009;19 Suppl 1:155–165.
29. Monnier P. *Pediatric Airway Surgery: Management of Laryngotracheal Stenosis in Infants and Children.* Berlin, Heidelberg, Germany: Springer-Verlag; 2010.
30. Schroeder JW, Jr., Bhandarkar ND, Holinger LD. Synchronous airway lesions and outcomes in infants with severe laryngomalacia requiring supraglottoplasty. *Arch Otolaryngol Head Neck Surg.* 2009;135:647–651.
31. Cohen SR, Eavey RD, Desmond MS, May BC. Endoscopy and tracheotomy in the neonatal period: a 10-year review, 1967–1976. *Ann Otol Rhinol Laryngol.* 1977;86:577–583.
32. Krashin E, Ben-Ari J, Springer C, Derowe A, Avital A, Sivan Y. Synchronous airway lesions in laryngomalacia. *Intl J Pediatr Otorhinolaryngol.* 2008;72:501–507.
33. Yuen HW, Tan HK, Balakrishnan A. Synchronous airway lesions and associated anomalies in children with laryngomalacia evaluated with rigid endoscopy. *Intl J Pediatr Otorhinolaryngol.* 2006;70:1779–1784.
34. Giannoni C, Sulek M, Friedman EM, Duncan NO, 3rd. Gastroesophageal reflux association with laryngomalacia: a prospective study. *Intl J Pediatr Otorhinolaryngol.* 1998;43:11–20.
35. Reinhard A, Sandu K. Laryngomalacia: principal cause of stridor in infants and small children. *Rev Med Suisse.* 2014;10:1816–1819.

36. Olney DR, Greinwald JH, Jr., Smith RJ, Bauman NM. Laryngomalacia and its treatment. *Laryngoscope*. 1999;109: 1770–1775.

37. Matthews BL, Little JP, McGuirt WF, Jr., Koufman JA. Reflux in infants with laryngomalacia: results of 24-hour double-probe pH monitoring. *Otolaryngol Head Neck Surg*. 1999;120:860–864.

38. Ulualp SO, Rodriguez S, Holmes-Wright CN. Flexible laryngoscopy-guided pharyngeal pH monitoring in infants. *Laryngoscope*. 2007;117:577–580.

39. Ulualp SO, Toohill RJ, Hoffmann R, Shaker R. Pharyngeal pH monitoring in patients with posterior laryngitis. *Otolaryngol Head Neck Surg*. 1999;120:672–677.

40. Hoff SR, Schroeder JW, Jr., Rastatter JC, Holinger LD. Supraglottoplasty outcomes in relation to age and comorbid conditions. *Intl J Pediatr Otorhinolaryngol*. 2010; 74:245–249.

41. Thompson DM. Laryngomalacia: factors that influence disease severity and outcomes of management. *Curr Opin Otolaryngol Head Neck Surg*. 2010;18:564–570.

42. Gonzalez C, Reilly JS, Bluestone CD. Synchronous airway lesions in infancy. *Ann Otol Rhinol Laryngol*. 1987; 96:77–80.

43. Weinstein JE, Lawlor CM, Wu EL, Rodriguez KH. Utility of polysomnography in determination of laryngomalacia severity. *Intl J Pediatr Otorhinolaryngol*. 2017;93:145–149.

44. O'Connor TE, Bumbak P, Vijayasekaran S. Objective assessment of supraglottoplasty outcomes using polysomnography. *Intl J Pediatr Otorhinolaryngol*. 2009;73: 1211–1216.

45. Powitzky R, Stoner J, Fisher T, Digoy GP. Changes in sleep apnea after supraglottoplasty in infants with laryngomalacia. *Intl J Pediatr Otorhinolaryngol*. 2011;75:1234–1239.

46. Simons JP, Greenberg LL, Mehta DK, Fabio A, Maguire RC, Mandell DL. Laryngomalacia and swallowing function in children. *The Laryngoscope*. 2016;126:478–484.

47. Shah UK, Wetmore RF. Laryngomalacia: a proposed classification form. *Intl J Pediatr Otorhinolaryngol*. 1998;46: 21–26.

48. Lyon J. Study questions use of acid suppressors to curb mild infant reflux. *JAMA*. 2017;318:1427–1428.

49. Kavanagh KT, Babin RW. Endoscopic surgical management for laryngomalacia. Case report and review of the literature. *Ann Otol Rhinol Laryngol*. 1987;96:650–653.

50. Solomons NB, Prescott CA. Laryngomalacia. A review and the surgical management for severe cases. *Intl J Pediatr Otorhinolaryngol*. 1987;13:31–39.

51. Zalzal GH, Collins WO. Microdebrider-assisted supraglottoplasty. *Intl J Pediatr Otorhinolaryngol*. 2005;69: 305–309.

52. Groblewski JC, Shah RK, Zalzal GH. Microdebrider-assisted supraglottoplasty for laryngomalacia. *Ann Otol Rhinol Laryngol*. 2009;118:592–597.

53. Roy S, Smith LP. Surgical fires in laser laryngeal surgery: are we safe enough? *Otolaryngol Head Neck Surg*. 2015;152:67–72.

54. Patel A, Nouraei SA. Transnasal humidified rapid-insufflation ventilatory exchange (THRIVE): a physiological method of increasing apnoea time in patients with difficult airways. *Anaesthesia*. 2015;70:323–329.

55. Humphreys S, Rosen D, Housden T, Taylor J, Schibler A. Nasal high-flow oxygen delivery in children with abnormal airways. *Paediatr Anaesthes*. 2017;27:616–620.

56. Preciado D, Zalzal G. A systematic review of supraglottoplasty outcomes. *Arch Otolaryngol Head Neck Surg*. 2012; 138:718–721.

57. van der Heijden M, Dikkers FG, Halmos GB. Treatment outcome of supraglottoplasty vs. wait-and-see policy in patients with laryngomalacia. *Eur Arch Otorhinolaryngol*. 2016;273:1507–1513.

58. Durvasula VS, Lawson BR, Bower CM, Richter GT. Supraglottoplasty in premature infants with laryngomalacia: does gestation age at birth influence outcomes? *Otolaryngol Head Neck Surg*. 2014;150:292–299.

59. Czechowicz JA, Chang KW. Catch-up growth in infants with laryngomalacia after supraglottoplasty. *Intl J Pediatr Otorhinolaryngol*. 2015;79:1333–1336.

60. Amin MR, Isaacson G. State-dependent laryngomalacia. *Ann Otol Rhinol Laryngol*. 1997;106:887–890.

61. Tauman R, Gulliver TE, Krishna J, Montgomery-Downs HE, O'Brien LM, Ivanenko A, et al. Persistence of obstructive sleep apnea syndrome in children after adenotonsillectomy. *J Pediatr*. 2006;149:803–808.

62. Mitchell RB. Adenotonsillectomy for obstructive sleep apnea in children: outcome evaluated by pre- and postoperative polysomnography. *Laryngoscope*. 2007;117:1844–1854.

63. Bhattacharjee R, Kheirandish-Gozal L, Spruyt K, et al. Adenotonsillectomy outcomes in treatment of obstructive sleep apnea in children: a multicenter retrospective study. *Am J Resp Crit Care Med*. 2010;182:676–683.

64. Richter GT, Rutter MJ, deAlarcon A, Orvidas LJ, Thompson DM. Late-onset laryngomalacia: a variant of disease. *Arch Otolaryngol Head Neck Surg*. 2008;134:75–80.

CHAPTER 3

Laryngeal Cleft

Sophie G. Shay, Douglas Sidell, and Dinesh Chhetri

INTRODUCTION

Laryngeal cleft is a rare congenital anomaly. The trachea and esophagus initially form as a common lumen which is then separated by the tracheoesophageal septum between 20 and 40 days' gestation.[1] Between the fifth and seventh gestational weeks, failure in the posterior fusion of the cricoid from the sixth branchial arch, abnormal development of the interarytenoid muscle or mucosa, or partial or complete failure to develop the tracheoesophageal septum leads to formation of a laryngeal or laryngotracheal cleft.[2] This developmental anomaly leads to communication between the gastrointestinal tract and airway, potentially leading to aspiration, airway obstruction, or both.

Most cases occur sporadically, though nonsyndromic associations with other airway anomalies have previously been reported (tracheoesophageal anomalies, subglottic stenosis, vocal cord immobility, laryngomalacia, tracheomalacia).[3] Laryngeal clefts can also occur as part of a syndrome, including Optiz–Frias (G) syndrome, Pallister–Hall syndrome, CHARGE (coloboma of the eyes, heart anomalies, choanal atresia, growth and mental retardation, genital anomalies, ear abnormalities), and VACTERL (vertebral anomalies, anal atresia, cardiac defects, tracheoesophageal fistula, ear anomalies, renal anomalies, and limb defects).[4] It is also critical to recognize potentially associated cardiac anomalies, including aortic coarctation, transposition of the great vessels, patent ductus arteriosus, and septal defects.

CASE 1

History

A 2-year-old male previously full-term infant without significant prenatal history was referred to the otolaryngology clinic for long-standing feeding difficulties. The patient also has a history of poor weight gain and recurrent respiratory infections requiring multiple hospitalizations.

Workup

Modified barium swallow study (MBSS) performed a year prior demonstrated deep laryngeal penetration and direct aspiration to thin liquids as well as nectar-thickened and syrup-thickened liquids with minimal cough response. Gastroenterology evaluation was notable for gastroesophageal reflux. Subsequently, the patient had a gastrostomy tube placed at an outside institution for feeding prior to evaluation with otolaryngology.

A flexible endoscopic evaluation of swallow (FEES) was performed during our clinical evaluation which continued to reveal laryngeal penetration and aspiration to thin liquids without evidence of aspiration to nectar-thickened liquids. After our clinical evaluation, the patient was started on an oral diet of nectar-thickened liquids.

Diagnosis

Microdirect laryngoscopy in the operating room revealed a deep interarytenoid notch consistent with a type I laryngeal cleft (Figure 3–1).

Management

The patient underwent endoscopic repair of the type I cleft under microsuspension laryngoscopy and insufflation technique (Figure 3–2). The larynx was topicalized with 2% lidocaine and oxymetazoline. The carbon dioxide laser was used in this case at 4 watts continuous mode to denude the mucosa in the interarytenoid space. Care was taken to remove the mucosa at the most inferior portion of the cleft without injuring the surrounding glottis or supraglottic structures. Microscissors were used to further develop interartyenoid mucosal flaps. A 5-0 polydioxanone suture (PDS) was then used in mass-closure technique as previously described.[5] The patient was left extubated at the end of the procedure.

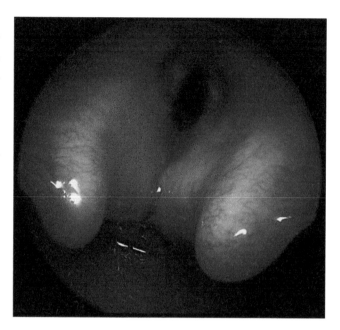

Figure 3–2. Type I laryngeal cleft following endoscopic surgical repair using the mass-closure technique.

Postoperative Course

The patient was admitted overnight to the pediatric intensive care unit for close airway monitoring postoperatively. On postoperative day 1, speech language pathology was consulted for a bedside swallow evaluation and the patient started on nectar-thickened liquids prior to discharge.

Follow-Up

The patient was seen for 6-week follow-up for a repeat FEES, which showed a healing surgical site and improved swallowing without evidence of aspiration or penetration to thin liquids.

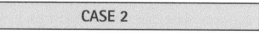

CASE 2

History

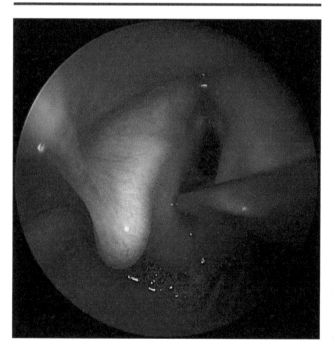

Figure 3–1. Type I laryngeal cleft extending to the level above the true vocal cords. A blunt right angle probe is seen splaying apart the interarytenoid space for endoscopic evaluation.

A neonate presented to an outside institution at 5 days of life with progressive respiratory distress and feeding difficulties.

Workup

A nasogastric feeding tube was placed, causing immediate worsening of respiratory distress. The patient was subsequently intubated. The patient was taken to the operating room and underwent diagnostic laryngoscopy, bronchoscopy, and tracheostomy. During the bronchoscopy, the patient was noted to have a type III laryngeal cleft. Shortly thereafter, the patient also had a gastrostomy tube placed.

Diagnosis

The patient was subsequently referred for further evaluation. The patient underwent another diagnostic laryngoscopy and bronchoscopy, which confirmed the presence of a type III laryngeal cleft, extending to the distal cervical trachea.

Management

Surgical repair of the laryngeal cleft was performed via an open transtracheal approach with laryngofissure. During the laryngofissure, the anterior commissure was carefully tagged, and reapproximated after cleft repair. The mucosa of the cleft was carefully denuded, taking special care to denude the apical mucosa. The cleft was repaired using a three-layer closure: (1) esophageal mucosa closure with knots in the esophageal lumen, (2) intervening sternal periosteum, (3) tracheal mucosa closure with knots in the tracheal lumen. The closure is performed up to the interarytenoid space. Due to the nature of the cleft, there is usually a redundancy of esophageal mucosa.

Postoperative Course

During hospitalization, the patient underwent a clinical bedside per os (PO) swallow trial, as well as an MBSS with esophageal follow-through to ensure that there was no contrast extravasation. The patient had follow-up bronchoscopies at 10 days, 6 weeks, and 3 months postoperatively, during which suture granulation tissue was trimmed.

CASE 3

History

A 3-month-old infant presented to the pediatric otolaryngology clinic for evaluation of mild inspiratory stridor without respiratory distress. The patient was tolerating a regular diet and thin liquids without a history of dysphagia.

Workup

In-office flexible fiberoptic laryngoscopy revealed significant mucosal redundancy in the interarytenoid space, suspicious for a laryngeal cleft. The patient was admitted to the pediatric intensive care unit, during which a nasogastric tube was placed, inciting respiratory distress and requiring intubation.

Diagnosis

The patient was taken to the operating room for a diagnostic laryngoscopy and bronchoscopy, which revealed a type III laryngeal cleft extending through the cricoid.

Management

The laryngeal cleft was repaired using the transoral, endoscopic mass-closure technique.[5] The cleft mucosa was denuded using cold steel, paying special attention to removing all of the mucosa at the apex prior to closure. A combination of 4-0 and 5-0 PDS was used, working distal to proximal, up to the interarytenoid space.

Postoperative Course

A nasogastric tube was kept postoperatively until the first bronchoscopy. A clinical bedside swallow evaluation and MBSS with esophageal follow-through were used to assess the integrity of the cleft repair. The patient was taken back to the operating room for bronchoscopy on postoperative day 10, at which time mildly redundant esophageal mucosa and suture granulation tissue were carefully removed using endoscopic techniques. Additionally, the patient was taken to the operating room at 6 weeks and 3 months postoperatively in order to continually assess the repair integrity and monitor for delayed repair breakdown.

EPIDEMIOLOGY

In 1792, Richter first described laryngeal cleft in an infant presenting with recurrent aspiration. However, to this day, laryngeal cleft still represents a diagnostic challenge and requires a high index of suspicion. The incidence of laryngeal cleft is likely underestimated in the literature, as the diagnosis of type I laryngeal clefts is relatively subjective; moreover, minor laryngeal clefts may be asymptomatic and go undiagnosed, and endoscopic diagnosis can be elusive when the diagnosis is not considered. Congenital anomalies of the larynx have been estimated to be between 1 in 10,000 to 1 in 50,000 live births, with laryngeal clefts representing 0.5 to 1.6% of these abnormalities. Among endoscopies performed for recurrent respiratory symptoms, the published incidence ranges from 0.2% to 7.6%.[6–12] On postmortem laryngeal examination, Moungthong and Hollinger[7] found a 7% incidence of submucous laryngeal cleft and 2.6% of laryngotracheoesophageal cleft among 115 cases. There is a slight male predominance, with a reported male:female ratio of 1.2:1 to 1.8:1.[13,14] There is currently no evidence to suggest a racial predominance.

CLASSIFICATION

Multiple classification schemes have been suggested based on the length of the laryngeal cleft.[15,16] The most commonly used system was developed in 1989 by Benjamin and Inglis, who described four types of cleft.[1] Type I is above the level of the true vocal cords, representing a supraglottic interarytenoid cleft. Type II extends into but not completely through the posterior cricoid lamina, below the level of the true vocal cords (Figure 3–3). Type III extends through the posterior cricoid lamina with or without extension into cervical tracheoesophageal wall. Type IV extends through the tracheoesophageal wall to the level of the carina. Additionally, Tucker and Maddalozzo[17] described an occult, submucous cleft consisting of a midline submucosal

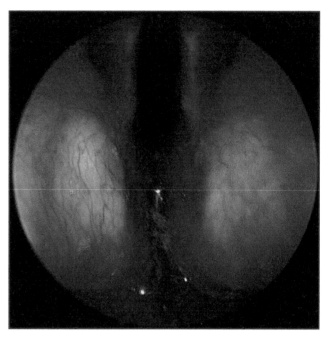

Figure 3–3. Type II laryngeal cleft extending past the true vocal cords and involving the cricoid cartilage.

defect of the posterior cricoid cartilage with intact overlying interarytenoid mucosa and musculature.

Sandu and Monnier[18] modified the Benjamin and Inglis classification to further stratify type III and type IV laryngeal clefts: type IIIa is a complete cleft of the cricoid plate, type IIIb involves the intrathoracic trachea no farther past the level of the sternal notch, type IVa extends into the intrathoracic trachea to the carina, and type IVb is an intrathoracic extension of the cleft involving one main bronchus.

PRESENTATION

Presenting symptoms of laryngeal clefts are often respiratory in nature, with severity of symptoms typically correlating with depth of the cleft. In a case series of 22 patients, Rahbar and colleagues[19] reported that 90% of patients with types I–III clefts had respiratory symptoms. Type I clefts can present subtly with mild feeding difficulties or recurrent pulmonary infections. Patients with type I and II clefts can also present with chronic cough, wheezing, stridor, hoarse cry, and pharyngeal hypersecretions, and may also have coughing, choking, dyspnea, and cyanosis while feeding. Rahbar and colleagues[20] also reported a 15% hospital admission rate for respiratory symptoms among patients with type I clefts and 25% for type II clefts. Chien et al[6] described 20 patients diagnosed with type I clefts in which the most common presenting symptoms were aspiration of thin liquids (90%), recurrent aspiration pneumonia (50%), and chronic cough (35%). Type I clefts often do not cause significant symptomology until the first several months of life, and are commonly diagnosed between 2 and 5 years of age; however, type I clefts may also be asymptomatic and only diagnosed incidentally when evaluating the airway for unrelated symptoms.[14] In a series of 31 patients with type I laryngeal cleft, van der Doef et al[21] reported that age at diagnosis ranged from 1 month to 13 years, with a mean age of 1 year and 10 months. Other studies have suggested that most patients are diagnosed between 2 and 5 years of age.[6,8,19] While one study found a 90% association of type I laryngeal cleft with congenital stridor, other studies have found a lower incidence between 8% and 41%.[4,21,22] Reported rate of associated laryngomalacia has ranged from 5% to 90% in the literature[16,21,23]; and it is important to note that both the diagnoses of laryngomalacia and of laryngeal cleft are rather subjective. On endoscopy, the findings of laryngomalacia and type I cleft can be similar, with the difficult distinction between tall arytenoids versus a deep interarytenoid notch further blurring the diagnoses.

Types III and IV clefts present with more severe respiratory symptoms, including hypoxia and apnea, often prompting earlier medical attention and diagnosis. These major clefts are often associated with other pulmonary and foregut anomalies and congenital abnormalities, which portend high mortality rates without prompt diagnosis and initiation of appropriate nutritional and respiratory care.[24] In particular, type IV clefts often lead to severe aspiration, excessive pulmonary mucus, and early respiratory distress requiring mechanical ventilation. In these patients, presentation usually occurs in the first few days of life.

DIAGNOSIS

When approaching a pediatric patient with postfeeding stridor, feeding difficulties, and/or recurrent pulmonary infections, it is important to include laryngeal cleft in the differential diagnosis. While other etiologies, including laryngomalacia, gastroesophageal

reflux disease, neuromuscular disorders, and reactive airway disease, are more common and may produce similar nonspecific symptoms, it is prudent to investigate for a laryngeal cleft during any diagnostic laryngoscopy. All patients with a suspected laryngeal cleft should undergo a careful history and physical examination, swallowing assessment for aspiration with MBSS, FEES, or both, and an operative laryngoscopy and bronchoscopy.

Endoscopy Under Sedation or Anesthesia

The gold standard for diagnosing a laryngeal cleft is palpation of the interarytenoid space during microlaryngoscopy. This is done under general anesthesia, and can be performed with suspension laryngoscopy to allow for palpation of the larynx, in conjunction with rigid bronchoscopy to evaluate the distal airways. A comprehensive evaluation of the airway is often performed in concert with a pulmonary flexible bronchoscopy, so as to allow for a dynamic evaluation of the trachea and bronchi under light anesthesia followed by a bronchoalveolar lavage when indicated. Endoscopy is performed with the patient spontaneously ventilating, to allow for a dynamic tracheobronchial evaluation. Topical lidocaine is applied to the vocal cords and either a microscope or Hopkins rod telescope is used to obtain a high-definition assessment of the glottis and supraglottis. The posterior glottis and interarytenoid space is palpated, often with a right-angled probe, to assess the presence of the interarytenoid muscle. In some cases of type I cleft, the interarytenoid muscle is present but atrophic, making the diagnosis of type I cleft somewhat subjective as the degree of atrophy can be variable.[25,26]

Radiographic Assessment

Plain chest radiographs may offer nonspecific signs of pulmonary infiltrates suggestive of chronic aspiration. Chronic aspiration may also be evident with pneumonia or peribronchial cuffing on plain films.[8] MBSS is helpful in preoperative assessment of aspiration and is noninvasive, but also is nonspecific regarding the etiology of aspiration, particularly in relation to laryngeal anatomy. In the evaluation of laryngeal clefts, MBSS often shows immediate aspiration of barium into the trachea. Johnston et al[8] reported that 75% of patients with type I and type II clefts will demonstrate aspiration on MBSS.

Non-Sedated Flexible Endoscopy

Flexible laryngoscopy may be done at bedside or in clinic for an initial airway assessment, and may be suggestive of a laryngeal cleft, but provides a poor view of the posterior glottis and does not allow for palpation of the airway; it should thus be considered unreliable for diagnosis.

FEES can be a helpful adjunct to laryngeal cleft workup and can be done at the time of flexible laryngoscopy during the initial clinical evaluation. While patient cooperation may make assessment difficult depending on patient age, FEES allows for dynamic evaluation of the larynx and pharynx and penetration and aspiration of various liquid and solid food textures, and may localize where the aspiration occurs. Chien et al[6] found that among 11 patients with type I laryngeal cleft who had both MBSS and FEES performed, 36% had an abnormal FEES with normal MBSS findings, suggesting that FEES may also be more sensitive. However, it is important to emphasize that both MBSS and FEES may have normal results in patients with subtle laryngeal clefts and intermittent aspiration. Additionally, it is important to review the MBSS/FEES prior to considering type I cleft repair, as the pattern of aspiration seen on the swallow studies may not involve the interarytenoid cleft and would not benefit from laryngeal cleft repair.

Neurologic Evaluation

It is becoming more apparent that the swallowing dysfunction associated with laryngeal cleft is a multifactorial challenge.[27,28] In particular, it appears that despite surgical management, a subset of patients continued to have persistent swallowing difficulties, with many of these patients having multiple medical comorbidities. Walker and colleagues[29] retrospectively reviewed 242 patients with laryngeal cleft and found that 38.4% had evidence of neuromuscular dysfunction or dyscoordination. Among patients who obtained brain imaging, abnormal findings were present in 64%. Furthermore, 4 patients were ultimately referred for neurosurgical intervention (3 with a diagnosis of Chiari malformation, and 1 patient with an intracranial tumor). Neuromuscular dysfunction likely plays a large role in the development and prognosis of patients with laryngeal cleft, and neurologic assessment may be indicated in the appropriate clinical setting. The relationship among laryngeal cleft, swallowing dysfunction, and neuromuscular disorders is likely complex and continues to be elucidated in the literature.

MANAGEMENT

Conservative/Medical Management

Patients with laryngeal cleft should be treated with appropriate medical management prior to surgical measures. Conservative measures include proton pump inhibitors for gastroesophageal reflux, feeding therapy, upright positioning when feeding, and a texture modification diet. Nasogastric tube feeds can be considered for severe swallowing difficulties. Parsons[23] and van der Doef[21] advocated for conservative management for type I laryngeal clefts, with the latter reporting 90% success with conservative management. However, Watters and Russell[30] and Chien et al[6] reported that 75–80% of patients with type I laryngeal cleft managed initially with conservative management required surgical intervention.

Surgery

The first successful surgical laryngeal cleft repair was reported by Pettersson in 1955.[15] Surgical intervention depends largely upon the severity of the laryngeal cleft.

Injection Laryngoplasty

The least invasive method of surgically managing a type I laryngeal cleft is with an endoscopic injection laryngoplasty of gelatin sponge,[31] sodium carboxymethylcellulose aqueous gel,[31] or hyaluronic-acid based gel.[33] This is done with suspension microlaryngoscopy either with visualization using an operating microscope or 0-degree Hopkins rod telescope. As outlined by Kennedy et al,[31] the injection of gelatin sponge is prepared by mixing 1 gram of gelatin sponge powder with 4 mL of sterile 0.9% saline and approximately 1 mL injected submucosally into the interarytenoid area. With either injection material, the injection is applied to the apex of the interarytenoid notch until fullness and blunting of the area is noted. Four of the 8 patients (50%) treated with gelatin sponge powder by Kennedy et al[31] had marked improvement of symptoms and did not require further interventions, while Cohen et al[32] reported that 9 of 16 patients (56%) had resolution of symptoms following injection laryngoplasty and Mangat and El-Hakim[33] reported a 72% success rate.

Horn and Parikh[34] investigated the role of injection laryngoplasty in children with chronic aspiration, both with and without anatomic evidence of type I laryngeal cleft. Interestingly, they found improvement of aspiration on MBSS following augmentation of the interarytenoid space regardless of the presence of a cleft, although noncleft patients were more likely to have recurrence of symptoms after an initial period of improvement. While type I laryngeal cleft remains a fairly subjective diagnosis, their findings suggest that in patients with multifaceted swallow dysfunction or uncoordinated swallowing, the interarytenoid space serves as the path of least resistance for aspiration.

Endoscopic Repair

For type I and type II laryngeal clefts, endoscopic repair is considered the gold standard, with success rates reported between 80% and 100%,[6,20,30] and can be done at the time of diagnostic laryngoscopy. Several variations of technique have been described. Endoscopic repair is performed with suspension microlaryngoscopy, usually with an infant or pediatric Lindholm suspension laryngoscope. In coordination with the anesthesiologist, the patient is induced with general anesthesia with spontaneous ventilation. The repair is most commonly performed with the patient spontaneously ventilating, using insufflation technique through the ventilating port of the laryngoscope or a cut endotracheal tube placed at the oral commissure. The interarytenoid space is then palpated to assess the laryngeal cleft and the submucosa injected with 1% lidocaine with epinephrine 1:100,000. Use of cold steel microflap or carbon dioxide (CO_2) laser reapproximation have both been advocated. In comparing microflap versus CO_2 laser techniques, Ketcham et al[35] did not find a difference in success rate between the two techniques. A diamond-shaped incision extending bilaterally to the edge of the cleft is made to denude the interarytenoid mucosa, and anterior and posterior flaps are formed. This incision exposes the remnant interarytenoid muscle. The anterior and posterior flaps are then reapproximated in the midline using resorbable sutures in a single layer.

Postoperative intubation has been controversial. The rationale for postoperative intubation is to maintain a secure airway in the postoperative period while the cleft repair heals. However, many authors have advocated for immediate postoperative extubation with close airway monitoring.[2,36,37] Even among those who advocate for postoperative intubation, there is no clear consensus on duration of postoperative intubation, ranging from 1 to 12 days.[6,19]

Following endoscopic repair, patients may need to undergo swallow evaluation prior to initiating oral feeding, depending on the preoperative assessment and depth of the cleft. This can be done with repeat MBSS or bedside swallow evaluation in the days and weeks following repair. Patients are given postoperative intravenous steroids for 24 hours, antibiotics, and proton pump inhibitors.

For type I or II laryngeal clefts, we recommend the endoscopic "mass closure technique"[5] with development of a cold-steel microflap followed by an interrupted submucosal everting closure with 4-0 or 5-0 PDS on an RB-2 needle (Figure 3–4). The key to this technique is removal of an adequate strip of mucosa at the repair site, ensuring that the mucosa is removed completely at the apex of the cleft, as breakdown in this area is probably the most common. Special attention is also given to placement of the apex stitch, which, for the same reasons, is most important to the integrity of the cleft repair. Author D.S. prefers to leave the patients extubated postoperatively. The majority of patients are discharged on postoperative day 1 with a soft diet for

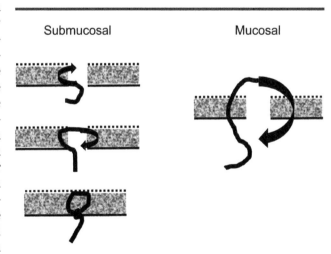

Figure 3–4. Endoscopic mass-closure technique as described by Balakrishnan et al (2015),[5] with both submucosal and mucosal techniques shown. Arrow depicts the direction of the suture, dotted lines represent tracheal mucosa, and solid lines represent esophageal mucosa.

2 weeks and follow-up with an MBSS versus FEES 6 weeks postoperatively.

Garabedian et al[37] reported the successful endoscopic repair of four patients with type III laryngeal cleft; two of the four patients required a second endoscopic procedure for additional supraglottic closure. Adil et al[38] described using a CO_2 laser for endoscopic management of six patients with type III laryngeal cleft, of whom five patients (83%) had resolution of aspiration symptoms at 3 months follow-up. However, the literature remains sparse regarding endoscopic repair for these larger clefts.

Open Repair

Balakrishnan and colleagues[5] compared endoscopic repair with open repair of types I, II, and III clefts and found that endoscopic repairs using the mass-closure technique[19] were associated with shorter operative time and reduced hospital stays than open approaches, although this was largely determined by the need for postoperative intubation in patients who underwent an open approach. There was no significant difference in effectiveness of open versus endoscopic approaches. However, for the more severe, deeper clefts, open approaches should certainly be considered. Open surgical approaches also allow for additional open airway reconstructive procedures to occur simultaneously, should they be indicated.

Compared with type I or II laryngeal clefts, types III and IV laryngeal clefts often present with more severe symptoms, and are more likely to be associated with other congenital foregut or pulmonary abnormalities. As such, the management of these rare and complex clefts requires multidisciplinary input. Many of these patients may require repair of a tracheoesophageal fistula, esophageal atresia, or microgastria.[8] These patients may benefit from gastrostomy tube placement for nutritional support and food diversion away from the surgical repair site. Nissen fundoplication may also be beneficial, particularly in children with recurrent aspiration pneumonia or increased laryngopharyngeal secretions. Tracheotomy is frequently required in children with severe laryngeal clefts for airway protection, pulmonary toilet, and management of concurrent tracheomalacia/tracheobronchomalacia prior to repair.

Repair of type III and type IV laryngeal clefts requires distinguishing two distinct lumens—the trachea and the esophagus, and thus requiring repair of two luminal walls. The pharyngoesophageal mucosa and the laryngotracheal mucosa are repaired either with symmetric or asymmetric flaps, which are then separated by an interposition graft. Asymmetric flaps are used to prevent overlapping suture lines, which may lead to fistulization or dehiscence of the repair. Garabedian and colleagues[39] described the use of tibial periosteum as an interposition graft, placed through an open anterior laryngofissure approach, and stretched and fixed laterally. In this approach, a rectangular piece of tibial periosteum is harvested from the anteromedial aspect of the tibia. In addition to tibial periosteum, the use of sternal periosteum and clavicular periosteum has also been described[40,41]; periosteum represents a strong and reliable graft for reconstructive purposes. Other sources for an interposition graft include auricular cartilage, temporalis fascia, pericardium, sternocleidomastoid muscle flaps, pleura, strap muscle, and jejunum.[8,19,42–44]

For extended clefts, open repair often requires a combination of cervical and thoracic approaches. Repair can be accessed through an anterior cervical incision with or without thoracic incisions. A lateral pharyngeal approach may also be advantageous in some cases, as the endotracheal tube does not directly obstruct the field of repair, although this technique may be associated with higher risk of recurrent laryngeal nerve injury, fistula formation, and poor exposure, and is not commonly performed.[44] Open repair can be accomplished with tracheal ventilation with an endotracheal tube placed distal to the repair. Some authors advocate for repair of the laryngeal cleft using extra corporeal membrane oxygenation (ECMO) or cardiopulmonary bypass in order to obtain an unobstructed view of the cleft without an endotracheal tube, particularly for patients with bronchial involvement of a type IV laryngeal cleft.[44,45]

In particular, type IV laryngeal clefts pose imminent mortality without early repair.[14,45] In a review of 85 patients, Roth et al[46] reported a 93% (13 of 14 patients) mortality rate for patients with type IV laryngeal cleft. The higher rate of mortality for these patients is associated with pulmonary complications, associated comorbidities, and feeding difficulties. Shehab and Bailey[24] reported a 33% mortality rate (2 of 6 patients) among those who underwent type IV laryngeal cleft repair, while a follow-up study at the same institution also demonstrated a 33% mortality rate.[45]

CONCLUSION

Laryngotracheal clefts remain uncommon diagnoses. However, among children with chronic aspiration, it is critical to have a high suspicion for laryngeal cleft. Despite increasing recognition as a diagnosis, type I laryngeal clefts likely remain underrecognized. Although clinical assessment and radiographic workup may suggest the presence of a laryngeal cleft, diagnosis can only be made endoscopically. Even with prudent investigation during endoscopy, the finding of type I clefts is quite subjective. Following diagnosis, laryngeal clefts often require surgical repair, either endoscopically for types I and II and some type III clefts or open surgical repair for the majority of types III and IV clefts. Nonetheless, the diagnosis of laryngeal cleft must be considered in the larger backdrop of the patient's other medical comorbidities, particularly neurologic or neuromuscular dysfunction. The presence of significant comorbidities may be strong predictors of the patient's postoperative swallowing prognosis, as not all patients return to normal swallowing function following surgical cleft repair.

REFERENCES

1. Benjamin B, Inglis A. Minor congenital laryngeal clefts: diagnosis and classification. *Ann Otol Rhinol Laryngol.* 1989;98(6):417–420. doi:10.1177/000348948909800603.

2. Bakthavachalam S, Schroeder JW, Holinger LD. Diagnosis and management of type I posterior laryngeal clefts. *Ann Otol Rhinol Laryngol.* 2010;119(4):239–248. doi:10.1177/000348941011900406.

3. Alarcón A de, Osborn AJ, Tabangin ME, et al. Laryngotracheal cleft repair in children with complex airway anomalies. *JAMA Otolaryngol Neck Surg.* 2015;141(9):828–833. doi:10.1001/jamaoto.2015.1419.

4. Watters K, Ferrari L, Rahbar R. Laryngeal cleft. *Adv Otorhinolaryngol.* 2012;73:95–100. doi:10.1159/000334452.

5. Balakrishnan K, Cheng E, de Alarcon A, Sidell DR, Hart CK, Rutter MJ. Outcomes and resource utilization of endoscopic mass-closure technique for laryngeal clefts. *Otolaryngol Neck Surg.* 2015;153(1):119–123. doi:10.1177/0194599815576718.

6. Chien W, Ashland J, Haver K, Hardy SC, Curren P, Hartnick CJ. Type 1 laryngeal cleft: establishing a functional diagnostic and management algorithm. *Int J Pediatr Otorhinolaryngol.* 2006;70(12):2073–2079. doi:10.1016/j.ijporl.2006.07.021.

7. Moungthong G, Holinger LD. Laryngotracheoesophageal clefts. *Ann Otol Rhinol Laryngol.* 1997;106(12):1002–1011. doi:10.1177/000348949710601203.

8. Johnston DR, Watters K, Ferrari LR, Rahbar R. Laryngeal cleft: evaluation and management. *Int J Pediatr Otorhinolaryngol.* 2014;78(6):905–911. doi:10.1016/j.ijporl.2014.03.015.

9. Pezzettigotta SM, Leboulanger N, Roger G, Denoyelle F, Garabédian E-N. Laryngeal cleft. *Otolaryngol Clin North Am.* 2008;41(5):913–933. doi:10.1016/j.otc.2008.04.010.

10. Narcy P, Bobin S, Contencin P, Le Pajolec C, Manac'h Y. [Laryngeal anomalies in newborn infants. Apropos of 687 cases]. *Ann Oto-Laryngol Chir Cervico Faciale Bull Soc Oto-Laryngol Hopitaux Paris.* 1984;101(5):363–373.

11. Fearon B, Ellis D. The management of long term airway problems in infants and children. *Ann Otol Rhinol Laryngol.* 1971;80(5):669–677. doi:10.1177/000348947108000508.

12. McIntoshNTOSH R, Merritt KK, Richards MR, Samuels MH, Bellows MT. The incidence of congenital malformations: a study of 5,964 pregnancies. *Pediatrics.* 1954;14(5):505–522.

13. Andrieu-Guitrancourt J, Narcy P, Desnos J, Bobin S, Dehesdin D, Dubin J. [Diastema or laryngeal or posterior laryngotracheal cleft. Analysis of 16 cases]. *Chir Pediatr.* 1984;25(4–5):219–227.

14. Myer CM, Cotton RT, Holmes DK, Jackson RK. Laryngeal and laryngotracheoesophageal clefts: role of early surgical repair. *Ann Otol Rhinol Laryngol.* 1990;99(2 pt 1): 98–104.

15. Pettersson G. Inhibited separation of larynx and the upper part of trachea from oesophagus in a newborn; report of a case successfully operated upon. *Acta Chir Scand.* 1955; 110(3):250–254.

16. Evans JN. Management of the cleft larynx and tracheoesophageal clefts. *Ann Otol Rhinol Laryngol.* 1985;94(6 pt 1):627–630. doi:10.1177/000348948509400620.

17. Tucker GF, Maddalozzo J. "Occult" posterior laryngeal cleft. *Laryngoscope.* 1987;97(6):701–704.

18. Sandu K, Monnier P. Endoscopic laryngotracheal cleft repair without tracheotomy or intubation. *Laryngoscope.* 2006;116(4):630–634. doi:10.1097/01.mlg.0000200794.78614.87.

19. Rahbar R, Rouillon I, Roger G, et al. The presentation and management of laryngeal cleft: a 10-year experience. *Arch Otolaryngol Head Neck Surg.* 2006;132(12):1335–1341. doi:10.1001/archotol.132.12.1335.

20. Rahbar R, Chen JL, Rosen RL, et al. Endoscopic repair of laryngeal cleft type I and type II: when and why? *Laryngoscope.* 2009;119(9):1797–1802. doi:10.1002/lary.20551.

21. van der Doef HP, Yntema JB, van den Hoogen FJ, Marres HA. Clinical aspects of type 1 posterior laryngeal clefts: literature review and a report of 31 patients. *Laryngoscope.* 2007;117(5):859–863. doi:10.1097/MLG.0b013e318033c2e9.

22. Kubba H, Bailey M, Gibson D, Hartley B. Techniques and outcomes of laryngeal cleft repair: an update to the Great Ormond Street Hospital series. *Ann Otol Rhinol Laryngol.* 2005;114(4):309–313. doi:10.1177/000348940511400410.

23. Parsons DS, Stivers FE, Giovanetto DR, Phillips SE. Type I posterior laryngeal clefts. *Laryngoscope.* 1998;108(3): 403–410.

24. Shehab ZP, Bailey CM. Type IV laryngotracheoesophageal clefts—recent 5 year experience at Great Ormond Street Hospital for Children. *Int J Pediatr Otorhinolaryngol.* 2001;60(1):1–9. doi:10.1016/S0165-5876(01)00464-5.

25. Delahunty JE, Cherry J. Congenital laryngeal cleft. *Ann Otol Rhinol Laryngol.* 1969;78(1):96–106. doi:10.1177/000348946907800108.

26. Lim TA, Spanier SS, Kohut RI. Laryngeal clefts: a histopathologic study and review. *Ann Otol Rhinol Laryngol.* 1979;88(pt 1):837–845. doi:10.1177/000348947908800619.

27. Ojha S, Ashland JE, Hersh C, Ramakrishna J, Maurer R, Hartnick CJ. Type 1 laryngeal cleft: a multidimensional management algorithm. *JAMA Otolaryngol Head Neck Surg.* 2014;140(1):34–40. doi:10.1001/jamaoto.2013.5739.

28. Osborn AJ, de Alarcon A, Tabangin ME, Miller CK, Cotton RT, Rutter MJ. Swallowing function after laryngeal cleft repair: more than just fixing the cleft. *Laryngoscope.* 2014;124(8):1965–1969. doi:10.1002/lary.24643.

29. Walker RD, Irace AL, Kenna MA, Urion DK, Rahbar R. Neurologic evaluation in children with laryngeal cleft. *JAMA Otolaryngol Neck Surg.* April 2017. doi:10.1001/jamaoto.2016.4735.

30. Watters K, Russell J. Diagnosis and management of type 1 laryngeal cleft. *Int J Pediatr Otorhinolaryngol.* 2003;67(6):591–596. doi:10.1016/S0165-5876(03)00058-2.

31. Kennedy CA, Heimbach M, Rimell FL. Diagnosis and determination of the clinical significance of type 1a laryngeal clefts by Gelfoam injection. *Ann Otol Rhinol Laryngol.* 2000;109(11):991–995. doi:10.1177/000348940010901101.

32. Cohen MS, Zhuang L, Simons JP, Chi DH, Maguire RC, Mehta DK. Injection laryngoplasty for type 1 laryngeal cleft in children. *Otolaryngol Neck Surg.* 2011;144(5):789–793. doi:10.1177/0194599810395082.

33. Mangat HS, El-Hakim H. Injection augmentation of type 1 laryngeal clefts. *Otolaryngol Neck Surg.* 2012;146(5):764–768. doi:10.1177/0194599811434004.

34. Horn DL, DeMarre K, Parikh SR. Interarytenoid sodium carboxymethylcellulose gel injection for management of pediatric aspiration. *Ann Otol Rhinol Laryngol.* 2014;123(12):852–858. doi:10.1177/0003489414539129.

35. Ketcham AS, Smith JE, Lee F-S, Halstead LA, White DR. Clinical course following endoscopic repair of type 1 laryngeal clefts. *Int J Pediatr Otorhinolaryngol.* 2008;72(8):1261–1267. doi:10.1016/j.ijporl.2008.05.008.

36. Chiang T, McConnell B, Ruiz AG, DeBoer EM, Prager JD. Surgical management of type I and II laryngeal cleft in the pediatric population. *Int J Pediatr Otorhinolaryngol.* 2014;78(12):2244–2249. doi:10.1016/j.ijporl.2014.10.023.

37. Garabedian E-N, Pezzettigotta S, Leboulanger N, et al. Endoscopic surgical treatment of laryngotracheal clefts: indications and limitations. *Arch Otolaryngol Head Neck Surg.* 2010;136(1):70–74. doi:10.1001/archoto.2009.197.

38. Adil E, Al Shemari H, Rahbar R. Endoscopic surgical repair of type 3 laryngeal clefts. *JAMA Otolaryngol Head Neck Surg.* 2014;140(11):1051–1055. doi:10.1001/jamaoto.2014.2421.

39. Garabedian E-N, Ducroz V, Roger G, Denoyelle F. Posterior laryngeal clefts: preliminary report of a new surgical procedure using tibial periosteum as an interposition graft. *The Laryngoscope.* 1998;108(6):899–902. doi:10.1097/00005537-199806000-00020.

40. Propst EJ. Repair of short type IV laryngotracheoesophageal cleft using long, tapered, engaging graft without need for tracheotomy. *Laryngoscope.* 2016;126(4):1006–1008. doi:10.1002/lary.25472.

41. Propst EJ, Ida JB, Rutter MJ. Repair of long type IV posterior laryngeal cleft through a cervical approach using cricotracheal separation. *Laryngoscope.* 2013;123(3):801–804. doi:10.1002/lary.23660.

42. Ferrari LR, Zurakowski D, Solari J, Rahbar R. Laryngeal cleft repair: the anesthetic perspective. *Pediatr Anesth.* 2013;23(4):334–341. doi:10.1111/pan.12119.

43. Kawaguchi AL, Donahoe PK, Ryan DP. Management and long-term follow-up of patients with types III and IV laryngotracheoesophageal clefts. *J Pediatr Surg.* 2005;40(1):158–165. doi:10.1016/j.jpedsurg.2004.09.041.

44. Geller K, Kim Y, Koempel J, Anderson KD. Surgical management of type III and IV laryngotracheoesophageal clefts: the three-layered approach. *Int J Pediatr Otorhinolaryngol.* 2010;74(6):652–657. doi:10.1016/j.ijporl.2010.03.013.

45. Mathur NN, Peek GJ, Bailey CM, Elliott MJ. Strategies for managing type IV laryngotracheoesophageal clefts at Great Ormond Street Hospital for Children. *Int J Pediatr Otorhinolaryngol.* 2006;70(11):1901–1910. doi:10.1016/j.ijporl.2006.06.017.

46. Roth B, Rose KG, Benz-Bohm G, Günther H. Laryngotracheo-oesophageal cleft. Clinical features, diagnosis and therapy. *Eur J Pediatr.* 1983;140(1):41–46.

CHAPTER 4

Laryngeal Webs

Hannah Burns

Laryngeal webs consist of abnormal fibrous tissue running between and connecting the vocal folds and can be congenital or acquired. Both offer challenging management dilemmas for clinicians.

INTRODUCTION

Congenital webs occur in 1 in 10,000 births. Laryngeal atresia represents the most severe form of congenital laryngeal web. Laryngeal embryology explains this spectrum of anomalies. The larynx forms from endoderm and mesoderm between the 4th and 6th branchial arches. At day 20 the laryngotracheal groove appears. By day 26 it has become a tube which is separated from the esophagus. This fusion occurs in a caudal to cranial direction and if incomplete leads to laryngeal clefts and tracheo-esophageal fistulae. By day 32 the 6th branchial arches have formed the mesenchymal arytenoid swellings at the cranial end of this tube. These swellings fuse to form the epithelium laminae which occlude the cranial portion of the primitive larynx. The hypobranchial eminence above this forms epiglottic and cuneiform cartilages. The thyroid cartilage develops from the 4th arch and cricoid and tracheal cartilages from the 6th. By day 44 the cricoid ring is complete. The epithelial lamina dissolves in a dorsal to ventral direction at around 8 weeks allowing re-canalization of the trachea. Failure to re-canalize results in the spectrum of pathology from atresia through to mild webs. Most webs are associated with a degree of subglottic stenosis (SGS): this association is explicable by the same mechanisms of abnormal branchial arch development.

Acquired webs can occur from laryngeal trauma, iatrogenic injury secondary to intubation, or laryngeal surgery, infection or radiation. Reflux has been discussed as a causative factor.[1] Connective tissue disorders such as Ehlers–Danlos syndrome (EDS), and autoimmune conditions such as granulomatosis with polyangitis (GPA, formerly Wegener's granulomatosis) may also predispose to web formation. Injury to the vocal folds results in inflammation, fibroplasia, and remodeling. Collagen is deposited and scar forms up to 12 to 20 weeks after the injury.[2]

A number of classification systems have been described for laryngeal atresia and webs.[3,4] Benjamin[5]

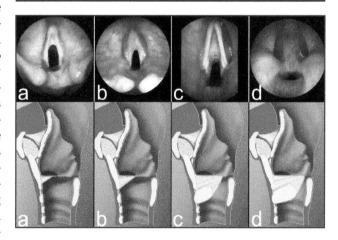

Figure 4–1. Cohen classification of laryngeal webs. **a)** Type 1, <35% **b)** Type 2, 35–50% **c)** Type 3, 50–75% **d)** Type 4, >75%
Source: Reproduced from Monnier P. *Pediatric Airway Surgery.* Dordrecht: Springer; 2011.

PERCENTAGE OF OBSTRUCTION BY ACTUAL ENDOTRACHEAL TUBE SIZE												
Patient age	Normal ID (mm)	Normal OD (mm)	Percentage of obstruction with actual endotracheal tube size									
			ID = 2.0	ID = 2.5	ID = 3.0	ID = 3.5	ID = 4.0	ID = 4.5	ID = 5.0	ID = 5.5	ID = 6.0	
Premature	2.0	2.8	0%									
	2.5	3.6	40%	0%								
	3.0	4.3	58%	30%	0%							
0–3 mo	3.5	5.0	68%	48%	26%	0%						
3–9 mo	4.0	5.6	75%	59%	41%	22%	0%					
9 mo to 2y	4.5	6.2	80%	67%	53%	38%	20%	0%				
2y	5.0	7.0	84%	74%	62%	50%	35%	19%	0%			
4y	5.5	7.6	86%	78%	68%	57%	45%	32%	17%	0%		
6y	6.0	8.2	89%	81%	73%	64%	54%	43%	30%	16%	0%	

ID – Inside diameter, OD – Outside diameter

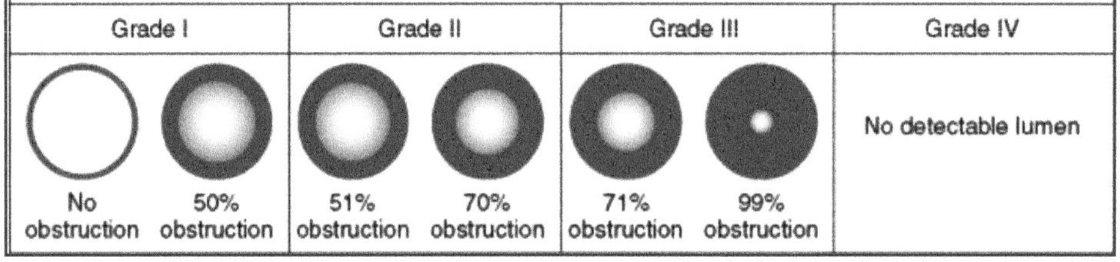

Grade I		Grade II		Grade III		Grade IV
No obstruction	50% obstruction	51% obstruction	70% obstruction	71% obstruction	99% obstruction	No detectable lumen

Figure 4–2. Cotton-Myer Subglottic stenosis grading system.

described webs by their level of laryngeal involvement, supraglottic, glottic, or subglottic. The most commonly used and perhaps most useful clinically was proposed by Cohen in 1985,[6] based on the percentage of vocal cords involved (Figure 4–1). The associated SGS is classically defined using the Myer–Cotton grading scale[7] (Figure 4–2).

Goals of treatment are two-fold, airway patency and improved voice quality.

CASE 1

A term baby is born via vaginal delivery at a regional hospital. Low Apgar's and respiratory distress lead to attempts to intubate which are unsuccessful. Bag mask ventilation improves oxygenation, the child is placed on continuous positive airway pressure (CPAP) ventilation and transferred to the neonatal intensive care at a tertiary institute.

Although stable on CPAP, all attempts to wean are unsuccessful and an ENT consultation is requested.

Further history from the family identifies normal antenatal screening but a maternal diagnosis of velocardiofacial syndrome. The genetic microarray on the neonate is pending and mildly dysmorphic features are recognized, including a bifid uvula. A low lymphocyte count prompts T-cell evaluation, which confirmed

a T-cell lymphopenia. Echocardiogram identified an atrial septal defect with no cardiovascular compromise.

Chest and neck plain films demonstrate no tracheal narrowing. CPAP is unable to be removed to listen for stridor or perform flexible nasendoscopy. The infant is too unstable to be moved for further imaging and after consultation with the parents and neonatologists, microlaryngoscopy and bronchoscopy under general anesthetic are arranged. The parents are consented for a tracheostomy if required.

With an experienced airway anesthetist, the neonate undergoes a gas induction and is kept spontaneously breathing. Judicious use of intravenous anesthetic agents allow the correct depth of anesthetic to allow examination of the airway. The anesthetist performs direct laryngoscopy which identifies a grade 1 view of the larynx and applies local anesthesia to the glottis. Due to the quick desaturation during this time, it is decided to perform flexible bronchoscopy via anesthetic mask to maintain saturations. Figure 4–3 identifies the glottic anatomy found.

A tracheostomy is performed without intubating. Normal tracheal cartilages are identified and once the airway is secured a formal suspension microlaryngoscopy is performed. This confirms a high Cohen type 4 laryngeal web, bordering on atresia with only a pinhole posterior airway. The smallest Hopkins rod (1.9 mm) cannot be passed through. A size 4 mm balloon is used to dilate the airway to allow the subglottis to be

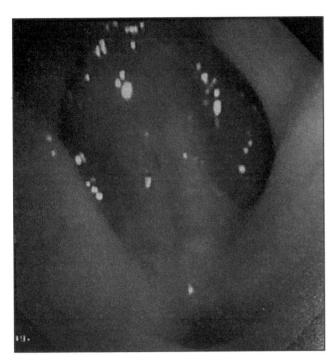

Figure 4–3. Type 4 laryngeal web. Pinhole posterior airway.

further examined. This confirmed SGS with abnormal cricoid cartilage. There is moderate tracheobronchomalacia, but no tracheoesphageal fistula is identified.

Microarray confirmed 22q11.2 deletion. Feeding continued to be difficult with significant vomiting despite transpyloric tube feeding and ultimately, at 18 months of age, a gastrostomy tube is placed and fundoplication performed. The child is managed by immunology due to T-cell deficiency and receives regular Intragam P (CSL, Australia) infusions. Although developmentally delayed, his progress is steady. At 3 years, airway reconstruction is discussed with the parents.

Management of High Grade Laryngeal Webs

Initial management of type 3 and 4 laryngeal webs in the neonate involves securing an airway. This acute management requires close and careful collaboration with a skilled anesthetist, and all possibilities must be discussed and planned for before the anesthetic is delivered. In Case 1, the pathology was unknown before the bronchoscopy. Alternative pathologies considered were subglottic stenosis, complete tracheal rings, and complete atresia with tracheo-esophageal fistulae.

The algorithms for treating these pathologies are different but must be planned for. Atresia may be diagnosed in the prenatal period with diagnosis of congenital high airway obstruction syndrome (CHAOS) and results in the need for an ex utero intrapartum treatment (EXIT) procedure with tracheostomy placement.[8] Fetoscopic division of the atretic plate has been reported to improve fetal cardiovascular function prior to EXIT procedure; however, long-term outcomes are still poor.[9–12]

Syndrome of 22q11.2 deletion is a relatively common genetic syndrome occurring in 1:4000 live births.[13] It is the unifying genetic abnormality for DiGeorge, velocardiofacial, autosomal dominant Opitz G/BBB, Sedlackova, Caylor cardiofacial, Shprintzen, and conotruncal anomaly face syndromes, all of which represent a variation of phenotypes for this one genotype. The synonym CATCH22 (Figure 4–4) is a useful pnemonic to assist ENT surgeons when managing these individuals, but represents only the most common clinical presentations. Features can be subtle. In a review of 104 22q patients who underwent review by otolaryngology for airway symptoms, 21% were diagnosed with glottic webs,[14] while 55% had more than one level of airway obstruction.

The affected region of chromosome 22 codes for approximately 40 genes, some of which are involved with formation of the branchial arch derivatives,[15] thus deletions in this region may affect laryngeal development in addition to other reported features, including thymic abnormalities. In a study from Cincinnati Children's Hospital,[16] 11/17 patients diagnosed with

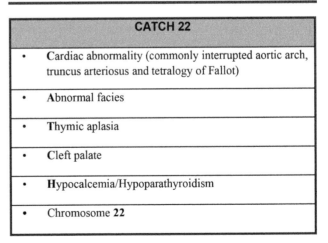

Figure 4–4. Common features in 22q11.2 deletion syndrome.

webs were found to be positive for 22q11.2 deletion, of which 5 had no other obvious features to predict this deletion, leading to the recommendation to routinely test for this deletion in all patients with webs.

Other syndromes have been associated with laryngeal webs, including Fraser syndrome[17] and VACTERL syndrome,[18] and thus a referral to genetics is recommended for all cases.

Definitive reconstruction of high grade webs is best managed with open techniques. Recognition of the associated subglottic stenosis has allowed laryngotracheal reconstructive (LTR) techniques using costal cartilage to be used to expand the subglottis and stent the divided web.[19–21] The decision for anterior only versus anterior and posterior graft depends on the grade of webbing and stenosis. Sorichetti et al,[18] described only a cricoid split and keel placement with a covering tracheostomy in a newborn with successful results. In certain circumstances cricotracheal resection in combination with stenting has also been used.[20] Combining an endoscopic division of the web prior to the external laryngofissure and costocartilage graft placement allows greater visualization of the glottic web component and may help prevent inadvertent division of the anterior commissure during the external component of the surgery.[20]

In the majority of cases these reconstructions are safest managed as a two-stage procedure with a covering tracheostomy. This allows for extended periods of stenting which improves success rates. The type of stent used is variable. A number of commercially marketed stents have been developed, such as the Rutter Suprastomal Stent, LT Mold™, but the availability of these are not universal and a fashioned ivory Silastic endotracheal tube is a readily available option.

Even in the best hands revision surgery is common—20% requiring at least 1 further open procedure in the Swiss experience, with a further 20% requiring endoscopic laser revision.[20] Wyatt and Hartley[19] reported 10% revision open surgery, although one of those had been operated on at a different center in the first instance.

Timing of reconstruction should be managed on a case by case base. Although open reconstruction has been described in the under 12-month-old,[18–20] the child's other premorbid conditions must be considered. Cardiac, respiratory, and gastrointestinal conditions should be optimized. Immunodeficiencies require management by specialist physicians. Multi-resistant *Staphylococcus aureus* (MRSA) and reflux both increase the risk of graft failure and require eradication and management in the lead-up to reconstruction. The goal of decannulation prior to starting school is a realistic expectation for most families.

CASE 2

A 12-year-old girl is referred to clinic with long-standing dysphonia. Although she has never presented with acute airway distress, she has a degree of limitation on exertion which had been previously treated as asthma.

Her antenatal/infancy period was unremarkable and she has reached normal developmental milestones. She has never been intubated or undergone surgery.

On examination, her voice is husky with no audible stridor. A flexible nasendoscopy is performed in clinic (Figure 4–5). Further evaluation in the operating theater confirms a Cohen high type 2 web (Figure 4–6). Use of a 30-degree endoscope can be beneficial to examine the subglottis distal to the web. As is the case in the majority of congenital webs, this confirms subglottic extension onto the anterior cricoid.

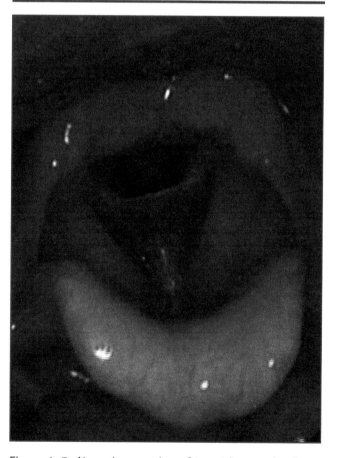

Figure 4–5. Nasendoscope view of type 2 laryngeal web.

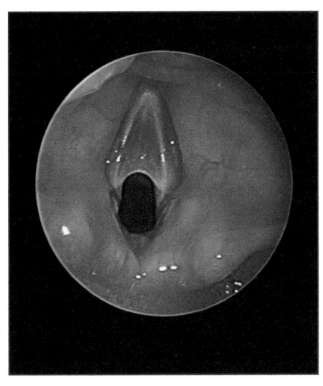

Figure 4–6. Microlaryngoscopy view of type 2 laryngeal web.

Management of Type 1 and 2 Webs

Unlike high grade webs, these milder forms may present later in life with dysphonia and without airway symptoms. Management options are more varied. Both endoscopic open and combined techniques have been described.

Endoscopic simple division of the web, with or without application of mitomycin C, although the easiest technique, is the least successful.[22] Restenosis invariably occurs and this technique poorly manages any coexisting SGS.

A variety of micro-endoscopic techniques in which flaps are elevated and the raw epithelium covered by the flap,[22–24] with or without very fine endoscopic sutures, have been described. Authors report success, but "touch up" surgery is often required and this technique also fails to manage any underlying SGS.

Division followed by keel placement is more successful.[22,23] Following cold steel or laser division a splint is inserted into the anterior commissure to prevent re-stenosis. The subglottic component can simultaneously be managed with balloon dilation. A range of materials have been described for the keel. Pre-prepared silastic keels are available, but a keel can also be fashioned from Silastic sheeting, with or without a central fine catheter to sit into the anterior commissure.[25,26] The use of a surgical tape has also been described.[27] The keel is then sutured into place endoscopically.

Endoscopic sutures can be placed either "inside out" or "outside in." The "outside in" technique requires passing the suture externally through the laryngeal cartilages, often via a large-bore cannula, delivery through the glottis, and back out of the mouth to be secured to the keel. The keel is pulled back into the anterior commissure via the external suture.[4] The "inside-out" technique is made easier with the use of the Lichtenberger endo-extralaryngeal needle carrier, which allows the needle to be passed from inside the larynx out through the cartilages to be secured either subcutaneously or over a button at the skin.[28–30] Both techniques can be challenging, especially when trying to manage a compromised airway.

Although usually placed into the anterior commissure, Hsueh et al[31] described a Silastic stent that is placed endoscopically around one vocal cord only and acts as a stent to prevent re-adhesion and lateralizes the cord.

Whichever technique is used, close liaison with the anesthetist is required. Unless a tracheostomy is in situ, the patient requires ventilation through a shared airway. Options include intermittent intubation with periods of extubation to allow suture placement, jet ventilation, spontaneous respiration with entrainment of O_2 from a pharyngeal catheter or more recently either apneic or spontaneously breathing combined with high flow nasal oxygenation.[32–34]

Duration of keel placement is variable and has been shown to be tolerated by adult patients for many weeks.[30,31,35] Paniello et al[30] described 5 complications in his series of 22 adults. Two extruded early due to suture breakage, which led to a change of suture to 2-0 Prolene and a reduction in the tension of the sutures to prevent tension during swallowing. One patient developed a granuloma after the keel was removed, one developed a small needle tract infection, and one had distal migration. No patient required a tracheostomy (although three already had one).

Keel placement has been described in children,[22,35] all with covering tracheostomies. There are no large pediatric cohort studies. Placement in very young children may not be viable due to the size of the airway, making this technically difficult and causing a risk of airway obstruction while in place. As stages 1 and 2, webs are most likely to present with voice symptoms and without acute airway difficulties, and postponing definitive surgery until late childhood or early adolescence would seem a sensible management plan and may allow keel placement without a tracheostomy. A short period of intubation without a keel following division may be an option in milder cases to prevent re-stenosis.

Removal of keels has been described both endoscopically under general anesthesia and in the office setting in the awake patient.[30]

Open repair of low grade webs carries a high success rate as illustrated by the Great Ormond St and Swiss experiences.[19,20] In children not requiring a tracheostomy, for airway obstruction, a one stage anterior graft LTR has been successful. One stage LTR, however, carries more risk than two stage, where the airway is protected by a tracheostomy and the stent can be left in for the standard 6 weeks, allowing better graft integration into the laryngeal framework. Success with one stage procedures is likely better in centers with high turnover of cases due to greater institutional experience of post-LTR care.

Regardless of the technique used re-adhesion rates are still relatively high, Alkan et al,[22] had an overall re-adhesion rate of 63% with a variety of techniques and a re-operation rate of 30%. Best results were with keel placement but total patient numbers were small. Lichtenberger,[29] who described his needle carrier technique, only had complete elimination of the web in 5/13 patients but all reported improved airway and voice. Paniello's series of 22 adult patients[30] treated with keels reported recurrence of webs in 3 patients—one due to early removal of stent secondary to suture rupture and patient declining revision, the second in a patient with severe granulomatosis with polyangitis who re-fibrosed, and the third due to distal migration of the keel. Chen[26] had reformation in 10/36 and found this was independent of web grade but dependent on web thickness.

Dysphonia is often the presenting symptom in patients with grades 1 and 2 webs. Very few papers, however, measure voice outcomes. Goudy[36] rated the postoperative voice outcomes in 18 patients subjectively; 80% of these families reported voice as adequate. De Trey[20] reported 46% normal to mild dysphonia in those treated with open reconstruction. In the early 1980s McGuirt[24] advocated the endoscopic flap as providing good voice outcomes; however, only 6/10 patients underwent pre- and post-surgical voice assessments, and no specific results are presented in this paper. Furthermore, patients underwent an undisclosed number of procedures to achieve these outcomes. The Voice

Handicap Index 10 (VHI-10) was used by Chen et al,[26] who found with keel placement a significant improvement in VHI-10 at 3 months. It should be remembered that those with 22q are likely to have other causes for voice problems, including palatal insufficiency and potential vocal cord palsy secondary to cardiac surgery.

CASE 3

EE is a 2-year-old female who presents in acute airway distress at age 14 months to a regional center. She requires intubation and is found to have recurrent respiratory papillomatosis (RRP). Following transfer to a tertiary hospital she undergoes microlaryngoscopy, bronchoscopy, and debridement of her papilloma (Figure 4–7). Her disease is extensive, involving epiglottis, false cords, anterior commissure, true cords, and pharynx. Initially her subglottis is not involved. Human papilloma virus (HPV) typing confirms type 11 and despite adjuvant cidofovir, monthly debridements are required to maintain a patent airway. The child receives vaccination with the quadrivalent HPV vaccine. Microdebrider, coblation, and cold steel are used. Despite care taken at the anterior commissure, at 20 months anterior glottic webbing has developed (Figure 4–8). Voice is poor and disease has now spread to the subglottis.

Treatment of Acquired Webs

RRP is caused by HPV, usually subtypes 6 and 11. Two distinct but clinically similar cohorts exist. Juvenile onset (JoRRP) secondary to vertical spread from a typi-

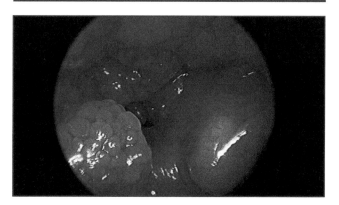

Figure 4–7. Extensive RRP involving larynx and including anterior commissure.

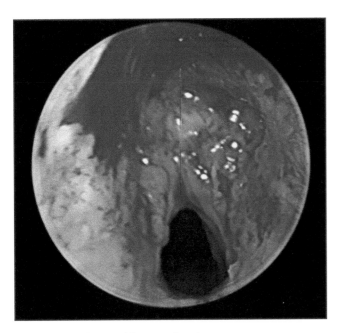

Figure 4–8. Acquired laryngeal web.

cally asymptomatic but infected mother to baby, and adult onset (AoRRP), where the infection may be sexually transmitted or reactivation of latent infection.[37] Since the widespread adoption of vaccination with Gardasil® and other multivalent HPV vaccines, the rate of infection has greatly diminished in the developed world[38,39] and resulted in a subsequent decrease in prevalence of JoRRP.[40] However, cases are still likely to appear in unvaccinated adults, children of unvaccinated mothers, and in countries without a vaccination program. Treatment typically involves mechanical debridement. Due to the common involvement of the anterior commissure by the papillomata and the numerous procedures required to remove disease, trauma at the commissure resulting in webbing is relatively common. Holland et al,[1] in a retrospective review of 31 patients with RRP, found 13 (42%) developed web formation. Acquired anterior laryngeal web in the presence of active RRP poses a very difficult management problem.

Prevention of acquired webbing is the preferred "treatment." Surgical technique influences the risk of mucosal trauma. Mucosal preservation is paramount, and avoidance of bilateral anterior vocal cord treatment is recommended but not always feasible, with airway obstructing lesions. All lasers can cause scarring due to thermal penetration, this can be mitigated by using the shortest possible time pulse and preventing areas of thermal overlap.[41] Patients with severe disease require more treatments and this is not surprisingly a risk factor for web formation.[1]

Laryngopharyngeal reflux (LPR) has been implicated in a wide range of airway disorders including airway stenosis.[1,42,43] Holland[1] described an association between reflux and RRP, and proposed active treatment with anti-reflux medication may reduce severity of the disease, thereby reducing complications. A recent review, however, has found insufficient evidence to prove that gastroesophageal reflux disease (GERD) does or does not aggravate the clinical course of RRP.[44] The theory of inflammation and irritation provoking higher viral numbers and growth is feasible. The role of acid in impairing mucosal healing is also logical, assuming refluxate may result in inflammation and thus fibrosis.

The ideal treatment for RRP would involve no mechanical debridement and instead systemic treatment of the virus. Adjuvant treatment with cidofovir (an anti-viral medication) and bevacizumab (a vascular endothelial growth factor inhibitor) has in some cases allowed less aggressive debridement and potentially less risk of scar formation. More recently bevacizumab has been used systemically in patients with very aggressive disease.[45] Results have been very promising and the long-term goal of finding a medical treatment for some of these patients may be close at hand.

Paniello et al[30] described preventing web formation in four cases identified as at greater risk of developing anterior webbing by placing a keel at the time of the anterior commissure surgery. One of these adult patients had active RRP. They also describe using an "outside-in" suture technique to prevent any chance of seeding the subcutaneous tissues with papilloma. This patient did not develop a web at this surgery but no information is provided about long term follow-up. In a large retrospective series from China, 18.6% developed anterior webbing if a keel was used prophylactically versus 54.5% of those managed without a keel and treated only with mitomycin C.[46]

As adhesions and thus webs form when two demucosalized surfaces come into contact, Xiao et al[47] have described an elegant technique to re-oppose the mucosal surfaces of the true vocal cord after the papillomata are removed by using an 8-0 absorbable suture. Although their patient still developed an adhesion, it was less than they had expected and repeat procedures over time were successful in treating both the web and the papillomata.

Topical treatment to prevent adhesions has been attempted in many otolaryngological settings with variable success. Fibrin glue has been used to prevent adhesions in patients undergoing phonomicrosurgery.[48] By spraying on first fibrinogen and then thrombin 10/17, patients developed no webbing, while the others developed webbing to less than 30% of their cord length.

CASE 4

A 17-year-old female presents with a year of worsening dysphonia and exercise intolerance. She has a family history of type VIII Ehlers Danlos syndrome (EDS) (also called periodontal EDS). She has never been intubated and as a child had a good singing voice. Office flexible nasendoscopy shows anterior glottic webbing, and a microlaryngoscopy confirms Cohen grade 1 web with extension into her subglottis with a grade 1 Cotton-Myer stenosis (Figure 4–9).

Vasculitic screen is negative and no organisms are grown from subglottic tissue. Histology confirms fibrosis and chronic inflammation. She is commenced on a proton pump inhibitor.

Initial treatment involves endoscopic division of the web, balloon dilation, and placement of a Silastic keel (Figure 4–10).

The keel is tolerated for 2 weeks and then endoscopically removed. Initial results are promising, with improved exercise tolerance, but at 6 months, further

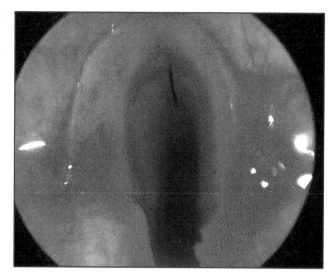

Figure 4–10. Silastic keel in situ following division and balloon dilation.

dilations are required due to worsening subglottic stenosis. Over the coming years stenosis of her whole larynx occurs both at subglottic and glottic levels, with fixation of her cricoarytenoid joints.

Immunosuppression is trialed in an attempt to prevent progressive fibrosis, first with methotrexate and then other immunomodulators. All fail to slow this process. Adjuvant steroid and mitomycin are used with limited improvement.

Eventually dilations are required at three monthly intervals. Anterior webbing has reformed, along with posterior glottic fixation and subglottic stenosis. To prevent tracheostomy, a one-stage LTR with posterior graft is proposed.

Since diagnosis the patient's aunt has been treated for posterior glottic web and her 14-year-old cousin diagnosed with grade 3 laryngeal web (Figures 4–11, 4–12).

Pathogenesis of Acquired Webs

This family illustrates a rare and poorly described form of acquired webbing and stenosis associated with a connective tissue disorder. EDS is a collection of connective tissue disorders unified by joint hypermobility, skin hyperextensibility, and tissue friability. Most, but not all subtypes have collagen abnormalities.[49]

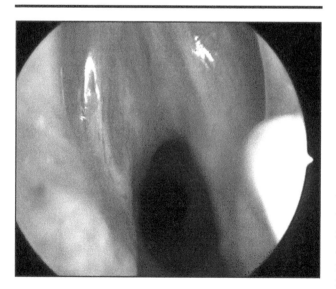

Figure 4–9. Type 1 laryngeal web and grade 1 SGS.

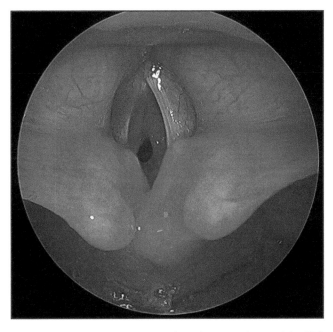

Figure 4–11. Type 4 acquired web in patient with EDS type VIII.

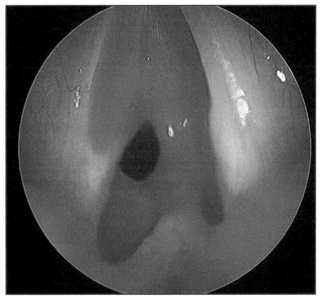

Figure 4–12. Close-up view of web showing fibrosis arising from deep surface of vocal cords.

Dysphonia has been described in EDS in the otolaryngology literature[50] and type VIII more specifically in the dermatology literature.[51] Only one paper has been found in the literature that has described laryngeal stenosis in EDS.[52] This paper describes a similar patient to Case 4, who ultimately underwent a posterior graft LTR for glottic stenosis.

Type VIII EDS has been mapped to chromosome 12p13 and encodes genes involved in the complement pathway.[53] These defects are hypothesized to interfere with pro-collagen and thus may result in abnormal wound healing. The acquired nature of the laryngeal stenosis in these individuals may reflect an abnormal tissue response to some form of laryngitis, such as infection, reflux, voice abuse, trauma, or other irritant. This wound response poses problems for management, with iatrogenic trauma occurring during treatment itself. Systemic treatment aimed toward the complement abnormality may offer an alternative treatment option.

Several autoimmune diseases are associated with acquired laryngotracheal stenosis, including granulomatosis with polyangitis, relapsing polychondritis and sarcoidosis.[54,55] These conditions often respond to immunosuppression.

Idiopathic SGS (iSGS) reflects an as yet undetermined pathological process which results in elevated IL-17a and ultimately airway fibrosis.[56] Recent studies have shown an association with mycobacterium and propose it may trigger this disease in patients with a pathological immune response.[57] Idiopathic SGS likely shares common pathways with EDS and autoimmune acquired SGS.

CONCLUSION

Congenital and acquired webs rarely present as isolated conditions. Congenital cases are often part of a syndrome and require management by a team of physicians, with the airway being only one part of the puzzle. Patients who develop acquired webs may have been intubated for extended periods due to significant illness, with laryngeal injury coming to light during their recovery. Infections, inflammation, autoimmune conditions, and genetics all interlace to result in abnormal tissue responses in the unlucky patient who develops a web.

The optimal treatment is prevention, but once established, a range of techniques are available to the otolaryngologist to manage this disorder.

REFERENCES

1. Holland B, Koufman J, Postma G, McGuirt W. Laryngopharyngeal reflux and laryngeal web formation in patients with pediatric recurrent respiratory papilloma. *Laryngoscope.* 2002;112(11):1926–1929.
2. Zapater E, Frías S, Pérez A, Basterra J. Comparative study on chronic tissue damage after cordectomies using either CO_2 laser or microdissection electrodes. *Head Neck.* 2009;31(11):1477–1481.
3. Smith I, Bain A. XXX Congenital atresia of the larynx. *Ann Otol Rhinol Laryngol.* 1965;74(2):338–349.
4. Zaw-Tun H. Development of congenital laryngeal atresias and clefts. *Ann Otol Rhinol Laryngol.* 1988;97(4):353–358.
5. Benjamin B. Congenital laryngeal webs. *Ann Otol Rhinol Laryngol.* 1983;92(4):317–326.
6. Cohen S. Congenital glottic webs in children. *Ann Otol Rhinol Laryngol.* 1985;94(6, suppl):2–16.
7. Myer C, O'Connor D, Cotton R. Proposed grading system for subglottic stenosis based on endotracheal tube sizes. *Ann Otol Rhinol Laryngol.* 1994;103(4):319–323.
8. Butler C, Maughan E, Pandya P, Hewitt R. Ex utero intrapartum treatment (EXIT) for upper airway obstruction. *Curr Opin Otolaryngol Head Neck Surg.* 2017;25(2):119–126.
9. Kohl T, Hering R, Bauriedel G, et al. Fetoscopic and ultrasound-guided decompression of the fetal trachea in a human fetus with Fraser syndrome and congenital high airway obstruction syndrome (CHAOS) from laryngeal atresia. *Ultrasound Obstet Gynecol.* 2005;27(1):84–88.
10. Kohl T, Van de Vondel P, Stressig R, et al. Percutaneous fetoscopic laser decompression of congenital high airway obstruction syndrome (CHAOS) from laryngeal atresia via a single trocar—current technical constraints and potential solutions for future interventions. *Fetal Diagn Ther.* 2009;25(1):67–71.
11. Saadai P, Jelin E, Nijagal A, et al. Long-term outcomes after fetal therapy for congenital high airway obstructive syndrome. *J Pediatr Surg.* 2012;47(6):1095–1100.
12. Martínez J, Castañón M, Gómez O, et al. Evaluation of fetal vocal cords to select candidates for successful fetoscopic treatment of congenital high airway obstruction syndrome: preliminary case series. *Fetal Diagn Ther.* 2013;34(2):77–84.
13. McDonald-McGinn D, Emanuel B, Zackai E. 22q11.2 deletion syndrome. *Ncbinlmnihgov.* 2017. from https://www.ncbi.nlm.nih.gov/books/NBK1523/. Retrieved October 14, 2017.
14. Sacca R, Zur K, Crowley T, Zackai E, Valverde K, McDonald-McGinn D. Association of airway abnormalities with 22q11.2 deletion syndrome. *Int J Pediatr Otorhinolaryngol.* 2017;96:11–14.
15. Marom T, Roth Y, Goldfarb A, Cinamon U. Head and neck manifestations of 22q11.2 deletion syndromes. *Eur Arch Oto-Rhino-Laryngol.* 2011;269(2):381–387.
16. Miyamoto R, Cotton R, Rope A, et al. Association of anterior glottic webs with velocardiofacial syndrome (chromosome 22q11.2 deletion). *Otolaryngol Head Neck Surg.* 2004;130(4):415–417.
17. Izadi F, Ahmadi A, Zobairy H, Bakhti S, Hirbod H, Safdarian M. Fraser syndrome with laryngeal webs: report of two cases and a review of the literature. *Int J Pediatr Otorhinolaryngol.* 2015;79(11):1959–1962.
18. Sorichetti B, Moxham J, Kozak F. Type IV congenital laryngeal web: case report and 15 year follow up. *Am J Otolaryngol.* 2016;37(2):148–151.
19. Wyatt M, Hartley B. Laryngotracheal reconstruction in congenital laryngeal webs and atresias. *Otolaryngol Head Neck Surg.* 2005;132(2):232–238.
20. de Trey L, Lambercy K, Monnier P, Sandu K. Management of severe congenital laryngeal webs—a 12 year review. *Int J Pediatr Otorhinolaryngol.* 2016;86:82–86.
21. Milczuk H, Smith J, Everts E. Congenital laryngeal webs: surgical management and clinical embryology. *Int J Pediatr Otorhinolaryngol.* 2000;52(1):1–9.
22. Alkan U, Nachalon Y, Vaisbuch Y, Katz O, Hamzany Y, Stern Y. Treating paediatric anterior glottic web: single-centre experience of 20 patients with comparison among techniques. *Clin Otolaryngol.* 2016;42(4):893–897.
23. Koltai P, Mouzakes J. The surgical management of anterior glottic webs. *Operat Tech Otolaryngol Head Neck Surg.* 1999;10(4):325–330.
24. McGuirt W, Salmon J, Black D. Normal speech for patients with laryngeal webs. *Laryngoscope.* 1984;94(9):1176–1180.
25. Parelkar K. A misdiagnosed laryngeal web: treated with an innovative self-made keel. *J Clin Diagn Res.* 2017 May;11(5):MD04
26. Chen J, Shi F, Chen M, Yang Y, Cheng L, Wu H. Web thickness determines the therapeutic effect of endoscopic keel placement on anterior glottic web. *Eur Arch Oto-Rhino-Laryngol.* 2017;274(10):3697–3702.
27. McGuire J, Govender R, Park-Ross P, Fagan J. Endolaryngeal anterior commissure stent-cheap and easy. *Laryngoscope.* 2017;127(8):1869–1872.
28. Lichtenberger G, Toohill R. The endo-extralaryngeal needle carrier. *Otolaryngol Head Neck Surg.* 1991;105(5):755–756.
29. Lichtenberger G, Toohill R. New keel fixing technique for endoscopic repair of anterior commissure webs. *Laryngoscope.* 1994;104(6):771–774.
30. Paniello R, Desai S, Allen C, Khosla S. Endoscopic keel placement to treat and prevent anterior glottic webs. *Ann Otol Rhinol Laryngol.* 2013;122(11):672–678.
31. Hsueh J, Stella Tsai C, Hsu H. Intralaryngeal approach to laryngeal web using lateralization with Silastic. *Laryngoscope.* 2000;110(10):1780–1782.

32. Humphreys S, Lee-Archer P, Reyne G, Long D, Williams T, Schibler A. Transnasal humidified rapid-insufflation ventilatory exchange (THRIVE) in children: a randomized controlled trial. *Br J Anaesth*. 2017;118(2):232–238.

33. Booth A, Vidhani K, Lee P, Thomsett C. Spontaneous respiration using intravenous anaesthesia and Hi-flow nasal oxygen (STRIVE Hi) maintains oxygenation and airway patency during management of the obstructed airway: an observational study. *Br J Anaesth*. 2017;118(3):444–451.

34. Humphreys S, Rosen D, Housden T, Taylor J, Schibler A. Nasal high-flow oxygen delivery in children with abnormal airways. *Pediatr Anesth*. 2017;27(6):616–620.

35. Sztanó B, Torkos A, Rovó L. The combined endoscopic management of congenital laryngeal web. *Int J Pediatr Otorhinolaryngol*. 2010;74(2):212–215.

36. Goudy S, Bauman N, Manaligod J, Smith R. Congenital laryngeal webs: surgical course and outcomes. *Ann Otol Rhinol Laryngol*. 2010;119(10):704–706.

37. Taliercio S, Cespedes M, Born H et al. Adult-onset recurrent respiratory papillomatosis. *JAMA Otolaryngol Head Neck Surg*. 2015;141(1):78.

38. Osborne S, Tabrizi S, Brotherton J et al. Assessing genital human papillomavirus genoprevalence in young Australian women following the introduction of a national vaccination program. *Vaccine*. 2015;33(1):201–208.

39. Chow E, Read T, Wigan R, et al. Ongoing decline in genital warts among young heterosexuals 7 years after the Australian human papillomavirus (HPV) vaccination programme. *Sex Transmit Infect*. 2014;91(3):214–219.

40. Novakovic D, Cheng A, Cope D, Brotherton J. Estimating the prevalence of and treatment patterns for juvenile onset recurrent respiratory papillomatosis in Australia pre-vaccination: a pilot study. *Sex Health*. 2010;7(3):253.

41. Yan Y, Olszewski A, Hoffman M, et al. Use of lasers in laryngeal surgery. *J Voice*. 2010;24(1):102–109.

42. Halstead L. Role of gastroesophageal reflux in pediatric upper airway disorders. *Otolaryngol Head Neck Surg*. 1999; 120(2):208–214.

43. Halstead L. Gastroesophageal reflux: a critical factor in pediatric subglottic stenosis. *Otolaryngol Head Neck Surg*. 1999;120(5):683–688.

44. San Giorgi M, Helder H, Lindeman R, de Bock G, Dikkers F. The association between gastroesophageal reflux disease and recurrent respiratory papillomatosis: a systematic review. *Laryngoscope*. 2016;126(10):2330–2339.

45. Zur K, Fox E. Bevacizumab chemotherapy for management of pulmonary and laryngotracheal papillomatosis in a child. *Laryngoscope*. 2016;127(7):1538–1542.

46. Chen J, Shu Y, Naunheim M, Chen M, Cheng L, Wu H. Prevention of laryngeal webs through endoscopic keel placement for bilateral vocal cord lesions. *Frontiers Med*. 2017.

47. Xiao Y, Wang J, Han D, Ma L. Stagewise treatment of anterior commissure laryngeal web and recurrent laryngeal papillomatosis under endoscope. *Am J Otolaryngol*. 2014;35(3):427–430.

48. Adachi K, Umezaki T. Effectiveness of fibrin coating in the management of web formation after laryngomicrosurgery. *Am J Otolaryngol*. 2017;38(1):1–6.

49. Brady A, Demirdas S, Fournel-Gigleux S, et al. The Ehlers-Danlos syndromes, rare types. *Am J Med Genet Part C: Semin Med Genet*. 2017;175(1):70–115.

50. Rimmer J, Giddings C, Cavalli L, Hartley B. Dysphonia—a rare early symptom of Ehlers–Danlos syndrome? *Int J Pediatr Otorhinolaryngol*. 2008;72(12):1889–1892.

51. George S, Vandersteen A, Nigar E, Ferguson D, Topham E, Pope F. Two patients with Ehlers-Danlos syndrome type VIII with unexpected hoarseness. *Clin Exp Dermatol*. 2016;41(7):771–774.

52. Arulanandam S, Hakim A, Aziz Q, Sandhu G, Birchall M. Laryngological presentations of Ehlers-Danlos syndrome: case series of nine patients from two London tertiary referral centres. *Clin Otolaryngol*. 2016;42(4):860–863.

53. Kapferer-Seebacher I, Pepin M, Werner R et al. Periodontal Ehlers-Danlos syndrome is caused by mutations in C1R and C1S, which encode subcomponents C1r and C1s of complement. *Am J Med Genet*. 2016;99(5):1005–1014.

54. Hall S, Allen C, Merati A, Mayerhoff R. Evaluating the utility of serological testing in laryngotracheal stenosis. *Laryngoscope*. 2016;127(6):1408–1412.

55. Guardiani E, Moghaddas H, Lesser J, et al. Multilevel airway stenosis in patients with granulomatosis with polyangiitis (Wegener's). *Am J Otolaryngol*. 2015;36(3): 361–363.

56. Gelbard A, Katsantonis N, Mizuta M, et al. Idiopathic subglottic stenosis is associated with activation of the inflammatory IL-17A/IL-23 axis. *Laryngoscope*. 2016;126(11): E356–E361.

57. Gelbard A, Katsantonis N, Mizuta M, et al. Molecular analysis of idiopathic subglottic stenosis for mycobacterium species. *Laryngoscope*. 2016;127(1):179–185.

CHAPTER 5

Pediatric Post-Intubation Airway Stenosis

Sarah N. Bowe and Christopher J. Hartnick

INTRODUCTION

Stridor is an abnormal, high-pitched sound produced by turbulent airflow in the larynx or trachea. The differential diagnosis can be refined by characteristics that reflect the level of the affected airway. Important historical features include age of onset, rate of progression, exacerbating and alleviating features, history of intubation, and prematurity status. The initial physical exam generally begins with a rapid assessment for respiratory distress. The respiratory rate should be assessed, as well as changes in the rate that may indicate fatigue. The patient should be observed for the presence of nasal flaring or use of accessory neck or chest muscles. If there is evidence of significant distress, further examination is best undertaken where equipment for endoscopic evaluation, airway intubation, and possible tracheotomy is readily available. Depending on resource capabilities, this may be the emergency room, pediatric intensive care unit, or operating room.

CASE PRESENTATION

A 6-month-old ex-24-week male presents on transfer from an outside hospital where he has been admitted to the pediatric intensive care unit (PICU) for stridor and increased work of breathing. He is currently stable without any respiratory distress, but has had multiple recent admissions for similar symptoms and there is no local pediatric otolaryngologist.

INITIAL ASSESSMENT

History of Present Illness

The patient was brought to his pediatrician by his mother because of stridor, tachypnea, and retractions. He was afebrile without any other upper or lower respiratory symptoms. The pediatrician referred the patient to the emergency department (ED). He was given an albuterol nebulizer treatment in the ED without any improvement. Due to his persistent respiratory distress, he was admitted to the PICU.

Past Medical History

The patient had a history of 3-month neonatal intensive care unit (NICU) stay with multiple intubations, pulmonary hemorrhage, retinopathy of prematurity, and grade 2 intraventricular hemorrhage. He required resuscitation at birth with continuous positive airway pressure support and eventual intubation with surfactant administration. He was intubated initially for 32 days, including 8 days of oscillator ventilation. In addition, he was re-intubated three times for increased work of breathing during the NICU stay.

Two weeks earlier, he was admitted to the PICU with a similar presentation in the setting of upper respiratory infection symptoms. At that time, he was treated with steroids and required hi-flow oxygen during the admission. A pulmonology follow-up was scheduled, but the patient re-presented to the ED prior to making the appointment.

Past Surgical History

None

Immunization History

Immunizations were up to date through the 4-month visit.

Medications

None

Physical Examination

No acute distress. Breathing comfortably, although mild subcostal retractions are present. Audible biphasic stridor present, softer inspiratory and louder expiratory breath sounds.

Imaging

Anteroposterior (AP) and lateral soft tissue views of the neck were performed at the outside hospital. Report on the AP view notes "soft tissue indentation arising from the right lateral wall of the trachea associated with narrowing of the trachea" and the lateral view notes "expected position of the vocal cords has an unusual appearance with a rounded contour concerning for an intraluminal soft tissue projection."

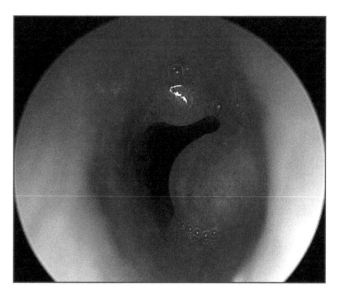

Figure 5–1. View through endoscope showing two small, round, fluid-filled masses present within the subglottis.

Diagnosis

Subglottic cysts

Management

Suspension laryngoscopy with placement of vocal fold distractors and marsupialization using microlaryngeal instruments (Figure 5–2).

SCENARIO 1	SCENARIO 2

Direct laryngoscopy and bronchoscopy are performed under general anaesthetic with spontaneous ventilation. An appropriately sized straight blade laryngoscope is placed into the vallecula to expose the larynx. A 0° 1.9 mm Hopkins rod-lens telescope with attached camera head, and size 2.5 mm endotracheal tube loaded in a Seldinger fashion, is brought into the field and used to evaluate the supraglottis, glottis, and subglottis. Two small, round, fluid-filled masses are noted in the subglottis (Figure 5–1).

Direct laryngoscopy and bronchoscopy are performed under general anaesthetic with spontaneous ventilation. An appropriately sized straight blade laryngoscope is placed into the vallecula to expose the larynx. A 0° 1.9 mm Hopkins rod-lens telescope with attached camera head, and size 2.5 mm endotracheal tube loaded in a Seldinger fashion, is brought into the field and used to evaluate the supraglottis, glottis, and subglottis. A narrowing of the subglottis beginning just underneath the vocal cords is noted (Figure 5–3).

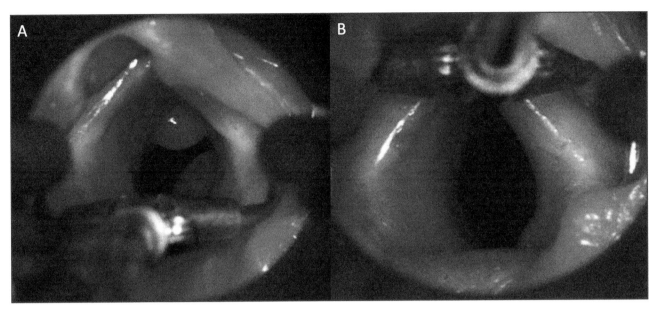

Figure 5–2. View through operating microscope following suspension laryngoscopy and placement of vocal fold distractors before (A) and after (B) marsupialization with microlaryngeal instruments.

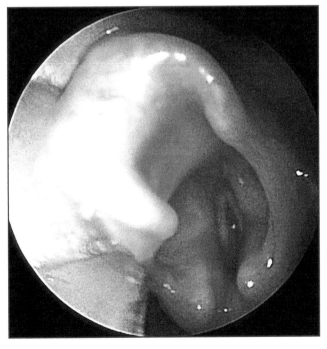

Figure 5–3. View through 0° 1.9 mm Hopkins rod-lens telescope viewing the glottis and subglottis.

Diagnosis

Subglottic stenosis (grade 3)

Management

Immediately secure the airway with available size 2.5 mm endotracheal tube (Figure 5–4). Then, proceed with pediatric tracheotomy using vertical skin incision, subcutaneous fat removal, stay suture placement, vertical tracheostomy incision, and stoma maturation.

SCENARIO 3

The following summer, the patient from Scenario 2, now 1.5 years old, has been unable to tolerate capping. Direct laryngoscopy and bronchoscopy are performed under general anaesthesia with ventilation provided by tracheostomy. An appropriately sized straight blade laryngoscope is placed into the vallecula to expose the larynx. A 0° 4.0 mm Hopkins rod-lens telescope with attached camera head is brought into the field and used to evaluate the supraglottis, glottis, and subglottis. A

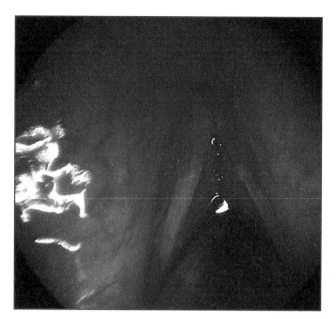

Figure 5–4. View through 0° 1.9 mm Hopkins rod-lens telescope after intubation with size 2.5 mm endotracheal tube.

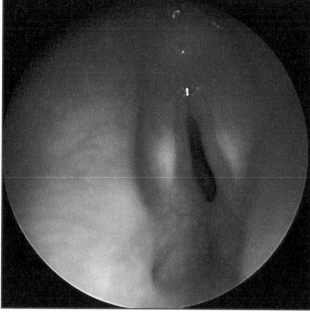

Figure 5–5. View through 0° 4.0 mm Hopkins rod-lens telescope viewing the glottis and subglottis.

persistent narrowing of the subglottis beginning just underneath the vocal cords is noted (Figure 5–5).

Diagnosis

Persistent subglottic stenosis (grade 3)

Management

Two primary techniques of open laryngotracheal reconstruction (LTR) with cartilage grafting have been described. Double-stage LTR (dsLTR) involves keeping the tracheostomy tube in place following reconstruction and placement of a suprastomal stent in order to maintain a patent airway lumen while healing occurs. In contrast, single-stage LTR (ssLTR) involves reconstructing the airway while decannulating the patient at the same time of surgery (when a tracheostomy is already present) or avoiding a tracheostomy altogether. In ssLTR, the endotracheal tube serves as the stent during healing.

In 2013, Setlur et al described a novel technique for LTR, called the hybrid or one-and-a-half-stage LTR (hLTR).[1] This technique combines aspects of both the ssLTR (nasotracheal intubation) and dsLTR (maintenance of tracheostomy) during reconstruction. Similar to dsLTR, those who undergo hLTR should be those

expected to remain tracheostomy dependent following the procedure, including patients with high-grade stenosis, multi-level stenosis, or other comorbidities preventing decannulation.[2]

Double-Stage Laryngotracheal Reconstruction

The patient from Scenario 3 underwent a dsLTR with costal cartilage harvest and anterior and posterior cricoid split with grafting. The stent was fashioned from a trimmed size 4.0 endotracheal tube (Figure 5–6).

The stent was removed at 1 week and direct laryngoscopy and bronchoscopy were performed. Expected postoperative mucosal edema was present without evidence of graft extrusion (Figure 5–7).

Direct laryngoscopy and bronchoscopy were performed again at 2 weeks. Resolving postoperative mucosal edema was noted without evidence of graft extrusion (Figure 5–8).

Advantages of Double-Stage Laryngotracheal Reconstruction

- Airway remains secure with tracheostomy in postoperative period
- Opportunity for prolonged stenting without the need for sedation/paralysis

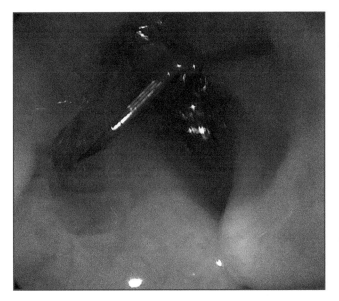

Figure 5–6. Endoscopic view showing suprastomal stent.

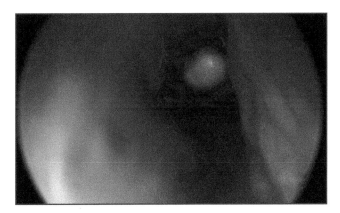

Figure 5–7. Endoscopic view at the time of stent removal.

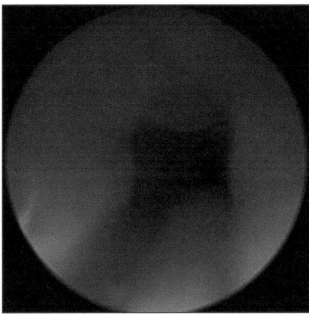

Figure 5–8. Endoscopic view two weeks after stent removal.

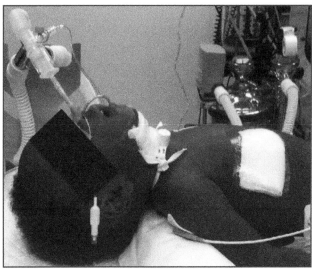

Figure 5–9. Hybrid laryngotracheal reconstruction with simultaneous placement of nasotracheal tube and tracheostomy tube.

Disadvantages of Double-Stage Laryngotracheal Reconstruction

- Risk of granulation tissue formation at the site of the stent
- Risk of stent migration and possible airway obstruction, predisposition to aspiration, or inadequate graft support

Hybrid (One-and-a-Half-Stage) Laryngotracheal Reconstruction

The patient from Scenario 3 could have undergone hLTR. Since 2013, hybrid LTR has become our option of choice for patients meeting criteria for dsLTR, as

mentioned previously. Costal cartilage harvest and anterior and posterior cricoid split with grafting proceed in a similar manner to other types of LTR. At the completion of the case, however, nasotracheal intubation with an age-appropriate size endotracheal tube is performed. Additionally, a 3.0 neonatal Shiley tracheostomy tube is replaced. This represents the blend of ssLTR and dsLTR techniques (Figure 5–9).

Advantages of Hybrid Laryngotracheal Reconstruction

- Airway remains secure with tracheostomy in postoperative period
- Decreased risk of granulation tissue formation with endotracheal tube serving as stent

Disadvantages of Hybrid Laryngotracheal Reconstruction

- Risk for ventilation difficulty due to peristomal air leak

SCENARIO 4

The following summer, the patient from Scenario 3, now 2.5 years old, has been unable to tolerate capping despite a patent subglottis (Figure 5–10A). Direct laryngoscopy and bronchoscopy are performed with ventilation provided by tracheostomy. An appropriately sized straight blade laryngoscope is placed into the vallecula to expose the larynx. A 0° 4.0 mm Hopkins rod-lens telescope with attached camera head is brought into the field and used to evaluate the supraglottis, glottis, and subglottis. The tracheostomy tube appears to be blocking a substantial portion of the airway (Figure 5–10B).

The tracheostomy tube is removed and marked to determine the ideal location to perform fenestration (Figure 5–11).

A Kerrison rongeur is used to fenestrate the tracheostomy tube. Then the tracheostomy tube is replaced and appropriate positioning of the fenestration is confirmed endoscopically (Figure 5–12).

SCENARIO 5

Despite fenestration, the patient from Scenario 4 is still unable to tolerate capping. Repeat evaluation by direct laryngoscopy and bronchoscopy is concerning for severe suprastomal collapse as the suspected cause (Figure 5–13).

Management Options for Suprastomal Collapse

To avoid primary resection and reanastamosis, several methods of repair have been reported, including[3–5]:

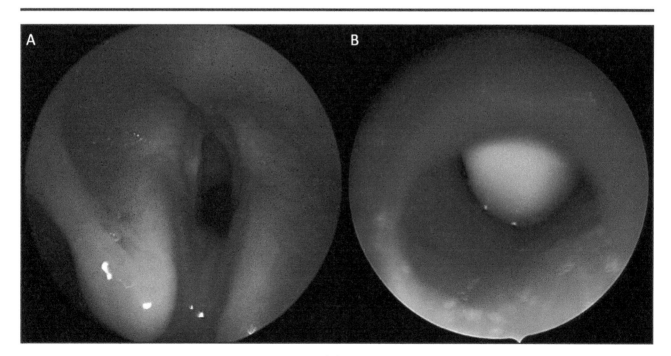

Figure 5–10. Endoscopic view showing a patent subglottis (A) and nearly complete airway obstruction by the tracheostomy tube (B).

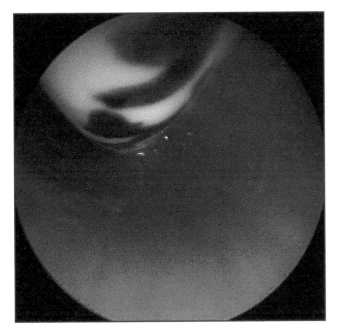

Figure 5–11. Tracheostomy tube marked with numbers 1, 2, and 3 along the shaft to aid determination of fenestration location.

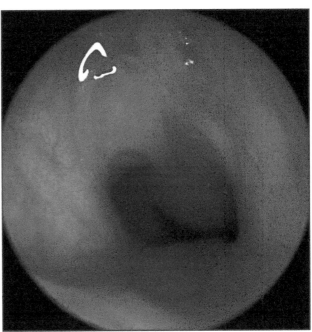

Figure 5–13. Endoscopic view showing severe suprastomal collapse.

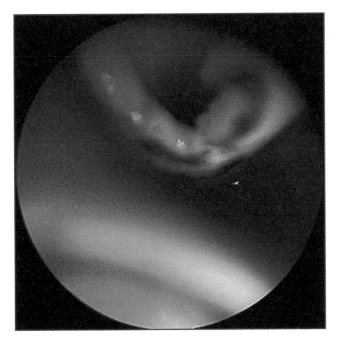

Figure 5–12. Endoscopic view confirming fenestration directed toward the tracheal lumen.

- Internal stenting with endotracheal tube placement
- Anterior cricotracheal suspension
- Autologous costal cartilage laryngotracheoplasty
- Suprastomal plate suspension with bioabsorbable microplates

The patient underwent suprastomal plate suspension (Figure 5–14) with nasotracheal intubation for 5 days.

The endotracheal tube was removed after 5 days and direct laryngoscopy and bronchoscopy revealed a patent airway without evidence of stent exposure (Figure 5–15).

Direct laryngoscopy and bronchoscopy were performed again after 2 weeks with continued airway patency without evidence of stent exposure (Figure 5–16).

The patient is now 15 months out from surgery and doing well without any airway symptoms.

DISCUSSION

Noisy breathing is the hallmark symptom prompting referral to a pediatric otolaryngologist for an airway

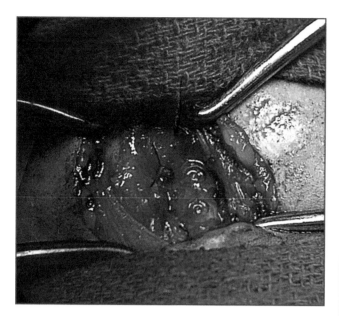

Figure 5–14. Bioresorbable suprastomal plate shown in situ just prior closure.

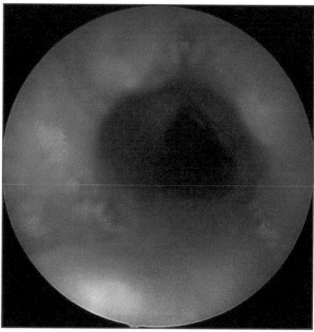

Figure 5–16. Endoscopic view two weeks after extubation from suprastomal plate suspension procedure.

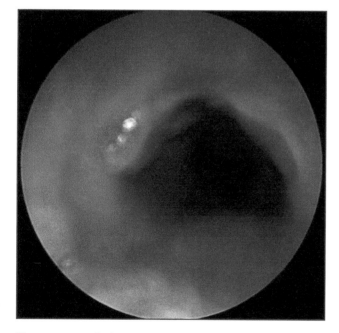

Figure 5–15. Endoscopic view one week after extubation from suprastomal plate suspension procedure.

evaluation. The presence of stridor indicates obstruction within the larynx or trachea. Prematurity status, age of onset, and history of intubation provide input to the differential diagnosis, particularly regarding concerns for subglottic cysts or subglottic stenosis. The ini-

tial physical exam must be directed toward a rapid assessment for respiratory distress, including respiratory rate, presence of nasal flaring, and use of accessory neck or chest muscles. If there is evidence of significant distress, further examination should be halted until equipment for endoscopic evaluation, airway intubation, and possible tracheotomy is readily available. This may be the emergency room, pediatric intensive care unit, or operating room, depending on institutional resource availability and accessibility.

Anesthesia and Airway Management

Dynamic evaluation of the larynx with flexible laryngoscopy can provide specific information about the configuration and function of laryngeal structures, but is not mandatory prior to operative endoscopy, especially if it could worsen respiratory status. In cases of unknown airway pathology, effective communication between the anesthesiologist and surgeon during preoperative planning and intraoperative management is paramount. The anesthetic technique may be modified depending on the child's age, suspected diagnosis, underlying impairment of oxygenation and ventilation, and potential treatment modalities. In nearly all cases, spontaneous ventilation is recommended. The patient maintains his/her own respiratory effort, resulting in an unobstructed operative field, aiding in diagnosis and management. Anesthesia can be induced with inhalation (sevofluorane) agents or possibly IV (sodium thiopental, ketamine, or propofol) agents if an established IV exists.[6] With inhalation techniques, the delivered concentration requires a delicate balance that is high enough to prevent coughing and laryngospasm, but also low enough to avoid cardiovascular depression and apnea. This can be difficult to achieve with short-acting agents. Thorough topical anesthesia with 2 to 4% lidocaine, delivered either by atomizer or syringe, can provide additional anesthesia and reduce systemic requirements. When using topical lidocaine, it is important to remain cognizant of the maximum dosage limits based on the child's weight. In addition, adjunctive agents, such as propofol infusion, may be used to reduce or replace the need for inhalational anesthesia.[6]

For patients with a potentially tenuous airway, there are several pieces of equipment we have deemed essential in the operation room.[7] Working from the simplest to the most complex, these include appropriately sized bag-mask ventilation devices, oropharyngeal airways, laryngeal mask airways, straight blade laryngoscopes, and ventilating bronchoscopes. In addition, we have a 0° 1.9 mm Hopkins rod-lens telescope and size 2.5 mm endotracheal tube loaded in a Seldinger fashion present (Figure 5–17). Finally, we have a percutaneous transtracheal needle insufflation device available and formal tracheotomy set open on the back table prior to induction[7] (Figure 5–18).

Subglottic Cysts

Pediatric subglottic cysts are a rare, but increasingly present, cause of respiratory complications in neonates. While congenital cases have been reported, subglottic cysts occur almost exclusively in premature infants

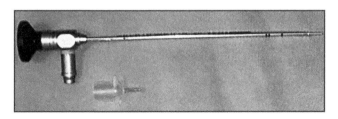

Figure 5–17. 0° 1.9 mm Hopkins rod-lens telescope with size 2.5 mm endotracheal tube loaded in a Seldinger fashion.

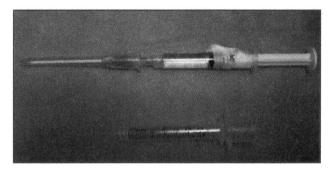

Figure 5–18. Percutaneous transtracheal needle insufflation device prepared and available prior to induction.

with a history of endotracheal intubation.[8] Following traumatic mucosal injury, the native mucous glands within the subglottis become obstructed due to subepithelial fibrosis, resulting in cyst formation.[9] In 1981, Couriel and Phelan managed three patients with subglottic cysts over a 12-month period.[10] They suspected that the increasing survival of very low-birth-weight infants following prolonged intubation and intermittent positive pressure ventilation would result in an increased incidence of subglottic cysts. As a result, they stressed the importance of adding subglottic cysts to the differential diagnosis of stridor in infants with past intubation history and the role for careful endoscopic examination in diagnosis. In particular, they noted that such cysts could be easily ruptured, relieving the airway obstruction and eliminating the need for more morbid procedures, such as tracheostomy.[10]

Subglottic cysts are now a well-known and recognized cause of respiratory distress in previously intubated infants, with over 130 cases presented in the literature to date.[11–12] The main treatment methods include observation, bronchoscopic rupture and decompression, and endoscopic marsupialization. Endoscopic marsupialization with cold steel instruments or CO_2 laser has been the most commonly reported method for subglottic cyst treatment, although despite proper surgical management, recurrence has been noted in 12.5–71% of cases.[11] In 2009, Ransom et al incorporated use of the microdebrider in a small series of 8 patients with subglottic cysts. They noted a symptomatic recurrence rate of 12.5%, which was managed with a repeat procedure, and otherwise disease-free follow-up among their patient with a mean follow-up of 21 months.[13] More recently, 16 patients with subglottic cysts underwent rupture and decompression with use of a Bugbee fulgurating electrode.[12] In this series, only 1 patient (6%) developed a symptomatic recurrence requiring repeat cyst lysis. These authors concluded that both microdebrider and cautery offer safe and effective alternatives to current techniques with potentially lower symptomatic recurrence rates than previously reported.

Due to the shared history of prior and often prolonged intubation, the most common associated laryngotracheal finding identified with subglottic cysts is subglottic stenosis.[12] This highlights the importance of a thorough endoscopic evaluation and postoperative follow-up to determine the relative contribution of co-existing pathologies.

Subglottic Stenosis

Laryngotracheal stenosis continues to remain a significant health issue within the pediatric population. With the introduction of prolonged endotracheal intubation for premature neonates, the incidence of subglottic stenosis reached a peak in the late 1970s and early 1980s.[14] With improvements in airway management, there has been a decline over the past few decades, although the incidence of subglottic stenosis still likely ranges from 0.63% to 2.0% of intubated neonates.[15–17] During the neonatal period, tracheostomy and anterior cricoid split are the typical treatment options for subglottic stenosis resulting in failed extubation.[18] Following the neonatal period, treatment options generally include tracheostomy, endoscopic airway surgery, or open airway reconstruction. While advances in endoscopic management have occurred, open techniques remain the mainstay for treatment, whether performed as a primary operation or following failure of endoscopic procedures.[19–23]

Operative endoscopy remains the standard for evaluation of airway stenosis. At the time of endoscopy, the stenosis is generally graded I to IV according to the Myer–Cotton classification system.[23] Severe cases (grades III and IV) of subglottic stenosis require a tracheotomy. Management is then individualized according to patient age and health status, as well as endoscopic findings including grade, location, and quality of stenosis.[24] The best chance for the patient lies in the first operation, thus the surgeon must be fully trained in pediatric airway endoscopy and laryngotracheal surgery.[25] Endoscopic techniques for isolated subglottic stenosis may be successful in grade I and occasionally grade II. Expansion laryngotracheal surgery, combining the use of laryngeal and cricoid splits, cartilage grafts, and stenting is very successful in grades II/III

stenosis and some grade IV stenosis. Surgical repair at the youngest age possible eliminates the morbidity and mortality associated with a tracheostomy and enhances opportunities for age-appropriate speech and language development.[25]

As noted, ssLTR compresses the prolonged stenting period of traditional LTR into a briefer period of endotracheal intubation. The optimal time for intubation has not been established and frequently varies depending on a variety of factors, including patient age and location of grafting sites. Certainly, advantages of this technique include decannulation at the time of surgery or possible tracheostomy avoidance altogether. On the other hand, disadvantages include the risk of extubation in the postoperative period, with concern for difficult re-intubation, as well as the effects of prolonged sedation and possible withdrawal syndrome.

With dsLTR, the tracheostomy remains in place following reconstruction, with decannulation planned for a later date in time. Persistence of the tracheostomy provides a stable airway throughout the postoperative period. When choosing stents, the surgeon has to consider the material, size, location, and duration. The senior author favors the following: cut Montgomery t-tube with superior end sutured closed, cut endotracheal tube with superior end sutured closed, and Aboulker stent. The stent is sized by extrapolating the outer diameter of an age-appropriate pediatric endotracheal tube. Disadvantages of this technique relate directly to stent complications, including granulation tissue formation. Additionally, there is the risk for stent migration with possible airway obstruction, predisposition to aspiration, or inadequate graft support.

In order to combine the advantages of both ssLTR and dsLTR, Setlur et al developed a novel technique deemed the hybrid LTR.[1] A case series of four patients with a combination of glottic and subglottic stenosis underwent open LTR, after which the airway was stented via nasotracheal intubation. The length of the patient's preexisting tracheostomy tube was measured and a size 3.0 endotracheal tube was cut to match with the external portion sutured closed. The endotracheal tube stent was placed into the tracheostoma and secured to the neck with cloth ties. The neck was then dressed to minimize air leakage. At postoperative day 7, the patients returned to the operating room for extubation and bronchoscopy. Once completed, the tracheostomal stent was removed and the patient's tracheostomy tube was easily replaced. The authors noted that single-stage procedures are generally considered better for patients with lower-grade stenosis;

however, the presence of the stent in to tracheostoma allows for emergent airway access during the postoperative period, thereby allowing ssLTR to become applicable to those patients with higher-grade and complex stenoses.[1]

In 2015, Raol et al further described the modifications to and outcomes from the hybrid LTR technique.[26] A disadvantage of the hLTR technique noted previously was the potential for peristomal air leakage in the postoperative period with ventilation difficulty.[1] In order to limit this risk, a 3.0 neonatal Shiley tracheostomy tube is inserted into the tracheostoma at the completion of the surgery, instead of the trimmed endotracheal tube.[26] The flanges allow the tube to rest against the neck and be secured by tracheostomy ties in the standard fashion. The tracheostomy tube and endotracheal tube occupy the airway simultaneously without issues (Figure 5–19). In addition, in the rare but possible event of accidental extubation in the postoperative period, the tracheostomy tube is already in place, allowing for maintenance of ventilation until otolaryngology personnel arrive to address the situation appropriately.

With respect to outcomes, since the hybrid LTR is useful in the same subset of patients who are candidates for dsLTR, decannulation rates should be similar if the technique is equally efficacious. Raol et al found an operation-specific decannulation rate of 69.2% and overall decannulation rate of 76.2%.[26] In the first report comparing outcomes in ssLTR versus dsLTR, Saunders et al found an operation-specific decannulation rate of 61.2% for the dsLTR group.[27] Hartnick et al examined 101 children who underwent dsLTR and noted operation-specific decannulation rates of 85%, 37%, and 50% for Myer–Cotton grades 2, 3, and 4, respectively.[28] The overall decannulation rates were 95%, 74%, and 86% for the same patient populations. Most recently, Smith et al reported their outcomes for ssLTR and dsLTR, demonstrating an operation-specific decannulation rate of 68% for dsLTR patients.[29] Thus, the initial results for the rate of decannulation for the hybrid LTR patients have proved comparable to the literature for dsLTR patients.[26]

Within our institution, in those patients who would traditionally be dsLTR candidates, the hybrid LTR has largely replaced the dsLTR primarily due to its safety, effectiveness, and overwhelming intensivist and parental support.

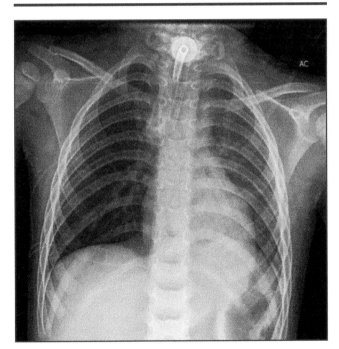

Figure 5–19. Chest x-ray in post-operative hybrid laryngotracheal reconstruction patient showing simultaneous occupation of the airway with endotracheal tube and tracheostomy tube.

Decannulation Considerations

The recent clinical consensus statement on tracheostomy care sought to reduce variations in practice when managing patients with a pediatric tracheostomy in order to minimize complications.[30] The following pertinent statements regarding decannulation achieved consensus:

- In children, prior to decannulation, a discussion with family regarding care needs and preparation for decannulation should take place.
- In children, prior to decannulation, no ventilator assistance should be needed where a tracheostomy would be required.
- In children, there should be no documented aspiration events that would preclude decannulation.
- In children, prior to decannulation, a flexible laryngoscopy should reveal at least one mobile vocal fold or a patent glottis.
- In children, prior to decannulation a bronchoscopy should be performed within a

few months to ensure a patent airway with no occluding suprastomal granuloma.

- For children, prior to decannulation, the tracheostomy tube should be capped all day and the cap removed at night for several weeks to determine whether the cap can remain on even when the child has an upper respiratory infection.
- Prior to decannulation, children with a tracheostomy should undergo a daytime capping trial (if they are older than 2 years and if the tracheostomy does not occupy so much of the trachea so as to preclude capping). If they pass such a capping trial, options prior to decannulation include a capped sleep study, a capped exercise test, or a nighttime capping trial while hospitalized and being observed.
- In a child who is either too young or too small to undergo a successful capping trial, decannulation protocols need to be individualized for the particular patient.

In younger and smaller patients, the tracheostomy tube may occupy most of the tracheal lumen, precluding a capping trial. In 1969, MacLachlan discussed several methods of decannulation, noting that the use of fenestrated tracheostomy tubes was "impracticable and dangerous since it is impossible to maintain the fenestra opposite the tracheal lumen."[31] Fortunately, endoscopy provides an opportunity to evaluate the tracheostomy tube in situ. Thus, the ideal location to perform fenestration can be identified and the correctness of that location confirmed once the tracheostomy is replaced. A fenestrated tracheostomy tube should never be left in place, as it poses a substantial risk for irritation of the tracheal mucosa and granulation formation. However, an overnight trial with a capped fenestrated tracheostomy can provide critical information prior to decannulation in younger and smaller patients, with minimal risk for adverse sequelae.[32]

Persistent failure to decannulate can be due to multiple causes, including suprastomal collapse, which can approach 20% in young children with long-standing tracheostomies.[33] In some cases, this obstruction is severe enough to limit decannulation. Several methods of repair have been reported, including internal stenting, anterior cricotracheal suspension, and autologous costal cartilage laryngotracheoplasty, with the method of choice depending on the degree of airway obstruction and the strength of the surrounding laryngotracheal complex.[33–34] While effective, these techniques

may lack rigid support, require prolonged stenting, or involve additional morbidity and operative time due to cartilage harvesting. Gorostidi et al utilized bioresorbable microplates to manage localized severe transverse, paramedian, and anteroposterior tracheal collapse allowing decannulation in patients who had experienced multiple previous failures.[35] In their case series, however, temporary endoluminal stenting of 3 to 6 months was performed prior to subsequent decannulation trials.

More recently, we incorporated the use of bioabsorbable microplates to manage suprastomal collapse limiting decannulation, providing rigidification to the weakened cartilage without the need for additional surgical procedures.[36] All three patients underwent a similar intraoperative technique for placement of the bioabsorbable plate in coordination with tracheocutaneous fistula closure. The initial two patients underwent 5 days of endotracheal stenting via nasotracheal intubation. As the technique proved safe and effective, when intraoperative bronchoscopy showed good reduction of the collapse in our third patient, she was extubated immediately postoperatively and monitored overnight in the pediatric intensive care unit. All three patients remain successfully decannulated at 13, 17, and 11 months following the suprastomal plate suspension procedure.

SUMMARY

Stridor is a frequent symptom prompting referral to a pediatric otolaryngologist for an airway evaluation. Prematurity status, age of onset, and history of intubation provide input to the differential diagnosis, particularly regarding concerns for subglottic cysts or subglottic stenosis. The initial physical exam must be directed toward a rapid assessment for respiratory distress with the need to determine the safest environment to proceed with further workup and management. When dealing with cases of unknown airway pathology in the operating room, effective communication between the anesthesiologist and surgeon during preoperative planning and intraoperative management is paramount. In addition, for patients with a potentially tenuous airway, the armamentarium of essential equipment must be ready prior to induction.

Pediatric subglottic cysts are a rare but increasingly present cause of respiratory complications in neonates. Fortunately, there are numerous surgical options for management that have proven successful. Due to the shared history of prior and often prolonged intubation, the most common associated laryngotracheal finding identified with subglottic cysts is subglottic stenosis. This highlights the importance of a thorough endoscopic evaluation and postoperative follow-up to determine the relative contribution of coexisting pathologies. Subglottic stenosis continues to remain a significant health issue within the pediatric population. While advances in endoscopic management have occurred, open techniques remain the mainstay for treatment, whether performed as a primary operation or following failure of endoscopic procedures. The specific technique (eg, ssLTR, dsLTR, hLTR) is then individualized according to patient age and health status, as well as endoscopic findings including grade, location, and quality of stenosis.

Ideally, patients undergoing LTR will eventually be ready for decannulation. In patients who are too young or too small to undergo a successful capping trial, decannulation protocols need to be individualized for the particular patient, which may incorporate a capped fenestrated tracheostomy overnight trial. In those patients with persistent failure to decannulate, suprastomal collapse is now a frequently recognized cause. Fortunately, suprastomal plate suspension with bioabsorbable microplates has shown promise in a small case series. Regardless, the most important consideration is to engage the family throughout the care pathway, including preparation for decannulation.

REFERENCES

1. Setlur J, Maturo S, Hartnick CJ. Novel method for laryngotracheal reconstruction combining single- and double-stage techniques. *Ann Otol Rhinol Laryngol*. 2013;122:445–449.
2. Liew L, Blaney SPA, Morrison GAJ. Surgical selection and outcomes in laryngotracheal reconstruction for subglottic stenosis. *Int Congr Ser*. 2003;1254:147–150.
3. Froehlich P, Seid AB, Morgon A. Suprastomal collapse complicating pediatric tracheotomy. *Op Tech Otolaryngol Head Neck Surg*. 1998;9:175–177.
4. Anton-Pacheco JL, Villafruela M, Lopez M, Garcia G, Luna C, Martinez A. Surgical management of severe suprastomal cricotracheal collapse complicating pediatric tracheotomy. *Int J Pediatr Otorhinolaryngol*. 2008;72:179–183.
5. Bowe SN, Colaianni A, Hartnick CJ. Management of severe suprastomal collapse with bioabsorbable microplates. *Laryngoscope*. 2017; 127/;2823–2826.
6. Swanson VC, Taneja PA, Gries H, Koh J. Anesthesia in pediatric otolaryngology. In: Lesperance MM, Flint PW, eds, *Cummings Pediatric Otolaryngology*. Philadelphia, PA: Elsevier Saunders; 2015:21–38.
7. Gallagher TQ, Setlur J, Maturo S, Hartnick CJ. Percutaneous transtracheal needle insufflation: a useful emergency airway adjunct simply constructed from common items found on your anesthesia cart. *Laryngoscope*. 2012; 122:1178–1180.
8. Bruno CJ, Smith LP, Zur KB, Wade KC. Congenital subglottic cyst in a term neonate. *Arch Dis Child Fetal Neonatal Ed*. 2009;94:F240.
9. Wigger HJ, Tang P. Fatal laryngeal obstruction by iatrogenic subglottic cysts. *J Pediatr*. 1968;72:815–820.
10. Couriel JM, Phelan PD. Subglottic cysts: a complication of neonatal endotracheal intubation. *Pediatrics*. 1981; 60:103–105.
11. Aksoy EA, Elsurer C, Serin GM, Unal OF. Evaluation of pediatric subglottic cysts. *Int J Pediatr Otorhinolaryngol*. 2012;76:240–243.
12. Richardson MA, Winford TW, Norris BK, Reed JM. Management of pediatric subglottic cysts using the Bugbee fulgurating electrode. *JAMA Otolaryngol Head Neck Surg*. 2014;140:164–168.
13. Ransom ER, Antunes MB, Smith LP, Jacobs IN. Microdebrider resection of acquired subglottic cysts: case series and review of the literature. *Int J Pediatr Otorhinolaryngol*. 2009;73:1833–1836.
14. Santos D, Mitchell R. The history of pediatric airway reconstruction. *Laryngoscope*. 2010;120:815–820.
15. Choi SS, Zalzal GH. Changing trends in neonatal subglottic stenosis. *Otolaryngol Head Neck Surg*. 2000;122:61–63.
16. Walner DL, Loewen MS, Kimura RE. Neonatal subglottic stenosis—incidence and trends. *Laryngoscope*. 2001; 111:48–51.
17. Thomas RE, Rao SC, Minutillo C, Vijayasekaran S, Nathan EA. Severe acquired subglottic stenosis in neonatal intensive care graduates: a case-control study. *Arch Dis Child Fetal Neonatal Ed*. 2018;103(4):F349–F354 .
18. Cotton RT, Seid AB. Management of the extubation problem in the premature child: anterior cricoid split as an alternative to tracheostomy. *Ann Otol Rhinol Laryngol*. 1980;89:508–511.
19. Dahl JP, Purcell PL, Parikh SR, Inglis AF Jr. Endoscopic posterior cricoid split with costal cartilage graft: a fifteen-year experience. *Laryngoscope*. 2017;127:252–257.
20. Sharma SD, Gupta SL, Wyatt M, Albert D, Hartley B. Safe balloon sizing for endoscopic dilatation of subglottic stenosis in children. *J Laryngrol Otol*. 2017;131:268–272.
21. Lee GS, Irace A, Rahbar R. The efficacy and safety of the flexible fiber CO2 laser delivery system in the endoscopic management of pediatric airway problems: our long term experience. *Int J Pediatr Otorhinolaryngol*. 2017;97:218–222.
22. Chen C, Ni WH, Tian TL, Xu ZM. The outcomes of endoscopic management in young children with subglottic stenosis. *Int J Pediatr Otorhinolaryngol*. 2017;99:141–145.
23. Myer CM 3rd, Hartley BEJ. Pediatric laryngotracheal surgery. *Laryngoscope*. 2000;110:1875–1883.

24. Zalzal GH, Cotton RT. Glottic and subglottic stenosis. In: Lesperance MM, Flint PW, eds, *Cummings Pediatric Otolaryngology*. Philadelphia, PA: Elsevier Saunders; 2015: 348–360.

25. Bailey M, Hoeve H, Monnier P. Paediatric laryngotracheal stenosis: a consensus paper from three European centres. *Eur Arch Otorhinolaryngol*. 2003;260:118–123.

26. Raol N, Rogers D, Setlur J, Hartnick CJ. Comparison of hybrid laryngotracheal reconstruction to traditional single- and double-stage laryngotracheal reconstruction. *Otolaryngol Head Neck Surg*. 2015;152:524–529.

27. Saunders MW, Thirlwall A, Jacob A, Albert DM. Single-or-two-stage laryngotracheal reconstruction: comparison of outcomes. *Int J Pediatr Otorhinolaryngol*. 1999;50:51–54.

28. Hartnick CJ, Hartley BE, Lacy PD, et al. Surgery for pediatric subglottic stenosis: disease-specific outcomes. *Ann Otol Rhinol Laryngol*. 2001;110:1109–1113.

29. Smith LP, Zur KB, Jacobs IN. Single- vs double-stage laryngotracheal reconstruction. *Arch Otolaryngol Head Neck Surg*. 2010;136:60–65.

30. Mitchell RB, Hussey HM, Setzen G, et al. Clinical consensus statement: tracheostomy care. *Otolaryngol Head Neck Surg*. 2013;148:6–20.

31. MacLachlan RF. Decannulation in infancy. *J Laryngol Otol*. 1969;83:991–1003.

32. Merritt RM, Bent JP, Smith RJH. Suprastomal granulation tissue and pediatric tracheotomy decannulation. *Laryngoscope*. 1997;107:868–871.

33. Anton-Pacheco JL, Villafruela M, Lopez M, Garcia G, Luna C, Martinez A. Surgical management of severe suprastomal cricotracheal collapse complicating pediatric tracheostomy. *Int J Pediatr Otorhinolaryngol*. 2008; 72:179–183.

34. Froehlich P, Seid AB, Morgon A. Suprastomal collapse complicating pediatric tracheotomy. *Op Tech Otolaryngol Head Neck Surg*. 1998;9:175–177.

35. Gorostidi F, Reinhard A, Monnier P, Sandu K. External bioresorbable airway rigidification to treat refractory localized tracheomalacia. *Laryngoscope*. 2016;126:2605–2610.

36. Bowe SN, Colaianni A, Hartnick CJ. Management of severe suprastomal collapse with bioabsorbable microplates. *Laryngoscope*. 2017;127(12):2823–2826.

CHAPTER 6

Long-Segment Tracheal Stenosis

Michael J. Rutter and Claudia Schweiger

INTRODUCTION

Long-segment tracheal stenosis is usually congenital, due to complete tracheal rings (CTRs), with or without associated vascular compression of the airway. The stenosis may be associated with Down syndrome or VACTERL (vertebral defects, anal atresia, cardiac defects, tracheo-esophageal fistula, renal anomalies, and limb abnormalities). If the stenosis is not severe, it may be a late presentation or an incidental finding, but most times it requires surgery in the first weeks or months of life.

We present here a patient with congenital long-segment tracheal stenosis and discuss the diagnosis and management of this condition.

CASE PRESENTATION

A 2-month-old boy with a history of hypoplastic left lung and left pulmonary artery stenosis presented mild biphasic stridor since birth. Difficulty during intubation for cardiac catheterization when he was 1 month old at an outside hospital prompted a bronchoscopy, which revealed a long segment of CTRs. The child was referred to our hospital for additional evaluation and repair. Symptomatically, he was getting worse, with retractions and requiring oxygen via nasal cannula since 1 month of age.

On the first bronchoscopy at our hospital, there were CTRs from the third or fourth tracheal ring down to the carina. His trachea was very narrow, and could not accommodate a 1.9 mm telescope. He was also found to have a hypoplastic left lung with abnormal blood supply consisting of a very tiny native left pulmonary artery and a collateral from the celiac plexus as well. He presented a large atrial septal defect and a left superior vena cava to a coronary sinus, and his shunting at the atrial level was all left to right by echocardiogram.

A surgical repair was planned. Patient was intubated with a 3.5 endotracheal tube, with the tip confirmed to be at the level of the subglottis, and placed on cardiopulmonary bypass. Slide tracheoplasty and subtotal closure of the atrial septal defect were carried out. Total cardiopulmonary bypass time was 117 minutes. The patient remained intubated at the end of the procedure, and was extubated 2 days later. Before the extubation, a flexible bronchoscopy was performed, in order to remove any mucus plugs and blood clots.

He did well in the following days after extubation, with no oxygen requirements, and was discharged home 3 weeks later. He developed a very mild figure-of-8 trachea that did not require any treatment. His last follow-up bronchoscopy was last year, at age 5 years. His airway sized with a 5.5 endotracheal tube with a leak at 5 cm H_2O. He was asymptomatic.

EVALUATION AND DIAGNOSTIC WORKUP

History

Children with long-segment tracheal stenosis due to CTRs typically present with progressive worsening of respiratory function over the first few weeks or months of life. Stridor, retractions, dying spells, and marked intermittent exacerbation of symptoms during upper respiratory tract infections are the typical presentation. Children may also present an expiratory grunting, barky, or brassy cough. Symptoms are exacerbated when the infant is agitated or when feeding.[1]

Because the growth of the trachea is not commensurate with the growth of the child over the first few months of life, decompensation frequently occurs around 4 months of age, with the child presenting respiratory failure. However, even in a neonate with a life-threatening tracheal stenosis, there may be surprisingly few symptoms.

Physical Exam

Stridor and retractions are almost always present. Patients with distal tracheal stenosis usually have a characteristic biphasic wet-sounding breathing pattern that transiently clears with coughing; this pattern is referred to as "washing machine breathing."[2]

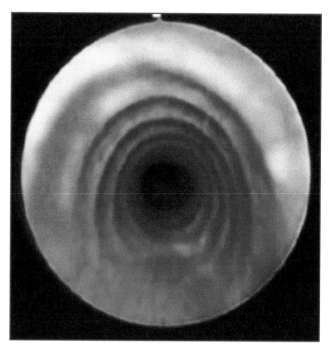

Figure 6–1. Tracheoscopy showing complete tracheal rings.

Differential Diagnosis

Many other conditions may mimic congenital long-segment tracheal stenosis. These conditions include short-segment stenosis, tracheal webs, tracheomalacia, tracheal tumors, and vascular compression. Vascular compression may be caused by the innominate artery, vascular rings such as a double aortic arch, and vascular slings.

Laryngeal pathology may also mimic tracheal stenosis by producing inspiratory or biphasic stridor and respiratory distress; examples include subglottic stenosis, vocal fold paralysis, and laryngeal masses.

Micro-Laryngotracheobronchoscopy and Flexible Airway Endoscopy

Rigid bronchoscopy is the gold standard for the diagnosis of tracheal stenosis.[2] In patients with CTRs, the cartilaginous rings appear circular and may affect varying lengths of the trachea; also, the trachealis muscle is absent (Figure 6–1). The diameter of the complete cartilage rings is always smaller than the trachea above the affected segment, although the severity of the stenosis may vary (Figure 6–2). Edema of the tracheal

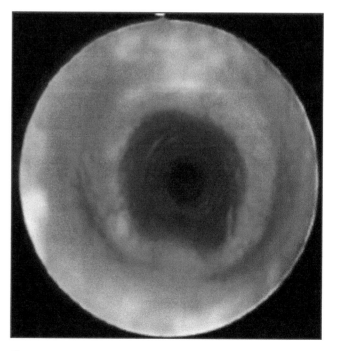

Figure 6–2. Complete tracheal rings appear as a narrow portion of the trachea just below normal trachea.

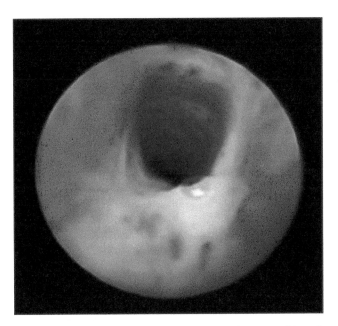

Figure 6–3. Post-intubation tracheal edema, making it difficult to identify the complete tracheal rings.

mucosa may obscure the contours of the rings, making them more difficult to identify (Figure 6–3). Also, differentiating absent tracheal rings from CTRs may be difficult by endoscopy alone, as the endoscopic findings in patients with absent rings may be similar to those in patients who have complete rings with mucosal edema.[3] Endoscopic findings in patients with acquired long-segment stenosis are more variable.

During endoscopy, one should determine the tracheal length that is involved in the stenosis and measure the diameter of the narrowest point of the stenosis. The diameter of the stenosis can be estimated by the size of the Hopkins rod telescope or endotracheal tube able to comfortably pass into the area of stenosis.[2] However, in patients with severe narrowing, it may not be possible to pass an endoscope through the stenosis to measure its diameter or to visualize the distal extent of the stenosis. In this situation, we prefer identifying only the proximal extent of the tracheal stenosis without fully evaluating the distal airway, rather than forcing a telescope through a narrow stenosis, to avoid the risk of respiratory decompensation. Dexamethasone (0.5 mg/kg) should be administered routinely on induction, to avoid edema of the airway.

Although rigid endoscopy provides excellent visualization of the airway, flexible bronchoscopy is a useful adjunct. It does not stent the airway as much as rigid endoscopy, thus allowing better identification of abnormal airway dynamics. A pulmonary artery sling, for example, may be more apparent with flexible bronchoscopy. Another benefit of flexible bronchoscopy is that it permits evaluation of the distal airways and a bronchoalveolar lavage, both of which identify infectious and inflammatory processes that may affect planning of a tracheal surgery.

Imaging Exams

In view of the high proportion of patients with other congenital anomalies, a thorough diagnostic investigation should include an echocardiogram and a contrast-enhanced computed tomography (CT) scan of the chest with three-dimensional reconstruction.

Echocardiography

Preoperative identification of cardiovascular malformations allows planning for operative management while the patient is on cardiopulmonary bypass for the tracheal repair. Echocardiography allows detection of myocardial dysfunction, valvular pathology, atrial and ventricular septal defects, and anomalies of the proximal great vessels.

CT Scan

For patients with congenital tracheal stenosis, a CT scan of the airway with fine cuts (0.5 mm–1 mm) and three-dimensional reconstruction is the imaging exam of choice. Simultaneous CT angiography of the chest and neck must be obtained in order to identify congenital anomalies of the cardiovascular system and points of vascular compression of the airway.

The most common cardiovascular anomaly is the pulmonary artery sling (PAS), though intracardiac anomalies and the presence of a persistent left superior vena cava draining to the coronary sinus with absence of the innominate vein are also common.

MANAGEMENT

The pediatric otolaryngologist typically coordinates the patient's care; however, the appropriate consulting services—cardiothoracic surgery, cardiology, pulmonology, anesthesiology and critical care, nutrition, and social work—must be involved in the patient care as early as possible. The evaluation of associated anomalies and assessment of the general status of the patient prior to definitive treatment is as important as the management of the tracheal obstruction itself.

If possible, the child should be kept extubated, as most children with CTRs maintain ventilation more effectively themselves than on a ventilator. To prevent mucus accumulation, saline may be regularly nebulized if required.

Approximately 50% of children with CTRs have a tracheal inner diameter of approximately 2 mm at the time of diagnosis. Therefore, the standard interventions for managing a compromised airway, such as intubation with a small endotracheal tube or performing a tracheotomy, are not applicable. If a child with CTRs requires intubation, we should remember that the smallest endotracheal tube (inner diameter 2.0 mm, outer diameter 2.9 mm) and the smallest tracheotomy tube (inner diameter 2.5 mm) cannot pass through the stenotic segment without severe damage to mucosa or tracheal rupture. Also, as the stenosis usually extends to carina in the long-segment tracheal stenosis, bypassing the stenosis risks bronchial intubation. This may leave extracorporeal membrane oxygenation (ECMO) as the only viable alternative for stabilizing the child in the event of decompensation.

In an effort to avoid ECMO in a child decompensating and poorly ventilating, intubation proximal to the complete rings may be attempted. The endotracheal tube should be sized to the cricoid, with the Murphy eye just below vocal fold level. Given that it is unusual for the proximal two tracheal rings to be complete, shallow intubation is achievable in most children with CTRs. A nasal intubation to allow tube stabilization is advisable. Ventilation requires a long inspiratory and even longer expiratory phase to allow air to pass the stenosis. Higher than typical ventilator pressures may be tolerated, as the stenosis ensures that the lungs are not exposed to the same pressures as the subglottis.

Maintenance of high humidity levels is key, as mucus accumulation may be lethal and is often heralded by rising CO_2 rather than low oxygen saturation. In a crisis, 1 mL of 1:10000 epinephrine delivered down the endotracheal tube may assist ventilation.

All patients with tracheostomy should undergo methicillin-resistant *Staphylococcus aureus* (MRSA) screening and treatment before the surgery. MRSA infection in open airway procedures can be a devastating complication, resulting in dehiscence and weakening of the cartilaginous structure of the laryngotracheal complex.[4]

Although gastroesophageal reflux disease (GERD) plays an important role in the pathogenesis and prognosis of laryngeal stenosis, its impact on children with tracheal or bronchial stenosis is insignificant.[1]

Observation and Serial Endoscopy

A select group of children with complete tracheal rings can be managed expectantly without surgical intervention.[5–7] Airway growth does occur in this population and can be monitored over time.

In our last published cohort, the 10 patients who initially underwent conservative management of CTRs fell into the following three categories: 5 patients were minimally symptomatic or asymptomatic, showed bronchoscopic evidence of progressive airway growth, and did not require tracheoplasty; 2 patients had worsening symptoms of exercise intolerance, showed minimal airway growth, and ultimately required tracheoplasty; and 3 patients were still being clinically observed and would eventually require tracheoplasty. Periods of observation varied from 1 year to over 12 years.[5]

A standardized method for sizing the unrepaired CTRs, usually with endotracheal tubes, allows for assurance of continued growth of the airway while following these patients. If growth does not occur as time goes by and the patient becomes increasingly symptomatic, then surgical repair is required.

Endoscopic Surgery

Endoscopic techniques such as balloon dilation rarely have a role in the treatment of congenital tracheal stenosis. More specifically, they are contraindicated in the initial management of CTRs, as the risk of tracheal rupture is high. Balloon dilation may, however, have a role after reconstruction if restenosis occurs.[6]

Slide Tracheoplasty

Slide tracheoplasty is a surgical technique originally designed by Goldstraw in the 1980s to repair congenital tracheal stenosis caused by complete tracheal rings.[8] This technique was popularized by both Grillo et al[9] and by our team at Cincinnati Children's Hospital.[2] It consists of overlapping stenotic segments of the trachea, shortening it but doubling the diameter of the narrowed area, and can be performed through a sternotomy or through the neck. It is currently the operation of choice for tracheal stenosis attributed to CTRs.[2,10–14]

This technique has a number of advantages relative to other methods. These advantages include immediate tracheal reconstruction with rigid, vascularized tissue with a normal mucosa; ability to extubate patients early in many cases; less postoperative granulation tissue formation; less risk of dehiscence; and growth potential of the reconstructed trachea.[9] The slide can extend into the membranous trachea or into the carina if required. The whole length of the trachea may be slid, even past the carina, which makes this a very useful technique for long-segment stenosis.

At Cincinnati Children's Hospital, we have performed slide tracheoplasty since 2001. Our experience has demonstrated that slide tracheoplasty with cardiopulmonary bypass support can be performed with very low mortality despite the complexity of this patient population. In our last cohort, including 80 patients, we found a mortality rate of only 5% (4 children).[15] This rate was much lower than the previously reported mortality rate of up to 24% in some series.[16,17] Also, the slide technique requires airway re-intervention less frequently than other techniques. When needed, re-intervention rarely involves more than balloon dilation, endoscopic resection of granulation tissue, or temporary stent placement.[15]

Successful surgical management depends upon close collaboration of the airway surgeon and the cardiovascular surgeon. Although current anesthetic methods, including jet ventilation, may allow for repair of distal and long-segment tracheal stenosis, these can create challenges in infants and younger children. Cardiopulmonary bypass is a safe alternative that allows partial deflation of the heart and lungs so that exposure of the complete trachea is optimized. Conversion of ECMO to cardiopulmonary bypass is also recommended for the procedure for this same reason.

Transthoracic Approach

If the distal one third of the trachea is involved or if there are coexistent cardiovascular anomalies that require repair, we recommend repair utilizing a transthoracic approach, with cardiopulmonary bypass. More than 90% of children requiring slide tracheoplasty for long-segment congenital tracheal stenosis fall into this category.

A sternotomy allows for exposure of the trachea, placement of atrial and aortic cannulae, and repair of any coexisting cardiovascular anomalies. The trachea is exposed by dissecting between the ascending aorta and the superior vena cava. In the process, removal of the right paratracheal lymph nodes facilitates tracheal exposure. The carina is identified deep to the right pulmonary artery and the anterior trachea is exposed from the carina to the upper aspect of the CTRs.

Intraoperative bronchoscopy is then performed to define the upper and lower limits of the complete tracheal ring segment. A 30-gauge needle is placed through the anterior tracheal wall as it is visualized by a 2.8 mm flexible bronchoscope to define the proximal and distal CTRs. At this point, with the patient stabilized on cardiopulmonary bypass, a more comprehensive evaluation of the distal airway can also be performed if desired.

The length of the stenosis is then measured and the trachea is transected at the midpoint of the segment of complete rings (Figure 6–4). Each end of the transected trachea is then mobilized. The lateral vascular attachments to the trachea are preserved in this process. The anterior wall of the proximal tracheal segment is incised vertically (Figure 6–5). The posterior wall of the distal segment is cut vertically toward the carina. Cartilage is then trimmed from the corners of the proximal and distal segments, and the segments then slid over each other. Depending upon the length of the stenotic segment, this requires additional tracheal mobilization from both superior and inferior attachments. The carina is displaced superiorly by temporary stay sutures.

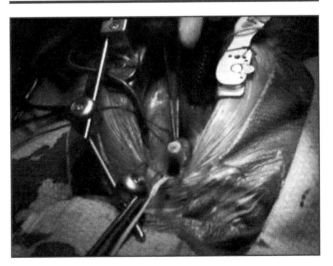

Figure 6–4. Transection of the trachea at the midpoint of the segment of complete rings.

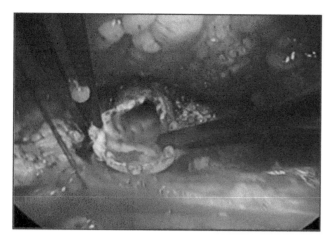

Figure 6–5. Vertical anterior incision of the proximal tracheal segment.

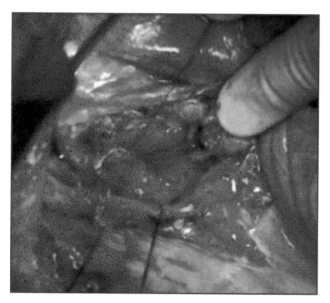

Figure 6–6. Double-armed 5.0 or 6-0 PDS.

The anastomosis is commenced from distal posterior (carinal) in a running fashion using appropriate sized double-armed polydioxanone sutures (5.0 or 6-0 PDS in infants) (Figure 6–6). Four to six throws of the suture are generally placed at the carina and tightened with a nerve hook. The anastomosis is then continued up the left and right sides of the trachea, with the sutures placed through cartilage and mucosa, therefore being exposed intraluminally. An effort is made to evert the lateral sides of the anastomosis to prevent internal bunching of the anastomotic lines (a "figure of 8" trachea). Before the anastomotic suture lines rejoin in the midline at the proximal anterior aspect of the repair, the trachea is suctioned clear and the patient is intubated with an age-appropriate endotracheal tube, and the tip of the tube positioned under direct visualization. The anastomosis is completed with a single proximal knot being thrown, leak tested (to 35 cm water pressure), and marked with Ligaclips applied to the proximal and distal ends of the anastomosis (to help identify the extent of the anastomosis on postoperative radiographs). Fibrin glue is then applied to the anastomosis. The patient is then removed from bypass, the chest closed, and the patient is transferred to the intensive care unit. At completion of the procedure, the airway is reevaluated with a flexible bronchoscope to ensure that the repair is adequate and that blood and secretions are suctioned.

Even with near full-length tracheal reconstruction, it is unusual to need a suprahyoid release or chin to chest sutures. Extension of the slide into a bronchus or cricoid cartilage has been performed successfully at our institution and may assist with repairing these concomitant stenoses. In children with an associated pig bronchus, a modified slide can also be performed, with the rings being split slightly oblique to the midline, so as not to compromise the orifice to the bronchus. The proximal extent of the slide should extend at least two rings into normal trachea beyond the pig bronchus.

Cervical Slide

If only the upper or mid-trachea is involved, repair may be performed with routine anesthesia through a cervical approach. This technique is very similar to the intrathoracic slide tracheoplasty described above. In older children with a more proximal stenosis, the risk of developing a "figure 8" trachea is higher, and a temporary silicone stent may be placed for a week or more if required.

In long-segment acquired cervical stenosis, part of the stenosis may be resected, and the remainder slid. If scarred trachea is slid into normal trachea, the outcome will be acceptable. If scarred trachea is slid into scarred trachea, the result is less predictable.

Cervical slide tracheoplasty has also been performed by airway surgeons at Cincinnati Children's since 2003. In our cohort published in 2012, we described 29 patients who underwent this procedure. Operation-specific success rate was 79% (23 of 29 patients), including all 10 patients with long-segment acquired tracheal stenosis. Lower operative success occurred in patients with concomitant subglottic stenosis, posterior glottic stenosis, and multilevel airway lesions. Four patients (14%) experienced complications: one patient had a minor wound infection; one had a dehiscence that was managed with a revision tracheoplasty; one had an innominate artery injury that was successfully treated intraoperatively without sequelae; and one had a symptomatic "figure 8" deformity that required revision therapy.[18]

POSTOPERATIVE CONSIDERATIONS

Following tracheal repair we aim to extubate a child within 24 to 96 hours. During this time we try to avoid positive pressure ventilation of over 30 cm of water so as not to threaten the anastomosis. Chest drains are left in place until after the extubation. Some children may preoperatively present extremely unstable and ventilated, and in very rare cases even on ECMO support. In this circumstance, postoperative ECMO may be required. The aim is to establish endotracheal ventilation and remove the child from ECMO as rapidly as possible.

Follow-up endoscopy to examine the repair is routinely performed 1 and 2 weeks after the operation. Balloon dilation is sometimes useful during the recovery phase if the figure-of-8 tracheal deformity at the repair is significant. This intervention helps prevent left and right lateral suture lines from coming into contact and adhering.[15] Children without cardiopulmonary anomalies are typically discharged from the hospital 2 to 3 weeks postoperatively.

Complications

While there are complications associated with slide tracheoplasty, these are mostly not of long-term consequence. The figure-of-8 trachea (lateral bunching of the anastomosis) seen in the majority of patients tends to spontaneously resolve over subsequent months in most patients and rarely causes obstruction or requires intervention (Figure 6–7A to C).

Recurrent laryngeal nerve palsy occurs in less than 20% of patients and is usually unilateral and transient. Restenosis is rare, as is anastomosis dehiscence. Restenosis is more likely to occur at the proximal end of a slide tracheoplasty when a tracheal bronchus is present at this apex; it may be prevented by extending the slide two or three rings higher, proximal to the tracheal bronchus, into normal trachea.[17]

Prognosis

Although three decades ago the diagnosis of long-segment tracheal stenosis carried a mortality rate as high as 50 to 80%, we now expect a survival rate exceeding 90%.

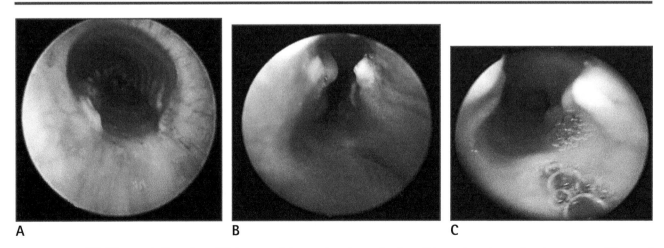

A   B   C

Figure 6–7. **(A)** "Figure of 8" trachea. **(B)** Aspect of the trachea 1 month after slide tracheoplasty, showing a severe "figure of 8" trachea. **(C)** Aspect of the trachea of the same patient 1 year later, showing improvement of the "figure of 8." The patient was asymptomatic.

Previously, outcomes were influenced by length of stenosis, severity of the stenosis, whether the carina was involved, and bronchial stenosis. Currently, it is no longer the trachea that is the primary determinant of outcome, but rather the overall health status of the child.[15] A significant proportion of children born with CTRs also have other significant health issues that a slide tracheoplasty does not address. These issues have become the dominant influence on long-term outcome. Bronchial stenosis, lung agenesis or hypoplasia, and complex cardiac disease are now the most significant issues affecting outcome.[19]

DISCUSSION AND PITFALLS

The incidence of congenital pediatric tracheal stenosis remains unclear. Diagnosis is frequently delayed because of the rarity of the lesion or because other more apparent associated malformations draw the attention of the clinician. For this reason, experience and a high level of clinical suspicion are essential in establishing an accurate diagnosis.[6]

Infants with congenital tracheal stenosis may present with varying degrees of respiratory distress. A history of mild respiratory complaints such as wheezing, persistent coughing, and accompanying feeding disorders are often present. The first few months of life may be riddled with frequent visits to the pediatrician for these complaints where reflux and reactive airway disease are often blamed. As increasing respiratory compromise ensues, respiratory distress is accompanied with retractions and distal airway sound. In particular, infants with complete tracheal rings and severe obstruction will present very early with distressing respiratory compromise.

A careful bronchoscopy for evaluation of the airway anatomy should be performed, taking care not to cause edema of the airway and to turn a stable airway into an emergency. It is better to "incompletely" assess the CTRs than to compromise the airway.

Optimal management of children with tracheal stenosis requires comprehensive evaluation prior to repair, avoiding the temptation to proceed straight to definitive repair. One should take care not to underestimate associated anomalies, since the tracheal obstruction is the most prominent symptom. Coexisting cardiac anomalies increase the risk of mortality in patients with congenital tracheal stenosis.[16]

Clearly, tracheotomy is rarely helpful, as the smallest CTRs tend to be more distal, and the smallest available commercial tracheotomy tube is 3.6 mm in outer diameter. In an airway compromised enough to consider tracheotomy, the stenotic segment is typically 2.0 to 2.5 mm in diameter, and therefore not amenable to tracheotomy placement. More importantly, tracheotomy may further compromise the options of subsequent operative repair.

In children with long-segment CTRs requiring intubation before surgery, a longer inhalation and exhalation time is recommended, and higher peak pressure may be tolerated. Mucus plugging is a concern, and maximal humidity is therefore recommended.

Slide tracheoplasty is currently the operation of choice for these children, either by a transthoracic approach or through the neck. Regarding the anesthetic technique, although current methods, including jet ventilation, may allow for repair of distal and long-segment tracheal stenosis, these can often be obtrusive and cumbersome for the surgeon. Cardiopulmonary bypass is a safe alternative that allows partial deflation of the heart and lungs so that exposure of the complete trachea is optimized. Conversion of ECMO to cardiopulmonary bypass is also recommended for the procedure for this same reason. Successful surgical management thus depends upon close collaboration of the airway surgeon and the cardiovascular surgeon. For the cervical slide tracheoplasty, endotracheal intubation should be used.

Postoperatively, the aim should be extubate as soon as possible, sometimes even at the table. If early extubation cannot be achieved, prevention of mucus plugging with saline down the endotracheal tube is critical.

Periodic postoperative airway evaluations are performed in the operating room utilizing primarily rigid bronchoscopy. This is initially performed weekly for the first 2 weeks postoperatively. In patients with persistent pulmonary secretions flexible bronchoscopy is added to address distal retained secretions. A figure-8 deformity is commonly found during surveillance endoscopy. This represents the natural tendency of the complete rings at their anastomosis to bend internally.

A good tracheal outcome at 3 months probably predicts an excellent long-term tracheal outcome. However, an excellent tracheal outcome does not guarantee an excellent overall outcome, due to the comorbidities usually presented by these children.

SUMMARY

Long-segment tracheal stenosis is usually due to complete tracheal rings. Optimal management of these children requires comprehensive evaluation prior to repair. Imaging studies and endoscopic evaluation are essential. To minimize the risk to the patient during these procedures, a high index of suspicion is strongly recommended.

In the current era of slide tracheoplasty for the management of long-segment tracheal stenosis due to CTRs, a patient's prognosis is less about the trachea than about other coexisting anomalies.

The slide tracheoplasty is clearly an operation with a learning curve, and the best results on treating patients with long-segment tracheal stenosis are achieved with a team approach at a center of excellence.

REFERENCES

1. Schweiger C, Cohen AP, Rutter MJ. Tracheal and bronchial stenoses. *J Thorac Dis*. 2017;8(11):3369–3378.

2. Rutter MJ, Cotton RT, Azizkhan RG, Manning PB. Slide tracheoplasty for the management of complete tracheal rings. *J Pediatr Surg*. 2003;38:928–934.

3. Rutter MJ, Vijayasekaran S, Salamone FN, Cohen AP, Manning P, Collins MH, Mortelliti A. Deficient tracheal rings. *Int J Pediatr Otorhinolaryngol*. 2006;70:1981–1984.

4. Statham MM, deAlarcon A, Germann JN, Tabangin ME, Cohen AP, Rutter MJ. Screening and treatment of methicillin-resistant Staphylococcus aureus in children undergoing open airway surgery. *Arch Otolaryngol Head Neck Surg*. 2012;138(2):153–157.

5. Rutter MJ, Willging JP, Cotton RT. Nonoperative management of complete tracheal rings. *Arch Otolaryngol Head Neck Surg*. 2004;130:450–452.

6. Anton-Pacheco JL, Cano I, Garcia A, Martinez A, Cuadros J, Berchi FJ. Patterns of management of congenital tracheal stenosis. *J Pediatr Surg*. 2003;38:1452–1458.

7. Wong KS, Lan RS, Liu HP, Lin TY. Congenital tracheal stenosis: report of 6 cases. *Changgeng Yi Xue Za Zhi*. 1995; 18:365–370.

8. Tsang V, Murday A, Gilbe C, et al. Slide tracheoplasty for congenital funnel shaped tracheal stenosis. *Ann Thorac Surg*. 1989;48:632–635.

9. Grillo HC, Wright CD, Vlahakes GJ, MacGillivray TE. Management of congenital tracheal stenosis by means of slide tracheoplasty or resection and reconstruction, with long-term follow-up of growth after slide tracheoplasty. *J Thorac Cardiovasc Surg*. 2002;123:145–152.

10. Grillo HC. Development of tracheal surgery: a historical review. Part 1: Techniques of tracheal surgery. *Ann Thorac Surg*. 2003;75:610–619.

11. Grillo HC. Development of tracheal surgery: a historical review. Part 2: Treatment of tracheal diseases. *Ann Thorac Surg*. 2003;75:1039–1047.

12. Hasaniya N, elZein CF, Mara S, Barth MJ, Ilbawi M. Alternative approach to the surgical management of congenital tracheal stenosis. *Ann Thorac Surg*. 2006;82: 2305–2307.

13. Koopman JP, Bogers AJ, Witsenburg M, Lequin MH, Tibboel D, Hoeve LJ. Slide tracheoplasty for congenital tracheal stenosis. *J Pediatr Surg*. 2004;39:19–23.

14. Herrera P, Caldarone C, Forte V et al. The current state of congenital tracheal stenosis. *Pediatr Surg Int*. 2007;23: 1033–1044.

15. Manning PB, Rutter MJ, Lisec A, Gupta R, Marino BS. One slide fits all: the versatility of slide tracheoplasty with cardiopulmonary bypass support for airway reconstruction in children. *J Thorac Cardiovasc Surg*. 2011;141: 155–161.

16. Chiu PL, Kim PC. Prognostic in the surgical treatment of congenital tracheal stenosis: a multicenter analysis of the literature. *J Pediatr Surg*. 2006;41:221–225.

17. Kocyildirim E, Kanani M, Roebuck D, Wallis C, McLaren C, Noctor C, et al. Long-segment tracheal stenosis: slide tracheoplasty and a multidisciplinary approach improve outcomes and reduce costs. *J Thorac Cardiovasc Surg* 2004;128:876–882.

18. de Alarcon A, Rutter MJ. Cervical slide tracheoplasty. *Arch Otolaryngol Head Neck Surg*. 2012;138(9):812–816.

19. Backer CL, Kelle AM, Mavroudis C, Rigsby CK, Kaushal S, Holinger LD. Tracheal reconstruction in children with unilateral lung agenesis or severe hypoplasia. *Ann Thorac Surg*. 2009;88(2):624–630.

CHAPTER 7

Subglottic Hemangioma

James Johnston and Jacqueline Allen

INTRODUCTION

The most common causes of congenital upper airway problems in infants and children are laryngomalacia, vocal fold hypomobility, laryngeal webs, subglottic stenosis, and subglottic hemangiomata (SGH). Subglottic hemangiomata account for around 1.5% of congenital anomalies of the trachea.[1] Symptoms generally occur during infancy, with the most common presenting symptom being biphasic stridor.[1] These tumors usually undergo an initial phase of proliferation in newborns, followed by a period of involution to around 1 year of age and then resolution by approximately 5 to 7 years of age.[1,2] Complications in infants include cardiac failure, respiratory distress, and hemoptysis. Although rare, SGH can also occur in the adult population. However, symptoms are usually more subtle and include dysphagia, dyspnea, recurrent infections, and cough.[1]

SGH that are in the proliferative phase can be histologically distinguished from other vascular anomalies by their lobular arrangement of capillaries with multi-laminated basement membranes.[3] Development of immunohistochemical markers such as glucose transporter type 1 (GLUT1) has allowed physicians to distinguish SGH from other vascular lesions with confidence.[3] GLUT1 is an antigen that has an unusual microvascular phenotype uniquely shared by SGH at all stages of their evolution.[3] This antigen is not expressed by the normal vasculature of skin or by benign vascular tumors that would otherwise be histologically similar to SGH, such as tufted angioma, kaposiform hemangioendothelioma, and pyogenic granuloma.[3] This is also true of granulation tissue and vascular malfor-

mations.[3] Imaging with magnetic resonance (MRI) and computed tomography (CT) is useful to determine the vascular nature of the lesion and appreciate the extent of tracheal involvement and depth of invasion.[1] Treatment was previously with surgery and corticosteroid therapy; however, it is currently based on the beta-blocker propranolol, which reduces the necessity for invasive techniques.[4]

DEFINITION

Subglottic hemangioma is a rare vascular tumor of the airway that is benign and shows a distinctive pattern of angiogenesis with tissue positivity to GLUT1 receptor. Typically infantile and self-regressing, this process may take several years and symptoms are produced by the obstructive nature of the lesion and associated vascular effects.

CASE PRESENTATION

A 3-month-old female infant presents with a 7-day history of worsening respiratory distress and biphasic stridor. Associated symptoms include decreased oral intake, dysphagia, and cough. Parents report concern that she is not sleeping normally and not gaining weight. They indicate their child is struggling to breathe and suck at the same time.

Birth history: Normal vaginal delivery without complication, full-term delivery

Medications: None

Nil known allergies

Initial Assessment

History

Red flag symptoms include biphasic or inspiratory stridor (this may be exacerbated by feeding, excitement, or upper respiratory tract infections and can lead to respiratory difficulty), a barking cough, cyanosis, dysphagia, hoarseness, hemoptysis, and failure to thrive.[5] Half of the patients have an accompanying cutaneous lesion.[5]

Examination

Examination consists of general observations and complete physical, including cardiovascular, respiratory, and head and neck examination (red flag findings: tachycardia, tachypnea, cyanosis, indrawing, tracheal tug, inspiratory or biphasic stridor, cutaneous hemangioma).

Investigations

A plain neck x-ray may reveal asymmetric subglottic narrowing. Transnasal flexible laryngoscopy should be performed to identify cause of the patient's symptoms if possible. This is a useful investigation to exclude

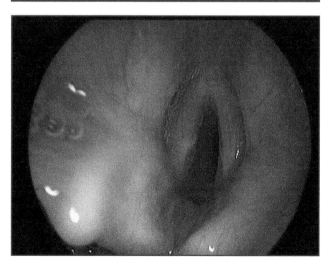

Figure 7–1. Endoscopic photomicrograph of subglottic mass showing typical vascular discoloration.

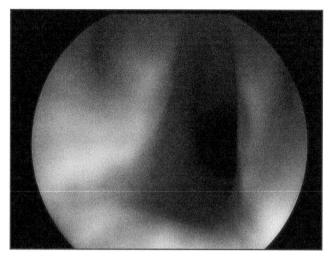

Figure 7–2. Endoscopic photomicrograph of larynx in closer magnification with typical erythematous discoloration of infraglottic surface of the left vocal fold.

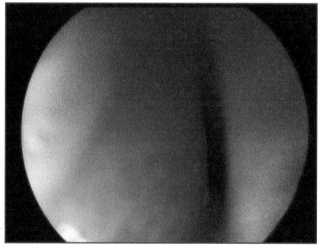

Figure 7–3. Endoscopic photomicrograph of subglottis distorted by large subglottic hemangioma (on left, red in color) occupying greater than 80% of the available airway.

vocal fold paralysis and laryngomalacia. Rigid endoscopy under general anesthesia must be performed to establish the diagnosis and assess mucosal quality. Diagnosis is confirmed with bronchoscopy via the observation of a soft, smooth, and eccentric lesion with a color ranging from blue to red depending on the extent of the submucosal vascular proliferation (Figures 7–1, 7–2, and 7–3).[1] Caution with biopsy should be exercised given the vascular nature of the lesions.

A CT scan using intravenous contrast medium is useful for evaluating abnormal vessels narrowing the trachea without requiring sedation.[5] CT is also helpful for revealing unrelated vascular anomalies and for assessing the distal airway in patients with total obstruction.[5] Once a patient's airway has been secured, an MRI of the head and neck can be useful to ensure that the hemangioma has not extended into the neck or skull.[5] SGH appear as solid tissues of moderate hyperintensity on T2-weighted spin-echo images and intermediate intensity on T1-weighted spin-echo images.[6]

Scenario 1

Examination reveals she was afebrile; pulse rate was 154 beats/min, and respiratory rate 56 breaths/min. There was no evidence of cutaneous hemangiomata. There were crepitations heard in both lungs, and intercostal retractions were observed. Under general anesthesia, laryngoscopy/bronchoscopy was performed and a reddish smooth sub-occlusive lesion in the left posterolateral subglottis obstructing 80% of the laryngotracheal airway was noted (see Figures 7–1, 7–2, and 7–3). Given the unstable clinical condition of the patient, a tracheostomy was performed.

Diagnosis

Subglottic hemangioma

Investigations

A T1-weighted MRI was performed while the patient was under general anesthetic and showed an isointense T1 subglottic lesion filling the laryngeal lumen with contrast enhancement on postcontrast T1-weighted MRI.

Management

Treatment was initiated with 1 mg/kg/day of oral propranolol for 7 days. This was increased to 2 mg/kg/day for 3 days, and the child was discharged on day 10 with the tracheostomy tube in situ. The child continued propranolol monotherapy for 9 months without any adverse effects and was weaned off it 1 year following discharge with no recurrence of air-

way symptoms. The tracheostomy tube was removed 10 months following insertion.

Scenario 2

Patient was afebrile with severe dyspnea and tachypnea, indrawing, and increased work of breathing. She demonstrated a dry "barking cough." Auscultation of her chest revealed bilateral crepitations and biphasic stridor, which was more evident in the inspiratory phase. No cutaneous hemangiomata were observed.

Diagnosis

Viral croup

Investigations

Chest x-ray showed normal pulmonary parenchyma and no cardiomegaly.

Neck x-ray (AP) revealed a steeple sign, which signifies subglottic narrowing.

Neck x-ray (lateral) revealed a distended hypopharynx during inspiration.

Management

- Hydration
- Reassurance
- Avoid smoking in the home
- Keep the child's head elevated
- At nighttime, parents/caregivers should stay close to the ill child so that they can immediately assist the child if he or she begins to have difficulty breathing.
- A single dose of dexamethasone (0.15–0.6 mg/kg)
- Single or multidose nebulized epinephrine
- Consider high flow nasal oxygen or heliox (helium and oxygen gas)
- Admit or review in 1 to 2 days depending on the clinical condition

At Review

If there is no symptomatic relief, then arrange additional investigations as appropriate.

Laryngoscopy can be performed in children who have no clinical improvement or where the clinical course is abnormal. The primary indication for performing this is to rule out an underlying congenital or anatomic abnormality. Options for laryngoscopy include:

1. Flexible transnasal laryngoscopy
2. Rigid laryngoscopy and bronchoscopy under general anesthesia

Further management may include intravenous antibiotics, non-invasive ventilatory support (CPAP or BiPAP, or high flow nasal oxygen), or intubation if needed. The child may require observation in the high dependency unit or pediatric intensive care if intubated.

Scenario 3

On examination, she had severe biphasic stridor with increased work of breathing and retrosternal retractions. She had a facial hemangioma in the "beard distribution."

Immediately: Emergent airway management is indicated with supportive oxygen (high-flow humidified nasal oxygen is ideal); call to pediatric intensive care and the operating room for definitive airway stabilization. If possible, perform an awake flexible laryngoscopy in the resuscitation bay. If unstable, then the child must go to the operating room for tracheostomy or intubation.

Investigations

Flexible laryngoscopy demonstrated red discoloration of the posterior pharyngeal wall with a glimpse of a circumferential subglottic hemangioma.

Under general anesthetic a rigid laryngoscopy and bronchoscopy revealed a subglottic hemangioma, with reddish color along the posterolateral tracheal wall to the carina.

A CT angiography and MR angiography showed an absence of right carotid and innominate arteries.

Diagnosis

Subglottic hemangioma in PHACE syndrome (*poste*rior fossa malformations, *h*emangiomas typically occurring on the head and neck, *a*rterial lesions involving abnormalities in the blood vessels of the head and neck, *c*ardiac abnormalities, and *e*ye abnormalities).[7]

DIFFERENTIAL DIAGNOSIS

There is a broad differential diagnosis when considering a pediatric airway obstruction. This ranges from the life-threatening pathology of subglottic hemangioma itself to the more common and relatively benign viral croup. The following are important differential diagnoses to consider:

Subglottic stenosis

Laryngo- and tracheomalacia

Laryngeal web, agenesis, and cleft

Viral or membranous croup

Vocal fold paralysis

Laryngotracheal papillomatosis

Compressive vascular aberrations (e.g., aberrant innominate artery)

Syndromes—DiGeorge, CHARGE, First arch (eg, Pierre Robin), Hunter

Adequate workup will require operative examination, appropriate imaging, and consideration of systemic involvement depending on the potential etiology.

MANAGEMENT

Typically, multidisciplinary involvement is useful for airway complaints with pediatric otorhinolaryngology surgeons, pediatricians, pediatric pulmonology/general/thoracic surgeons, speech language therapy, and radiology all involved. Parental counselling is important in explaining the diagnosis, natural history, prognosis, and the close monitoring necessary to manage these lesions.

Stabilization

If needed in newly identified SGH, initial airway stabilization may be required such as oxygen treatment, monitoring, or tracheostomy. Management of distal airway obstructive problems may also be needed during the period of involution (eg, pneumonia, bronchitis, secretions).

Propranolol

Propranolol has revolutionized the treatment of subglottic hemangiomata. It provides a non-invasive treatment option for a potentially life-threatening disease process. To date, there are no widely accepted guidelines regarding optimal dosing or treatment duration of propranolol, but a starting dose of 2 mg/kg/day is common.[2] A recent systematic review by Schwartz et al showed that 88% of patients exhibited complete symptom resolution within 24 hours of being administered propranolol. Interestingly, five of six treatment failures received concurrent systemic steroids at the time of propranolol initiation.[2] It is unclear whether simultaneous oral steroid usage affects the success rate of propranolol in treating airway hemangiomata. A recent literature review by Hardison et al suggested that combined therapy is associated with an increased incidence of treatment failure.[8] Therefore, decision to treat with both propranolol and systemic steroids should be made with caution.

Rebound rate for SGH treated with propranolol is reported to be around 9%.[2] This is lower than the reported rate of 17% in cutaneous hemangiomata. However, it is likely that the rebound rate in SGH is underestimated given that visualization of the lesion requires bronchoscopy and this is unlikely to be indicated unless symptoms are ongoing.[2] Even though there is limited evidence supporting a dosing regime in the treatment of subglottic hemangioma, propranolol has an extensively characterized safety profile. Minimal complications occur with doses between 1 and 4 mg/kg/day.[2] Two mg/kg/day is generally considered the most common starting dose, increasing the dose to 3 mg/kg/day, and resolved the majority of ongoing respiratory symptoms and rebound growth.[2] Side effects of propranolol include hypoglycemia, hypotension, bronchoconstriction, bradycardia, somnolence, rash, and gastroesophageal reflux.[9]

Opinions vary as to the necessity for regular laryngoscopy/bronchoscopy to ensure stability or regression of these lesions.[10] In general, its use should be based on patient's symptoms and clinical judgment. If the first follow-up endoscopy after treatment reveals an absence of subglottic hemangioma, then repeat endoscopy is not warranted unless new symptoms arise.[2] Given that propranolol is a beta-blocker and will affect the patient's cardiovascular system, the clinician must always consider the possibility of PHACE syndrome in these children.[2] It is important to note that despite widespread use, the rarity of this condition has limited previous studies to small series and case reports.[8] Therefore, no evidence-based guidelines exist as yet for the correct use of propranolol in the treatment of subglottic hemangioma.[8]

Steroids

Before the frequent use of propranolol in the treatment of SGH, systemic steroids were the mainstay of therapy.[11] Although they exhibit some success in the reduction of lesion size, only one in four patients noticed a complete resolution of symptoms with this modality alone.[6] Greater efficacy was seen with intralesional steroid injection, with up to 77% of patients obtaining full resolution.[12] However, this process would often result in 30 to 50 days of intubation time while the patient underwent serial injections.

Interferon Alpha-2a

Interferon inhibits angiogenesis by decreasing the concentration of angiogenic factors.[11] The dose of interferon given in the treatment of SGH is 2 to 3 million units/m^2 injected subcutaneously every day.[11] Treatment duration is usually between 6 and 12 months.[6] Interferon has an efficacy rate of up to 71%. However, the many side effects, including fever, transient neutropenia, myalgia, spastic diplegia, and anemia, make it a therapy of last resort.[13]

Radiation Therapy

External beam radiation was used in the early to mid-1900s to treat subglottic hemangiomata. However, given the significant concerns associated with damage to the normal airway and the potential to develop secondary malignancy, this procedure was abandoned in the 1970s.[6]

Cryotherapy

This treatment modality was used in several patients in the 1970s but quickly lost favor. Despite some initial promise, the unpredictability of the depth of tissue destruction when performing cryotherapy could result in significant complications such as subglottic stenosis. For this reason, this method is not recommended.

Endoscopic Laser Resection

Before the widespread use of propranolol in the treatment of SGH, endoscopic laser resection was a key player. The carbon dioxide (CO_2) laser is the most commonly used, followed by the potassium titanyl phosphate (KTP) laser, neodymium:yttrium-aluminium-garnet (Nd: YAG) laser, and pulsed dye laser.[11] There is some advantage in using the KTP laser, as its wavelength of light (532 nm) is preferentially absorbed by hemoglobin and thus may target the vascular hemangioma more specifically.[14] While laser resection has a high overall success rate of 89%,[11] there are some undesirable side effects, such as a high rate of subglottic stenosis, risk of anterior glottic web, and a high recurrence rate necessitating multiple surgical procedures.[15] Laser ablation can also aggravate obstruction of the airway due to postoperative tissue edema and reaction.[16] Furthermore, most patients require at least two treatments to achieve stabilization of the airway. Most available information on laser use in the treatment of subglottic hemangiomata is based on case studies and small case series. Therefore, larger series are required before laser use can be deemed a safe modality for the treatment of this condition. It is important to note that larger prospective studies may not be ethically viable given the high efficacy and lesser invasiveness of treatment with propranolol.

Microdebrider

Treatment of SGH with a surgical microdebrider is a relatively new technique that has been utilized for removal of laryngeal lesions since 1999.[17] This technique has several advantages, including rapid debulking and precise resection, a clearer surgical field secondary to the suction system on the device, prevention of thermal injury compared with laser techniques, and a less invasive procedure than open excision.[16] This technique has been widely used in the excision of laryngeal papillomata, but few cases have been reported using this technique to treat subglottic hemangiomata.[16]

Open Surgical Excision

While this is the most extensive of the surgical options, it is useful in those patients with a bilateral or circumferential lesion who would otherwise require a tracheostomy.[11] This procedure has also translated directly to a decreased number of surgeries needed for a cure.[6]

This procedure begins with a diagnostic rigid laryngoscopy and bronchoscopy to assess the extent of disease. Following diagnosis, the patient undergoes orotracheal intubation, and a skin incision is made over the cricoid cartilage. An incision is made in the midline of the cricoid, and the incision extended inferiorly through the first two tracheal rings and superiorly to the thyroid cartilage. At this point, the orotracheal tube is removed, and an endotracheal tube is inserted into the inferior aspect of the incision. The cut cricoid is retracted, and under microscope guidance, a submucosal flap is raised, and the hemangioma is carefully dissected away. Following excision, a thyroid cartilage graft is utilized to increase the size of the subglottic laryngeal framework.[11]

Following the operation, the patient requires careful monitoring in the pediatric intensive care unit. Postoperative management including corticosteroids, proton pump inhibitors, intravenous antibiotics, and paralysis is maintained for 24 hours following surgery.[11] The patient is extubated in theater under endoscopic guidance only if the airway is deemed adequate. Any respiratory symptoms, such as respiratory distress, poor feeding, and stridor, are investigated by additional rigid laryngoscopy and bronchoscopy.[11] Compared with other surgical treatment options, open excision is more invasive and requires many days in the intensive care unit. Therefore, this option is reserved for severe bulky, obstructive disease and limited to surgeons experienced in this procedure with access to a pediatric intensive care unit.

Tracheostomy and Observation

Subglottic hemangiomata were traditionally treated with tracheostomy and observation with the knowledge that the natural history of the disease is for the tumor to regress and resolve. It remains a viable alternative to resection, especially in centers that do not have access to other described surgical and medical modalities. It is currently utilized much less often due to the introduction of relatively inexpensive and highly effective propranolol treatment. It is important to consider that prolonged tracheostomy is associated with significant morbidity and a 1% mortality rate.[11]

WHAT IS THE CAUSE?

Subglottic hemangiomata are errors of embryonic development and are present at birth. They have a standard rate of endothelial cell turnover and grow proportionally with the child. Subglottic hemangiomas contain mast cells, interstitial cells, fibroblasts, and pericytes. The life cycle of SGH has been characterized by electron and light microscopy as well as immunohistochemical techniques.[6] The first phase in the life cycle is the proliferative phase and is characterized by increased levels of vascular endothelial growth factor and basic fibroblast growth factor.[6] The involution phase is characterized by apoptosis of the endothelial cells and decreased angiogenesis. In this phase there is increase in tissue inhibitor metalloproteinases and the accumulation of mast cells.[6]

Currently, the mechanism that drives the proliferation and regression of subglottic hemangioma is unknown. GLUT1 is an erythrocyte-type glucose transporter that is expressed in the endothelium of blood—tissue barriers.[18] GLUT1 is an immunohistochemical marker that is highly expressed in subglottic hemangiomata at all stages, and it is not observed in other vascular malformations or vascular tumors.[18] It is known that SGH and the placenta both express GLUT1. This may explain why children of women who undergo chorionic villus sampling have a 10 times higher risk of developing a hemangioma.[6] This has also led to speculation that subglottic hemangiomata may result from angioblasts that derive from embolized placental cells or differentiate toward a placental phenotype.[18] Other theories that have been postulated to explain the development of subglottic hemangiomata include genetic alterations and viral origin.[6]

SUBGLOTTIC HEMANGIOMA AND PHACE SYNDROME

PHACE syndrome[7] is commonly associated with congenital vascular anomalies, including abnormalities of the arteries of the head, neck, and chest.[7] It is widely accepted that the syndrome represents a defect in development that occurs early in gestation, with the hemangioma usually appearing on the same side of any structural abnormalities. It affects females more commonly than males and is most common in Caucasian children.[9] Those affected with PHACE syndrome are more likely to be born at term with normal birth weight. This is in contrast to those with non-PHACE subglottic hemangiomas, which are more likely to be born premature and underweight.[9] The incidence of airway hemangioma in children with PHACE syndrome and large facial hemangiomas is around 24%.[19,20]

Caution must be taken when considering using propranolol in children with PHACE syndrome. This is because of the potential risk of stroke and hypotension in these children, who often have associated cerebral vascular anomalies.[21] In fact, cerebral vascular anomalies are the most common extracutaneous manifestation of PHACE syndrome.[9] No guidelines exist in regard to the airway evaluation of children with PHACE syndrome. However, most of the literature supports rigid laryngoscopy and bronchoscopy by a pediatric otolaryngologist for children with PHACE and airway symptoms and asymptomatic PHACE children with large cutaneous hemangiomas in the "beard distribution."[9] Given the high rate of asymptomatic children with PHACE syndrome who undergo airway evaluation and have subglottic hemangiomas, one should have a low threshold for performing airway evaluation.[9] This is particularly true of children who are not already receiving systemic therapy for their cutaneous hemangiomas.[9]

SUMMARY

Subglottic hemangiomata are the most common benign vascular tumor of the infant airway and have the potential to be life-threatening.[6] Many forms of surgical and medical treatments have been proposed, and although propranolol appears to yield the best overall results, no single treatment modality is acceptable for all patients. The physician must always balance the natural history of disease and its gradual involution versus the risk of causing additional iatrogenic morbidity to the patient.[6] A treatment regime should be tailored to each patient and take into account the presenting symptoms, the extent of the subglottic hemangioma, presence or absence of other hemangiomata, as well as the facilities and surgical experience available at your institution.[6]

REFERENCES

1. Robitaille C, Fortin M, Trahan S, Delage A, Simon M. Subglottic hemangioma. *J Bronchology Interv Pulmonol.* 2016;23(3):232–235.
2. Schwartz T, Faria J, Pawar S, Siegel D, Chun RH. Efficacy and rebound rates in propranolol-treated subglottic hemangioma: a literature review. *Laryngoscope.* 2017; 127(11):2665–2672.

3. Badi AN, Kerschner JE, North PE, Drolet BA, Messner A, Perkins JA. Histopathologic and immunophenotypic profile of subglottic hemangioma: multicenter study. *Int J Pediatr Otorhinolaryngol*. 2009;73(9):1187–1191.

4. Ajmi H, Mama N, Hassayoun S, et al. Life-threatening subglottic hemangioma in an infant successfully treated with propranolol. *Arch Pediatr*. 2018;25(5):331–333.

5. Wu L, Wu X, Xu X, Chen Z. Propranolol treatment of subglottic hemangiomas: a review of the literature. *Int J Clin Exp Med*. 2015;8(11):19886–19890.

6. Rahbar R, Nicollas R, Roger G, et al. The biology and management of subglottic hemangioma: past, present, future. *Laryngoscope*. 2004;114(11):1880–1891.

7. Petrauskas LA, Vaitaitis VJ, Mundinger G, Sheahan C, Poole J, Kanotra SP. Open resection and laryngotracheal reconstruction in a case of subglottic hemangioma in PHACE syndrome. *Int J Pediatr Otorhinolaryngol*. 2018; 108:186–189.

8. Hardison S, Wan W, Dodson KM. The use of propranolol in the treatment of subglottic hemangiomas: a literature review and meta-analysis. *Int J Pediatr Otorhinolaryngol*. 2016;90:175–180.

9. Durr ML, Meyer AK, Huoh KC, Frieden IJ, Rosbe KW. Airway hemangiomas in PHACE syndrome. *Laryngoscope*. 2012;122(10):2323–2329.

10. Mahadevan M, Cheng A, Barber C. Treatment of subglottic hemangiomas with propranolol: initial experience in 10 infants. *ANZ J Surg*. 2011;81(6):456–461.

11. O-Lee TJ, Messner A. Subglottic hemangioma. *Otolaryngol Clin North Am*. 2008 Oct;1(5):903–911–viii–ix.

12. Hoeve LJ, Küppers GLE, Verwoerd CDA. Management of infantile subglottic hemangioma: laser vaporization, submucous resection, intubation, or intralesional steroids? *Int J Pediatr Otorhinolaryngol*. 1997;42(2):179–186.

13. Pransky SM, Canto C. Management of subglottic hemangioma. *Curr Opin Otolaryngol Head Neck Surg*. 2004;12(6): 509–512.

14. Kacker A, April M, Ward RF. Use of potassium titanyl phosphate (KTP) laser in management of subglottic hemangiomas. *Int J Pediatr Otorhinolaryngol*. 2001;59(1):15–21.

15. Bitar MA, Moukarbel RV, Zalzal GH. Management of congenital subglottic hemangioma: trends and success over the past 17 years. *Otolaryngol Head Neck Surg*. 2005; 132(2):226–231.

16. Jia H, Huang Q, Lü J, et al. Microdebrider removal under suspension laryngoscopy: an alternative surgical technique for subglottic hemangioma. *Int J Pediatr Otorhinolaryngol*. 2013;77(9):1424–1429.

17. Myer CM, Willging JP, McMurray S, Cotton RT. Use of a laryngeal micro resector system. *Laryngoscope*. 1999;109 (7 pt 1):1165–1166.

18. North PE, Waner M, Mizeracki A, Mihm MC Jr. GLUT1: A newly discovered immunohistochemical marker for juvenile hemangiomas. *Hum Pathol*. 2000;31(1):11–22.

19. Haggstrom AN, Skillman S, Garzon MC, et al. Clinical spectrum and risk of PHACE syndrome in cutaneous and airway hemangiomas. *Arch Otolaryngol Head Neck Surg*. 2011;137(7):680–687.

20. Haggstrom AN, Garzon MC, Baselga E, et al. Risk for PHACE syndrome in infants with large facial hemangiomas. *Pediatrics*. 2010;126(2):e418–426.

21. Metry DW, Garzon MC, Drolet BA, et al. PHACE syndrome: current knowledge, future directions. *Laryngoscope*. 2009:381–398.

CHAPTER 8

The Drooling Child

Silvia G. Marinone-Lares and Murali Mahadevan

INTRODUCTION

Drooling is abnormal in children over the age of 4 and frequently occurs in those with developmental delay and neuromuscular abnormalities, with the most commonly cited pathology associated with problematic drooling being cerebral palsy (CP).[1-3] The prevalence of drooling in this group is not well established, with reports in the literature ranging from 10% to 58%.[1-4]

While children with CP may have a range of other health and quality of life issues, drooling can be problematic in a number of ways, such as causing social embarrassment for the child and his or her caregivers, local irritation of the skin, dehydration, interference with speech and feeding, soiling of clothing and objects, to the most severe end of the spectrum where it can cause aspiration pneumonia.[1-3,5]

The cause of drooling in children with CP is believed to be poor muscle tone and motor coordination resulting in poor posture, particularly of the head, as well as oromotor dysfunction leading to an open-mouth posture.[6] Many other contributing factors may also be present, such as nasal obstruction and associated mouth breathing, orthodontic abnormalities, side effects of medications and swallowing disorders; the latter are highly prevalent in severely neurologically impaired children,[7,8] and aspiration is the most frequent cause of death in this group.[7]

The above highlights the importance of a multidisciplinary approach to managing the drooling child, ideally with the involvement of experts in fields such as developmental pediatrics, pediatric neurology, otolaryngology, dental health, and speech-language therapy. Other disciplines such as physiotherapy and occupational therapy may also play a role. The cooperation of teachers and others involved in the care of the child is also beneficial.[2,4,5]

The senior author employs a multidisciplinary approach in his Saliva Control Clinic comprising a specialist pediatric otolaryngologist, a dentist with special interest in pediatrics, and a pediatric speech-language pathologist.

DEFINITION

Drooling can be defined as the unintentional spillage of saliva from the mouth.[1,5] It can be further characterized as anterior, when there is loss of saliva from the mouth, or posterior, which may contribute to soiling of the lungs by way of aspiration.[1,4,9,10]

CASE PRESENTATION

A 6-year-old boy presents with drooling on most days, both day and night, but often worse during upper respiratory tract infections. He has a diagnosis of mild CP, has normal cognition, and attends local primary school. He is a known mouth breather, sleeps poorly with frequent awakening and restlessness in bed, is a loud snorer, and has frequent apneas lasting seconds rather than minutes, as described by his parents. He is noted to have nasal obstruction and snotty nose since the age of 3 years, well before he started attending regular preschool and daycare. He has had an allergy review with a local allergist and no significant allergies were detected.

Social history: No smokers or pets at home.

Medications: Recent trial of steroid-based nasal sprays (fluticasone propionate 1 spray each nostril b.i.d.) with nil improvement.

Allergies: Nil.

Initial Assessment

This particular child has mild CP, with normal cognition.

History

Is the snoring and obstruction benign? Does this need further questioning (are there behavioral or developmental issues, bed wetting, tantrums, swallowing difficulties or choking, failure to thrive, small for age concerns)? Any oximetry or sleep study? Feeding history—can he feed normally without aspiration? Feeds himself, but clumsy and takes a long time to finish his meals.

Examination

Nasal and oropharyngeal exam included grade of tonsils, adenoids, size of tongue, presence of ankyloglossia, health of teeth and gums, anterior nasal obstruction, turbinate size, septal deviation, polyps, nasal and/or oropharyngeal masses or cysts.

SCENARIO 1

This 6-year-old presents with a history suggestive of obstructive sleep apnea with snoring, apneas, nighttime awakening, restless sleep, bedwetting, difficulty swallowing solids, gagging with solids, failure to thrive with percentile in height and weight having dropped from the 50th to the 3rd percentile. Examination shows grade 3/4 tonsils and grade 3/4 adenoids without any significant anterior nasal obstruction. Drooling severity and frequency score of 4/4, respectively, according to the Thomas-Stonell and Greenberg classification of drooling (Figure 8–1).

Diagnosis

Adenotonsillar hypertrophy. See Figure 8–2.

Investigations

Flexible nasendoscopy if patient tolerates procedure or lateral neck x-ray for evaluation of adenoidal size. See Figure 8–3.

Assessment of drooling

Frequency

    1 - No (or rare) drooling
    2 - Occasional drooling (not every day)
    3 - Frequent drooling (every day but all the time)
    4 - Constant drooling - always wet

Severity

    1 - Dry - never drools
    2 - Mild - only the lips are wet
    3 - Moderate - wet on the lips and chin
    4 - Severe - drools to the extent the clothes get damp and need changing
    5 - Profuse - clothing, hands and objects become wet

Figure 8–1. Drooling Frequency and Severity Scale.

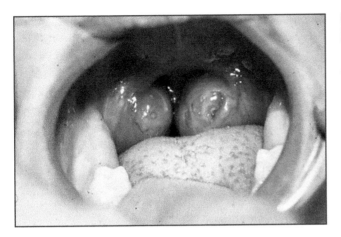

Figure 8–2. Tonsillar hypertrophy.

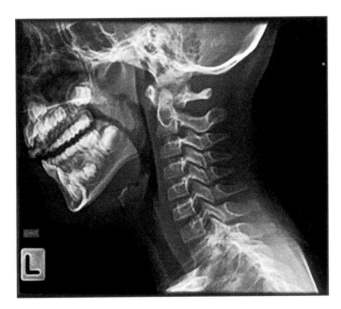

Figure 8–3. Lateral neck x-ray demonstration of adenoidal hyperplasia.

Management

First line of treatment is adenotonsillectomy. Intensive speech and swallowing therapy may also be required to re-learn swallowing and breathing following adenotonsillectomy, along with behavioral therapy (making him aware of saliva on lips and chin and smartphone/ computer program for prompting to swallow). Posture, head positioning, and situational factors (concentrating at school, drawing/writing with head down) that contribute to "head down" positioning should also be addressed, especially in wheelchair-bound children.

Adenotonsillar tissue grade 1/4, moderate nasal obstruction and rhinitis due to allergic rhinitis and moderate ankyloglossia (tongue tie) with restricted anterior-posterior and lateral tongue movement. There is also evidence of early dental caries with gum ulceration and inflammation.

Diagnosis

Multifactorial: anterior nasal obstruction with turbinate hypertrophy, poor tongue mobility with ankyloglossia, and dental and gum disease.

Management

Allergy testing for inhaled and food allergens. Avoidance therapy, trial of combination of non-sedating antihistamines (cetirizine) and nasal corticosteroid (fluticasone propionate) therapy. Consider desensitization therapy by either sublingual or subdermal immunotherapy for selected patients (difficult in severely neurologically compromised children on multiple medications). Division of tongue tie along with intensive oromotor function-targeted speech therapy to improve tongue mobility.

Dental caries and fissures should be treated along with a robust ongoing dental hygiene program. As this child has near normal cognition, pharmacotherapy with short courses of scopolamine patches (1.5 mg 1 patch per 3 days in patients over 25 kg, 1/2 patch in patients 10–20 kg, contraindicated in children under 3 years of age) or glycopyrrolate oral solution (0.02 mg/ kg/dose, maximum dose 1.2 mg) may enable us to render them dry for short periods of time, hence enabling us to offer biofeedback techniques. Side effects and drug interactions with current medications are a common reason for not tolerating these medications in the long term.

In children with good dentition, intraoral appliance therapy such as a modified Castillo Morales prosthesis is likely to improve tongue mobility, swallowing, and oropharyngeal sensation. Castillo Morales prosthesis is easier to implement after eruption of permanent dentition, as less adjustments and remodeling of the appliance are required, given mandibular and dental growth plateau after arrival of permanent dentition, hence best introduced in children older than 8 years of age.

A 6-year-old with severe CP, with known aspiration to solids and fluids, entirely gastrostomy fed with normal oropharynx, normal tonsils, and adenoids. The child continues to drool most days and all through the day with poor response to glycopyrrolate and scopolamine patches over the last 6 months.

Investigations: Most CP children are under the care of a developmental pediatrician. A Gross Motor Function Classification System (GMFCS) score is useful in determining level of function. If the degree of aspiration and dysphagia is unknown, a speech pathologist–assisted videofluoroscopic swallowing study would be useful to determine the stage and site of dysphagia.

Management

This child is unable to swallow his own saliva safely, and the likely issue here is an inability to initiate and coordinate the swallow rather than overproduction of saliva.

Medical and surgical treatments reduce the amount of saliva in the oral cavity and oropharynx, hence enabling them to manage smaller volumes.

Botulinum toxin injection to the submandibular gland (SMG) or parotid gland under ultrasound guidance is a reasonable therapeutic measure for this child. The typical dosage in our center is 20 units of botulinum toxin to each SMG. A therapeutic effect is seen at 3 to 4 days and lasts 3 to 6 months. Injections can serve as a gauge to assess the reduction in drooling should the treatment be escalated to SMG excision in future.

For severe cases of drooling with frequency/severity grade of 4/5, and CP disability grades of GMFCS III and higher, a more permanent solution such as excision of bilateral SMG and ligation of bilateral parotid gland ducts may be required.

Prior to removal of both SMG and ligation of parotid ducts, which eliminates 80 to 90% of resting and post-prandial saliva, patients require counseling regarding the change in saliva consistency that follows, becoming thicker and occasionally developing a pungent smell when dehydrated, which occurs often in these children. This can be alleviated by a regular dental hygiene program, good hydration, and mouth washes.

Regular 3-month dental follow-up is recommended. Dental assessment under general anesthetic may be required in these children, in which case it can be performed every 6 months.

MANAGEMENT OF THE DROOLING CHILD

History and Physical Examination

Given the wide range of abnormalities that can contribute to drooling, the initial assessment of the child should include a thorough history including the degree of disability, medications taken, history of aspiration pneumonia, swallowing difficulties, symptoms of gastroesophageal reflux, posture, position and tone of the mouth, lips, and orofacial musculature, dental status, and craniofacial abnormalities in order to tailor management to the individual's needs.[3–5]

In our center, all children referred for assessment of problematic drooling are reviewed by a multidisciplinary team, as described above. The speech-language therapist plays a key role in assessing lip and jaw position, motion of the tongue, and speech and feeding ability.[2,5] The dentist will determine the status of the teeth and gingiva, as well as abnormalities such as malocclusion that may be amenable to orthodontic treatment. Finally, the otolaryngologist will perform a full head and neck examination, taking particular care to look for signs suggestive of dysphagia, aspiration, and nasal and oropharyngeal obstruction.

Measurement of Drooling

After one has obtained relevant data from the history and performed a physical examination, subjective and objective measures of drooling can be helpful to assess the severity of the problem and the impact on the patient and the caregivers' quality of life.

Subjective measurement of drooling includes the Thomas-Stonell and Greenberg classification of drooling (also known as the Drooling Frequency and Severity Scale) (see Figure 8–1), the Teacher Drooling Scale, visual analogue scales and, more recently, the Drooling Impact Scale.[1,3,4,10–13]

Objective measures include the number of bib changes required per day, the Drooling Quotient, which measures the amount of time a patient drools during two separate sessions of 10 minutes duration, and the salivary flow rate, which is determined by measuring the weight of saliva collected on a cotton ball.[3,9,10,12,13]

While objective measures of drooling can be useful for research purposes, the senior author's preference is to use a subjective measure of drooling that illustrates the impact on the patient and caregivers' quality of life, as most often the latter is the main motivation for seeking treatment. The Thomas-Stonell and Greenberg classification is used in the Saliva Control Clinic for this purpose. This classification estimates the frequency and severity of drooling on a 9-point scale obtained by adding the individual frequency and severity scores.[11] Patients attending the Saliva Control Clinic will typically complete the form at baseline and 3 months following treatment. A reduction of 2 or more points on the scale is considered clinical improvement, as this cutoff seems to correlate with subjective impression of improvement, as rated by the caregiver.[14]

Treatment

Treatment for drooling typically begins with the least invasive method and progresses in a stepwise fashion to more aggressive treatments when required.[4,15] These treatments are described below.

Conservative

These include behavioral therapy such as positive and negative reinforcement, cueing, and self-management techniques such as increasing the frequency of swallowing and wiping the chin.[1,3–5] In this scenario, a sufficient degree of cognition is required.[12]

Other conservative measures such as speech-language therapy and oromotor rehabilitation aim to improve oromotor function by improving tone and position of the lips, jaw, and tongue, thereby encouraging a closed-mouth posture and improving chewing and deglutition. Techniques include straw drinking and blowing tasks to improve lip function.[1,2,5]

Malocclusion may be addressed by orthodontic treatment. Children with permanent teeth may benefit from intraoral appliances such as the Innsbruck Sensorimotor Activator and Regulator[1,16] and the modified Castillo Morales intraoral plate. The latter, as initially described by Castillo Morales, is used in conjunction with manual therapy to improve orofacial function. Over time, modifications to the original appliance have been made, with the addition of a bead in the palate that stimulates tongue movement, encouraging a dorsal-cranial shift of the tongue, and vestibular wires to stimulate lip movement and tone, resulting in improved position at rest with a closed mouth posture and thus reducing the severity of drooling (Figure 8–4).

In our center, the modified Castillo Morales appliance is offered to selected children. It is typically used three times a day for 30 minutes for a minimum of 3 months. Formal orofacial therapy as described initially by Castillo Morales is not employed, although some children may receive simultaneous speech-language therapy input. Our pediatric dentist has used this approach for many years, and reduction in drooling can be seen in up to 72% of children who undergo this treatment[17] (Figure 8–5).

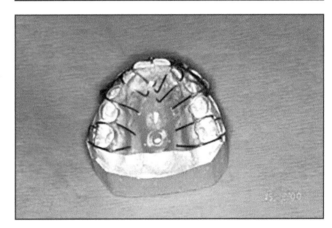

Figure 8–4. Castillo Morales intraoral plate with central palatal button and vestibular wires.

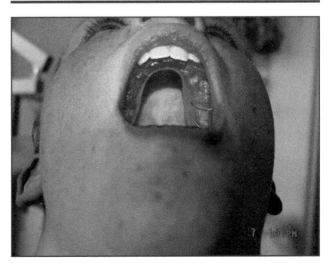

Figure 8–5. Castillo Morales intraoral plate in a patient.

Pharmacotherapy

The mainstay of pharmacotherapy for drooling is systemic antimuscarinic drugs, which can be administered transdermally, transorally, parenterally, or via nebulization. These include scopolamine, tryhexyphenidyl, atropine, benztropine, and glycopyrrolate. Side effects of these drugs are well known and are due to their systemic nature and inability to selectively target the salivary glands. They include dry mouth, thick secretions, urinary retention, constipation, and vision changes. They are often severe enough that patients discontinue treatment. Their use is also limited due to potential drug interactions, as well as contraindications to the use of anticholinergic drugs.[1–3,5,18,19]

Recently, there has been increased interest in the use of glycopyrrolate, as the Food and Drug Administration in the United States has approved the use of an oral solution for the treatment of drooling in children with neurologic abnormalities.[19]

It is speculated that anti-reflux medication reduces stimulation of the esophagosalivary reflex and in turn reduces the severity of drooling.[2] This has not been extensively studied. In nine patients who underwent evaluation of drooling during a clinical trial of treatment with ranitidine and cisapride versus placebo, only one child with severe esophagitis had reduction of drooling while on anti-reflux medication.[20] Thus, it is the authors' opinion that anti-reflux should not be a first-line treatment for drooling, rather it is indicated only if there are coexisting symptoms or signs of gastroesophageal reflux, in particular if reflux is thought to be contributing to aspiration.

Intraglandular Injection of Botulinum Toxin

In the last two decades, botulinum toxin injection into the salivary glands has gained popularity among clinicians who treat children with problematic drooling.[9,12] In 2010, an International Consensus Statement on the use of botulinum toxin for drooling in adults and children was published with recommendations including indications and contraindications, timing of intervention, technique, and monitoring. These recommendations were largely based on expert opinion; dosage and technique vary across centers and the best technique and dosage have yet to be established.[4]

Botulinum toxin A and botulinum toxin B can be used for this purpose. Most clinicians favor botulinum toxin A, as indicated by a systematic review published in 2012.[9] Regardless of the neurotoxin used, the mechanism of action is the same: blocking the release of acetylcholine at the neuromuscular junction and possibly directly at the neuroglandular junction, thus inhibiting salivary flow.[2,21]

Botulinum toxin can be applied to the submandibular glands, the parotid glands, or both, under local or general anesthetic. Clinicians may choose to inject one or all four glands[10,22] by identifying anatomical landmarks or using ultrasound guidance.[4,21] Although there is currently not a consensus for dosing or technique, there is a trend toward injecting all four glands with equal dose distribution to each one, as well as using ultrasound guidance to increase precision of the injection and reduce the risk of complications.[10,21]

Not all patients respond to botulinum toxin injection, but there is a positive effect in 70 to 75% of patients. The reason for this is unknown. Non-responders to botulinum toxin A may respond to botulinum toxin B.[10,21] The duration of the effect can vary with a wide range of time of reported benefit, from 5 to 16 months.[12,21] Injections may be repeated as required. Interestingly, it has been suggested that repeated botulinum toxin injections may provoke atrophy of the salivary glands secondary to prolonged denervation, thus reducing the volume of drooling permanently.[11,14]

In our center, intraglandular botulinum toxin injections are performed under general anesthesia. Ultrasound guidance is provided by an interventional radiologist in order to reduce the risk of injection into the surrounding musculature and thus complications such as dysphagia. The injection is performed by a pediatric otolaryngologist and only the SMGs are addressed. Botulinum toxin type A is used at a concentration of 100 U/mL in 0.9% saline solution and the usual dose is 20 units per gland for patients weighing more than 25 kg or 15 units per gland for patients weighing less than 20 kg. A good clinical outcome is achieved in 60.4% of patients.[14]

Reported complications of intraglandular botulinum toxin injection include xerostomia, thickened saliva, dysphagia which is usually transient (although a small number of severe cases requiring hospital admission and nasogastric tube feeding have been reported), and pneumonia. The complication rate has been shown to decrease when injections are performed with ultrasound guidance.[2,9,12,19,21]

Surgery

There are a number of surgical treatments available for the management of drooling in children with cerebral palsy. Clearly, a surgical intervention is by far the most invasive form of treatment and is usually reserved for patients who have had no or limited response to less invasive treatments. Surgical options include tympanic neurectomy, rerouting and ligation of the submandibular and parotid ducts, excision of the sublingual glands, excision of the submandibular glands, or a combination of the aforementioned procedures.[2,5,15] When mouth breathing is thought to be a contributing factor, adenotonsillar and turbinate surgery are often employed.[2,5]

Submandibular and parotid duct transposition are minimally invasive surgical techniques that reposition the salivary ducts posterior to the tongue base in order to redirect saliva posteriorly into the pharynx.[2] Both techniques are performed intraorally and can be done simultaneously. It is the decision of the surgeon whether to address the submandibular ducts, the parotid ducts, or both. It is not appropriate for children with a disordered pharyngeal swallowing phase and is contraindicated in those with a history of aspiration pneumonia.[2,23] Complications include ranula formation, transient swelling of the glands, damage to the lingual nerve, and aspiration pneumonia.[2]

Submandibular and parotid duct ligation may be performed in those with history of previous aspiration.[24] Salivary duct ligation is also performed intraorally and one may address only one set of ducts or perform four-duct ligation. Following ligation procedures, one expects that the salivary glands will atrophy over time.[23] Complications include buccal abscess, sialocele, increased risk of submandibular calculi formation, ranula, and parotid duct fistula.[2,23]

Sublingual gland excision, unilateral or bilateral, may be performed in conjunction with submandibular gland excision or duct transposition. Sublingual gland excision is now seldom performed in this fashion, as it increases postoperative morbidity and does not appear to improve control of drooling compared with submandibular gland excision or duct transposition done in isolation.[2,24]

Submandibular gland excision is typically performed transcervically under general anesthetic. Complications include damage to the lingual nerve, the hypoglossal nerve, and the mandibular branch of the facial nerve. The complication rate is low, however.[25] In our center, we perform bilateral excision through two separate horizontal incisions two or three fingerbreadths inferior to the mandible, alone or in conjunction with parotid duct ligation. A drain is typically not required. The child may be discharged when comfortable and tolerating diet, usually the day following the procedure.

While submandibular gland excision is more often performed transcervically, excision via a transoral route is also possible.[26,27] Advantages of this technique are avoidance of a scar in the neck, reduction in the risk of damage to the hypoglossal, lingual, and marginal mandibular nerves, and a lower incidence of postoperative mucoceles and stone formation, the latter given that the entirety of the duct is removed in the transoral approach.[26–28] A case series of 10 pediatric patients who underwent this procedure for various indications has recently been reported with good results.[28] A meta-analysis of surgical treatment for drooling suggests that the most effective of these procedures is bilateral submandibular gland excision with simultaneous parotid duct ligation or rerouting.[15] Several groups have reported that it efficiently controls drooling and reduces the frequency of aspiration.[7,8,29]

DISCUSSION

All children drool in some stage of their development but the key is to identify those who drool excessively. In a child with normal neurologic status and cognition, control of saliva and swallowing is well established by age 4. In this group if drooling is encountered, a small proportion have excessive salivation due to oropharyngeal infections, dental caries, and teething. In contrast, the majority of troubled patients have upper airway obstruction due to adenotonsillar hyperplasia/ obstruction or poor lip and tongue sensorimotor dysfunction affecting the oral preparatory and initiation phases of swallowing as their cause for excessive drooling. Children with speech impediments can be assisted with intensive speech therapy, and speech improvement will parallel the drooling severity improvement.

Conversely, children with neurologic dysfunction, syndromic anomalies and CP have normal salivary production. In this group, the main issues are difficulty controlling normal volumes of saliva within their oral cavity and swallowing safely without incoordination or aspiration. The severity of their swallowing disability is often dictated by their global motor and neurocognitive ability.

Areas that can be targeted to improve drooling in these children include posture, oral hygiene, malocclusion, lip, chin, and oral sensation, tongue and lip movement and suck, behavioral therapy with biofeedback regarding awareness of wetness of lip and chin, and more recently reminders via smartphone/ tablet applications. These therapies require moderate patient cooperation and participation. In severely handicapped children this is not always possible due to their cognitive and communication deficit. In these children a more aggressive treatment option should be considered.

The aim of pharmacotherapy and surgery is to reduce the amount of saliva and make the volume/ amount of saliva more manageable within their oral cavity. Pharmacotherapy may offer a good short-term solution but does have significant side effects. Few patients are able to tolerate them as a permanent solution.

In the senior author's experience, botulinum toxin has temporary improvement in 60.4% of patients treated with SMG injections and has a therapeutic effect for 3 to 6 months. As the SMGs produce 65 to 70% of saliva at rest, only these glands are injected.[14]

SMG removal with simultaneous parotid duct ligation has now become the largely accepted and advocated surgical option for severe drooling. While reducing approximately 90% of saliva, it does increase the risk of developing dental caries. There are a group of patients who are initially dry for 1 to 2 years but relapse after the procedure, which may be due to compensation of intraoral sublingual and minor salivary glands. In this case, the sublingual glands can be removed via an intraoral approach should drooling again become troublesome.

IMPACT ON QUALITY OF LIFE

To the majority of patients with drooling and their caregivers, it is reassuring to know that there are a number of options for reducing saliva. Many of these children have multiple comorbidities and their families are well versed with numerous interactions with many subspecialty pediatric and developmental health care practitioners over the years. They tend to be realistic and practical when it comes to choosing yet another intervention for their child. They are often looking for small but significant changes in drooling patterns and are able to cope with other situations adequately when drooling is more pronounced—for instance, at meal times or when concentrating on a tablet. For many older high school children, social acceptance by peers is paramount, especially when they are integrated into normal schools. The confidence to manage a normal school day without significant soiling is a major plus. It also appears that positive dry periods promote more dry periods.

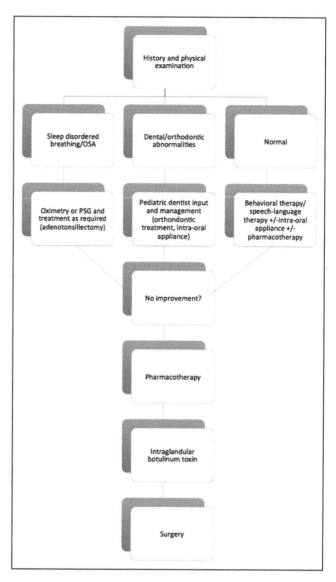

Figure 8–6. Suggested treatment algorithm for management of the drooling child.

SUMMARY

Drooling management should be tailored to an individual patient with a careful history with emphasis on situational factors, severity/frequency, impact on home and school life, family concerns, and previous management. A stepwise progression of management strategies from simple to complex should be employed—for example, from physical therapy and/

or speech therapy to pharmacotherapy and surgery. Some children require more than one modality to control drooling (Figure 8–6).

REFERENCES

1. Rating GD. Challenges in managing drooling in children. *Drug Ther Bull.* 2015;53(6):66–68. doi:10.1136/dtb.2015.6.0331.
2. Walshe M, Smith M, Pennington L. Interventions for drooling in children with cerebral palsy. Walshe M, ed. *Cochrane Database Syst Rev.* 2012;(11):1–52. doi:10.1002/14651858.CD008624.
3. Chaléat-Valayer E, Porte M, Buchet-Poyau K, et al. Management of drooling in children with cerebral palsy: a French survey. *Eur J Paediatr Neurol.* 2016;20(4):524–531. doi:10.1016/j.ejpn.2016.04.010.
4. Reddihough D, Erasmus CE, Johnson H, Mckellar GMW, Jongerius PH. Botulinum toxin assessment, intervention and aftercare for paediatric and adult drooling: international consensus statement. *Eur J Neurol.* 2010;17:109–121. doi:10.1111/j.1468-1331.2010.03131.x.
5. Montgomery J, McCusker S, Lang K, et al. Managing children with sialorrhoea (drooling): experience from the first 301 children in our saliva control clinic. *Int J Pediatr Otorhinolaryngol.* 2016;85(2016):33–39. doi:10.1016/j.ijporl.2016.03.010.
6. Reid SM, Mccutcheon J, Reddihough DS, Johnson H. Prevalence and predictors of drooling in 7- to 14-year-old children with cerebral palsy: a population study. *Dev Med Child Neurol.* 2012;54(11):1032–1036. doi:10.1111/j.1469-8749.2012.04382.x.
7. Manrique D, Sato J. Salivary gland surgery for control of chronic pulmonary aspiration in children with cerebral palsy. *Int J Pediatr Otorhinolaryngol.* 2009;73(9):1192–1194. doi:10.1016/j.ijporl.2009.05.002.
8. Noonan K, Prunty S, Ha JF, Vijayasekaran S. Surgical management of chronic salivary aspiration. *Int J Pediatr Otorhinolaryngol.* 2014;78(12):2079–2082. doi:10.1016/j.ijporl.2014.09.008.
9. Rodwell K, Edwards P, Ware RS, Boyd R. Salivary gland botulinum toxin injections for drooling in children with cerebral palsy and neurodevelopmental disability: a systematic review. *Dev Med Child Neurol.* 2012;54(11):977–987. doi:10.1111/j.1469-8749.2012.04370.x.
10. Porte M, Chaleat-Valayer E, Patte K, D'Anjou MC, Boulay C, Laffont I. Relevance of intraglandular injections of botulinum toxin for the treatment of sialorrhea in children with cerebral palsy: a review. *Eur J Paediatr Neurol.* 2014;18(6):649–657. doi:10.1016/j.ejpn.2014.05.007.
11. Thomas-Stonell N GJ. Three treatment approaches and clinical factors in the reduction of drooling. *Dysphagia.* 1988;3(2):73–78. doi:10.1007/BF02412423.
12. Scheffer ART, Erasmus C, Van Hulst K, Van Limbeek J, Jongerius PH, Van Den Hoogen FJ. Efficacy and duration of botulinum toxin treatment for drooling in 131 children. *Arch Otolaryngol Neck Surg.* 2010;136(9):873–877. doi:10.1001/archoto.2010.147.
13. Rashnoo P, Daniel SJ. Drooling quantification: correlation of different techniques. *Int J Pediatr Otorhinolaryngol.* 2015;79(8):1201–1205. doi:10.1016/j.ijporl.2015.05.010.
14. Mahadevan M, Gruber M, Bilish D, Edwards K, Davies-Payne D, van der Meer G. Botulinum toxin injections for chronic sialorrhoea in children are effective regardless of the degree of neurological dysfunction: a single tertiary institution experience. *Int J Pediatr Otorhinolaryngol.* 2016;88:142–145. doi:10.1016/j.ijporl.2016.06.031.
15. Reed J, Mans CK, Brietzke SE. Surgical management of drooling: a meta-analysis. *Arch Otolaryngol Head Neck Surg.* 2009;135(9):924–931. doi:10.1001/archoto.2009.110.
16. Johnson HM, Reid SM, Hazard CJ, Lucas JO, Desai M, Reddihough DS. Effectiveness of the Innsbruck Sensorimotor Activator and Regulator in improving saliva control in children with cerebral palsy. *Dev Med Child Neurol.* 2004;46(2004):39–45. doi:10.1017/S0012162204000076.
17. Marinone S, Gaynor W, Johnston J, Mahadevan M. Castillo Morales appliance therapy in the treatment of drooling children. *Int J Pediatr Otorhinolaryngol.* 2017. doi:10.1016/j.ijporl.2017.10.020.
18. Jongerius PH, van Tiel P, van Limbeek J, Gabreëls FJM, Rotteveel JJ. A systematic review for evidence of efficacy of anticholinergic drugs to treat drooling. *Arch Dis Child.* 2003;88(10):911–914. doi:10.1136/adc.88.10.911.
19. Eiland LS. Glycopyrrolate for chronic drooling in children. *Clin Ther.* 2012;34(4):735–742. doi:10.1016/j.clinthera.2012.02.026.
20. Heine RG, Catto-Smith AG, Reddihough DS. Effect of antireflux medication on salivary drooling in children with cerebral palsy. *Dev Med Child Neurol.* 1996;38(11):1030–1036. doi:10.1111/j.1469-8749.1996.tb15063.x.
21. Lungren MP, Halula S, Coyne S, Sidell D, Racadio JM, Patel MN. Ultrasound-guided botulinum toxin type a salivary gland injection in children for refractory sialorrhea: 10-year experience at a large tertiary children's hospital. *Pediatr Neurol.* 2016;54:70–75. doi:10.1016/j.pediatrneurol.2015.09.014.
22. Lin YC, Shieh JY, Cheng ML, Yang PY. Botulinum toxin type A for control of drooling in Asian patients with cerebral palsy. *Neurology.* 2008;70(4): 316–318. doi:70/4/316 [pii]\r10.1212/01.wnl.0000300421.38081.7d.
23. Becmeur F, Schneider A, Flaum V, Klipfel C, Pierrel C, Lacreuse I. Which surgery for drooling in patients with cerebral palsy? *J Pediatr Surg.* 2013;48(10):2171–2174. doi:10.1016/j.jpedsurg.2013.06.017.
24. Glynn F, O'Dwyer TP. Does the addition of sublingual gland excision to submandibular duct relocation give better overall results in drooling control? *Clin Otolaryngol.* 2007;32(2):103–107. doi:10.1111/j.1365-2273.2007.01388.x.

25. Delsing CPA, Viergever T, Honings J, van den Hoogen FJA. Bilateral transcervical submandibular gland excision for drooling: a study of the mature scar and long-term effects. *Eur J Paediatr Neurol.* 2016;20(5):738–744. doi:10.1016/j.ejpn.2016.05.001.

26. Hong KH, Kim YK. Intraoral removal of the submandibular gland: a new surgical approach. *Otolaryngol Head Neck Surg.* 2000;122(6):798–802. doi:10.1067/mhn.2000.99034.

27. Brown JJ, Yao M. Trans-oral submandibular gland removal. *Oper Tech Otolaryngol-Head Neck Surg.* 2009;20(2):120–122. doi:10.1016/j.otot.2009.06.001.

28. Hughes CA, Brown J. Pediatric trans-oral submandibular gland excision: a safe and effective technique. *Int J Pediatr Otorhinolaryngol.* 2017;93:13–16. doi:10.1016/j.ijporl.2016.11.026.

29. Stern Y, Feinmesser R, Collins M, Shott SR, Cotton RT. Bilateral submandibular gland excision with parotid duct ligation for treatment of sialorrhea in children: long-term results. *Arch Otolaryngol Head Neck Surg.* 2002;128(0886-4470 (Print)):801–803. doi:10.1001/archotol.128.7.801.

CHAPTER 9

Supraglottic Cystic Lesion

Georgina Harris

INTRODUCTION

The supraglottis is the upper division of the larynx, extending from the upper limit of the laryngeal inlet (free edge of the epiglottis and aryepiglottic folds, and back to the arytenoid cartilages) to a horizontal line through the apex of the laryngeal ventricle. It is further divided into subsites: suprahyoid and infrahyoid epiglottis, aryepiglottic folds (laryngeal aspect), false vocal cords, and arytenoids.

Most laryngeal supraglottic lesions are mucosal based and the most common tumor is squamous cell carcinoma. Mucous retention cysts are quite common and easily recognized; however, there are a variety of less common submucosal supraglottic lesions that can occur. As these lesions are all deep to the mucosa, and therefore deep to an endoscopy view, computed tomography (CT) and magnetic resonance imaging (MRI) are important adjuncts in accurately assessing a supraglottic lesion.

CASE PRESENTATION 1

A 39-year-old woman presents with a 6-month history of dysphonia. Her voice quality has changed and she describes it as constantly hoarse. Associated symptoms include a foreign body sensation. These symptoms had a gradual onset and are slowly progressing. She denies fevers, pain, dysphagia, stridor, or any hemoptysis.

She is an ex-smoker with a 15-pack-year history. She ceased smoking 6 years ago and has only minimal alcohol. Her only other medical history is that of gastric reflux for which she takes pantoprazole 40 mg daily. She is married with three young children.

Initial Assessment

Clinical examination revealed a hoarse, slightly breathy voice with reasonable projection and range. Neck examination did not reveal any masses or tenderness. Flexible nasal endoscopy revealed bilateral smooth cystic lesions in the supraglottis (Figure 9–1), much larger on the right-hand side. The lesion on the right was clearly cystic and was centered on the false cord, obscuring most of the underlying true vocal cord. The lesion on the left was less clearly defined, but was more of a fullness of the anterior left false cord. The underlying

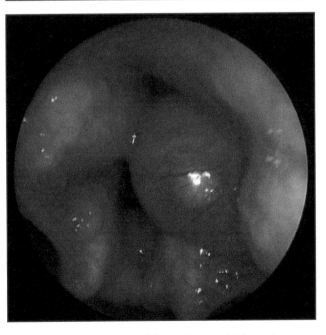

Figure 9–1. Demonstrates bilateral supraglottic cysts.

true vocal cords appeared to have full movement. The rest of the endoscopic examination was unremarkable. Valsalva revealed a transient increase in the side of the lesion on the right. A definition CT scan of the larynx, with contrast, confirmed the cysts were fluid filled and confined to the supraglottis.

DIFFERENTIAL DIAGNOSES OF SUPRAGLOTTIC LESIONS

Most supraglottic lesions are mucosa based—either related to inflammation (from bacterial/viral infection or radiation induced) or neoplastic, of which squamous cell carcinomas are by far the most prevalent.

Given the mucosa overlying the lesions is intact and looks healthy, a submucosal lesion is more likely in this given scenario.

Submucosal lesions are much less common and can be divided anatomically into lesions that arise in the submucosal layer, lesions that arise from the spaces of the supraglottic larynx (pre-epiglottic and paraglottic spaces), and lesions from the cartilage skeleton.

The differential diagnosis for this clinical scenario would include:

- Submucosal neoplasm
  - Minor salivary gland tumors
    - Adenoid cystic carcinoma
    - Adenocarcinoma
    - Mucoepidermoid
  - Oncocytic cystadenomas

- Lesions from mesenchymal elements within the spaces of the supraglottic larynx
  - Neurogenic lesions
    - Schwannoma
    - Neurofibroma
  - Hemangioma or vascular malformations
  - Paraglangliomas
  - Lymphoma
  - Granulomatous disease
    - Sarcoid
    - Wegener's
    - Amyloid
  - Ductal cyst
  - Saccular disorder (congenital or acquired)
    - Laryngocele
    - Saccular cyst
    - Laryngopyocele

- Lesions from or involving cartilage skeleton
  - Chondroma/chondrosarcoma

- Congenital
  - Thyroglossal duct cyst
  - Branchial cleft cyst

In this patient, given the submucosal nature of the lesions and their location, a saccular disorder is most likely. Whenever we consider saccular pathology, we need to consider the possibility of a mass obstructing the orifice of the saccule, which could be a neoplasm.

LARYNGEAL SACCULE AND SACCULAR DISORDERS

The laryngeal saccule is a blind outpouching of the laryngeal ventricle at its anterior end. Known as the saccule or laryngeal appendix, it was first described by Hilton in 1837[1] but is a structure often overlooked in anatomy discussions. They are blind pouches that ascend in the loose areolar tissue of the pre-epiglottic space, between the false vocal cord and the inner surface of the thyroid cartilage (Figure 9–2). There is a large variation in their normal size, ranging from 6 mm to 15 mm in length.[2]

The saccules are lined by pseudostratified columnar epithelium and contain both mucous and serous glands in the submucosa. As the saccules are protected, they fail to undergo the metaplasia to stratified squamous epithelium that is often seen in other more exposed parts of the larynx.[1] Lymphocytic infiltration and lymphoid follicles within the saccule are often seen in children but only seen in adults in pathological conditions such as carcinoma.[3]

Functionally, they appear to be an evolutionary remnant from our higher primate ancestors. In simian animals such as gorillas, complicated air sacs arising from the saccule are thought to increase resonance and speed of phonation. In humans, however, the sole function appears to be lubricating the ipsilateral vocal cord. Thin portions of the thyroepiglottic and aryepiglottic muscles surround the saccule (forming the compressor sacculi laryngis) and theoretically can compress the saccule.

Clinical presentation of patients with saccular disorders is variable. The most common complaint is dysphonia,[4,5] but other symptoms described include foreign body sensation, snoring, dysphagia, and cough. Soft lateral cervical neck masses are present if the saccule

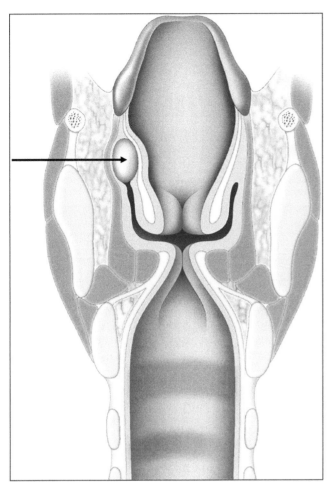

Figure 9–2. Coronal view of larynx demonstrating the blind pouch ascending from the left laryngeal ventricle (*arrow*).

saccule. Some authors[4,5,8] suspect this has been overstated, as a large proportion of reported patients did not have such occupations and a number of studies have shown no predisposing factors at all. Previous trauma and surgery have been indicated[9] as possibly precipitating enlargement of the saccule as well as preceding upper respiratory tract infections[10] and a smoking background.[5]

What is more clear is the relationship with laryngeal carcinomas and the increased incidence of laryngoceles in these patients. Up to 20% of patients who underwent surgery for laryngeal carcinoma were found to have enlarged saccules extending to the level of thyroid or beyond[10,11] as compared with only 2% in patients who had surgery for extralaryngeal malignancies. Of note is the fact that the saccule can be found on the contralateral side to the tumor, therefore the possible ball valve effect of an obstructing lesion near the saccule inadequately explains this. A more likely suggestion is altered laryngeal physiology that may increase intralaryngeal pressures such as coughing or altered neuromuscular mechanics.[12]

Looking at it from a different perspective, Canalis found 4% of occult laryngeal malignancies in patients who present with symptomatic laryngoceles.[13] Either way, the relationship is sufficient to warrant a high degree of suspicion in any patient who presents with a saccular disorder.

CLASSIFICATION

Classification of laryngeal cysts can be confusing but a simple way is to consider the contents of the saccule. De Santo and Holinger et al differentiated cysts on the basis of communication with the laryngeal lumen.[14] If it is air-filled, with open communication to the laryngeal lumen, the term laryngocele is used, or large saccule. If there is distention of the saccule with a blocked orifice and accumulation of mucus, an epithelial lined cyst is formed and it is referred to as a saccular cyst.

This is in comparison to a ductal cyst, which is synonymous with mucus retention cysts. This more common laryngeal cyst[3] is due to obstruction of a mucous gland, is found within the mucous membrane, and is therefore more superficial. These ductal cysts are found at any subsite within the larynx where mucosal glands are found—this excludes the free edge of the vocal cords.

Laryngoceles are abnormal dilations of the saccules, extending above the level of the thyroid cartilage.

herniates through the thyrohyoid membrane. Very occasionally, they may enlarge enough to present with life-threatening symptoms such as dyspnea, stridor, and airway obstruction. Saccular cysts and laryngopyoceles have been reported as causes of death in a small number of cases,[6] though this is exceedingly rare and most likely related to superimposed infection causing rapid enlargement.

The etiology of saccular disorders has yet to be clearly defined. In neonates, they appear congenital and are thought to be failures of the obliterated ventriculosaccular opening to recanalize (during embryology, this opening obstructs with mesenchyme but then recanalizes).[7]

Acquired factors, such as glass blowing or playing wind instruments, have long been discussed as possible causes for gradual enlargement of the laryngeal

De Santo classifies laryngoceles as symptomic large saccules, while others define them more anatomically, based on whether or not they ascend to above the level of the thyroid cartilage.

If the saccule remains deep to the thyrohyoid membrane, it is termed internal. If it herniates, typically where the superior laryngeal bundle pierces the membrane, to have an external component as well, it is termed combined (Figure 9–3). These patients present with a compressible, lateral neck mass that can change with the Valsalva maneuver. In recent times, we have moved away from the three classifications of internal, external, and combined. This is because by definition, an internal component must always be present in an external laryngocele.

Saccular cysts are also classified according to their location. Anterior saccular cysts appear as rounded, fluid-filled masses arising from the anterior ventricle and extend medially and posteriorly into the lumen of the larynx. They therefore protrude into the laryngeal lumen between the true and false vocal cords. Lateral saccular cysts expand more postero-superiorly, within the paraglottic space, and appear similar to laryngoceles, as submucosal fullness of the false vocal fold or aryepiglottic folds.

According to De Santo's classification, obstructed laryngoceles can become laryngomucoceles or saccular cysts, and superimposed infections result in laryngopyocele or saccular pyocele. Despite this spectrum of development and overlap in terminology, laryngoceles and saccular cysts remain separated when discussing management and treatment in most literature.[14]

IMAGING

Radiologic investigation plays a critical role in finding the diagnosis as well as treatment, and is often used to evaluate the submucosal and deep tissues of the larynx which cannot be assessed by direct visualization on laryngoscopy. Preoperative planning is critical for successful management of saccular disorders, and imaging should attempt to differentiate between saccular cysts and solid tumors, infected from non-infected lesions, and should accurately outline the anatomic boundaries of the lesion.

CT is the cross-sectional imaging modality of choice, with 2 mm axial images sufficient to exclude unexpected cystic extension, ascertain the contents of the cyst (air or mucus), and look for any occult laryngeal lesion.[15] Laryngoceles appear as well circumscribed lesions with low density (–1000 HU) identifying the air within the lumen. Saccular cysts or laryngopyoceles have densities ranging between those of water and soft tissue, with the more purulent material having a higher density. The rapidity of image acquisition in CT means that it is less susceptible to artefacts caused by swallowing and breathing.

MRI, however, provides excellent soft tissue discrimination and is superior to CT in distinguishing neoplastic disease from mucus and inflammation, and therefore should always be considered, especially to help with surgical planning when a neoplastic lesion is already suspected. The lack of ionizing radiation is an obvious other benefit. Saccular cysts will show a high signal intensity on T2-weighted images and low signal intensity on T1-weighted images, although this will increase if the protein content is high.

Imaging features that suggest a laryngopyocele include enhancement of the periphery seen after contrast in both CT and MRI and presence of air-fluid levels.

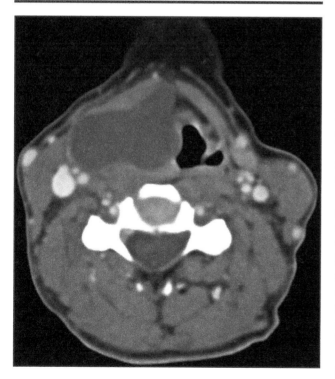

Figure 9–3. Axial CT scan of larynx demonstrating a combined laryngocele.

CASE 1 MANAGEMENT

The CT scan demonstrated bilateral laryngoceles. The lesion on the right was a low density cystic lesion that communicates with the laryngeal ventricle, consistent with a laryngocele. Superiorly there is extension between the hyoid bone and the thyroid cartilage into the lateral soft tissues consistent with a combined laryngocele. The laryngocele on the left also protruded through the thyrohyoid membrane but was smaller than the contralateral side. There was no evidence of any occult tumor masses.

The patient was taken to surgery for microlaryngoscopy and endoscopic resection of both lesions with the carbon dioxide (CO_2) laser. The author's preferred anesthetic technique is to have no endotracheal tube because of the risk of a fire. This can be achieved using either supraglottic or subglottic jet ventilation techniques. Laser "safe" tubes may be preferred by some, but each tube has a component that may be ignited by the laser. The transnasal humidified rapid insufflation ventilator exchange (THRIVE) technique[16] is relatively contraindicated because of the increased risk of fires with the laser.

After the patient is anesthetized, a wide lumen laryngoscope (Lindholm pattern by Storz) is inserted and suspended. The laryngeal ventricle was carefully inspected using both 0-degree and 30-degree Hopkins telescopes to exclude any neoplastic lesions.

The CO_2 is the preferred laser in this situation and can be used with a defocused beam for hemostasis and a focused beam for gentle dissection around the sac wall. The underlying true vocal cords are protected with wet neurosurgical patties. A technique similar to that described by Devesa is used[17]—careful dissection to completely mobilize the internal component, gradual traction with dissection to draw the external component back into the larynx, remembering to identify and preserve, if possible, the superior laryngeal bundle as it pierces the thyrohyoid membrane. Both laryngoceles were resected (Figure 9–4).

Following surgery, the patient recovered well and her voice quality dramatically improved. Her postoperative follow-up was unremarkable and no recurrence has been identified.

TREATMENT OF SACCULAR DISORDERS

Management of these lesions is surgical and has evolved over time from needle aspiration and decompression

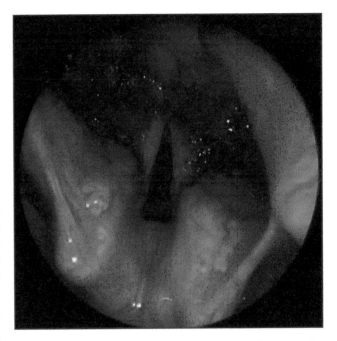

Figure 9–4. Removal of bilateral supraglottic cysts/laryngocoeles at the time of surgery.

to external excision and now endoscopic laser interventions. Size and location of saccular cysts and laryngoceles, as well as surgical experience are the two main considerations when planning for surgery. Small asymptomatic lesions may be observed, after a secondary pathology at the saccule orifice has been ruled out by clinical examination and imaging.

Traditionally the external approach has been the mainstay of treatment, for both combined and internal lesions. Three main techniques have been described for the external approach; trans-thyrohyoid membrane, thyrotomy with resection of the upper part of the thyroid cartilage, and V-shaped lateral thyrotomy.[7,8,18] These procedures have the advantage of excellent access and broad exposure to the laryngocele and low recurrence rates but with associated morbidity, the possible need for a covering tracheostomy, and prolonged hospital stay.

Mobashir et al[8] argue that their V-shaped lateral thyrotomy approach provides direct access and good exposure of the paraglottic space, thereby allowing dissection along the plane between the laryngocele and the paraglottic tissue. As the endolarynx is only entered through the ventricle, there is very little morbidity to the surrounding tissue and no tracheostomy is needed.

Recent advances in endoscopic technique and the increased use of the CO_2 laser in laryngeal surgery have enabled a shift toward endoscopic management for internal laryngoceles and saccular cysts, and this is now the accepted gold standard. This technique, compared with the open approaches, is quicker and a safe alternative, with fewer complications. It allows for good functional recovery and earlier discharge from hospital and avoids the need for tracheostomy.

Dursun et al recommended CO_2 laser resection for internal laryngoceles and an external approach for combined laryngoceles,[19] and this has been the management paradigm for many years.

The combined laryngocele, with its lateral component, remains a surgical challenge. Some surgeons advocate for a combined approach when treating combined laryngoceles.[5] In this approach, the lateral component of the laryngocele is dissected out and traced to where it herniates through the thyrohyoid membrane. Here it is tied off and the external component of the laryngocele excised. The internal component is then removed via the endoscopic approach.

As our experience with endoscopic microsurgery and the CO_2 laser improves, more authors are attempting to remove the entire lesion endoscopically (Figure 9–5). In the case report by Szwarc and Kashima, the first to use endoscopic surgery for a combined laryngocele, the external component was not dissected out, as no isthmus could be found nor was any fluid able to be expressed on lateral neck pressure. Despite this incomplete resection, no recurrence was identified clinically or on MRI up to 5 years later.[20]

Devesa et al reported 12 cases of laryngocele (3 combined) managed endoscopically with the CO_2 laser.[17] After identifying the internal component, the external component was able to be completely resected, following the cyst wall over the thyroid cartilage and gently pulling it back into the laryngeal lumen using traction and blunt dissection. The superior laryngeal vessels and nerves were able to be easily identified and preserved. No recurrence was observed.

The main limitation with endoscopic surgery, whether used in combination with an external approach or not, is the need for direct line of sight technique. Transoral robotic surgery (TORS) is a growing field in laryngeal surgery that allows for better visualization of the lateral areas. The use of robotic surgery for endolaryngeal resection of a combined laryngocele was first reported in 2013[21] and then again in 2015 when it was used in combination with the endoscopic laser approach after the sac ruptured.[22] More recently Kayhan et al published a case series of six patients with laryngoceles (four combined, two internal), all treated by transoral robotic approach.[23] There were no documented recurrence in the 2-year follow-up period.

Regardless of the approach used, it is important to aim for complete resection, in order to minimize the chance of recurrence. Aspiration and marsupialization are associated with very high recurrence rates up to 80%,[4] as were the earlier case reports of endoscopic laser excision. Young, in the largest series of endoscopically resected saccular cysts, including one with extension into the neck laterally, had a recurrence rate of 15%.[10] The two patients who had a recurrence

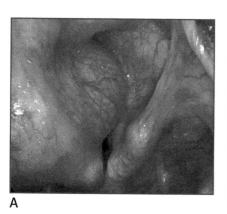 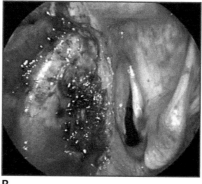 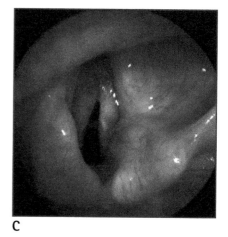

A   **B**   **C**

Figure 9–5. Left sided combined laryngocele (**A**), resected endoscopically with the CO_2 laser (**B**) and a view 4 weeks later (**C**).

remained asymptomatic and were treated conservatively; it is not clear if this included the patient with the lateral extension. As our experience with various techniques grows, the documented recurrence rates are reducing to more acceptable figures.[17–19]

This second case is of a 42-year-old female, presenting with progressively worsening dysphonia of 4 months duration. She had no other medical history. Endoscopic laryngeal examination, in the clinic, revealed a fullness in the left supraglottis with a medial extension beyond the midline (Figure 9–6).

The CT scan revealed a well-circumscribed cystic mass in the left supraglottis. There were scattered nodular lesions in the subglottis and trachea, as well as a small lesion in the area of the right ventricle. The remainder of the imaging was unremarkable; in particular there was no cervical lymphadenopathy.

This scenario highlights the importance of looking for an occult lesion as the primary cause for the enlarged saccule.

The patient was taken to surgery for suspension microlaryngoscopy and endoscopic resection with the CO$_2$ laser. The Lindholm laryngoscope was carefully inserted and suspended. A 0- and 70-degree Hopkins

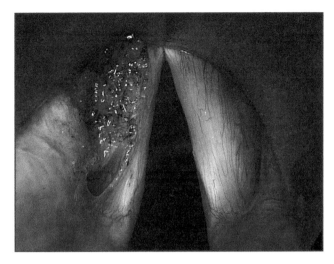

Figure 9–7. Left ventricular cyst removed to reveal a yellow infiltrate into the superior aspect of the left fold.

rod telescope was used to further access the larynx and the trachea.

After cyst removal, a yellowish mass was noticed infiltrating the superior aspect of the left vocal fold (Figure 9–7). This was debulked with the laser, avoiding radical surgery until proven necessary, with the intention of improving the voice. Small yellowish non-ulcerated submucosal nodules were visualized in the right ventricle, as well as the subglottis and farther into the trachea. Cupped forceps were used to take multiple biopsies from the various subsites and were sent for histopathological examination. The patient recovered well following her surgery and had a normal voice.

Histopathology of the specimen revealed a cyst with respiratory epithelium and a partly obstructing mass. This tissue from this mass, the subglottis, and trachea showed typical characteristics of amyloidosis. The patient was followed up and all investigations for systemic amyloidosis were negative. She was therefore diagnosed with localized laryngotracheal amyloidosis. She will be followed closely with endoscopic examinations as well as imaging.

Amyloidosis is a group of diseases characterized by the extracellular deposition of insoluble proteins, causing damage to tissues. These deposits are primarily made up of protein fibers known as amyloid fibrils, formed

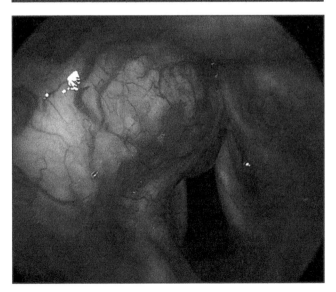

Figure 9–6. A fullness on the left supraglottis with an extension across the midline anteriorly.

when normally soluble body proteins misfold and become insoluble, aggregating in either a localized or systemic fashion.

These deposits can occur in any tissue and histologically give characteristic "apple-green" birefringence under polarized light when stained with Congo red (Figure 9–8). Amyloidosis is classified according to the type of precursor protein which forms the amyloid fibrils, and more than 20 precursor proteins have been described so far.[24]

Localized laryngeal amyloidosis is very rare (Figure 9–9), with most literature being either case reports or small case series. Localized laryngeal amyloidosis is usually associated with amyloid protein of the light chain (L) and therefore classified AL.[25] Of all benign laryngeal tumors, amyloid accounts for approximately 1% and has also been associated with laryngoceles in previous case reports.[26–28]

It affects both sexes equally and has been found in almost all subsites of the larynx, with the supraglottis and glottis more commonly affected.[29] More recent studies have described a multifocal pattern which can extend down into the tracheobronchial tree or upward into the upper aerodigestive tract.[29,30] Of the patients with localized laryngeal amyloid, 18% had involvement of a second organ in the study by Rudy et al.[26]

Although uncommon, the larynx can be affected in systemic amyloid.[26,31] As this diagnosis carries a dif-

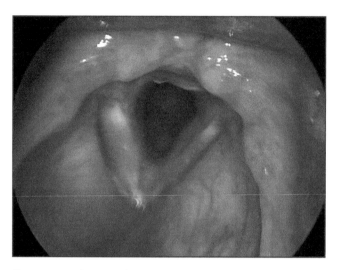

Figure 9–9. Laryngeal amyloid involving the vocal cords and extending into the paraglottic space on the right.

ferent treatment regime and significantly worse prognosis, any diagnosis of laryngeal amyloid should ensure appropriate workup to rule out systemic disease. Multiple myeloma and other blood cell dyscrasias need to be excluded.

At present, there is no consensus on what series of investigations should be carried out, but at a minimum should include blood and urine analysis, especially looking for monoclonal proteins as well as imaging of commonly affected organs such as the heart. Tissue biopsies have historically had low yield in patients with laryngeal amyloidosis; however, given the low morbidity of fine needle aspiration of abdominal fat and its high specificity,[32] it should at least be considered. Radiolabeled serum amyloid P component (SAP) scintigraphy is a specific imaging technique that helps to localize large amyloid deposits in the body but is only available in a few centers.[24]

Once systemic amyloidosis has been ruled out, treatment is often symptom driven and typically involves microlaryngeal surgery with laser or cold steel excision. There is no convincing literature that shows any cases progressing from localized to systemic amyloidosis, but progression to other subsites or recurrence is quite common.[26,29,30] In Hazenberg's long-term follow-up of laryngeal amyloidosis patients, 61% needed follow-up surgery due to recurrence, half of them within 12 months of their initial surgery. Revision surgery after more than 10 years is rarely indicated,[30,33] as the local progression of amyloid appears to slow down. This is possibly due to exhaustion of the underlying clonal

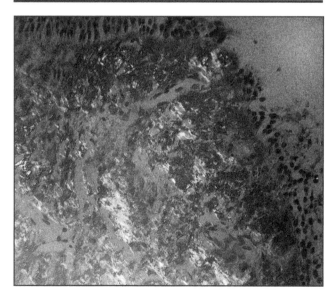

Figure 9–8. Pathology specimen from amyloid tissue demonstrating "apple-green" birefringence on Congo red staining.

plasma cells. Follow-up is therefore recommended for at least 10 years from the initial diagnosis. With more aggressive local or diffuse laryngotracheal disease, external beam radiotherapy has been shown to reduce further protein deposition.

REFERENCES

1. Porter PW, Vilensky JA. The laryngeal saccule: clinical significance. *Clin Anat.* 2012;25(5):647–649.
2. Broyles EN. Anatomical observations concerning the laryngeal appendix. *Ann Otol Rhinol Laryngol.* 1959;68(2):461–470.
3. Wenig B. Atlas of head and neck pathology. 3rd ed. Philadelphia, PA: Elsevier; 2016.
4. Flint PW, Cummings CW, Phelps T. *Cummings Otolaryngology Head & Neck Surgery.* 5th ed. Philadelphia, PA: Mosby/Elsevier; 2010.
5. Cohen O, Tzelnick S, Galitz YS, et al. Potential causative factors for saccular disorders: association with smoking and other laryngeal pathologies. *J Voice.* 2017;31(5):621–627.
6. Silingardi E, Sola N, Santunione AL, Trani N. Lateral saccular laryngeal cyst and unexpected asphyxial death. *Forensic Sci Int.* 2011;206(1–3):e17–e19.
7. Thabet MH, Kotob H. Lateral saccular cysts of the larynx. Aetiology, diagnosis and management. *J Laryngol Otol.* 2001;115(4):293–297.
8. Mobashir MK, Basha WM, Mohamed AE, Hassaan M, Anany AM. Laryngoceles: concepts of diagnosis and management. *Ear Nose Throat J.* 2017;96(3):133–138.
9. Marom T, Roth Y, Cinamon U. Laryngocele: a rare long-term complication following neck surgery? *J Voice.* 2011;25(3):272–274.
10. Young VN, Smith LJ. Saccular cysts: a current review of characteristics and management. *Laryngoscope.* 2012;122(3):595–599.
11. Alvi A, Weissman J, Myssiorek D, Narula S, Myers EN. Computed tomographic and magnetic resonance imaging characteristics of laryngocele and its variants. *Am J Otolaryngol.* 1998;19(4):251–256.
12. Harney M, Patil N, Walsh R, Brennan P, Walsh M. Laryngocele and squamous cell carcinoma of the larynx. *J Laryngol Otol.* 2001;115(7):590–592.
13. Canalis RF. Observations on the simultaneous occurrence of laryngocele and cancer. *J Otolaryngol.* 1976;5(3):207–212.
14. Heyes R, Lott DG. Laryngeal cysts in adults: simplifying classification and management. *Otolaryngol Head Neck Surg.* 2017;157(6):928–939.
15. Huang BY, Solle M, Weissler MC. Larynx: anatomic imaging for diagnosis and management. *Otolaryngol Clin North Am.* 2012;45(6):1325–1361.
16. Patel A, Nouraei SA. Transnasal humidified rapid-insufflation ventilatory exchange (THRIVE): a physiological method of increasing apnoea time in patients with difficult airways. *Anaesthesia.* 2015;70(3):323–329.
17. Martinez Devesa P, Ghufoor K, Lloyd S, Howard D. Endoscopic CO2 laser management of laryngocele. *Laryngoscope.* 2002;112(8 pt 1):1426–1430.
18. Zelenik K, Stanikova L, Smatanova K, Cerny M, Kominek P. Treatment of laryngoceles: what is the progress over the last two decades? *Biomed Res Int.* 2014;2014:819453.
19. Dursun G, Ozgursoy OB, Beton S, Batikhan H. Current diagnosis and treatment of laryngocele in adults. *Otolaryngol Head Neck Surg.* 2007;136(2):211–215.
20. Szwarc BJ, Kashima HK. Endoscopic management of a combined laryngocele. *Ann Otol Rhinol Laryngol.* 1997;106(7 pt 1):556–559.
21. Ciabatti PG, Burali G, D'Ascanio L. Transoral robotic surgery for large mixed laryngocoele. *J Laryngol Otol.* 2013;127(4):435–437.
22. Lisan Q, Hoffmann C, Jouffroy T, Hans S. Combined laser and robotic approach for the management of a mixed laryngomucocele. *J Robot Surg.* 2016;10(1):81–83.
23. Kayhan FT, Güneş S, Koç AK, Yiğider AP, Kaya KH. Management of laryngoceles by transoral robotic approach. *J Craniofac Surg.* 2016;27(4):981–985.
24. Jacques TA, Giddings CEB, Hawkins PN, Stearns MP. Head and neck manifestations of amyloidosis. *Otorhinolaryngologist.* 2013;6(1):35–40.
25. Bartels H, Dikkers FG, van der Wal JE, Lokhorst HM, Hazenberg BP. Laryngeal amyloidosis: localized versus systemic disease and update on diagnosis and therapy. *Ann Otol Rhinol Laryngol.* 2004;113(9):741–748.
26. Rudy SF, Jeffery CC, Damrose EJ. Clinical characteristics of laryngeal versus nonlaryngeal amyloidosis. *Laryngoscope.* 2018;128:670–674.
27. Aydin O, Ustündağ E, Işeri M, Ozkarakaş H, Oğuz A. Laryngeal amyloidosis with laryngocele. *J Laryngol Otol.* 1999;113(4):361–363.
28. Cankaya H, Egeli E, Unal O, Kiris M. Laryngeal amyloidosis: a rare cause of laryngocele. *Clin Imaging.* 2002;26(2):86–88.
29. Harris GA, Hawkins PN, Lachmann HJ, Sandhu G. Laryngeal amyloidosis—clinical update with 103 cases. in press.
30. Hazenberg AJ, Hazenberg BP, Dikkers FG. Long-term follow-up after surgery in localized laryngeal amyloidosis. *Eur Arch Otorhinolaryngol.* 2016;273(9):2613–2620.
31. Ginat DT, Schulte J, Portugal L, Cipriani NA. Laryngotracheal involvement in systemic light chain amyloidosis. *Head Neck Pathol.* 2017.
32. Halloush RA, Lavrovskaya E, Mody DR, Lager D, Truong L. Diagnosis and typing of systemic amyloidosis: The role of abdominal fat pad fine needle aspiration biopsy. *Cytojournal.* 2010;6:24.
33. Kennedy TL, Patel NM. Surgical management of localized amyloidosis. *Laryngoscope.* 2000;110(6):918–923.

CHAPTER 10

Pediatric Pharyngoesophageal Trauma Leading to Phagophobia

Mandy Henderson and Anna Miles

INTRODUCTION

Inhalation or esophageal lodgment of food or foreign bodies is common in young children. It can be life threatening or at the very least traumatic for parent and child. A choking incident/aspiration can result in acute temporary odynophagia (pain on swallowing) or respiratory distress. In extreme cases, there may be temporary or long-standing traumatic damage at the site of lodgment or caused during medical extraction. Interestingly, in some cases, the traumatic event or its sequelae may lead to phagophobia—a conditioned fear of eating in the absence of long-term physical impairment. A multidisciplinary approach is needed to facilitate a child (with the support of family) to return to enjoyable, nutritionally complete mealtimes.

DEFINITION

Phagophobia is the conditioned fear of eating; commonly occurs following a traumatic event associated with choking or the neck, for example, strangulation.

CASE PRESENTATION

An 18-month-old boy presented to the emergency department with a 4-hour history of crying associated with choking on a peanut.

Initial Assessment

History

Choked on a peanut given to him by his sibling 4 hours ago. Has been crying since incident. Nil previous medical history. Achieving developmental milestones appropriately. Appropriate growth, with weight and height tracking along the 50th percentile. Tolerating an age-appropriate diet of standard family foods. No previous history of aspiration or foreign body ingestion.

Examination

Distressed and crying. Parents also distressed. No audible stridor or increased work of breathing, but reduced air entry on right. Oxygen saturations 99% on air. Afebrile. Chest x-ray identified hyperinflation of the right side of chest, displacement of heart and mediastinum to left side on expiration.

Laryngoscopy and Bronchoscopy

Peanut located and retrieved from right main bronchus. Minimal surrounding edema and granulation, no pus.

Diagnosis

Peanut inhalation with localized edema.

101

Discharge

Postoperative recovery unremarkable. Afebrile. Oxygen saturations 99% on air. No increased work of breathing or audible upper airway sounds. No longer crying and is accepting sips of water from mother. Parents keen to take child home.

Represented 24 Hours Later

History

Vomiting and inability to keep any food down. Nil complications evident postoperatively. Well overnight at home post discharge. In the morning, vomited milk feed and continued to vomit for remainder of the day. Mild fever suspected by parents.

Examination

No increased work of breathing, good air entry in all zones, no crackles or wheeze. Afebrile. Oxygen saturations 99% on air.

Diagnosis

Possible vomiting in reaction to anesthesia versus throat pain post-bronchoscopy

Discharge

Child settled, accepted and tolerated milk feed with mother. No follow-up required. Recommendations to parents included regular paracetamol and plenty of fluids with monitoring of hydration. If any concerns to re-present to the emergency department or follow up with general practitioner.

Re-presented Six Months Later

History

Re-presented to otorhinolaryngology outpatient clinic 6 months later (age 2 years) with continued history of difficulty swallowing and breathing distress since the aspiration event. Child refusing to eat and drink, with minimal oral intake and subsequent weight loss. Weight dropped to the 25th percentile, with length still tracking along the 50th percentile. Mealtimes have become a battle, with parents stressed about reduced weight and oral intake. Parents report resorting to an extensive array of forceful strategies. Distraction, such as an iPad, is being used during mealtimes in an attempt to increase the volume the child accepts. Mealtimes typically lasting approximately 1 hour.

Action

Referral to speech-language therapy for assessment of eating and drinking. Referral to dietitian for analysis of intake and growth.

Examination

Clinical feeding evaluation completed by speech-language therapist in the child's home. Child having four 250 mL bottles a day of milk. No problems while drinking, but often gags following this and has increased work of breathing. Family foods are still being offered at mealtimes; however, child refuses and gags with all solid foods. Stressed behaviors evident with crying, pushing food away and refusing to sit in his highchair. Oral motor examination normal. Unable to fully assess chewing maturity or pharyngeal phase of swallowing secondary to minimal volumes accepted by child. Gagging after drinking observed. Clear breath sounds throughout and no changes to vocal quality associated with feed.

Action

Clinical feeding evaluation inconclusive, therefore instrumentation assessment recommended given history of gagging with oral intake and possible risk of airway compromise. Nasogastric tube inserted following dietitian assessment secondary to poor oral intake and weight loss.

Diagnosis

Unknown. Differential diagnosis (Table 10–1).

Table 10–1. Differential Diagnosis for Phagophobia

Diagnosis	Assessment	Possible Assessment Findings
Oral sensorimotor delay/ disorder	Clinical feeding evaluation Videofluoroscopic study of swallowing	Reduced bilabial seal resulting in anterior spillage of the bolus
		Reduced lateral tongue movements
		Decreased/immature vertical jaw movements (chewing)
		Finger manipulation required to move bolus within oral cavity
		Prolonged/poorly coordinated bolus preparation & transfer
		Premature/poorly controlled spillage of the bolus into the pharynx pre-swallow Oral residue post swallow
Pharyngeal sensorimotor delay/disorder	Clinical feeding evaluation Videofluoroscopic study of swallowing and/or flexible endoscopic evaluation of swallowing	Premature/poorly controlled spillage of the bolus into the pharynx pre-swallow Poor pharyngeal constriction
		Pharyngeal residue post swallow
		Aspiration of residue material post-swallow
Pharyngoesophageal segment opening impairment	Clinical feeding evaluation Videofluoroscopic study of swallowing Barium meal	Pyriform sinus residue
		Reduced pharyngoesophageal segment opening
		Poorly timed or shortened pharyngoesophageal segment opening
Esophageal impairment	Barium meal	Abnormal emptying of the esophagus
		Redirection/regurgitation/reflux of bolus in the esophagus
Airway compromise	Clinical feeding evaluation Videofluoroscopic study of swallowing and/or flexible endoscopic evaluation of swallowing	Penetration
		Aspiration
		Poor respiratory-swallow coordination
		Poor airway closure
Phagophobia	Clinical feeding evaluation Videofluoroscopic study of swallowing Video observations MDT assessment	No anatomical or physiological cause identified on other assessments
		Distressed behaviors associated with feeds despite no cause
		Precipitating stressful event around feeding/swallowing

VIDEOFLUOROSCOPIC SWALLOW STUDY

Child assessed with a range of food and drink, including milk via his usual bottle, yogurt, sandwich, and cookie. Remarkably, child was cooperative for the study and a full assessment was completed. No gagging behaviors observed. Appropriate oral, pharyngeal, cricoesophageal phases of swallowing (Figure 10–1). No abnormalities detected with any consistency. No airway compromise evident.

Diagnosis

No physiological abnormalities found on assessment. Phagophobia likely cause of gagging.

Action

To the Feeding Assessment Clinic for multidisciplinary management of eating and drinking difficulties. This specialized clinic includes input from a pediatrician,

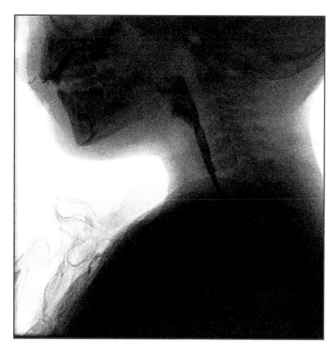

Figure 10–1. Videofluoroscopic study of swallowing within normal limits.

psychologist, dietitian, occupational therapist, and speech-language therapist (Table 10–2). Following initial multidisciplinary team assessment, the child was considered appropriate for the intensive tube weaning treatment program offered at the Children's Hospital. At this facility, this intensive approach includes a 3-week outpatient/day-stay program with the aim to decrease anxiety associated with mealtimes, increase oral intake, and reduce/eliminate nasogastric tube feeds.

Intensive Tube Weaning Treatment Program

Week 1

Daily input was provided by a speech-language therapist at each meal every 2 hours throughout the day (breakfast, morning tea, lunch, afternoon tea, dinner). Parents were supported by the psychologist to observe interactions between their child and the speech-language therapist during each mealtime and learned successful behavioral strategies. Daily occupational therapy input addressed sensory concerns regarding food, including sensory food play. Ongoing monitoring from

dietitian and prescription of enteral nutrition occurred with purposeful reductions in enteral feeds made to provoke hunger. Daily oversight from the pediatrician ensures the child remained medically stable and copes with the reduction in enteral feeds.

Week 2

Enteral feeds stopped by the end of week 1. There was an increase in range and volume of oral intake. However, stressed behaviors continued, such as refusal, pushing the food away, and gagging. Parents were reintroduced into the feeding sessions by the end of week 2. Modelled feeding skills were maintained by the parents, and they demonstrated an ability to generalize these techniques into environments outside the clinic room.

Week 3

Weight was maintained from pre-treatment, hence all nasogastric feeds were stopped and the nasogastric tube was removed by discharge from the program. Guidance provided for the transition home. Referrals were made to the community team to continue sensory desensitization and progressive introduction of new food types.

One-Month Review

Child continued to manage a full oral diet, with an increasing range of new foods accepted. Growth was maintained. Parents reported family mealtimes had become enjoyable again, and they were able to eat out at restaurants successfully for the first time as a family.

DISCUSSION

Inhalation or esophageal lodgment of food or foreign bodies is common in children and is the most common cause of otorhinolaryngology emergencies.[1] It can be life threatening or at the very least traumatic for parent and child.[2] It is most common in children between 1 and 4 years old where oral exploration and immature dentition, chewing, and cognition combine to increase risk.[2–4] Commonly inhaled materials include nuts, seeds, dried fruit, toys, and lithium button batteries, leading to coughing, choking, stridor, wheeze, and distress. To avoid respiratory complications, urgent bronchoscopy should be actioned.

Table 10–2. Roles and Responsibilities of the Team Members in Phagophagia

Profession	Assessment	Treatment
Primary consultant	General medical observations Full medical history Assessment of active and past medical issues Developmental history Full blood count and general chemistry Syntheses assessments from all disciplines Referral to other specialties/for further investigations if indicated, eg, barium meal, Otorhinolaryngologist, Respiratory physician	Medical management and oversight during treatment Monitoring of hydration Monitoring of overall well-being response to hunger provocation Medical support as needed
Speech-language therapist	Feeding history Oral sensorimotor assessment Clinical evaluation of the child eating and drinking Analysis of videoed mealtime from parents Consideration of instrumental assessment, eg, videofluoroscopic study of swallowing and flexible endoscopic evaluation of swallowing Recommendations regarding progression of oral motor-sensory skills	Participation in five mealtimes per day with child Recommendation of food consistencies appropriate for child Recommendation of any utensils or positioning changes to assist oral intake Determines mealtime duration for expected volume of intake Ongoing monitoring of child's oral motor and sensory skills and adaption of food consistencies as appropriate Modelling of appropriate feeding skills/behaviors Behavior management as required with support from psychologist Feedback and modeling to parents
Occupational therapist	Sensory assessment Recommendations to advance sensory integration skills	Daily sensory food play session Exploration and advancement of texture tolerance Feedback to team regarding appropriate food consistencies to use during mealtimes
Psychologist	Parental stress assessment Paediatric behavioral feeding assessment Observation of parent–child behavior and interaction	Participation in five mealtimes per day with speech-language therapist and child, or observing session with parents Behavior management strategies recommended to speech-language therapist and modelled to child during mealtimes Education to parents during observations regarding behavior management strategies Psychological support and intervention for parental anxiety
Dietitian	Anthropometric measures Assessment of daily food and fluid intake Review and prescribe volume of enteral feeds dependent on medical condition and nutritional requirements	Weekly weight review Daily intake review Determines energy, nutrition and fluid goals Assessment of oral food and fluid intake and reduction in tube feed volume as appropriate Support family

Foreign bodies lodged in the pharynx/esophagus should also be taken seriously.[2,5] In non-verbal children, detection may be difficult and any suspicion should be acted upon. Symptoms may include gagging, drooling and food refusal, odynophagia, and dysphagia. Chest x-ray should be ordered, as coins are the most commonly swallowed foreign object. Suspected button batteries need urgent removal, as esophageal injury occurs within 2 hours.[6] Interestingly, dysphagia is the most prevalent symptom in children who ingest button batteries, with a prevalence of 30%, followed by cough and fever at 26%.[6] A recent qualitative study interviewing caregivers of children post chemical or button battery ingestion injury found significant challenges for parents regarding altered oral intake as well as managing the psychological stress of the traumatic event.[7]

Phagophobia is the fear of eating and is a direct conditioned fear. In children, it is often a consequence of a choking event or traumatic ingestion of a foreign body.[8] Typical symptoms of phagophobia are food refusal and weight loss, and children often describe a feeling of throat constriction or pain.[9]

While an enteral tube ensures essential adequate nutrition and hydration in children with both physical dysphagia and phagophobia, it can interrupt the progress of normal feeding development by decreasing oral experiences and the child's hunger-driven motivation to eat. Children who receive nutrition via an enteral tube can develop tube dependency. Tube dependency is becoming increasingly identified as an unintended result of tube feeding[10,11] and in many cases is considered preventable or treatable. It is characterized by noninterest, avoidance, refusal, gagging, vomiting, and other oppositional/aversive behaviors in response to oral experiences. Active food refusal prevents infants from making the transition from tube to oral feeding and from learning to eat in the absence of medical indication for continuation of enteral feeding. Caregivers may develop an intense drive to feed the child orally, leading to intrusive and frustrating feeding attempts which can exacerbate the problem more, impacting on the quality of life of the parents, child, and the entire family.

Transition from enteral feeding to oral feeding, and establishing normal eating behavior in children who have phagophobia can be challenging due to the complex interaction of biological, psychological, and environmental factors that combine to disrupt healthy infant development. Feeding is a highly integrated multisystem skill and often more than one contributing factor may be at work. The multifactorial causes of phagophobia involve a substantial behavioral compo-

nent. Therefore, a multidisciplinary approach to tube weaning and reintroduction of an age-appropriate diet are recommended for children with severe behavioral feeding difficulties.[12–16] The literature clearly supports multidisciplinary teams in the belief that tube-fed children with the potential to eat should be helped to do so as soon and as effectively as possible.[12–16]

Treatment may include biofeedback, psychoeducation, cognitive restructuring, and aversion and distraction techniques to induce normalized swallowing.[9] Other techniques involve education to child and parents, relaxation and family anxiety management techniques, and in some cases structured desensitization programs.[8] Intensive desensitization treatment approaches generally include appetite manipulation (rapid reduction of tube feeds), implementation of mealtime structure and a feeding schedule, child and parental anxiety reduction, behavioral modification, and parent training.[12–15] As well as weaning the child from the tube, goals are to increase the range and volume of food the child will accept and help the child accept new foods. Tube feeds are reduced with guidance from the dietitian in order to provoke hunger and motivate the child to eat. Food is offered every 2 hours, and the child may only have water to drink between these times. Feeding sessions are completed with the speech-language therapist five times throughout the day. These sessions are supported by the psychologist, who may be present in the feeding room or observing the feed via video link with the parents to provide education on the behavioral strategies. Each feeding session begins with anxiety reduction specific to the child. This may include handwashing/water play, blowing tasks, gross motor activities, or music. The child is then offered food choices including both preferred and non-preferred items. Modeling is provided by the speech-language therapist, as well as contingent reinforcement. Further behavioral strategies as prescribed by the psychologist are implemented depending on the child and her/his response to the feeding sessions. Behavior management strategies may include positive reinforcement (verbal praise, rewarding desired behavior), social modelling (teaching the social experience of eating), shaping (gradually changing a behavior through small steps toward the desired behavior), differential attention (reinforcing the behavior we want to increase), and redirection (changing the child's focus of attention). The parents will observe the feeding sessions in the first instance and learn the behavioral strategies through education and support from the psychologist and speech-language therapist. Once confident with the strategies, the parents are reintroduced into the room, with the gradual removal of the therapists from the feeding sessions. The goal is to generalize the feeding skills to beyond the treatment room by the end of the 3-week program. Given the intensive nature of this treatment approach, there are strict criteria for entry into the program. These include a cognitive level above 2 years in order to respond to the behavioral approach, absence of anatomic impairment precluding safe oral feeding, and consent and engagement from the family. The engagement from the family is particularly pertinent given the known stress parents feel following such a traumatic event in the first instance, followed by the altered feeding behaviors of the child and consequent disruption to the parent–child and wider family dynamics.[7]

Intensive treatment approaches have been shown to be highly successful, with an increase in the amount of oral intake children will consume, while having no adverse effect on their weight.[14] Over half the children admitted to an intensive multidisciplinary program will be discharged no longer requiring enteral nutrition.[17] Furthermore, improvements in eating are seen to be maintained long term, with children who have completed an intensive multidisciplinary tube-weaning program demonstrating maintenance of feeding skills 1 year post treatment.[12]

SUMMARY

Inhalation or esophageal lodgment of food or foreign bodies is common in pre-school children and can lead to phagophobia beyond the acute phase. In worse cases, weight loss and nutritional status can be compromised. A physical swallowing difficulty must be ruled out through instrumental assessment (preferably with both videofluoroscopic study of swallowing and flexible endoscopic evaluation of swallowing) to thoroughly assess anatomy and physiological function. A multidisciplinary treatment program must aim to wean a child from tube feeding (if tube feeding has been initiated) and support the child and parents to actively work toward a healthy, balanced age-appropriate diet as soon as possible.

REFERENCES

1. Khan AR, Arif S. Ear, nose and throat injuries in children. *J Ayub Med Coll Abbottabad*. 2005;17:54–56.
2. Berdan E, Sato TT. Pediatric airway and esophageal foreign bodies. *Surg Clin North Am*. 2016;97:85–91. doi:10.1016/j.suc.2016.08.006
3. Buttazzoni E, Gregori D, Paoli B, Soriani N, Baldas S, Rodriguez H, Lorenzoni G. The Susy Safe Working Group. *Int J Pediatr Otorhinolaryngol*. 2015;79:220–2207.
4. Rodriquez H, Passali GG, Gregori D, et al. Management of foreign bodies in the airway and oesophagus. *Int J Pediatr Otorhinolaryngol*. 2012;76S:S84–S91.
5. McKinney OW, Heaton PA, Gamble J, Paul SP. Recognition and management of foreign body ingestion and aspiration. *Nurs Stand*. 2017;23:42–52.
6. Yardeni D, Yardeni H, Coran AG. Severe esophageal damage due to button battery ingestion: can it be prevented? *Pediatr Surg Int*. 2004;207:496–501.
7. Follent AM, Rumbach AF, Ward EC, Marshall J, Dodrill P, Lewindon P. Dysphagia and feeding difficulties post-pediatric ingestion injury: perspectives of the primary caregiver. *Int J Pediatr Otorhinolaryngol*. 2017;103:20–28.
8. Okada A, Tsukamoto C, Hosogi M, et al. A study of psycho-pathology and treatment of children with phagophobia. *Acta Medica Okayama*. 2007;615:261–269.
9. Thottam PJ, Silva RC, McLevy JD, Simons JP, Mehta DK. Use of fiberoptic endoscopic evaluation of swallowing FEES in the management of psychogenic dysphagia in children. *Int J Pediatr Otorhinolaryngol*. 2014;79:108–110.
10. Dunitz-Scheer M, Levine A, Roth Y, et al. Prevention and treatment of tube dependency in infancy and early childhood. *ICAN Infant Child Adolesc Nutr*. 2009;1; 73-82.
11. Dunitz-Scheer M, Marinschek S, Beckenbach H, Kratky E, Hauer A, Scheer P. Tube dependence: a reactive eating behavior disorder. *ICAN Infant Child Adolesc Nutr*, 2011; 34:209–215.
12. Brown J, Kim C, Lim A, Brown S, Desai H, Volker L, Katz M. Successful gastrostomy tube weaning program using an intensive multidisciplinary team approach. *J Pediatr Gastroenterol Nutr*. 2014;586:743–749.
13. Byars KC, Burklow KA, Ferguson K, O'Flaherty T, Santoro K, Kaul A. A multicomponent behavioural program for oral aversion in children dependent on gastrostomy feedings. *J Pediatr Gastroenterol Nutr*. 2003;34:473–480.
14. Cornwell P, Kelly C, Austin C. Pediatric feeding disorders: effectiveness of multidisciplinary inpatient treatment of gastrostomy-tube dependent children. *Children's Health Care* 2010;393:214–231.
15. Kindermann A, Kneepkens CM, Stok A, van Dijk EM, Engels M, Douwes AC. Discontinuation of tube feeding in young children by hunger provocation. *J Pediatr Gastroenterol Nutr*. 2008;47:87–91.
16. Krom H, de Winter J, Kindermann A. Development, prevention, and treatment of feeding tube dependency. *Eur J Pediatr*. 2017;1766:683–688.
17. Silverman AH, Kirby M, Clifford LM, et al. Nutritional and psychosocial outcomes of gastrostomy tube-dependent children completing an intensive inpatient behavioral treatment program. *J Pediatr Gastroenterol Nutr*. 2013;57:668–672.

CHAPTER 11

Caustic Substance Ingestion in Children: New Management Strategies Versus Traditional Approaches

Ibrahim Uygun

INTRODUCTION

Caustic substances (also known as corrosive agents) are chemicals that can cause tissue damage upon direct contact. Ingestion of caustic substances continues to be a life-threatening problem worldwide, especially in developing countries, and particularly in subjects aged less than 6 years.[1–12] Sadly, in developing countries, legal sanctions are either insufficient or not effectively applied; generic caustics are sold as grease cleaners, pickling vinegar (undiluted acetic acid), or battery acid in ordinary bottles that can be easily opened by children (Table 11–1).[2,3,5] Although caustic ingestion is usually intentional in adults, it is usually accidental in children. However, it is difficult to accept that caustic ingestion accidents in developing countries are truly accidental, as they in fact reflect extreme negligence.[2] In fact, there is a consensus that these unacceptable accidents would be reduced if caustic substances were sold in their original childproof containers, highlighting the need for preventive and adult education programs.[1–6] The conventional management of caustic ingestion—based on initial endoscopic grading, starvation, total parenteral nutrition, late barium study after 21 days, later commencement of dilation for esophageal stricture, and gastrostomy—should cease.[2,5,6] Endoscopic grading within 48 hours after caustic ingestion is not necessary anymore. Now in its place there is a new prognostic scoring for all caustic patients: the DROOL Score (Table 11–2).[2,5,6] Addition-

ally, there is strong evidence that early diagnosis and dilation within 10 to 14 days in patients suffering from esophageal stricture after caustic ingestion improves treatment success (Figure 11–1).[2,3,5,6,8,12] Herein, some real cases with different histories and clinical features are presented with different managements and therapeutic approaches.

CASE PRESENTATIONS

Case 1

An 8-month-old girl was admitted because of caustic substance ingestion. Injuries occurred when her mother accidentally applied drops of an unlabeled wart solution containing acid instead of vitamin D_3 to the child's mouth; the cover was opened and the entire acid solution was poured into the girl's mouth and on her face and body. On physical examination, oral and oropharyngeal lesions (edema, hyperemia, friability, exudates, whitish membrane) and second-degree burns on the face, neck, and chest were seen (Figure 11–2). Child abuse investigation was normal. She was drooling saliva and had an aversion to eating. The white blood cell count was in the normal range for age (12,500 cells/mm^3). She did not have fever. Chest x-ray was normal. Drooling saliva and appetite recovered within 12 hours. Fortunately, the DROOL Score, as a

Table 11–1. Common Caustic Substances Ingested[3,5]

Caustic Substance Type	Commercial Form
Acids	
Sulphuric	Batteries
	Industrial cleaning agents
	Metal plating
Oxalic	Paint thinners, strippers
	Metal cleaners
Hydrochloric	Solvents
	Metal cleaners
	Lime solvents
	Toilet and drain cleaners
	Muriatic acid
	Anti-rust compounds
Acetic	Pickling vinegar
Phosphoric	Toilet cleaners
Alkali	
Sodium hydroxide	Grease cleaners
	Drain cleaners
Potassium hydroxide	Oven cleaners
	Washing powders
Sodium carbonate	Soap manufacturing
	Fruit drying on farms
Ammonia	
Commercial ammonia	Household cleaners
Ammonium hydroxide	Dirt solvents
Detergents, bleach	
Sodium hypochlorite	Household bleach
Sodium polyphosphate	Household cleaners
Condy's crystals	
Potassium permanganate	Disinfectants, hair dyes

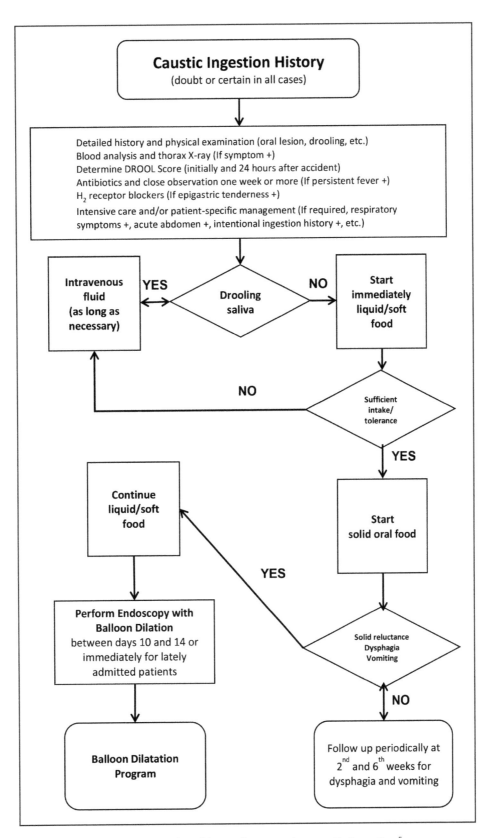

Figure 11–1. Flow chart, developed by us, for managing caustic ingestion.[5]

Table 11–2. The Five Criteria of the DROOL Score for the Assessment of Patients with Caustic Ingestion

THE DROOL CAUSTIC INGESTION SCORE				
Component of Acronym	**Signs and Symptoms**	**Score of 0**	**Score of 1**	**Score of 2**
Drooling	Drooling saliva	≥12 hours	<12 hours	No
Reluctance	Reluctance to eat, dysphagia, or food intolerance	≥24 hours	<24 hours	No
Oropharynx	Oral and oropharyngeal burns	Severe lesions*	Edema hyperemia	No
Others	No. of other signs/symptoms: persistent fever, hematemesis, abdominal tenderness, retrosternal pain, dyspnea, dysphonia	≥2	1	No
Leukocytosis	High white blood cell count	≥20,000	<20,000	No

* Friability, hemorrhage, erosion, blisters, whitish membrane, exudates, ulcer, or necrosis.

new prognostic tool instead of endoscopic grading for predicting esophageal stricture, was not low (score 6) (see Table 11–2).[5,6] Based on this and according to our management protocol, we commenced early feeding by the next day, and the child tolerated both soft and solid food (see Figure 11–1). After caring for her skin burns, she was discharged on the fourth day. On follow-up, she had no swallowing symptoms, and no further imaging (endoscopy or barium study) was needed. Her skin burns healed to almost scarless within 3 months (Figure 11–2).

Case 2

A 3-year-old boy was brought with caustic ingestion, having cut off the treatment from the other hospital by the parents. Three days previously he had drunk Siirt's Vinegar (pickling vinegar), a substance used for home-made regional pickles and containing concentrated acetic acid (Figures 11–7A and 11–7B), and which is sold in a non-childproof container, in his grandmother's house, where he was a guest. He drooled saliva for 2 days, and had starved for 3 days at the other hospital. Leukocytosis (20,560 cells/mm³) and persistent fever were observed. The DROOL Score, calculated retrospectively, was very low (score 1) (see Table 11–2). At admission to our hospital, he was reluctant to eat only solid food. Therefore, we began feeding him liquids and soft foods, according to our management protocol for preventing starvation (see Figure 11–1). Persistent

dysphagia continued. Therefore, at 14 days after caustic ingestion, according to our protocol based on early diagnosis and early starting of dilation of the esophageal stricture, an endoscopy was carried out, and two esophageal strictures in the upper and the middle esophagus were seen and dilated fluoroscopically via balloon dilator (15 mm, at 6 atm) in the same anesthesia (see Figure 11–1). Then, his esophageal strictures were dilated using balloons of gradually increasing diameter up to 20 mm over consecutive sessions on the balloon dilation program. After five dilations in only 3.5 months, he is now well and has been swallowing all food without dysphagia for 2 years (Figure 11–3).

Case 3

A 3-year-old girl was brought by her parents with esophageal stricture due to ingesting grease cleaner from a non-original container (stored in a 500 mL water bottle) 8 months earlier. She had undergone an esophageal dilation program consisting of 17 bouginages at another center. Her esophageal stricture was long (4 cm) and at the middle of the esophagus. After eight balloon dilations, her parents accepted the esophageal replacement by gastric pull-up, which was then carried out. After the gastric pull-up operation, followed by four balloon dilations for esophagogastric anastomotic mild stricture, she is well now without any symptoms and has been swallowing all food without dysphagia for 3 years (Figure 11–4).

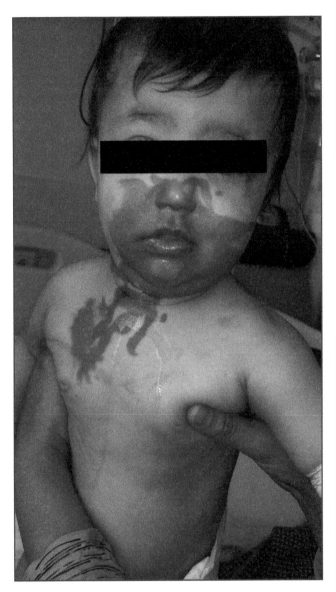

Figure 11–2. Clinical photograph of child with superficial dermal acid burns demonstrating spill pattern around mouth and nose and onto upper chest.

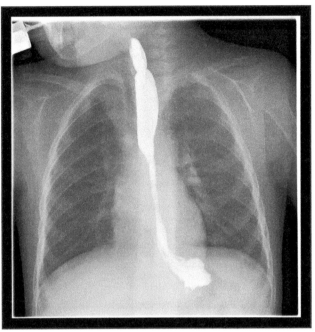

Figure 11–3. Postero-anterior chest fluoroscopic x-ray image demonstrating stenosis of the mid esophagus following caustic ingestion.

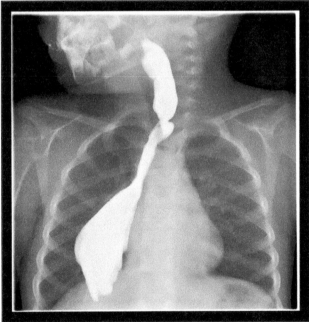

Figure 11–4. Fluoroscopic image demonstrating gastric pull-up configuration used to replace a strictured esophageal segment.

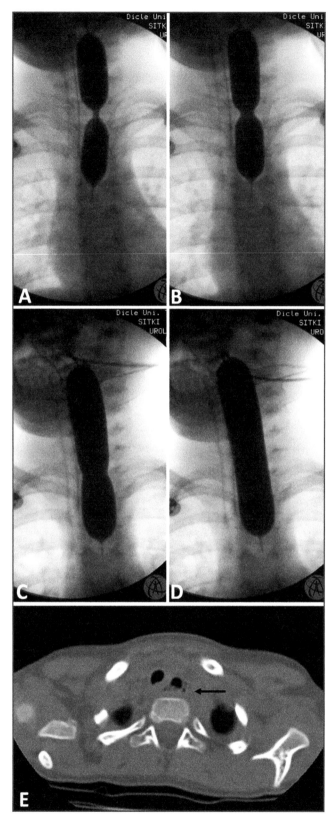

Figure 11–5. Figures A–D demonstrate fluoroscopic images of balloon dilation of the short esophageal stricture. Frame E illustrates free air around the esophagus after a perforation caused during balloon dilation. Eventually this stricture was resected to provide long-term relief of symptoms.

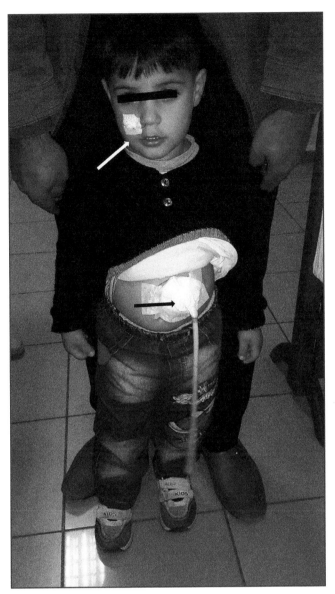

Figure 11–6. Clinical photograph demonstrating a gastrostomy tube with a nasal fastening rope from the right nares. This was able to be removed after balloon dilation program was undertaken at the tertiary treating hospital.

Case 4

A 4-year-old girl with esophageal stricture was referred for balloon dilation by a pediatric gastroenterologist. She drank pickling vinegar from an ordinary bottle, with the intention of drinking "zamzam" water 35 days earlier. The DROOL Score, calculated retrospectively, was very low (score 2) (see Table 11–2). After undergoing a management protocol at another center (initial endoscopy for prediction, starvation, late barium study after ≥21 days, and finally, starting of esophageal dilation), we immediately dilated her esophageal stricture first by way of balloon dilator (13.5 mm, at 4.5 atm) (see Figure 11–1). Her stricture was short (2 cm) but severe in the upper esophagus. During her third balloon dilation her esophagus perforated. This was diagnosed early via chest tomography, which was taken because of a persistent postoperative fever, before starting oral feeding, and was treated conservatively via nasojejunal feeding and antibiotics for 9 days. After eight balloon dilations, her parents accepted stricturectomy for her short resistant esophageal stricture, which was then carried out via a right cervical incision. After the operation and nine balloon dilations for mild anastomotic stricture, she is now well and has been swallowing all food without dysphagia for 4 years (Figure 11–5).

CASE 5

A 3-year-old boy with caustic esophageal stricture was brought by parents because of the continuing esophageal dilation program after 12 ineffective bouginages of another center. He had drunk grease cleaner from an ordinary container (a 500 mL water bottle) 9 months earlier. He had a gastrostomy tube and a thick rope fixed to his nose; its other end was tied to the gastrostomy tube (nose rope) as residues of the conventional habitual treatment (Figure 11–6). The gastrostomy tube and rope were removed in the first balloon dilation. After 11 dilations with 20 mm balloon dilators in one year, he is now well and has been swallowing all food without dysphagia for 1 year.

GENERIC CASE PRESENTATION

Case

The case is commonly a child under the age of 6, with a mean age of 3 years (see Cases 1–5). A sufferer may be a 1-month-old baby who accidentally is given bleach/acidic drug by a mother/babysitter, or, very rarely, an 18-year-old adolescent intentionally drinking battery acid.[2,3,5]

The cause is obvious; caustic agents are extremely neglected by adults. Because legal sanctions are either insufficient or not effectively applied, especially in developing countries, generic caustics are sold in ordinary non-original bottles that can be opened easily by children (Figure 11–7).

The caustics most commonly ingested by children are, approximately, bleach (30%), grease cleaner (30%), followed by other various agents (see Table 11–1 and Figure 11–7).[2–8] Fortunately, caustic ingestion injuries are usually limited to the oroesophageal mucosa, and do not feature massive necrosis or stricture development. The pH of ingested caustics greatly affects both the site and severity of tissue damage; pH values >12 and <1.5 are associated with massive caustic injuries.[2–5,8] Strong alkalis (pH values >12) sold in liquid form as grease cleaners (crystalline concentrated sodium hydroxide) are the major causes of severe esophageal damage (see Cases 3 and 5). They usually pass quickly through the oropharynx and cause extremely severe injuries to the upper, middle, and lower segments of the esophagus. Such caustics are particularly dangerous because they are transparent (like water) and are sold as generic grease cleaners in open transparent bottles (especially 500 mL water containers) that can be easily accessed by children in developing countries (see Figure 11–7).[5] In contrast to these, strong acids commonly cause damage to the gastric antrum, particularly if the stomach is empty. However, it must be kept in mind that all acids can cause damage in the esophagus (see Cases 2 and 4).[2–5,8]

History

The primary assessment of caustic ingestion patients should include taking a detailed medical history, to determine the time of contact, the amount and chemical nature of the caustic, the form of the container, and whether the container was original or not. Suicide and non-accidental injury need to be ruled out. The possibility of toxic effects, apart from caustic injury, should also be considered. All history and physical examination signs and symptoms must be recorded, and the caustic patient must be reported initially as a forensic patient.[2,3,5]

Recent clinico-epidemiological studies have shown that caustic ingestion accidents occur more often in boys (57–64%), in children of a mean age of 3 years, mostly in summer (38.1%) and spring (31.7%), mostly in the family home, and usually in the kitchen (51.5%).[5,7,10] Notably, a considerable number (22–23%) of caustic ingestion accidents occur during family visits (thus in the homes of grandparents and relatives).[2,5,7]. The caustics are mostly liquids sold in non-original con-

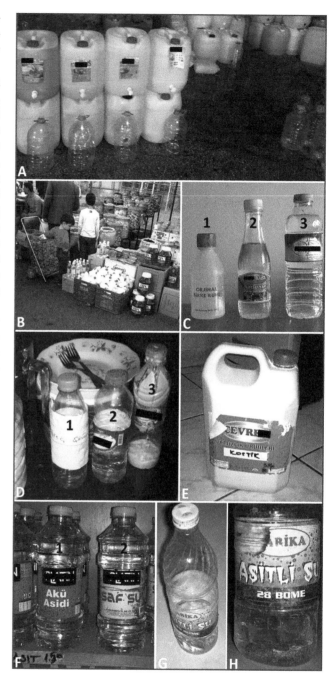

Figure 11–7. Image of variety of containers and vessels used to house caustic substances and how closely they resemble water containers leading to confusion and accidental ingestion.

tainers (69–93%), particularly transparent water bottles (38%), which are often 500 mL containers, or plastic carbonated-drink bottles (23%), both lacking warning labels (72–83%) and childproof safety caps (83–93%)

(see Cases 2–4).[5,7] Almost all ingestions by children are accidental; their intention is usually to drink water (82%) (see Cases 2–5).[5,7] However, it is difficult to accept that caustic ingestion accidents in developing countries are truly accidental, as they in fact reflect extreme negligence. In addition, most parents are poorly educated (mother, 88–96%; father, 62–80%) and have low incomes (see Figure 11–6).[5,7,10] One recent study found that children ingesting caustics were more impulsive than others; hyperactivity was also recognized as a risk factor for caustic ingestion in children younger than 5 years of age).[10] Caustic ingestion in adults is usually a deliberate suicide attempt[13]; this is rare (0–0.6%) in the case of children).[5,7,10]

Physical Examination

A detailed physical examination focusing on airway evaluation and hemodynamic stabilization is required. In some patients, urgent endotracheal intubation or surgical airway procedures may be needed. If an airway is severely compromised, emergency endotracheal intubation, cricothyroidotomy, or tracheostomy may be required. Persistent fever, peritonitis, chest pain, and/or hypotension may indicate visceral perforation.[3,5,8]

After caustic ingestion, patients may be either asymptomatic or may exhibit a variety of initial signs and symptoms, including drooling, a reluctance to eat, dysphagia/odynophagia, oral/oropharyngeal/skin/eye/other organ burns/lesions, retrosternal or abdominal pain, hematemesis, vomiting, fever, leukocytosis, epigastric pain, chest or abdominal tenderness/pain, agitation, tachycardia, and dyspnea. Most of these symptoms are mild, lasting only for several hours.[2,3,5]

Saliva is drooled because esophageal edema renders swallowing impossible; drooling disappears as the edema resolves (see Case 1). A reluctance to eat is associated with drooling. Appetite improves after drooling stops, but a reluctance to eat may persist (see Figure 11–1). Even if oral lesions are absent, esophageal injury cannot be excluded with full confidence.[3] A long duration of drooling (<12 h) and a reluctance to eat (>24 h) likely signal the presence of an esophageal injury.[5]

Laboratory

A hemogram is sufficient for almost all patients. However, in severe cases—such as those caused by intentional ingestion, those with airway symptoms, or those involving large amounts of ingestion—further laboratory investigations, such as blood gas analyses or biochemical tests, may be required.

No strong correlations are evident between blood counts or blood gas data and caustic ingestion outcomes. A leukocyte count >20,000/mL, an arterial pH below 7.22, and a base excess greater than −12 are indicative of severe esophageal injury.[5,14]

Imaging

A standing chest x-ray is required to rule out the presence of free air in the mediastinum, pulmonary involvement, or peritoneum. Fortunately, most of them are normal. Lateral neck radiographs should be obtained for patients exhibiting stridor or hoarseness. A contrast barium study (esophagogram) is not needed during initial assessment. However, if perforation is suspected, computerized tomography is recommended.[3,5,6]

Initial Management (0–14 days)

The management of patients with caustic ingestion depends on several factors, such as the severity of symptoms, the nature of the caustics, intention of ingestion, airway involvement, organ perforation, etc. (see Figure 11–1).[3,5,8]

Patients who intentionally drink caustics in suicide attempts (fortunately very rare among children) require special attention, as they are more likely to have ingested large amounts compared with those who have ingested caustic substances accidentally.[3,5,7,8,10] In addition, patients with signs and symptoms of an acute abdomen, mediastinitis, airway obstruction, or any perforation require specific careful management under intensive care conditions (see Figure 11–1).[2,3,5,6,8]

Patients with caustic ingestion who have no or mild signs and symptoms should be observed for a few hours or one night in an emergency room, during which time they should be offered clear liquids, then soft and solid foods, and finally discharged home (if they can swallow all food) after instructing the family to seek medical advice if dysphagia or a reluctance to eat develops. Follow-up after 10 days is appropriate. All other patients should be hospitalized (see Figure 11–1).[2,3,5,6,8]

The management of these patients is entirely symptomatic, and the main guide is drooling saliva (see Figure 11–1). If the patients have no drooling, they should be immediately fed liquids first, such as water and milk, followed by soft foods such as yogurt. If they have drooling, oral feeding should not be given until drooling stops. When drooling stops, liquid and soft foods should be started. If the patients can swallow liquids and soft foods, then solid foods should also be started within the same day. Intravenous plain fluid should be given for all patients who have inadequate oral intake. If they can eat solid foods without dysphagia or reluctance to eat, they should be discharged. However, if they cannot, hospitalization or close observation as outpatients at home with daily follow-up should be continued, and liquids and soft foods should be maintained (see Figure 11–1).[2,5,6]

No starvation. Many positive impacts of nutrition and saliva on surgical wound healing have been shown. An empirical study of caustic ingestion in rats has shown that sugar and honey have favorable effects on caustic burns.[5] Some historical reports recommend that patients with moderate or severe burns be left nil by mouth for more than 1 week. These proposed, without objective criteria, that foods impacting the esophagus increased the risk of infection.[15] However, we did not detect any food impaction, contrary to this claim, during endoscopy at 10 to 14 days after caustic ingestion in the esophagus of any symptomatic patient who fed with soft and solid foods (see Figure 11–1).[5,6]

Endoscopy grading within 48 hours after caustic ingestion is redundant, and this traditional approach should be abandoned.[2,5,6] It does not make any significant contribution to diagnosis, prediction, treatment, management, or guidance. To explain, endoscopy displays only the esophageal mucosa, not the muscle layer whose burns and necrosis trigger stricture formation. As a matter of fact, the esophageal stricture frequency varies for 25 to 90% of cases, even in children with bad endoscopic graded caustic burns.[2,4,5] The treatment and management of caustic patients are symptomatic; endoscopy does not guide treatment and hospitalization (see Figure 11–1). In addition, it is an invasive procedure of concern to parents. Endoscopy is contraindicated for perforated patients, and is not indicated for asymptomatic patients.[2,5,11,16] Now in its place there is a new prognostic scoring for all caustic patients: the DROOL Score (see Table 11–2).[2,5] The DROOL system (D, drooling saliva [<12 h]; R, reluctance to eat [>24 h]; O, oral and oropharyngeal burns; O, other signs/symptoms; L, leukocytosis [≤20,000/mL]), developed by us, is a simple and noninvasive scoring method (like scoring by APGAR [appearance, pulse, grimace, activity, and respiration]) that is based on the duration and severity of all symptoms (see Table 11–2).[2,5] Our recent, detailed, clinico-epidemiological study of 202 patients revealed that a DROOL Score ≤4 was highly predictive (100% sensitivity, 96.63% specificity, 85% positive predictive value, 100% negative predictive value) of esophageal stricture development ($p < 0.001$).[5] The DROOL Score should be preferred to endoscopic grading for all children who ingest caustic substances.[2,5,6]

At 10 to 14 days after caustic ingestion, if any symptom (mild, severe, or suspicious), such as a reluctance to eat, dysphagia, or vomiting, persists in outpatients or hospitalized patients, endoscopy must be performed promptly to diagnose any esophageal stricture, and fluoroscopic esophageal balloon dilation at the same anesthesia must be commenced simultaneously (see Figure 11–1).[2,5] Endoscopy is essential at this time (10–14 days after caustic ingestion) for only persistent symptomatic patients; not for the first day and not for all patients.[2,5,6] A recent study in adults, supporting our approach, demonstrated that endoscopic grading on day 5 is a better predictor of esophageal stricture than day 1 endoscopic grading.[17] Esophageal stricture then can be detected usually upon endoscopy. Additionally, fluoroscopic esophageal balloon dilation yields more detailed data on esophageal stricture location, length, and severity when used to screen the distal regions of serious stenoses and less severe lesions not detected by endoscopy, and treats them.[2,5,6,18]

Historically, a barium study was requested in all patients at 21 days or more after caustic ingestion.[9,15] However, this traditional approach usually further delays both esophageal stricture diagnosis and commencement of balloon dilation treatment.[2,5] It also delays diagnosis of patients with mild esophageal stricture, especially in the early period, and does not enable proper assessment of the distal part of the esophageal stricture because of slow flow.[5] In addition, if the barium study is normal it does not eliminate the necessity for endoscopy and dilation for patients with dysphagia. However, a barium study may be taken subsequently during a balloon dilation program to diagnose additional disorders, such as refluxing, presence of foreign bodies, motility disorders, fistula, total obstruction, swallowing discordance, etc.

Vomiting should not be induced, to avoid reexposing injured tissues to the caustic. If a patient exhibits persistent vomiting, a nasogastric tube should be inserted gently. Charcoal administration is not recommended, as charcoal does not adsorb caustics.[3,5]

Dilution therapy (water or milk) has also been recommended by some authors; however, no evidence supports such therapy in humans, and it is best avoided, as it may induce vomiting, perforation, or aspiration.[8]

Steroids have been suggested by some authors as a component of the management of caustic ingestion patients, to prevent stricture formation. However, other studies have suggested that steroids could be harmful. A meta-analysis of studies performed over 15 years concluded that steroids did not decrease the incidence of stricture formation after caustic ingestion, and were thus not useful.[2,5,6,19]

The routine prescription of antibiotics to caustic ingestion patients remains controversial. Theoretically, antibiotics are indicated to manage respiratory sepsis, persistent fever, or any suspect perforation. Prophylactic antibiotics should be indicated during dilation procedures; cerebral abscesses have developed following repeated esophageal dilation.[2,3,5,6,8,20]

Long-Term Treatment

Esophageal stricture development is a major complication after caustic ingestion by children (1.72–15%).[4,6,10,18] Esophageal dilation is the first treatment for esophageal stricture. Early esophageal dilation of esophageal stricture between 10 and 14 days after caustic ingestion improves treatment success.[2,3,5,6,8,12] Our study showed that starting balloon dilation early (10–14 days) has highly satisfactory treatment outcomes in comparison with late-dilation (≥21 days) patients who were referred lately to our clinic with esophageal stricture. In early-treatment patients, treatment duration (5 vs 18 months) and number of dilation (7 vs 22 sessions) were very significantly lower ($p < 0.001$) than in late-treatment patient.[5] Although early esophageal dilation (10–14 days) also has been proposed for many years in the main textbooks and in many publications, it unfortunately is still noteworthy that in some centers patients traditionally were still admitted at 3 weeks after caustic ingestion. The conventional management based on the initial endoscopic grading, starvation, total parenteral nutrition, late barium study after 21 days, later commencement of dilation for esophageal stricture, nose rope and gastrostomy should be avoided (see Cases 3–5).[2,5,6]

Various methods can be used for esophageal dilation, including using mercury-filled or flexible graded bougies for blind bouginage, guidewire-directed metal olives, or various balloon dilators. Modern balloon dilators, especially radially expandable balloons (Controlled Radial Expansion™, CRE fixed-wire 8-cm long balloon dilators, Boston Scientific Corp., Galway, Ireland), have several advantages; they are safe, efficacious, lack the shearing longitudinal force associated with other techniques, and do not require gastrostomies or nose ropes (see Case 5) (see Figure 11–6).[2,3,5,6,8,18]

Fluoroscopically-guided esophageal balloon dilation is appropriate for treatment of caustic esophageal stricture. This technique appears to be safe, with a low rate of complications and a high success rate, and in particular with superior image control, in that it allows the esophageal stricture to be visualized in its entirety (in terms of location, injury severity, length, rigidity, and shape).[5,6,21] However, balloon dilation programs should be begun sooner (10–14 days), and in children should be performed gently using balloons of gradually increasing diameter (approximately 18–20 mm) over consecutive sessions (see Cases 1–5).[2,5,6,18,21] In summary, esophageal stricture can be predicted accurately by using the simple new prognostic DROOL Score (≤4) instead of endoscopic grading, reduced by immediate feeding instead of starvation, diagnosed earlier (10–14 days) by endoscopy only for patients with persistent dysphagia instead of relying on a late classical barium study (≥21 days), and treated well by starting fluoroscopic balloon dilation earlier (see Table 11–2 and Figure 11–1).[2,5,6]

Although the major complication of esophageal dilation is esophageal perforation, the risk is relatively low (0–31%), especially with balloons. In our studies, the rate of perforation during fluoroscopically guided esophageal balloon dilations with large balloons (18–20 mm) was noticeable lower (1.6%) (see Case 4).[5,6] If perforation occurs, treatment is usually conservative (immediate nasojejunal feeding, antibiotics, and/or a tube thoracostomy if required); the mortality rate in children over the last decade has been close to zero. However, early diagnosis is important (see Case 4).[2,5,6,18,21–23] Esophageal perforation can be prevented by inserting and inflating balloon dilators gently and slowly.[5,6,18,21,22] It is essential to take particular care during the first session, which is associated with a more significant risk of perforation.[6,18,21]

Local steroid injection (triamcinolone acetate) into short esophageal strictures has yielded some success when combined with dilation, but has not been prospectively evaluated.[22] Similarly, mitomycin-C (an inhibitor of fibroblast proliferation) has also been used.[24]

Esophageal stents, partial esophagectomy, and esophageal replacement surgery are alternative methods.[1,3,5,6,8,25,26] Esophageal stents are not often placed in children, because such stents may trigger erosion of the trachea or bronchus.[26] Although balloon dilation treatments for short strictures are significantly shorter than for long strictures, a partial esophagectomy may be a suitable alternative to a short esophageal stricture treatment (see Case 4).[25] However, the entire esophagus must first be carefully assessed, both endoscopically and fluoroscopically, during balloon inflation to confirm that the stricture is indeed localized, because histologically a fibrotic injury may be much more extensive than radiography suggests. In addition, it must be kept in mind that a burned esophagus may be shortened and tethered, and thus a partial esophagectomy (stricturectomy) may be difficult.[3,5,6,8] Some authors prefer esophageal replacement surgery that uses the colon or stomach as a component of a long-term balloon dilation program.[1,2,8] Millar et al[3] have suggested that, should a dilation program or stenting fail after 12 weeks, replacement surgery should be performed. The two most common esophageal replacement surgeries are colonic interposition and gastric transposition; the latter seems to be associated with fewer complications and higher comfort (see Case 3).[1,2,3]

As is true also of benign esophageal strictures, the incidence and severity of gastroesophageal reflux must be investigated, and reflux must be excluded as contributing to a persistent stricture. It should be managed medically or surgically, if necessary.[2,3,5,6]

The esophagus is the organ most commonly affected after caustic ingestion.[3,5,8] Clinically significant gastric injury is relatively uncommon in children. Gastric outlet obstruction and pyloric stenosis are the gastric complications most frequently reported after caustic ingestion by children. Gastric perforation is very rare in children.[2,27]

Esophageal carcinoma is a late but serious complication of severe caustic injury. Its incidence after caustic ingestion has ranged from 2% to 30% in various patient series; carcinoma develops 1 to 3 decades after ingestion.[4] Unfortunately, in one case, lethal squamous cell carcinoma of the esophagus developed only 1 year after injury in a 14-year-old boy.[28] Dysplasia screening is recommended after a severe episode of caustic ingestion, to facilitate early detection of precancerous changes. Unfortunately, balloon dilation, esophageal stenting, and esophageal bypass surgery without esophagectomy do not prevent the development of esophageal carcinoma after caustic ingestion.[4,8] The incidence of esophageal carcinomas in patients who ingest caustics is 1,000-fold that of control patients of similar age, highlighting the need for enforcement of sanctions.[4]

SUMMARY

- Caustic substance ingestion remains a major health issue, particularly in developing countries, where safety laws are not effectively enforced.

- The unacceptable incidence of these accidents could be reduced by way of legal sanctions and the requirement that corrosive materials be sold in their original childproof containers.
- Strong alkalis, particularly crystalline grease cleaners (concentrated sodium hydroxide), are the principal causes of severe esophageal damage.
- The conventional management of caustic ingestion, based on initial endoscopic grading, starvation, total parenteral nutrition, late barium study after 21 days, later commencement of dilation for esophageal stricture, gastrostomy, and nose rope should be ceased.
- Using a new management protocol, esophageal stricture can be predicted with high accuracy by using the simple new prognostic DROOL Score (≤4) instead of endoscopic grading. Care protocol should include immediate oral feeding as soon as the patient can swallow saliva instead of starvation, endoscopy at 10–14 days in patients with persistent dysphagia instead of late barium study (≥21 days), and early fluoroscopic balloon dilation beginning at the same anesthesia.
- Fluoroscopically-guided esophageal balloon dilatation with large balloons (18–20 mm) seems to be safe, with a low frequency of complications and a high success rate. If dilation fails after a few months, esophageal replacement surgery should be performed.

REFERENCES

1. Spitz L. Esophageal replacement: overcoming the need. *J Pediatr Surg*. 2014;49:849–852.
2. Uygun I. Caustic oesophagitis in children: prevalence, the corrosive agents involved, and management from primary care through to surgery. *Curr Opin Otolaryngol Head Neck Surg*. 2015;23:423–432.
3. Millar AJ, Cox SG. Caustic injury of the esophagus. *Pediatr Surg Int*. 2015;31:111–121.
4. Kay M, Wyllie R. Caustic ingestions in children. *Curr Opin Pediatr*. 2009;21:651–654.
5. Uygun I, Aydogdu B, Okur MH, et al. Clinico-epidemiological study of caustic substance ingestion accidents in children in Anatolia: the DROOL score as a new prognostic tool. *Acta Chir Belg*. 2012;112:346–354.

6. Uygun I, Arslan MS, Aydogdu B, et al. Fluoroscopic balloon dilatation for caustic esophageal stricture in children: an 8-year experience. *J Pediatr Surg*. 2013;48:2230–2234.

7. Sanchez-Ramirez CA, Larrosa-Haro A, Vasquez-Garibay EM, et al. Socio-demographic factors associated with caustic substance ingestion in children and adolescents. *Int J Pediatr Otorhinolaryngol*. 2012;76:253–256.

8. Millar AJ, Numanoglu A. Caustic strictures of the esophagus. In: Coran AG, ed, *Pediatric Surgery*. 7th ed. Philadelphia, PA: Elsevier Saunders; 2012:919–938.

9. Kucuk G, Gollu G, Ates U, et al. Evaluation of esophageal injuries secondary to ingestion of unlabeled corrosive substances: pediatric case series. *Arch Argent Pediatr*. 2017;115:e85–e88.

10. Cakmak M, Gollu G, Boybeyi O, et al. Cognitive and behavioral characteristics of children with caustic ingestion. *J Pediatr Surg*. 2015;50:540–542.

11. Kaya M, Ozdemir T, Sayan A, et al. The relationship between clinical findings and esophageal injury severity in children with corrosive agent ingestion. *Ulus Travma Acil Cerrahi Derg*. 2010;16:537–540.

12. Tiryaki T, Livanelioglu Z, Atayurt H. Early bougienage for relief of stricture formation following caustic esophageal burns. *Pediatr Surg Int*. 2005;21:78–80.

13. Poley JW, Steyerberg EW, Kuipers EJ, et al. Ingestion of acid and alkaline agents: outcome and prognostic value of early upper endoscopy. *Gastrointest Endosc*. 2004;60:372–377.

14. Chen TY, Ko SF, Chuang JH, et al. Predictors of esophageal stricture in children with unintentional ingestion of caustic agents. *Chang Gung Med J*. 2003;26:233–239.

15. Baskin D, Urganci N, Abbasoglu L, et al. A standardised protocol for the acute management of corrosive ingestion in children. *Pediatr Surg Int*. 2004;20:824–828.

16. Crain EF, Gershel JC, Mezey AP. Caustic ingestions. Symptoms as predictors of esophageal injury. *Am J Dis Child* 1984;138:863–865.

17. Kochhar R, Ashat M, Reddy YR, et al. Relook endoscopy predicts the development of esophageal and antropyloric stenosis better than immediate endoscopy in patients with caustic ingestion. *Endoscopy*. 2017;49:643–650.

18. Temiz A, Oguzkurt P, Ezer SS, et al. Long-term management of corrosive esophageal stricture with balloon dilation in children. *Surg Endosc*. 2010;24:2287–2292.

19. Rosenberg N, Kunderman PJ, Vroman L, et al. Prevention of experimental esophageal stricture by cortisone. II. Control of suppurative complications by penicillin. *AMA Arch Surg* 1953;66:593–598.

20. Angel C, Wrenn E, Lobe T. Brain abscess: an unusual complication of multiple esophageal dilatations. *Pediatr Surg Int*. 1991;6:42–43.

21. Blount KJ, Lambert DL, Shaffer HA Jr, et al. Fluoroscopically guided balloon dilation of the esophagus. *Semin Intervent Radiol*. 2010;27:232–240.

22. Bicakci U, Tander B, Deveci G, et al. Minimally invasive management of children with caustic ingestion: less pain for patients. *Pediatr Surg Int*. 2010;26:251–255.

23. Gun F, Abbasoglu L, Celik A, et al. Early and late term management in caustic ingestion in children: a 16-year experience. *Acta Chir Belg*. 2007;107:49–52.

24. Sweed AS, Fawaz SA, Ezzat WF, et al. A prospective controlled study to assess the use of mitomycin C in improving the results of esophageal dilatation in post corrosive esophageal stricture in children. *Int J Pediatr Otorhinolaryngol*. 2015;79:23–25.

25. Malek MM, Shah SR, Katz AL, et al. Multimedia article: endoscopically guided thoracoscopic esophagectomy for stricture in a child. *Surg Endosc*. 2010;24:219.

26. Kramer RE, Quiros JA. Esophageal stents for severe strictures in young children: experience, benefits, and risk. *Curr Gastroenterol Rep*. 2010;12:203–210.

27. Ceylan H, Ozokutan BH, Gunduz F, et al. Gastric perforation after corrosive ingestion. *Pediatr Surg Int*. 2011;27:649–653.

28. Jain R, Gupta S, Pasricha N, et al. ESCC with metastasis in the young age of caustic ingestion of shortest duration. *J Gastrointest Cancer*. 2010;41:93–95.

SECTION II

VOICE AND AIRWAY

CHAPTER 12

Phonotrauma Management

C. Blake Simpson and Raymond Brown

INTRODUCTION

Caring for the professional voice user with dysphonia presents unique challenges for the laryngologist. The differential diagnosis is broad and the underlying pathology is often subtle, requiring a keen eye and ear and, in some cases, sophisticated diagnostic equipment to detect. Even slight voice changes that are nearly imperceptible to most may cause significant distress and dysfunction in the voice professional. Decisions regarding treatment and performance cancellation may have long-lasting effects on the patient's career and livelihood. A team approach is essential for optimal workup and management, and the laryngologist should work closely with a speech-language pathologist and vocal pedagogue in all aspects of care.

DEFINITIONS

Professional voice user: Anyone who depends on the use of his/her speaking or singing voice for a livelihood. This includes singers and actors as well as teachers, salespeople, attorneys, clergy, and telephone operators. Between 25% and 35% of the workforce in the United States can be considered professional voice users.[1]

Dysphonia: Disorder of voice. Can be structural or functional.

Hoarseness: General term for abnormal voice quality. A symptom.

CASE

History

A 25-year-old female soprano presents with a 5-month history of difficulty with her speaking and singing voice. She describes an intermittent raspy quality to her voice as well as increased effort and vocal fatigue. She has aspirations to become a professional pop singer and had been performing regularly with her band. She has not been able to perform recently due to her voice issues. She has difficulty with her transitional register and after her break, which is around D5, her voice is weak and uncomfortable. She is unable to hit the high notes that she could previously reach with ease.

Past medical and surgery history: None

Social: She does not smoke or drink alcohol but is often exposed to secondhand smoke.

Medications: Denies

Allergies: No known drug allergies

Initial Assessment

History

A complete history should include questions about the patient's vocal style and performance setting, prior vocal training and voice therapy, professional goals, and performance schedule. The medical history should include questions regarding gastroesophageal reflux risk factors, the use of medications that may alter the voice (eg, antihistamines), pulmonary status, asthma, allergies, endocrinopathies, environmental exposure (eg, stage or cigarette smoke), musculoskeletal injuries that may affect posture, temporomandibular joint dysfunction, history of endotracheal intubation, and prior laryngeal or thyroid surgery.

Questionnaires

Several validated subjective voice assessment instruments are available, including the Voice-Related Quality of Life (V-RQOL), Voice Handicap Index-10 (VHI-10), and the more recently developed Singing Voice Handicap Index 10 (SVHI-10).[2] Both the VHI-10 and the V-RQOL evaluate the effects of dysphonia on functional, physical, and social-emotional domains, and the results of each questionnaire are strongly correlated.[3] The SVHI-10 is more specific for measurement of self-perceived handicap associated with singing voice problems.[2] These instruments have become an essential component of the evaluation and management of voice professionals and are especially useful for monitoring the response to treatment.[2,3]

The Reflux Symptom Index (RSI) is a validated self-administered questionnaire designed to assess symptoms in patients suspected of having laryngopharyngeal reflux (LPR), which may be a contributing factor to dysphonia. A score of 13 or higher is considered abnormal and may indicate underlying LPR.[4] However, other conditions such as upper respiratory infections and atopic disease can cause elevated RSI scores as well.

Physical Exam

Evaluation of the patient with dysphonia should include a complete head and neck examination. The quality, volume, pitch, and prosody of the patient's speaking voice should be noted. The larynx and anterior neck musculature should be palpated and assessed for any tenderness or tension. The neurologic exam should include assessment of cranial nerves, gait and muscle tone, and tremor in the head or extremities.

Endoscopy

Laryngeal examination can be performed using a flexible rhinolaryngoscope and/or a transoral rigid laryngoscope. Newer flexible laryngoscopes utilize a camera at the distal tip of the scope, which allows

for a higher resolution and brighter image when compared with older fiberoptic systems containing the camera in the eyepiece. Rigid laryngoscopes provide a more illuminated and magnified image, making them the superior choice for characterization of vocal fold lesions. Videostroboscopy should be utilized in the evaluation of all patients with dysphonia. It provides a composite "slow-motion" view of mucosal cover layer of the vocal folds, which allows for the detection of small lesions and subtle changes in vocal fold mucosal wave and amplitude, findings that are often missed on continuous-light laryngoscopy.[5]

Voice Evaluation

Treating the vocal professional should ideally be a team effort, involving a laryngologist, speech-language pathologist (SLP), and in many cases a vocal pedagogue. In our practice, the initial history and examination for a patient with dysphonia is performed by the laryngologist and SLP in tandem. This allows for a more comprehensive history and often a more thorough and comfortable laryngeal examination. Voice analysis, including acoustic and aerodynamic measures of the speaking and singing voice, when appropriate, should be performed by the SLP as part of the initial examination. These measures may provide helpful information in the case of ambiguous clinical presentations (eg, paresis) and are useful in monitoring response to treatment.

Scenario 1

Exam

The head and neck examination is normal. Rigid videostroboscopy reveals normal true vocal fold position and mobility bilaterally. A right vocal fold midmembranous cystic lesion and left vocal fold midmembranous reactive lesion are seen. On the right, amplitude is normal and mucosal wave is moderately decreased at the site of the lesion. On the left, amplitude and mucosal wave are mildly decreased at the site of the lesion[6]. There is an hourglass vocal fold closure pattern at modal and high pitch and with unloading.

Diagnosis

Right vocal fold cyst and left vocal fold reactive lesion.

Investigations

No additional investigations are required.

Management

Proceed with initial trial of voice therapy. Generally, 6 to 8 sessions over a 2- to 3-month period is necessary. If voice improvement is inadequate, take to operating room for direct microlaryngoscopy and microflap excision of vocal fold cyst[7–10]. Also consider excision of contralateral reactive vocal fold lesion.

Scenario 2

Exam

The head and neck examination reveals excess tension in the paralaryngeal muscles and submental area. Flexible videostroboscopy shows anterior-posterior supraglottic compression as well as lateral compression of the false vocal folds on phonation. With unloading, complete closure is noted. True vocal fold position and mobility is normal bilaterally.

Diagnosis

Muscle tension dysphonia (MTD)

Investigations

- Elucidate any contributing factors (e.g., stressful life events, recent upper respiratory infection, poor vocal hygiene, poor breath support).
- Acoustic and aerodynamic measures by SLP.

Management

- Any factors contributing to the development of MTD should be addressed. This may include optimization of vocal hygiene, diet and lifestyle modifications for reflux, and referral to a therapist for treatment of underlying psychological factors[11–13]
- Flow phonation and resonant voice therapy is the primary treatment modality. Circumlaryngeal manual therapy can also be considered.

Scenario 3

Exam

The head and neck examination is significant for excess tension in the paralaryngeal muscles and focal tenderness at the level of the right thyroid cartilage. Rigid videostroboscopy reveals normal true vocal fold position and mobility bilaterally. Bilateral symmetric mid-membranous vocal fold lesions are seen. There is an hourglass closure pattern and the mucosal wave is intact bilaterally.

Diagnosis

- Vocal fold nodules
- Muscle tension dysphonia

Investigations

- Elucidate any contributing factors (eg, poor vocal hygiene, excessive vocalization, hard glottal attacks, glottal fry, poor breath support, "laryngeal focus" of phonation).
- Acoustic and aerodynamic measures by SLP.

Management

- Initial treatment of vocal fold nodules should always consist of voice therapy. The majority of patients will return to a functional voice quality. Surgical excision should only be considered in cases refractory to a complete 2- to 3-month trial of voice therapy.
- MTD should be treated as discussed previously. In most cases, it is expected to improve with voice therapy as the nodules resolve.[14]

Scenario 4

Exam

The head and neck examination is normal. Flexible videostroboscopy reveals excess thick mucus, inter-arytenoid and true vocal fold edema and erythema, and pseudosulcus (infraglottic edema). True vocal fold position, mobility, amplitude, and mucosal wave are normal.

Diagnosis

Laryngopharyngeal reflux

Investigations

- If the history and flexible laryngoscopy are consistent with LPR, a trial of a proton pump inhibitor (PPI) can be diagnostic and therapeutic and no additional investigations are typically needed.
- Esophageal pH monitoring (dual channel, to detect laryngopharyngeal reflux events) is considered by many to be the gold standard for diagnosis of esophageal reflux and LPR, and should be considered when reflux is strongly suspected but there is a poor response to empiric PPI treatment.
- High resolution manometry can detect motility disorders that may be contributing to reflux.
- Multichannel intraluminal impedance testing can detect nonacid reflux.

Management

- Diet and lifestyle modifications: Avoid spicy foods, chocolate, alcohol, caffeine, and other foods that subjectively worsen symptoms. Keep head of bed elevated while sleeping, don't eat within 3 hours of bedtime, eat smaller meals before bed, and work on losing excess abdominal fat.
- Medications: PPI ± H2 blocker, alginates.
- Surgery: In cases of refractory LPR or if patients cannot tolerate or do not wish to be on long-term PPI, Nissen fundoplication may be considered. Newer minimally invasive procedures such as Stretta and Linx are also available.

Scenario 5

Exam

The head and neck examination is normal. A complete neurologic examination is normal. Flexible videostroboscopy reveals mild bowing of the left vocal fold, prolonged open phase, increased vibratory amplitude on the left, and "chasing" mucosal wave propagation. The right vocal fold has normal mobility and normal mucosal wave and amplitude.

Diagnosis

Left vocal fold paresis

Investigations

- When the etiology is apparent based on the history (eg, recent intubation, upper respiratory infection [URI] preceding dysphonia) no additional workup is necessary.
- Consider laryngeal electromyography to confirm the diagnosis and provide prognostic information.
- Imaging studies to evaluate the course of the vagus/recurrent laryngeal nerve are usually not necessary in cases of stable vocal fold paresis, but one should consider imaging to evaluate for a compressive lesion if paresis worsens or the vocal fold becomes immobile.
- Consider neurology referral if there are any concerns that vocal fold paresis is a manifestation of an underlying neurological disorder (ie, if there are abnormalities on the neurologic exam). Parkinson's Disease may present with hypophonia and non-motor symptoms such as altered smell, mood or weight change.

Management

- Observation: Vocal fold mobility often recovers over time.
- Voice therapy: Should consider a trial of voice therapy prior to surgical management.
- Surgery: Surgical management includes injection augmentation of the vocal fold(s) and laryngeal framework surgery. Cases of recently diagnosed idiopathic paresis/paralysis with associated significant dysphonia or dysphagia should be managed with injection augmentation using a temporary substance such as hyaluronic acid, which resorbs after approximately 3 to 4 months. If the paresis/paralysis persists, medialization laryngoplasty should be considered.

DIFFERENTIAL DIAGNOSIS

The differential diagnosis for dysphonia in the voice professional is broad and is not limited to laryngeal pathology. Successful management of dysphonia requires consideration of all possible causes, including neurologic, psychological, pulmonary, and medication-related. However, a thorough history, physical examination, and videostroboscopic exam in the office will provide the diagnosis in most cases. In some instances, the diagnosis cannot be made definitively without microlaryngoscopy and possibly excisional biopsy. The causes of dysphonia are the same in voice professionals and nonprofessionals, but increased voice use and certain lifestyle factors (eg, secondhand smoke, reflux risk factors) place the professional at higher risk of voice dysfunction.

INFLAMMATORY/INFECTIOUS

- Inflammatory and infectious causes of dysphonia can range from a self-limited laryngitis associated with a viral upper respiratory infection or allergies to chronic reflux to more rare infectious granulomatous laryngitis (eg, tuberculosis).
- Laryngopharyngeal reflux (LPR)
  - LPR is retrograde flow of stomach contents into the larynx and pharynx. LPR causes disease through two pathways. In the direct pathway, the refluxate bathes laryngeal mucosa, causing inflammation, edema, and mucus production. In the indirect pathway, refluxate irritates the esophagus, which triggers a vagally mediated response.[15] Common LPR symptoms include dysphonia, dysphagia, cough, throat clearing, and globus. Most patients with LPR do not have heartburn.[15] Singers may have vocal fatigue, decreased vocal range and clarity, voice breaks, and anterior neck tightness.[16] There is some evidence that singing may predispose to LPR,[17] and performers with other reflux risk factors such as obesity and alcohol use may be at especially high risk. Laryngoscopy may reveal arytenoid, post-cricoid, and vocal fold edema and erythema, pseudosulcus, and thick endolaryngeal mucus, but these signs

are not specific to LPR. Patients with signs and symptoms of LPR should be started on a PPI as well as diet and lifestyle modifications. Long-term use of PPIs has been shown to have multiple adverse effects including increased risk of clostridium difficile colitis, pneumonia, hip fractures, renal disease, dementia, and platelet inhibition, and these medications should not be continued if there is no improvement in symptoms after an adequate trial (eg, 3 months).

- Acute laryngitis
  - Laryngitis is nonspecific and refers to inflammation of the larynx. The cause can be viral, bacterial, fungal, chemical, or traumatic. Acute laryngitis is characterized by symptom duration of less than 3 weeks. Patients will often have other URI symptoms, such as rhinorrhea, nasal congestion, and cough. Videostroboscopy will typically reveal laryngeal edema and erythema with impaired vocal fold vibration. Patients will report a deeper and raspier voice and singers may have difficulty transitioning into higher registers due to the mass effect on the vocal folds. Patients may also have throat pain, dysphagia, odynophagia, and odynophonia in more severe cases.
  - Treatment depends on the etiology and the severity of edema, but some degree of voice rest is always indicated. Mild laryngitis thought to be associated with a viral URI can be treated with vocal hygiene (eg, increased hydration), conservative voice rest (eg, limited voice use between performances), and a short course of systemic corticosteroids. Patients should be advised that voice use must be limited during treatment with steroids, since the risk of vocal fold hemorrhage and mucosal injury remains even if the voice feels normal. The risks of systemic steroids, including avascular hip necrosis, mood changes, and gastrointestinal ulcers, should be discussed with the patient. Severe laryngitis requires absolute voice rest and cancellation of upcoming performances. Videostroboscopy should be repeated before returning to full voice use.
  - Most cases of infectious laryngitis are caused by viral organisms such as

rhinovirus, influenza and para-influenza. Less frequently, acute laryngitis may be caused by bacteria such as *Moraxella catarrhalis, Haemophilus influenzae,* and *Streptococcus pneumoniae*. There are no criteria that can reliably differentiate between viral and bacterial etiologies.[18] Treatment for viral laryngitis is conservative, as discussed previously. Antibiotics do not appear to be effective in the treatment of most cases of acute laryngitis.[18] However, culture-directed antibiotic therapy can be considered if a laryngeal exudate is identified and can be collected for culture.

- Fungal laryngitis is most commonly caused by *Candida albicans* and often seen in immunocompromised patients (eg, DM, post-transplant, HIV positive). However, otherwise healthy, immunocompetent patients with certain risk factors such as prior radiation therapy, diabetes, smoking, and the use of systemic or inhaled steroids can also develop fungal laryngitis. Laryngoscopy will typically reveal scattered white plaques (often midmembranous) on the vocal folds and laryngeal mucosa with surrounding edema and erythema. However, erythematous, inflamed vocal folds may be the only laryngoscopic finding, so the diagnosis may be easily missed. Empiric treatment consists of fluconazole 200 mg daily for 2 to 4 weeks. Patients using inhaled steroids should be weaned off or switched to an alternative asthma medication if possible.
- Laryngitis may result from voice overuse or misuse. Voice rest and vocal hygiene along with voice therapy to correct the underlying cause is the cornerstone of treatment.
- Voice professionals may be exposed to environmental laryngeal irritants such as theatrical stage smoke and secondhand cigarette smoke, which can cause laryngitis.

BENIGN VOCAL FOLD LESIONS

- A variety of benign vocal fold lesions may cause dysphonia. The majority are phonotraumatic (ie, result from voice overuse or misuse). The most common vocal fold lesions are nodules, cysts, and polyps[8,9]. Phonotraumatic lesions typically occur in the midmembranous region of the vocal fold, which is the area of maximal collisional forces. These lesions reside within the lamina propria and the overlying epithelium is typically normal or thickened. It is common to see a reactive lesion in the midmembranous area of the contralateral vocal fold. These reactive lesions typically resolve spontaneously after treatment of the primary lesion.

- Nodules
  - Vocal fold nodules are, by definition, bilateral and typically symmetrical. Stroboscopy shows a normal or near normal mucosal wave and hourglass closure pattern. They are almost exclusively seen in adult females and children and they almost always respond to voice therapy.[8,10] Surgery is rarely required and only considered in patients with significant dysphonia after maximal nonsurgical management.
- Cyst
  - Vocal fold cysts are encapsulated, sac-like, midmembranous lesions within the lamina propria. Subepithelial cysts are superficial and associated with a normal or near normal mucosal wave and hourglass closure pattern on stroboscopy. Ligamentous cysts are located within the deep layer of the lamina propria closely associated with the vocal ligament.[10] Stroboscopy reveals a significant reduction in mucosal wave and hourglass closure. Vocal fold cysts typically do not resolve with voice therapy and usually require surgery.
- Fibrous mass
  - A fibrous mass is an accumulation of fibrous material within the lamina propria in the midmembranous vocal fold. These lesions are typically diffuse and ill-defined, which differentiates them from cysts, which have a distinct boundary.[8–10] Stroboscopy shows a severely reduced mucosal wave and a broadly based fullness at the midmembranous vocal fold. Treatment usually requires surgery.
- Polyp
  - Vocal fold polyps are exophytic midmembranous lesions with thin

overlying mucosa and often have a maroon hue due to their hemorrhagic nature. The polyp is sometimes associated with a feeding varix.[8–10] Stroboscopy reveals a slightly dampened mucosal wave and an hourglass closure pattern. The etiology is likely recurrent acute hemorrhage. These lesions usually respond poorly to voice therapy and require surgery. Polyps are usually removed using a microflap approach, but more exophytic lesions with a narrow stalk may be truncated. The feeding varix can be addressed with a potassium titanyl phosphate (KTP) laser. In select cases, a vocal fold polyp may be treated under local anesthesia in a clinic setting, using a KTP laser fiber passed through the side channel of a flexible laryngoscope.[7]

- Granuloma
  - Vocal fold granulomas are unilateral or bilateral lesions located near the vocal process of the arytenoid cartilage. Trauma to the arytenoid perichondrium leads to formation of an inflammatory mass.[8–10] Causes include endotracheal intubation, LPR, chronic cough/throat clearing, vocal misuse, and glottal incompetence. Symptoms may include globus, odynophagia, odynophonia, dysphagia, and dysphonia. Large lesions may obstruct the airway and cause dyspnea. Most lesions resolve spontaneously as long as reflux is controlled. Lesions that do not resolve can be treated with inhaled corticosteroids, injection of corticosteroids, botulinum toxin injections, or laser partial ablation.

MALIGNANT AND PREMALIGNANT VOCAL FOLD LESIONS

Malignancy must be kept in the differential diagnosis, especially when certain risk factors (eg, tobacco, alcohol, middle age-elderly, male) and red flag symptoms (eg, odynophagia, otalgia, neck mass) are present. Greater than 90% of glottic cancers are squamous cell carcinoma, but other cancers such as adenocarcinoma and sarcoma may arise in the glottis. Leukoplakia and erythroplakia are premalignant lesions that should be biopsied and monitored closely.

VOCAL TRAUMA

- Vocal fold trauma can result from voice overuse or misuse leading to vocal fold varices, hemorrhage, or scar. It can also result from occupational exposure (ie, inhalation or caustic injury), cigarette smoking (Reinke's edema), and intubation for surgery.
- Vocal fold hemorrhage/varices
  - A history of sudden, significant change in voice, especially while performing, should lead one to investigate for vocal fold hemorrhage.[16–18] This occurs due to tearing of microvasculature within the superficial lamina propria, which results in accumulation of blood within Reinke's space.[18] Predisposing factors include the use of anticoagulants or antiplatelet therapy, laryngitis, poor vocal technique, perimenstrual period, and vocal fold varices or ectasias. Videostroboscopy in the acute period will reveal a red, edematous, stiff vocal fold with decreased amplitude and wave. Like any bruise, the color will change from red to yellow over time as the blood is metabolized.[17] Treatment consists of strict voice rest and cancellation of any performances until the hemorrhage resolves. Systemic steroids should be used with caution as they may mask symptoms and lead to inappropriate voice use. Continued voice use and vocal performance in the presence of vocal fold hemorrhage may lead to scarring and permanent voice changes. However, recent evidence suggests that long-term voice outcomes after resolution of vocal fold hemorrhage are favorable, even with repeat episodes.[19] For repeated vocal fold hemorrhage, voice therapy and direct microlaryngoscopy to evaluate for and treat any underlying vocal fold vascular lesions may be helpful.
- Vocal fold scar and sulcus vocalis
  - Vocal fold scar is deposition of fibrous tissue within the lamina propria, whereas sulcus

vocalis is characterized by absence of lamina propria, resulting in a deep groove along the free edge of the vocal fold. Both lesions can cause significant dysphonia secondary to impaired vocal fold pliability. In many cases, the etiology is phonotraumatic and associated with prolonged voice misuse or overuse. Nonsurgical therapy including reflux management and voice therapy should be maximized prior to considering surgery. Surgical management may involve vocal fold augmentation, fat graft reconstruction of the vocal fold, and/or excision of the scar/sulcus.

- Polypoid corditis (Reinke's edema)
  - Polypoid corditis is characterized by accumulation of gelatinous fluid within the superficial lamina propria (Reinke's space) of the vocal fold and usually results in a low-pitched, gravelly voice. Nearly all patients with polypoid corditis are smokers. Usually, both vocal folds are affected and the entire length of the vocal fold is affected. Asking the patient to perform a quick inspiratory breath during stroboscopy reveals inferior prolapse of the excess vocal fold mucosa. Treatment involves smoking cessation (halts progression, but does not cause resolution of disease), reflux control, and voice therapy. Microlaryngeal surgery with removal of gelatinous material from the superficial lamina propria can be considered if there is inadequate response to nonsurgical management.

NEUROLOGIC/PSYCHOLOGIC

- A variety of neurologic and psychologic conditions can present with dysphonia.
- Muscle tension dysphonia
  - MTD is characterized by increased tension in paralaryngeal musculature associated with excessive or abnormal laryngeal movements during phonation. It is commonly seen with organic vocal fold pathology (eg, midmembranous vocal fold lesions), but can also be a primary voice disorder associated with voice misuse or overuse, LPR, and prior upper respiratory

infection. The voice is typically low-pitched and strained with frequent glottal attacks. The cornerstone of treatment is flow phonation and resonant voice therapy and circumlaryngeal manual therapy in addition to treatment of any underlying vocal fold pathology.[14,22]

- Vocal fold paresis and paralysis
  - Impairment of vocal fold mobility may be idiopathic or caused by malignancy, iatrogenic trauma (eg, thyroidectomy), endotracheal intubation, and neurologic disease. Vocal fold paralysis is readily apparent on flexible laryngoscopy, but vocal fold paresis may be more subtle and often requires videostroboscopy for diagnosis. Stroboscopic findings of paresis include reduced or sluggish vocal fold movement, asymmetry of the mucosal wave, increased vibratory amplitude, and vocal fold atrophy. Imaging to rule out a compressive lesion affecting the vagus/recurrent laryngeal nerve should be considered, especially in cases of vocal fold paralysis. Referral to neurology is appropriate if there are any concerning findings on the neurologic exam (eg, tongue fasciculations). Management depends on the severity of the paresis as well as the etiology and time course. Subtle paresis may be effectively managed with voice therapy alone, whereas more significant vocal fold mobility impairment with associated dysphagia requires early surgical intervention. Almost 70% of patients with idiopathic vocal fold paresis/paralysis recover vocal function spontaneously, usually within 6 months,[23] so expectant management is appropriate in some cases. Surgical management includes injection augmentation of the vocal fold(s) and laryngeal framework surgery. Injection augmentation with a temporary filler material (eg, hyaluronic acid) is preferred in newly diagnosed cases of paresis, when recovery of function is still possible. In long-standing cases of vocal fold paresis (ie, greater than 9 months), medialization laryngoplasty with Gore-Tex or Silastic with or without and arytenoid adduction is an excellent option. A trial injection augmentation with a short-acting substance

(eg, saline or carboxymethylcellulose) may be performed prior to medialization to predict the response to surgery.

- Spasmodic dysphonia
  - Spasmodic dysphonia (SD) is a focal dystonia characterized by laryngeal spasms that are vocal task specific. Adductor SD is the most common type (80% of cases) and is associated with strained-strangled speech caused by premature and excessive glottal closure. Abductor SD is characterized by breathy speech due to inappropriate glottal opening during speech. Treatment involves chemical denervation of the affected laryngeal muscles by injecting botulinum toxin into the posterior cricoarytenoid muscle in abductor SD and the thyroarytenoid-lateral cricoarytenoid muscle complex in adductor SD. Although the singing voice is typically spared in most cases of SD, variants exist where the first presentation occurs in the singing voice (and may be entirely limited to singing tasks).
- Dysphonia may be the presenting symptom in more severe neurologic conditions such as Parkinson's disease and amyotrophic lateral sclerosis (ALS). Up to one-third of patients with essential tremor have a vocal tremor.
- Anxiety and stage fright can cause dysphonia. Referral to a behavioral therapist and beta-blockers may be helpful in these situations.

RHEUMATOLOGIC/CONNECTIVE TISSUE DISEASE

Rheumatologic and connective tissue diseases such as rheumatoid arthritis (RA) and systemic lupus erythematosus (SLE) can cause dysphonia through the development of vocal fold lesions (eg, bamboo nodules seen in RA) and laryngeal joint ankylosis. Granulomatosis with polyangiitis (Wegener's disease) typically affects the subglottis, but may cause inflammation of the glottis as well.

MEDICATION–RELATED

Common medications, both prescription and over-the-counter, can lead to dysphonia through a variety of mechanisms, most commonly from drying effects.

OTHER

Pulmonary disease can result in poor breath support and a weak voice. Vocal fold atrophy is a common cause of dysphonia in aging voice professionals. Poor vocal hygiene (ie, inadequate water intake, excessive caffeine and alcohol) can result in drying and irritation of laryngeal mucosa and increased viscosity of laryngeal mucus, leading to dysphonia. Insufficient hydration and/or consumption of alcohol and caffeine, which act as diuretics, can result in drying and irritation of laryngeal mucosa and increased viscosity of laryngeal mucus, which may cause dysphonia. The touring schedule and lifestyle of a professional vocalist may predispose to poor vocal hygiene.[24,25] See Table 12–1.

MANAGEMENT

Management of dysphonia in the voice professional varies significantly depending on etiology and patient factors (ie, occupation, work/touring schedule). Appropriate referrals should be placed to pulmonology, neurology, rheumatology, or endocrinology for further workup and treatment of extralaryngeal causes of dysphonia. Medications thought to be contributing to dysphonia should be adjusted when possible. Treatment of laryngeal causes of dysphonia ranges from simple lifestyle modifications to voice therapy and vocal training to microlaryngeal surgery.[12,13,24,25]

Of particular concern to the voice professional is when to cancel a performance. This can be a difficult and stressful decision and is often complicated by professional and financial factors. It should be a joint decision between the voice professional and the laryngologist. However, certain findings such as vocal fold hemorrhage, large varix, or significant mucosal trauma should prompt a strong recommendation from the laryngologist of complete voice rest to prevent permanent, potentially career-ending damage.

PITFALLS

- Evaluation without the use of videostroboscopy may lead to an incorrect diagnosis by missing more subtle findings (eg, paresis, sulcus, small lesions).

Table 12–1. Differential Diagnosis of Dysphonia

Inflammatory/infectious
Laryngopharyngeal reflux
Laryngitis (viral, bacterial, fungal, chemical)
Upper respiratory infection
Allergic rhinitis (postnasal drip)

Benign vocal fold lesions
Laryngeal papilloma
Vocal fold cyst
Vocal fold polyp
Vocal fold nodules
Vocal fold granuloma
Fibrous mass
Polypoid corditis (Reinke's edema)

Malignant vocal fold lesions
Squamous cell carcinoma
Adenocarcinoma
Sarcomas
Spindle cell carcinoma
Leukoplakia and erythroplakia (premalignant)

Trauma
Vocal fold varices
Vocal fold hemorrhage
Vocal fold scar/sulcus
Vocal fold web
Inhalation or caustic injury
Intubation trauma

Neurologic/psychologic
Muscle tension dysphonia
Vocal fold paresis/paralysis
Multiple sclerosis
Myasthenia gravis
Guillain–Barre syndrome
Cerebrovascular accident
Parkinson's disease, Parkinson's plus syndromes
Amyotrophic lateral sclerosis, Multisystem atrophy
Spasmodic dysphonia
Anxiety
Essential tremor
Tic disorder
Myoclonus

Table 12–1. (*continued*)

Rheumatologic/connective tissue disease
Rheumatoid arthritis
Systemic lupus erythematosus
Granulomatosis with polyangiitis (Wegener's disease)

Medication-related (21)
Anticoagulants - vocal fold hemorrhage
Angiotensin-converting enzyme inhibitors (ACEI) - cough
Bisphosphonates - chemical laryngitis
Antihistamines, anticholinergics, diuretics - drying effect on mucosa
Antipsychotics - laryngeal dystonia
Inhaled steroids - fungal laryngitis, mucosal irritation

Other
Vocal fold atrophy
Poor vocal hygiene
Irritable larynx syndrome
Hypothyroidism
Pulmonary disease

- Attributing dysphonia to LPR or allergies without considering other possible causes. These are common incorrect or incomplete diagnoses that are often revised after thorough evaluation by a subspecialist.[26]
- Over-resection of epithelium and violation of vocal ligament during surgical management.

SUMMARY

Dysphonia in the professional voice user is distressing and debilitating for the patient and presents a challenging problem for the treating laryngologist. As illustrated in the case scenarios, dysphonia may result from a variety of etiologies and is often multifactorial. Pathology can range from a self-limited URI only requiring improved vocal hygiene and voice rest to complex phonotraumatic vocal fold lesions that require microlaryngeal surgery. A broad differential diagnosis should be considered and a diagnosis should not be made without videostroboscopy. Diagnosis and treatment of dysphonia is often complex and an interdisciplinary team is essential for optimal outcomes. Patient concerns about the effect of the voice disorder and its treatment on his/her livelihood and professional identity may lead to anxiety and reticence to undergo procedures, which could ultimately result in permanent voice alterations or limitations. Likewise, consideration of the technical skill required for microlaryngeal surgery and the implications of a surgical misstep may cause apprehension on the part of the surgeon. Therefore, a thoughtful risk-benefit analysis should be undertaken by both the patient and the surgeon, and a joint decision regarding treatment should be made. Following a systematic and thorough approach to the history and physical, utilizing available diagnostic and therapeutic instruments, and working as a team along with SLPs and vocal pedagogues will lead to excellent outcomes in most cases.

REFERENCES

1. Titze I, Lemke J, Montequin D. Populations in the U.S. workforce who rely on voice as a primary tool of trade: a preliminary report. *J Voice*. 1997;11:254–259.

2. Cohen SM, Statham M, Rosen CA, Zullo T. Development and validation of the Singing Voice Handicap-10. *Laryngoscope*. 2009;119(9):1864–1869. doi:10.1002/lary.20580.

3. Romak JJ, Orbelo DM, Maragos NE, Ekbom DC. Correlation of the Voice Handicap Index-10 (VHI-10) and Voice-Related Quality of Life (V-RQOL) in patients with dysphonia. *J Voice*. 2014;28(2):237–240. doi:10.1016/j.jvoice.2013.07.015.

4. Belafsky PC, Postma GN, Koufman JA. Validity and reliability of the Reflux Symptom Index (RSI). *J Voice*. 2002;16(2):274–277. doi:10.1016/S0892-1997(02)00097-8.

5. Scherer RC, Gould WJ, Titze IR, Meyers AD, Sataloff RT. Preliminary evaluation of selected acoustic and glottographic measures for clinical phonatory function analysis. *J Voice*. 1988;2(3):230–244. doi:10.1016/S0892-1997(88)80081-X.

6. Cho J-H, Choi Y-S, Joo Y-H, Park Y-H, Sun D-I. Clinical significance of contralateral reactive lesion in vocal fold polyp and cyst. *J Voice*. March 2017. doi:10.1016/j.jvoice.2017.02.011.

7. Rosen CA, Simpson CB. *Operative techniques in laryngology*. Berlin, Germany: Springer; 2008.

8. Johns MM. Update on the etiology, diagnosis, and treatment of vocal fold nodules, polyps, and cysts. *Curr Opin Otolaryngol Head Neck Surg*. 2003;11(6):456–461.

9. Rosen CA, Gartner Schmidt J, Hathaway B, et al. A nomenclature paradigm for benign midmembranous vocal fold lesions. *Laryngoscope*. 2012;122(6):1335–1341. doi:10.1002/lary.22421.

10. Altman KW. Vocal fold masses. *Otolaryngol Clin North Am*. 2007;40(5):1091–1108–viii. doi:10.1016/j.otc.2007.05.011.

11. Daniilidou P, Carding P, Wilson J, Drinnan M, Deary V. Cognitive behavioral therapy for functional dysphonia: a pilot study. *Ann Otol Rhinol Laryngol*. 2007;116:717–722.

12. Salturk Z, Kumral TL, Aydoğdu I, et al. Psychological effects of dysphonia in voice professionals. *Laryngoscope*. 2015;125(8):1908–1910. doi:10.1002/lary.25319.

13. Siupsinskiene N, Razbadauskas A, Dubosas L. Psychological distress in patients with benign voice disorders. *Folia Phoniatr Logop*. 2011;63(6):281–288. doi:10.1159/000324641.

14. Altman KW, Atkinson C, Lazarus C. Current and emerging concepts in muscle tension dysphonia: a 30-month review. *J Voice*. 2005;19(2):261–267. doi:10.1016/j.jvoice.2004.03.007.

15. Koufman JA. Laryngopharyngeal reflux is different from classic gastroesophageal reflux disease. *Ear Nose Throat J*. 2002;81(9 suppl 2):7–9.

16. Phyland DJ, Oates J, Greenwood KM. Self-reported voice problems among three groups of professional singers. *J Voice*. 1999;13(4):602–611. doi:10.1016/S0892-1997(99)80014-9.

17. Franco RA, Andrus JG. Common diagnoses and treatments in professional voice users. *Otolaryngol Clin North Am*. 2007;40;5:1025–1061–vii. http://doi.org/10.1016/j.otc.2007.05.008

18. Klein AM, Johns MM. Vocal emergencies. *Otolaryngol Clin North Am*. 2007;40(5):1063–1080–vii. doi:10.1016/j.otc.2007.05.009.

19. Kerwin LJ, Estes C, Oromendia C, Christos P, Sulica L. Long-term consequences of vocal fold hemorrhage. *Laryngoscope*. 2017;127(4):900–906. doi:10.1002/lary.26302.

20. Boltežar IH, Bahar MŠ, Kravos A, Mumović G, Mitrović S. Is an occupation with vocal load a risk factor for laryngopharyngeal reflux: a prospective, multicentre, multivariate comparative study. *Clin Otolaryngol*. 2012;37;5:362–368. http://doi.org/10.1111/coa.12006

21. Reveiz L, Cardona AF. Antibiotics for acute laryngitis in adults. *Cochrane Database Syst Rev*. 2015(5):CD004783. doi:10.1002/14651858.CD004783.pub5.

22. Van Houtte E, Van Lierde K, Claeys S. Pathophysiology and treatment of muscle tension dysphonia: a review of the current knowledge. *J Voice*. 2011;25(2):202–207. doi:10.1016/j.jvoice.2009.10.009.

23. Husain S, Sadoughi B, Mor N, Levin AM, Sulica L. Time course of recovery of idiopathic vocal fold paralysis. *Laryngoscope*. 2018;128(1):148–152. doi:10.1002/lary.26762.

24. Echternach M, Burk F, Burdumy M, et al. The influence of vocal fold mass lesions on the passaggio region of professional singers. *Laryngoscope*. 2016;5:120. doi:10.1002/lary.26332.

25. Zeitels SM, Hillman RE, Desloge R, Mauri M, Doyle PB. Phonomicrosurgery in singers and performing artists: treatment outcomes, management theories, and future directions. *Ann Otol Rhinol Laryngol Suppl*. 2002;190:21–40.

26. Keesecker SE, Murry T, Sulica L. Patterns in the evaluation of hoarseness: time to presentation, laryngeal visualization, and diagnostic accuracy. *Laryngoscope*. 2015;125(3):667–673. doi:10.1002/lary.24955.

CHAPTER 13

Phonotrauma

VyVy N. Young

Dysphonia, or hoarseness, is a common otolaryngologic presenting symptom.[1] In the United States, for example, approximately 6 to 7% of adults report a current voice problem[2-4] and up to 30% of the population experiences dysphonia at some point in their lifetime.[2,5] Nearly 18 million US adults every year report a voice problem.[6] Voice difficulties have a negative impact on quality of life,[7-9] affecting the social, psychological, financial, physical, or emotional aspects of patients' lives. To address these issues effectively, it is important to recognize that the etiology and treatment of voice problems can be quite varied.[1,3,10]

One cause of dysphonia relates to voice use. This phenomenon was previously labeled voice "abuse," "misuse," or "overuse," but use of these terms has declined over time due to their negative connotations. Gillespie and Verdolini Abbott showed that use of these terms decreased patients' self-efficacy, or their belief in their own ability to demonstrate a specific behavior,[11] which in turn may have a negative impact on treatment outcomes. Thus, the term "phonotrauma" has been proposed to clarify more specifically the etiology of the voice symptoms. These patients may develop voice difficulties related to vocal technique or inefficiency of voice production (eg, muscle tension dysphonia). Alternatively, some patients develop benign, midmembranous vocal fold lesions. In situations which relate to significant voice use, these growths are often referred to as "phonotraumatic" in nature. There are many potential scenarios in which phonotraumatic lesions and their associated symptoms may develop, such as:

- Teaching
- Coaching (sports, etc)
- Cheerleading
- Singing and/or acting (musical theatre, etc)
- Bartending/waitressing
- Working in a call center or as a cashier
- Preaching/ministry

The common underlying theme in many of these situations is a high degree of vocal demand, with or without an unfavorable environment (eg, background noise).[3,9,12-14] The presence of voice difficulties, especially in these situations, can have negative psychological, social, and financial consequences.[1,2,15,16]

A 29-year-old female professional singer presents with gradually worsening hoarseness over the last 9 months. This symptom began after an acute upper respiratory infection. She continued to work through her illness and noticed changes to her voice that have not resolved. She describes her speaking voice as raspy, effortful, and easily fatigued. In her singing voice specifically, she has lost some of her upper range and reports that her singing voice is occasionally breathy and strained. She is the lead singer of a heavy metal band and performs four or five shows per week, often in smoky environments (eg, bars). She is otherwise healthy and does not take any medications. She acknowledges smoking cigarettes (1 pack per day × 15 years) and occasionally marijuana as well. She drinks three cups of coffee and one bottle of water daily.

INITIAL ASSESSMENT

Critical information to guide treatment is obtained from a thorough history. A multidisciplinary approach including both a laryngologist and speech language pathologist (ideally, simultaneously) is advocated to optimize the patient's evaluation and development of the best treatment plan.[17,18] This approach has been shown to improve outcomes, including patients' adherence to voice therapy.[18]

- History of the presenting illness

  - Ask specifically about onset of symptoms—was the change gradual or sudden? What circumstances surrounded this time (eg, illness, stress, change in environment)? How have the symptoms progressed since that time? What treatments has the patient tried thus far and were they successful?

- Voice change characteristics

  - Ask about the exact nature of the changes to the patient's voice. These details should be clarified separately for both the speaking voice and the singing voice. Do these changes impact the sound of the voice, the feel of the voice, or both? Examples of adjectives that may be used to describe the voice changes include the following: raspy, effortful, strained, painful, fatigued, inconsistent, or breathy. Patients may also describe breaks in their voice. Specific changes to the singing voice including changes in range and alterations in clarity or quality of voice should be noted.

- Voice history

  - Has the patient had a similar episode in the past? If so, what treatment was tried and was it successful?
  - What kind of voice training has the patient had? (ie, number of teachers, years of training, type of training)
  - What style of music is the patient performing? Has this changed recently?

- Prior evaluation and/or treatment

  - Has the larynx been examined previously?
  - What treatment has been tried? Was it successful or not? Was a full course of treatment completed?

- Occupational demands

  - How long are the performances? How frequent are the performances? What is the environment in which performances occur? (ie, size of venue, use of amplification, presence of other background noise)
  - What type of music is being performed? Is it familiar or unfamiliar to the singer? Is it easy or challenging material?
  - What are the sets like? (ie, nonstop screaming or singing for hours, breaks built into the set, mixture of singing and instrumental intervals)
  - What additional voice use does the patient have outside of performances? (eg, waitressing, bartending, parenting, cantoring/singing at church)

- Laryngeal irritants

  - This patient has a known history of smoking (both cigarettes as well as marijuana) but it is important to clarify the details of this history (quantity, duration, etc).
  - Are there other potential irritants, such as laryngopharyngeal reflux, allergic rhinitis, or post nasal drip? It can be important to ask about these potential factors explicitly, as patients may not consider hay fever for which they take an over-the-counter antihistamine occasionally as a "medical condition" or a "medication" to report, although either of these factors could possibly affect their voice symptoms.
  - Environmental factors (eg, exposure to secondhand smoke or allergens, background noise) that may impact the larynx should be identified and ameliorated.
  - Hydration status (ie, caffeine vs water intake) is commonly overlooked but can significantly affect the voice, especially in the presence of dehydrating medications.

QUALITY OF LIFE MEASURES

The importance of collecting and serially tracking quality of life measures over time cannot be overemphasized. These questionnaires play a vital role in helping clinicians understand the impact of the voice symptoms on the patient's functionality as well as allow monitoring of response to treatment over time. Currently several validated, voice-specific questionnaires are available, including the Voice Handicap Index (VHI),[19] the shortened Voice Handicap Index 10 (VHI-10),[20] and Voice Related Quality of Life (VR-QOL).[21] The VHI and VHI-10 have been translated and validated into more than 10 different languages each for use worldwide; fewer translations of the VR-QOL are available.[22,23]

PHYSICAL EXAM

A standard head and neck examination should be performed as with any patient, but with special attention paid to the presence of any neck masses or signs of recent trauma (eg, bruising) or surgery (eg, scarring). Physical examination alone—without stroboscopic laryngeal exam—is unlikely to determine the etiology for the dysphonia.

INVESTIGATIONS

Stroboscopy (either flexible or rigid) is the fundamental evaluation tool in the assessment of dysphonia. Details of the basics of stroboscopy are beyond the scope of this chapter and the reader is referred elsewhere for that information.[24–26] The question of whether flexible or rigid stroboscopy is better for dysphonia assessment is commonly debated. Proponents of rigid stroboscopy highlight its superior magnification (although the difference compared with chip-tip flexible stroboscopy instrumentation is relatively minimal), whereas advocates for flexible (particularly chip-tip) stroboscopy tout its ability to allow closer vocal fold inspection and its better tolerance by many patients compared with rigid stroboscopy. Additionally, flex-

ible stroboscopy permits evaluation of tasks, including connected speech, singing, etc, whereas rigid stroboscopy is limited to sustained phonation (typically /i/). For the evaluation of vocal fold lesions, rigid stroboscopy likely allows better visualization, but certainly either or both methodologies may be useful in select situations.

Another controversial issue associated with stroboscopy relates to the nomenclature used to describe and identify benign, midmembranous vocal fold lesions. A recent report by Rosen et al defined specific characteristics to describe nine categories of benign vocal fold lesions: vocal fold nodules, fibrous mass (both subepithelial and ligamentous), cyst (again, both subepithelial and ligamentous), polyp, pseudocyst, reactive lesion, and non-specific vocal fold lesion.[27] These authors advocated that use of such a standardized classification system would improve communication between clinicians as well as with patients and suggested that this development would also aid clinical research. A 2016 follow-up study demonstrated that voice outcomes were directly related to the type of lesion present.[28] Deeper lesions (termed "ligamentous" by these authors) were associated with worse voice outcomes, attributed to the deeper extent of the lesion and associated surgical excision[28] which may be related to an increased risk of scarring postoperatively.

Auditory-perceptual evaluations as well as acoustic and aerodynamic measures related to voice are often assessed by the speech-language pathologist and can provide additional information about the nature and extent of the voice dysfunction.[29] The Consensus Auditory Perceptual Evaluation–V (CAPE-V) was developed by the American Speech-Language Hearing Association to describe the severity of patients' voices and includes assessment of connected speech using six specifically selected sentences as well as a sustained vowel.[30,31] Acoustic measures historically had relied upon jitter, shimmer, and noise-to-harmonic ratio (NHR), but more recently these measures have fallen out of favor due to their limitations.[32] In recent years, evaluation of cepstral peak prominence (CPP) and cepstral spectral index of dysphonia (CSID) has increased due to their reliability in connected speech measurements.[33,34] Correlation between these acoustic measures and auditory-perceptual assessments of voice has previously been shown, particularly among specific voice disorders.[35,36] Aerodynamic measures include mean airflow during phonation, estimated subglottal pressure, and laryngeal airway resistance and may also demonstrate disorder-specific patterns.[37]

INITIAL MANAGEMENT

1. Discontinue all forms of smoking as well as alcohol.
2. Optimize hydration (eg, decrease caffeine and increase water intake).
3. Assess work demands (performance schedule, logistics, etc).

   a. Does the patient need to stop working during treatment?
   b. Does the patient need voice rest?
   c. How can the patient's situation be optimized? (increase amplification, decrease background noise, cancel performances, shorten performances, change performance material if possible, etc.)

4. Provide voice therapy, if appropriate.

   a. It is essential that the patient be assessed by a speech-language pathologist initially regarding his/her candidacy (or stimulability) for voice therapy.[38–42] This evaluation reveals if the patient can achieve immediate voice improvements following clinician instructions or models. The clinician is also able to determine the patient's motivation to change as well as to observe any cognitive or physical limitations that may hinder successful voice therapy participation. This type of examination performed at the time of the initial assessment has been shown to increase patient adherence to therapy[17,18] and voice outcomes after therapy[18] and thus avoids wasting time, resources, and money.

5. Reassess for progress.

   a. Timeline for reassessment is controversial and can vary.
   b. Typically, this author schedules patients for follow-up reevaluation approximately 4 weeks after completion of voice therapy. The additional time after completion of therapy allows patients to assess their voice symptoms and functionality after a short period of return to "normal" life.
   c. This follow-up appointment could occur earlier if there was a clinician concern (worries about compliance, progression of symptoms, etc) or if clinically indicated (eg, patient has an upcoming performance and wants to reassess to see if they are ready to proceed or if they need to cancel the performance).

ADDITIONAL MANAGEMENT

The next step(s) of treatment of this patient will be determined based on the patient's responses to the initial treatment plan.

SCENARIO 1: PATIENT'S SYMPTOMS AND LARYNGEAL EXAM ARE IMPROVED/RESOLVED

By definition, vocal fold nodules are bilateral, mid-membranous vocal fold lesions which resolve with voice therapy.[27] Subsequently, the voice improves and often even returns to normal.[28] In the presence of resolution of voice symptoms as well as of the vocal fold lesions, no further treatment is indicated. However, the patient should be counseled about the importance of maintaining adequate hydration and avoiding laryngeal irritants (tobacco, allergens, reflux, etc). The patient should also be instructed about prompt return for reevaluation in the event of recurrence of symptoms.

SCENARIO 2: PATIENT'S SYMPTOMS ARE IMPROVED BUT LARYNGEAL EXAM IS UNCHANGED

Occasionally, patient's symptoms respond well to medical and/or behavioral intervention even though vocal fold lesions may remain. In this situation, further active intervention may not be required, if the patient's functional and occupational needs are adequately met. If, in future, the patient has recurrence or progression of voice symptoms, then reevaluation may need to be performed to determine what, if any, additional treatment is indicated.

SCENARIO 3: NEITHER PATIENT'S SYMPTOMS NOR LARYNGEAL EXAM ARE IMPROVED

If the patient does not have a favorable response to medical and/or behavioral intervention(s), it is important to determine what factors might have impacted this response. Was the patient adherent to the treatment plan? Are all medical issues (eg, reflux, allergies, pulmonary disease) adequately controlled? Would a repeat (so-called refresher) course of voice therapy be helpful? All modifiable factors should be optimized, prior to deciding to proceed to surgical removal of the lesion(s).

If all medical and behavioral aspects have been addressed, then a detailed discussion should be undertaken regarding the risks versus benefits of surgical intervention. Some patients may decide to pursue other alternatives (ie, career changes) rather than undergo a surgical procedure. In selected patients, other "less invasive" procedures can be considered. These may include steroid injection (potentially, serially) or laser treatment (often using the 532-nm pulsed potassium-titanyl-phosphate [KTP] laser). Outcomes data on the use of these modalities for these lesions have focused on short-term results,[43–47] so these techniques are not commonly utilized as first-line treatment of phonotraumatic lesions at present in the US, except in select cases. If surgical removal of the lesion(s) is indicated, thorough conversation with the patient about all considerations about surgery including both risks and benefits should be pursued to guide patient's expectations appropriately.

SPECIAL CONSIDERATIONS ABOUT SURGERY

Specific details regarding surgical techniques for removal of these lesions are beyond the scope of this chapter and the reader is referred to other resources for that information.[48] However, there are many aspects of surgical treatment of vocal fold lesions which remain poorly defined and controversial. These topics are highlighted here for the reader's consideration.

1. Unilateral versus bilateral surgery

   a. If bilateral lesions are symmetric, often they may be treated identically.
   b. If the lesions are significantly asymmetric (e.g., a unilateral lesion with a contralateral reactive lesion),[27] then staged removal may be considered. Removal of the larger lesion (with or without additional treatment of the reactive lesion, such as with steroid injection) could result in resolution of the contralateral reactive lesion and/or voice symptoms, and thus avoidance of surgical excision (with its attendant risks) of the contralateral side. If, however, the lesion and/or its symptoms persist, then a second surgery

may need to be undertaken. Clearly, simultaneous removal of bilateral lesions eliminates this latter concern but is associated with increased operative time, longer duration of anesthesia, and potential risk of scarring to both vocal folds.
   c. If there is concern about non-adherence to treatment (ie, postoperative voice therapy), then staged removal of the lesions may be prudent.

2. Timing of surgery

   a. Surgical removal of vocal fold lesions is almost universally elective in nature. Therefore, it is vital to consider the timing of any surgical intervention. Are there important events (eg, performances, auditions, presentations, family events) in the near future? Does the patient have adequate time off to recover from surgery, including any postoperative voice rest period as well as postoperative voice therapy sessions? Adequate expectations are again crucial to this decision-making process.

3. Use of steroid injection as an adjunct to surgical excision

   a. Data on the use and impact of adjunctive steroid injection are sparse.[10] This treatment may be more helpful for lesions that extend more deeply into the vocal fold, as their removal carries a higher risk of postoperative stiffness and scarring.

4. Use of laser therapy as an adjunct to surgical excision.

   a. There is very limited information on the addition of laser therapy in this situation.[10] A 532-nm pulsed KTP laser (more often used than carbon dioxide [CO_2; 10600-nm] or pulsed dye laser [PDL, 585-nm]) may be targeted toward blood vessels presumed to "feed" the lesion and foster its continued growth.

5. Timing of postoperative follow-up

   a. There are no data about the optimal timing for postoperative assessment. Initial postoperative examinations can vary from 1 to 30 days after surgery. This author believes that 5 to 7 days is a reasonable duration of time to allow initial healing but also to perform early identification and potential treatment of any suboptimal healing (eg, early steroid injection for significant stiffness).

6. Postoperative voice rest

   a. Similar to the timing of postoperative follow-up, there are few data about the optimal duration for postoperative voice rest.[49,50] The range of prescribed voice rest has varied widely, from none up to sometimes more than 4 to 6 weeks. Typically, many laryngologists may prescribe 3 to 7 days of voice rest but the data supporting any of these choices are poorly clarified.[51] Preliminary results from Kiagiadaki et al showed no significant difference between 5 versus 10 days voice rest after phonomicrosurgery in a small cohort of patients.[52] However, Kaneko and colleagues found evidence of improved wound healing after 3 days of voice rest as opposed to 7 days, leading them to suggest that early, "appropriate" stimulation could improve healing and functional outcomes.[53]

   b. The use of absolute versus relative voice rest remains similarly debated. Absolute voice rest may facilitate healing by avoiding any potential traumatic impact from even normal vocal fold vibration[54]; however the early introduction of gentle phonation (eg, humming) may decrease the inflammatory response, which may also expedite healing.[50,55] Evidence for either of these options remains limited, and results may be further limited by a low rate of patient adherence to voice rest.

   c. Known low rates of patient adherence to voice rest instructions likely also impact voice outcomes. Rousseau et al found a 35% overall compliance rate with voice rest, even among a patient cohort that comprised mostly singers.[56]

7. Patient adherence

   a. This factor is a critically important consideration in the decision of the surgeon to proceed with surgery but can be highly controversial. Often, patients with voice disorders are highly motivated to improve and thus will stop smoking, drink more water, adhere to voice therapy, and other inducements. However, not all patients follow their recommended treatment plans. The challenge arises when a patient is nonadherent to treatment recommendations (eg, refuses to stop smoking, does not attend voice

therapy), yet pushes for surgery. Occasionally a patient may list various excuses for not coming to preoperative voice therapy (cost, timing, transportation, etc).[57,58] but make assurances about adhering strictly after surgery. It can be very difficult to refuse patient's requests in this situation, but poor adherence before surgery may be predictive of the same after surgery, and the patient's outcome may be best optimized by waiting for a more conducive time to pursue this elective procedure. This situation is where patient counseling and guidance of appropriate expectations are most critical.

8. Addition and duration of postoperative voice therapy

   a. The addition of postoperative voice therapy can be helpful in guiding the patient's voice during the healing process, particularly if the patient is resuming voice use after any type of voice rest. Education, counseling, and instruction about appropriate vocal techniques are also thought to be beneficial in preventing recurrence of the lesions.[10,49,52,58]

CONCLUSION

Benign vocal fold lesions (especially phonotraumatic lesions) are a common cause of dysphonia.[1,27] A combination of medical and behavioral intervention can be highly successful at resolving at least the voice symptoms associated with these lesions, if not the lesions themselves. However, in the case of persistent symptoms and/or lesions, surgical intervention may be required. Fortunately, judicious application of appropriate treatment often results in significant improvement in voice, with restored functionality and improved quality of life.[28]

REFERENCES

1. Cohen SM, Kim J, Roy N, Asche C, Courey M. Prevalence and causes of dysphonia in a large treatment-seeking population. *Laryngoscope*. 2012;122(2):343–348.
2. Roy N, Merrill RM, Gray SD, Smith EM. Voice disorders in the general population: prevalence, risk factors, and occupational impact. *Laryngoscope*. 2005;115(11):1988–1995.

3. Roy N, Merrill RM Thibeault S, Parsa RA, Gray SD, Smith EM. Prevalence of voice disorders in teachers and the general population. *J Speech Lang Hear Res.* 2004; 47(2):281–293.

4. Bainbridge KE, Roy N, Losonczy KG, Hoffman HJ, Cohen SM. Voice disorders and associated risk markers among young adults in the United States. *Laryngoscope.* 2017;127(9):2093–2099.

5. Ramig LO, Verdolini K. Treatment efficacy: voice disorders. *J Speech Lang Hear Res.* 1998:41(1):S101–S116.

6. Bhattacharyya N. The prevalence of voice problems among adults in the United States. *Laryngoscope.* 2014; 124(10):2359–2362.

7. Krischke S, Weigelt S, Hoppe U, Köllner V, Klotze M, Eysholdt U, Rosanowski F. Quality of life in dysphonic patients. *J Voice.* 2005;19(1):132–137.

8. Wilson JA, Deary IJ, Millar A, MacKenzie K. The quality of life impact of dysphonia. *Clin Otolaryngol Allied Sci.* 2002;27(3):179–182.

9. Verdolini K, Ramig L. Review: occupational risks for voice problems. *Logoped Phoniatr Vocol.* 2001;26(1):37–46.

10. Sulica L, Behrman A. Management of benign vocal fold lesions: a survey of current opinion and practice. *Ann Otol Rhinol Laryngol.* 2003;112(10):827–833.

11. Gillespie AI, Abbott K. The influence of clinical terminology on self-efficacy for voice. *Logoped Phoniatr Vocol.* 2011;36(3):91–99.

12. Fritzell P. Voice Disorders and Occupations. *Logoped Phoniatr Vocol.* 1996:21:7–12.

13. Titze IR, Lemke J, Montequin D. Populations in the US workforce who rely on voice as a primary tool of trade: a preliminary report. *J Voice.* 1997:11(3):254–259.

14. Jones K, Sigmon J, Hock L, Nelson E, Sullivan M, Ogren F. Prevalence and risk factors for voice problems among telemarketers. *Arch Otolaryngol Head Neck Surg.* 2002;128(5):571–577.

15. Cohen SM, Dupont W, Courey M. Quality-of-life impact of non-neoplastic voice disorders: a meta-analysis. *Ann Otol Rhinol Laryngol.* 2006;115(2):128–134.

16. Roy N, Merrill RM, Thibeault D, Gray SD, Smith EM. Voice disorders in teachers and the general population: effects on work performance, attendance, and future career choices. *J Speech Lang Hear Res.* 2004;47(3):542–551.

17. Starmer HM, Liu Z, Akst LM, Gourin C. Attendance in voice therapy: can an interdisciplinary care model have an impact? *Ann Otol Rhinol Laryngol.* 2014;123(2):117–123.

18. Litts JK, Gartner-Schmidt JL, Clary MS, Gillespie AI. Impact of combined laryngologist and speech-language pathologist co-assessment on treatment outcomes and billing revenue. *Laryngoscope,* 2015;125:2139–2142.

19. Jacobson BH, The Voice Handicap Index (VHI): development and validation. *Am J Speech Lang Pathol.* 1997:6(3): 66–70.

20. Rosen CA, Lee AS, Osborne J, Zullo T, Murry T. Development and validation of the Voice Handicap Index-10. *Laryngoscope.* 2004;114(9):1549–1556.

21. Hogikyan ND, Sethuraman G. Validation of an instrument to measure voice-related quality of life (V-RQOL). *J Voice.* 1999;13(4):557–569.

22. Seifpanahi S, Jalaie S, Nikoo MR, Sobhani-Rad D. Translated Versions of Voice Handicap Index (VHI)-30 across languages: a systematic review. *Iran J Public Health.* 2015; 44(4):458–469.

23. Gilbert M, Gartner-Schmidt J, Rosen C. The VHI-10 and VHI item reduction translations—are we all speaking the same language? *J Voice.* 2017;31(2):250e1–250e7.

24. Young VN, Rosen C. Videostroboscopy: USA perspective. In: Yiu M, ed, *Handbook of Voice Assessments.* San Diego, CA: Plural Publishing; 2011:99–112.

25. Carroll TL, Wu YH, McRay M, Gherson S. Frame by frame analysis of glottic insufficiency using laryngovideostroboscopy. *J Voice.* 2012;26(2):220–225.

26. Woo P. *Stroboscopy.* San Diego, CA: Plural; 2010.

27. Rosen CA, Gartner-Schmidt J, Hathaway B, Simpson CB, Postma GN, Courey M, Sataloff RT. A nomenclature paradigm for benign midmembranous vocal fold lesions. *Laryngoscope.* 2012;122(6):1335–1341.

28. Akbulut S, Gartner-Schmidt JL, Gillespie AI, Young VN, Smith LJ, Rosen CA. Voice outcomes following treatment of benign midmembranous vocal fold lesions using a nomenclature paradigm. *Laryngoscope.* 2016;126(2):415–420.

29. Behrman A. Common practices of voice therapists in the evaluation of patients. *J Voice.* 2005;19(3):454–469.

30. Kempster GB, Gerratt BR, Verdolini Abbott K, Barkmeier-Kraemer J, Hillman RE. Consensus auditory-perceptual evaluation of voice: development of a standardized clinical protocol. *Am J Speech Lang Pathol.* 2009;18(2):124–132.

31. Zraick RI, Kempster GB, Connor NP, Thibeault S, Klaben BK, Bursac Z, et al. Establishing validity of the Consensus Auditory-Perceptual Evaluation of Voice (CAPE-V). *Am J Speech Lang Pathol.* 2011;20(1):14–22.

32. Carding PN, Wilson JA, MacKenzie K, Deary IJ. Measuring voice outcomes: state of the science review. *J Laryngol Otol.* 2009;123(8):823–829.

33. Awan SN, Roy N, Jetté ME, Meltzner GS, Hillman RE. Quantifying dysphonia severity using a spectral/cepstral-based acoustic index: comparisons with auditory-perceptual judgements from the CAPE-V. *Clin Linguist Phon.* 2010;24(9):742–758.

34. Awan SN, Roy N, Zhang D, Cohen SM. Validation of the Cepstral Spectral Index of Dysphonia (CSID) as a screening tool for voice disorders: development of clinical cut-off scores. *J Voice.* 2016;30(2):130–144.

35. Gillespie AI, Dastolfo C, Magid N, Gartner-Schmidt J. Acoustic analysis of four common voice diagnoses: moving toward disorder-specific assessment. *J Voice.* 2014.

36. Gillespie AI, Gartner-Schmidt J, Lewandowski A, Awan SN. An examination of pre- and posttreatment acoustic versus auditory perceptual analyses of voice across four common voice disorders. *J Voice.* 2017.

37. Dastolfo C, Gartner-Schmidt J, Yu L, Carnes O, Gillespie AI. Aerodynamic outcomes of four common voice

disorders: moving toward disorder-specific assessment. *J Voice*. 2016;30(3):301–307.

38. Powell TW, Miccio A. Stimulability: a useful clinical tool. *J Commun Disord*. 1996:29(4):237–253.

39. Gillespie A, Gartner-Schmidt J. Immediate effect of stimulability assessment on acoustic, aerodynamic, and patient-perceptual measures of voice. *J Voice*. 2015.

40. Bonilha H, Dawson A. Creating a mastery experience during the voice evaluation. *J Voice*. 2012;26(5):665.e1–e7.

41. Dejonckere PH, Lebacq L. Plasticity of voice quality: a prognostic factor for outcome of voice therapy? *J Voice*. 2001;15(2):251–256.

42. Gartner-Schmidt J. Voice therapy for voice disorders. In: Johnson J, Rosen C, eds, *Bailey's Head and Neck Surgery–Otolaryngology*. Philadelphia, PA: Wolters Kluwer/Lippincott Williams & Wilkins; 2013.

43. Wang CT, Liao LJ, Lai MS, Cheng PW. Comparison of benign lesion regression following vocal fold steroid injection and vocal hygiene education. *Laryngoscope*. 2014;124(2):510–515.

44. Lee SH, Yeo JO, Choi JI, Jin HJ, Kim JP, Woo SH, Jin SM. Local steroid injection via the cricothyroid membrane in patients with a vocal nodule. *Arch Otolaryngol Head Neck Surg*. 2011;137(10):1011–1016.

45. Hsu YB, Lan M, Chang S. Percutaneous corticosteroid injection for vocal fold polyp. *Arch Otolaryngol Head Neck Surg*. 2009;135(8):776–780.

46. Sridharan S, Achlatis S, Ruiz R, Jeswani S, Fang Y, Branski RC, Amin MR. Patient-based outcomes of in-office KTP ablation of vocal fold polyps. *Laryngoscope*. 2014;124(5):1176–1179.

47. Wang CT, Huang TW, Liao JL, Lo WC, Lai MS, Cheng PW. Office-based potassium titanyl phosphate laser-assisted endoscopic vocal polypectomy. *JAMA Otolaryngol Head Neck Surg*. 2013;139(6):610–616.

48. Rosen C, Simpson C. Phonomicrosurgical voice procedures. In: *Operative Techniques in Laryngology*. Berlin, Germany: Springer; 2008:99–139.

49. Behrman A, Sulica L. Voice rest after microlaryngoscopy: current opinion and practice. *Laryngoscope*. 2003;113(12):2182–2186.

50. Koufman JA, Blalock P. Is voice rest never indicated? *J. Voice*. 1989;3(1):87–91.

51. Kaneko M, Hirano S. Voice rest after laryngeal surgery: what's the evidence? *Curr Opin Otolaryngol Head Neck Surg*. 2017;25(6):459–463.

52. Kiagiadaki D, Remacle M, Lawson G, Bachy Y, Van der Vorst S. The effect of voice rest on the outcome of phonosurgery for benign laryngeal lesions: preliminary results of a prospective randomized study. *Ann Otol Rhinol Laryngol*. 2015;124(5):407–412.

53. Kaneko M, Shiromoto O, Fujiu-Kurachi M, Kishimoto Y, Tateya I, Hirano S. Optimal duration for voice rest after vocal fold surgery: randomized controlled clinical study. *J Voice*. 2017;31(1):97–103.

54. Cho SH, Kim HT, Lee IJ, Kim MS, Park HJ. Influence of phonation on basement membrane zone recovery after phonomicrosurgery: a canine model. *Ann Otol Rhinol Laryngol*. 2000;109(7):658–666.

55. Branski RC, Perera P, Verdolini K, Rosen CA, Hebda PA, Agarwal S. Dynamic biomechanical strain inhibits IL-1beta-induced inflammation in vocal fold fibroblasts. *J Voice*. 2006.

56. Rousseau B, Cohen SM, Zeller AS, Scearce L, Tritter AG, Garrett CG. Compliance and quality of life in patients on prescribed voice rest. *Otolaryngol Head Neck Surg*. 2011;144(1):104–107.

57. Hapner E, Portone-Maira C, Johns 3rd M. A study of voice therapy dropout. *J Voice*. 2009;23(3):337–340.

58. van Leer E, Connor N. Patient perceptions of voice therapy adherence. *J Voice*. 2010;24(4):458–469.

CHAPTER 14

Dysphonia and Hemorrhage in Singers

Kristina Piastro

Dysphonia, while trivial to some, poses significant distress to a professional voice user. A singer's livelihood depends on the health of the larynx. Even minor complaints deserve the physician's full attention.

The most feared source of dysphonia in a performer is vocal fold hemorrhage, a source of great anxiety. Increased vascularization and associated lesions are not uncommonly seen in this population. Hemorrhage from the vessels may occur through phonotrauma and is usually sudden in onset (Figure 14–1). If the singer does not present in a timely fashion and continues to sing, resorption of the lesion may be hampered. A vascular or hemorrhagic polyp may form at the "striking zone" of the vocal fold, further complicating treatment.

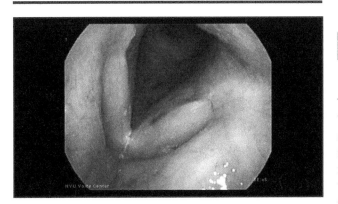

Figure 14–1. Left vocal fold hemorrhage at medial vocal fold edge.

CASE PRESENTATION

A 41-year-old male presents with a 2-week history of dysphonia. He noted an abrupt vocal change during a performance. At that time he was also suffering from an upper respiratory infection. At onset he recalled something "snapping" with his voice and loss of his upper range and resultant dysphonia. He reports increased variability in his singing; however, his speaking voice is intact. He also reports variability in the amount of effort and strain employed to sing. He denies odynophonia. He is in otherwise good health and denies any prior history of voice issues.

Social: Former smoker (quit 2006), social alcohol intake

Medications: None, no herbal or over-the-counter (OTC) supplements

INITIAL ASSESSMENT

History

Vocal fold hemorrhage usually is abrupt in onset with a notable decline in vocal quality. A precipitating event is usually noted. Events precipitating vocal fold hemorrhage not only include vocal strain but also coughing, vomiting, Valsalva, and weight lifting, among other causes[1]. The hemorrhage itself is not painful and should not cause difficulty with breathing or swallowing. Very rarely is the patient completely aphonic. The level of hoarseness is variable. Hoarseness may be obvious in the speaking voice or it may be subtle and only noted as a change in the singing voice.

Examination

Standard head and neck exam. Avoid pressing the patient for a perceptual vocal exam until visual laryngeal exam complete. Inquire about any blood thinning agents and/or OTC supplements as well as family history of bleeding disorders. If appropriate discuss menses.

Endoscopy

Transnasal or transoral fiberoptic laryngoscopy with stroboscopy should be performed.

EXAM FINDINGS

Office head and neck exam is normal. The patient presents with a constant dysphonia in both speaking and singing voice. He is found to have a yellow hemosiderin stained resolving hemorrhage at the anterior right vocal fold as well as bilateral internal laryngoceles (Figure 14–2). The vibration of the right vocal fold is dampened. The laryngoceles, at particularly higher pitches, appear to rest on the superior surface of the vocal folds.

Diagnosis

Resolving vocal fold hemorrhage

Management

Additional voice rest and follow-up with laryngeal exam to ensure hemorrhage resorption. Ensure that the patient is not currently taking any supplements that may cause a propensity to bleed. Consider voice therapy at resolution of hemorrhage. The therapy should be designed to improve laryngeal mechanics and prevent further strain leading to hemorrhage.

RECURRENT HEMORRHAGE

The patient ultimately has documented resorption of the hemorrhage and resolution of vibratory abnormality. He is able to return to performance. Four months later he presents again with similar symptoms. However, despite his dysphonia, he continued to perform and now has noted further decline in both his singing and speaking voice. He has been referred by his vocal coach and has an upcoming performance which he is eager to undertake. His speaking and singing voice are affected.

Exam Findings

The patient is noted to have a right-sided hemorrhagic polyp with surrounding hemorrhage (Figure 14–3). The

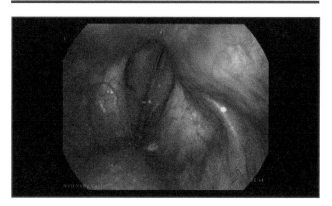

Figure 14–2. Right vocal fold resolving hemorrhage with yellow hemosiderin staining most prominent anteromedially.

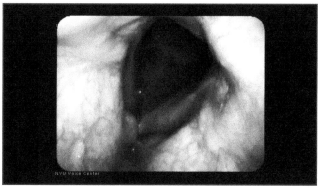

Figure 14–3. Right vocal fold hemorrhagic polyp and surrounding hemorrhage.

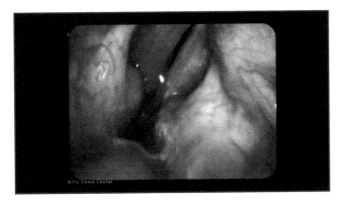

Figure 14–4. Right vocal fold hemorrhagic polyp and surrounding hemorrhage through the length of the medial vocal fold. Polyp prevents full glottis closure.

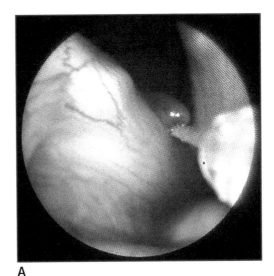

A

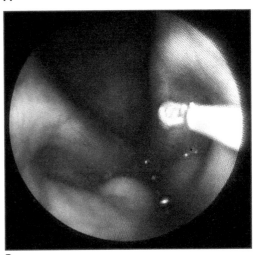

B

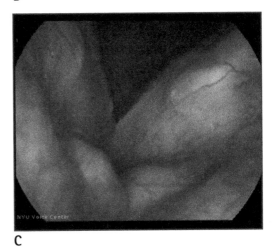

C

Figure 14–5. (**A** and **B**) Successful application of KTP laser therapy, with resolution of hemorrhagic polyp. (**C**) Patient at 6-week follow-up.

polyp prevents complete glottal closure (Figure 14–4). The right side mucosal wave is reduced.

Management

Hemorrhagic polyps, unlike hemorrhage alone, are unlikely to self-resolve. There are a variety of approaches at managing excision. Operative as well as in-office procedures may be offered, based on patient comfort, tolerance, and preference. We opt to use the potassium-titanyl-phosphate (KTP) laser in these presentations, as the polyp is small and in an easily accessible area despite presence of laryngoceles. KTP laser therapy was successfully performed in the office setting (Figure 14–5). The patient was cautioned to return to care should he experience any acute voice change. He was advised to avoid blood thinners and vocal strain until follow-up confirmed resolution and healing of the laser area. Ultimately he went on to recur with hemorrhage at the same right anterior vocal fold surface. This time it was felt that the laryngocele placed additional strain and dampens vibration of the right vocal fold. The recommendation is a direct laryngoscopy with ablation of the laryngocele to prevent further hemorrhagic recurrence and evaluate for underlying pathology.

DISCUSSION

Microvascular perturbations within the vocal fold have been described as varices, capillary ectasias, papillary ectasias, spider telengiectasias, and venous lakes. The anatomic variations are subtle on examination, with varices demonstrating a dilated, tortuous venous appearance and ectasias resembling coalescent hemangiomas. Varices and ectasias have been implicated in benign vocal fold lesions, including nodules and polyps as well as hemorrhage.

Histopathologic evaluation reveals that these blood vessels course through the superficial lamina propria (SLP), mainly adhering to a longitudinal direction. The vessels demonstrate many arteriovenous connections, allowing patency and circulation within the SLP during high-pressure vocal tasks. The undulating nature of the vasculature within the cover of the vocal fold allows for flexibility during changes in length, tension, and shearing stress during oscillation. The majority of ectasias and varices have been identified on the superior vocal fold edge and middle musculomembranous area, known as the striking zone, which is the area of greatest force during phonation.[2]

The etiology of vascular lesions remains uncertain and true prevalence is difficult to ascertain; however, it remains a fairly common finding in a laryngology practice[1]. An incidence of 3.5% was identified in a cohort of 800 patients.[3] In the professional voice user population, a much higher prevalence is observed, with 14% of female professional singers demonstrating vascular aberration. This leads many authors to believe that the root cause is related to repeat vocal trauma and inflammation as well as hormonal variations.

Menstruation-related hormone level variations cause laryngeal fluid retention, venous dilation, and edema of the interstitial tissues during the premenstrual period. Estrogen causes a mass effect on the vocal fold. Estrogens increase mucous flow and capillary permeability. Progesterone acts as an antagonist to estrogen and clamps down vessel permeability, trapping fluids and causing edema. The phenomenon is coined *dysphonia premenstrualis*, causing vocal fatigue, decreased vocal efficiency, unsteady pitch, and loss of range and high notes. At ovulation the fundamental frequency is noted to be higher.[4] Female singers tend to display dilation of varices in the premenstrual period and are at risk for hemorrhage during this time. Authors have suggested that there is vocal decline in the days leading up to menstruation and ovulation, during which performance is discouraged.[5] In fact some women performers are offered contractual "grace days." Data to support hormonally associated changes include evidence of laryngeal estrogen and progesterone receptors,[6] and observation of cervical and vocal fold thinning in post-menopausal women.[7] The afore-

mentioned studies have small sample sizes, and the effect of hormones continues to be disputed. A recent study looked at the vibratory characteristics of healthy premenopausal females without vocal complaints using high speed digital imaging. The study concluded that overall hormonal fluctuation during the menstrual cycle had no effect on the vibratory function of the vocal folds.[8] Estrogen peaks at ovulation, which precedes menstruation by 10 to 15 days, and it has the most effect on vascular dilation, yet no studies have demonstrated an increased risk of hemorrhage during this time. A firm recommendation to avoid heavy vocal use at this time remains the discretion of the medical professional.

Vocal fold varices may remain completely asymptomatic. However, the presence of varices has been noted to result in a 10-fold increase in risk of hemorrhage.[10] The vessels within the SLP are designed to withstand significant inertial stress. However, varices are known to be fragile and prone to rupture. Rupture may result in vocal fold hemorrhage, which easily spreads through the low resistance layer of the lamina propria, resulting in alteration of mucosal wave and amplitude and thus producing dysphonia. The onset is sudden and often temporally related to vocal trauma such as coughing, singing, yelling, etc.

Hemorrhage has also been associated with antiplatelet and anticoagulative medication, including coumadin/warfarin and heparin.[10] The use of aspirin and nonsteroidal anti-inflammatory drugs (NSAIDs) is considered to increase the risk and is discouraged in professional voice users. Anticoagulants and antiplatelet medications remain a mainstay of therapy for many conditions, and use must be weighed against risks and benefits. Many newer antithrombotic agents are not reversible and bleeding may be severe, resulting in an airway-compromising condition. The treating laryngologist should be familiar with these classes of medications and have a low threshold for close observation.

Recurrent hemorrhage may be seen in patients with high vocal demands, secondary to rupture of ectasias or varices. A leading hypothesis is that vocal fold phonotrauma as seen in professional singers, and sometimes in those with a vocal fold paralysis or a mucosal lesion would predispose to hemorrhage. However, a study by Tang et al in 513 professional voice users did not support an association with hemorrhage.[9] It has been proposed that hemorrhage would likely occur at the very lateral edge of the membranous vocal fold where the mucosal wave decelerates and begins to reverse course at the closing phase of oscillation. The same study revealed that location of a varix also appears not to increase predisposition to rupture. Tang concluded that the hemorrhage probability is over 60% in those with varices and approximately 5% in those without, at 50-month follow-up.

Hemorrhage is regarded as a devastating occurrence in the professional singer's career, resulting in performance cancellations and potential loss of income. It is generally believed that hemorrhage results in some element of scarring of the lamina propria.[11,12] Some authors recommend prompt hemorrhage evacuation to prevent scar and fibrosis.[11] However, there is a paucity of literature attributing scar formation to vocal fold hemorrhage. A recent study reviewed 41 patients who experienced vocal fold hemorrhage. It found at 40 months follow-up that there was no significant difference in patient perceptual or subjective vocal quality.[13] However, with recent media attention to famous pop stars and hemorrhage leading to tour canceling consequences, dysphonia leads to great anxiety in the professional voice user. The most common presenting symptom of hemorrhage is sudden onset of hoarseness (72%), decreased vocal range (16%), and vocal fatigue (12%).[3]

Treatment usually includes rest until resolution of hemorrhage is demonstrated endoscopically. If absolute voice rest is not possible, then intensity, frequency, and duration of voice used should be limited. Considering modifying mechanisms of glottal attacks such as cough and throat clearing is paramount. It is also important to address any other inflammatory conditions such as reflux, allergy, upper respiratory infection (URI), or laryngeal infection. In patients who avoid vocal misuse, recurrence is a rare phenomenon, with no recurrences in 11 patients reported at 4.5 years.[3] However, those with varices may experience a 48% rate of re-hemorrhage[14].

An asymptomatic varix does not need surgical or medical intervention. The patient should receive education about the possibility of hemorrhage and vocal change. In case of voice change the patient should observe strict voice rest until presentation for stroboscopic evaluation. The patient may resume vocal activities once the hemosiderin within the SLP has been resorbed. A patient who presents for evaluation will undergo a comprehensive voice evaluation as well as exam. These should include acoustic and aerodynamic testing as well as endoscopy with and without stroboscopy. If there are clinical findings of reflux, this should be addressed aggressively, with diet and behavior modification as well as blocking agents such as alginates, or anti-acids such as histamine receptor antagonists (H2RAs) or proton pump inhibitors (PPIs).

It is important to increase hydration, and some authors have advocated utilizing a mucolytic.[3] Discuss with the patient any anticoagulant medication use. Both prescribed and over-the-counter/herbal preparations should be evaluated for anticoagulant properties. If applicable, the discussion of any hormone therapies or noting the time within the menstrual cycle may be relevant.

Initial presentation with vocal fold hemorrhage should prompt immediate voice rest for 7 to 14 days as well as addressing some of the modifiers mentioned above. If a significant hematoma persists, some authors have advised a superiorly based cordotomy and gentle suction evacuation followed by an additional week of voice rest.[15] Once resolution is demonstrated, the patient should be counseled on potential recurrence, seen in follow-up with consideration of voice therapy.

Recurrent hemorrhage in the setting of an underlying varix is an indication for surgical intervention. The treatment in professional voice users and the lay public is the same. Timing of intervention is crucial for the performer, as post-treatment may require prolonged voice rest (1–2 weeks). Care and appropriate counseling must occur when discussing intervention for varices, as surgery itself may result in scar, reduced pliability, and an unacceptable vocal outcome. If there are multiple lesions, decision should be made in regard to staging interventions. If the lesions approximate each other at the medial edge of the vocal folds, to avoid postoperative webbing, a two-staged approach should be considered.

The offending vessel may be treated by either ablation or excision. Cold instrumentation was the preferred method of removal until the advent of laser therapies. Initially the CO_2 laser was popularized as it was felt to avoid excising healthy epithelium. However, it causes significant thermal injury, reduces pliability of the vocal fold mucosa, and may lead to scar formation. Cold excision is still employed at times for lesions that were difficult to access with laser or in instances of removing additional vocal fold pathology. Cold approach is performed microsurgically. Epithelial cordotomies are made overlying the varix and the varix is dissected free from the surrounding lamina propria.

The advent of angiolytic lasers sought to resolve the above CO_2 laser concerns. Using a flexible fiber delivery system, angiolytic lasers, such as KTP (532 nm) and pulsed-dye laser (PDL) (585 nm), target oxyhemoglobin. It is now possible to target the vessel at the subepithelial level. PDL and KTP lasers were studied concomitantly in 39 patients.[16] PDL laser was found to cause more subepithelial bleeding compared with KTP ablation. This required incision and drainage to avoid the absorbance of laser energy by the additional blood within the SLP, as well as to improve postoperative healing. There were no episodes of recurrent hemorrhage and all patients were able to return to singing without subjective vocal complaints. No patient was observed to have decreased mucosal wave function in the area of photoangiolytic laser treatment. Operative time was also noted to be shorter than similar lesions previously addressed with a cold knife technique. PDL was noted to cause more heating of the tissues, and the KTP was able to be adjusted to distribute laser energy over a longer time period, thus avoiding vessel rupture. Those treated with KTP were less likely to have hemosiderin present within the SLP at 2 weeks and thus could undertake a more rapid return to vocal function.

Recently Woo demonstrated the use of hyaluronidase injection in three cases of acute vocal fold hemorrhage. Noting that hyaluronidase is approved for accelerating reabsorption in vitreous hemorrhage, it was applied to the vocal fold in an off-label fashion. He noted the absence of the usual hemosiderin and edema generally present at one week post rupture. At follow-up, none of the three patients experienced rehemorrhage and all have been able to perform successfully and avoid surgical intervention.

Long-term follow-up of vocal fold hemorrhage in a group of 41 patients treated with voice rest did not demonstrate negative subjective or perceptual voice decline.[13]

REFERENCES

1. Lin PT, Stern JC, Gould WJ. Risk factors and management of vocal cord hemorrhages: an experience with 44 cases. *J Voice.*1991;5(1):74–77.

2. Hochman I, Sataloff RT, Hillman RE, Zeitels SM. Ectasias and varices of the vocal fold: clearing the striking zone. *Ann Otol Rhinol Laryngol.* 1999;108(1):10–16.

3. Postma GN, Courey MS, Ossoff RH. Microvascular lesions of the true vocal fold. *Ann Otol Rhinol Laryngol.* 1998;107(6):472–476.

4. Bryant G, Haselton M. Vocal cues of ovulation in human females. *Biol Lett.* 2009;5:12–15.

5. Chae SW, Choi G, Kang HJ, Choi JO, Jin SM. Clinical analysis of voice change as a parameter of premenstrual syndrome. *J Voice.* 2001;15(2):278–283.

6. Newman SR, Butler J, Hammond EH, Gray SD. Preliminary report on hormone receptors in the human vocal fold. *J Voice.* 1998;14(1):72–81.

7. Caruso S, Roccasalva L, Sapienza G. Laryngeal cytological aspects in women with surgically induced menopause who were treated with transdermal estrogen replacement therapy. *Fertil Steril.* 2000;74:1073–1079.

8. Kunduk M, Vansant MB, Ikuma T, McWhorter A. The effects of the menstrual cycle on vibratory characteristics of the vocal folds investigated with high-speed digital imaging. *J Voice.* 2017; 31:182–187.

9. Tang CG, Askin G, Christos PJ, Sulica L. Vocal fold varices and risk of hemorrhage. *Laryngoscope.* 2016;126: 1163–1168.

10. Neely JL, Rosen C. Vocal fold hemorrhage associated with coumadin therapy in an opera singer. *J Voice.* 2000; 14: 272–277.

11. Abitbol J. Vocal cord hemorrhages in voice professionals. *J Voice.* 1988;2:261–266.

12. Hsiung MW, Kang BH, Su WF, Pai L, Wang HW. Clearing microvascular lesions of the true vocal fold with the KTP/532 laser. *Ann Otol Rhinol Laryngol.* 2003:112: 534–539.

13. Kerwin LJ, Estes C, Oromendia C, Christos P, Sulica L. Long-term consequences of vocal fold hemorrhage. *Laryngoscope.* 2017;127:900–906.

14. Lennon CJ, Murry T, Sulica L. Vocal fold hemorrhage: factors predicting recurrence. *Laryngoscope.* 2014;124(1): 227–232.

15. Spiegel JR, Sataloff RT, Hawkshaw M, et al. Vocal fold hemorrhage. *Ear Nose Throat J.* 1996;75:784–789.

16. Zeitels SM, Akst LM, Burns JA, Hillman RE, Broadhurst MS, Anderson RR. Pulsed angiolytic laser treatment of ectasias and varices in singers. *Ann Otol Rhinol Laryngol.* 2006;115:571–580.

CHAPTER 15

Vocal Fold Scar

Lesley F. Childs and Ted Mau

INTRODUCTION

Vocal fold scar and sulcus represent some of the most challenging laryngologic entities. These lamina propria disorders involve a loss of normal vocal fold vibratory properties and can cause significant dysphonia. Many therapeutic strategies have been proposed, but a widely accepted and reliable treatment remains elusive.

DEFINITION

Vocal fold scarring occurs when a reparative response to injury produces fibrous tissue that is by nature stiff and lacks the vibratory properties of the native lamina propria. Sulcus is a congenital or acquired thinning or focal deficiency of lamina propria with epithelial invagination to the deeper part of the lamina propria.

CLINICAL CASE

A 36-year-old male call center employee notes progressive raspiness in his voice over the past 18 months. His voice quality initially would fluctuate; however, over the past year it has been persistently abnormal and strained. Prior to working at the call center, he served in the military as a drill sergeant.

Past medical history: allergic rhinitis

Social history: non-smoker, occasional alcohol

Medications: fluticasone propionate daily, fexofenadine prn

Allergies: no known drug allergies (NKDA)

INITIAL ASSESSMENT

History

His vocal demands professionally, both as a military drill sergeant and now a call center employee, predispose him to phonotraumatic vocal fold injury. The progressive nature of his dysphonia and the persistence of his symptoms imply a pathologic process that has been increasing in severity over time.

Examination

Subjectively, his voice is severely dysphonic, marked by breathiness and a strained quality. A comprehensive head and neck examination reveals thyrohyoid space tenderness and increased upper body tension.

SCENARIO 1

Laryngeal videostroboscopy: Laryngeal videostroboscopy reveals a focal, linear area of tethering with associated stiffness (or reduced amplitude of vibration) and hypervascularity along the leading edge of the left true vocal fold vibratory surface. Diffuse glottic edema is noted as well as glottic insufficiency and compensatory supraglottic hyperfunction.

Diagnosis: Left true vocal fold type 3 sulcus (sulcus vocalis)

Management: Voice therapy to assist with laryngeal unloading given the compensatory hyperfunctional activity present followed by a composite thyroid ala perichondrium flap.

SCENARIO 2

Laryngeal videostroboscopy: Reveals stiffness and thickening of the anterior one-third of the right true vocal fold vibratory surface. Glottic insufficiency and compensatory supraglottic hyperfunction are severe.

Diagnosis: Right vocal fold scar

Management: Voice therapy to assist with laryngeal unloading followed by an autologous temporalis fascia implant

DIFFERENTIAL DIAGNOSIS

Without the addition of videostroboscopy, inspection with a continuous light source would not reveal stiffness, therefore it is possible that only glottic insufficiency or even simply hyperfunction would be apparent. This may mistakenly lead to a diagnosis of atrophy, paresis, or primary muscle tension dysphonia. With the addition of stroboscopy, however, the stiffness underlying the glottic insufficiency indicates either scar or sulcus as the underlying etiology. Furthermore, the linear tethering in the first scenario confirms a sulcus and the surrounding inflammation points to a type 3 variety.

PITFALLS

As mentioned previously, the key is evaluating the vocal folds using videostroboscopy, without which an accurate diagnosis would not be possible. Even though videostroboscopy indicates stiffness and thus a high suspicion of scar or sulcus follows, diagnostic confirmation may require a diagnostic microsuspension laryngoscopy.

DISCUSSION

Scar Versus Sulcus

Although treatment options for both scar and sulcus overlap, histopathologically they differ. Ford and colleagues described three types of sulcus. Type 1 is termed "physiologic" and is significant for the presence of a medial concavity during some phase of vibration but without obvious histopathologic aberrance in the lamina propria. Types 2 and 3 sulci are associated with vocal fold stiffness and a loss of functional lamina propria, hence their determination as "pathologic" varieties.[1] Type 2 is referred to as "sulcus vergeture" and is believed to have a congenital or hereditary basis.[2,3] Additionally, type 2 sulci extend the length of the membranous vocal fold to the depth of the intermediate or deep layers of the lamina propria; these are without associated glottic inflammation. In contrast, a type 3 sulcus or "sulcus vocalis" is often described as a focal, pit-like deficit involving the vocal ligament or muscle with associated glottic inflammation. A "mucosal bridge" presents as two parallel sulci on the medial and superior surface of a vocal fold with normal-appearing mucosa in between. The etiology of a mucosal bridge is thought to be a ruptured cyst.

Whereas a type 3 sulcus is a relatively specific sequela of injury, vocal fold scar is a common product of injury to the vocal fold mucosa when the entire depth of the superficial lamina propria is injured or removed. The resultant fibrotic healing response leads to reduced vocal fold mucosal pliability, contracture with glottic insufficiency, and often dysphonia that is severe. In human vocal folds, excessive and disorganized collagen deposition is notable in areas of scar, especially in cases associated with deeper levels of injury.[4] The failure to restore vibratory function to the vocal folds is the single most common finding in patients with persistent dysphonia following laryngeal surgery.[5] Furthermore, post-surgical scarring following excision of a vocal fold lesion is likely poorly recognized in settings where videostroboscopy is not consistently performed.[6]

assessment for vocal fold vibrations by HSDI than by videostroboscopy.[9]

Diagnostic Considerations

A history of prolonged hoarseness is typical in cases of scar and sulcus. Specifically, with sulcus vergeture, hoarseness will most often be lifelong. The dysphonia is often both breathy and rough with an overlying straining pattern; the breathiness is secondary to the glottal insufficiency, the roughness is a result of aperiodic vibrations, and the straining pattern is consistent with compensatory hyperfunction. Eliciting a history of phonotrauma, previous vocal fold surgery (including laser treatment), radiation, or a traumatic intubation can help to clarify a diagnosis of sulcus vocalis or scar.

Perceptual, aerodynamic, and acoustic testing assists with estimating the dysphonia severity and helps serve as a comparison post-treatment.

Given that sulcus and scar both represent pathologic lamina propria manifesting as a loss of normal vibration, laryngoscopy with a continuous light source is insufficient for diagnostic purposes. As described by Hirano,[4] the presence of a mucosal wave indicates adequate functional separation of the vocal fold body and cover; histologically this requires an intact superficial lamina propria.[1] Thus, videostroboscopy is critical and will reveal stiffness or reduced amplitude of vibration and mucosal wave in the region of the scar or sulcus. More specifically, a linear tethering (unilateral or bilateral) or groove in the region of stiffness with a spindle-shaped glottal insufficiency indicates the presence of a sulcus.[7] Stroboscopically, the preservation of a mucosal wave has been reported to distinguish type 2 (sulcus vergeture) from type 3 (sulcus vocalis).[8] Frequently an overlay of compensatory supraglottic hyperfunction is present in patients with both sulcus and scar.

In patients with severe dysphonia, stroboscopic synchronization failure can occur due to the absence of a stable fundamental frequency resulting in less vibratory information. Similarly, limited methods of analyses applicable to stroboscopic data make quantitative comparisons more difficult. High-speed digital imaging (HSDI) uses a high frame rate to characterize vocal fold vibrations through entire cycles and improves the assessment of patients with severe dysphonia where the vibrations are highly aperiodic. Yamauchi et al compared videostroboscopy to HSDI for sulcus vocalis and noted that 1.6 times more patients could undergo

TREATMENT OPTIONS

Voice Therapy

Behavioral intervention, in the form of voice therapy, is particularly useful for purposes of laryngeal unloading, or decreasing the compensatory hyperfunction often present with both sulcus and scar. By optimizing and coordinating the unaffected vocal subsystems such as breath support and resonance, sound source abnormalities may become less obvious. Additionally, in cases with a phonotraumatic etiology, preventing further trauma to the lamina propria is ideal. In fact, prevention of the development of sulcus and scar is the most important intervention of all.

Surgery

The various surgical options to treat sulcus or scar address either the glottic insufficiency or the lamina propria itself. As mentioned earlier, no surgery at all is a valid treatment option given that complete normalization of voice quality is rarely achieved from surgical intervention.

Surgical Options to Reduce Glottal Gap

The glottal gap left by sulcus or scar can be reduced by injection augmentation (as an office-based procedure or under a general anesthetic) or a type I thyroplasty (most often performed under a local anesthetic with sedation-analgesia). A trial injection augmentation (especially if performed in an office setting) provides a convenient way to assess the level of vocal improvement and may help to inform the decision-making process when considering a permanent intervention in the form of thyroplasty. An injection augmentation (either transoral or transcervical) involves the injection of a filler agent into the paraglottic space, with resultant medial shifting of the vocal fold edge and reduction of the glottal gap. The commercially available injectables in the Americas are non-permanent by nature, whereas some permanent synthetic injectables are available in Europe and Asia. Fat, the oldest material, requires a harvest but provides more durable results. A type I thyroplasty or medialization laryngoplasty involves placement of a non-absorbable implant into the paraglottic space via a window created in the thyroid cartilage in order to medialize the vocal fold edge.

It is important to recognize that these options do not address the mucosal pliability problem, so while they may result in a reduction in perceived breathiness or vocal fatigue, the voice quality will remain abnormal.

Surgical Options to Target Scar

The pathologic lamina propria in sulcus and scar can be addressed via excisions, superficial injections, or laser treatment. Excisions of pathologic tissue through microdissection techniques require separating adherent tissue from the vocal ligament, with difficulty achieving coaptation of non-diseased edges and the potential for further scarring.[1] Pontes described a mucosal slicing technique with the surgical goal of disrupting the longitudinal tension of the scar. Postoperative recovery times of up to a year have been described following this technique.[10] Steroid injections into the superficial lamina propria of scarred vocal folds are based on successful treatment of hypertrophic cutaneous scar and keloids. Steroids also possess anti-inflammatory effects and decrease collagen synthesis. In a case series by Young et al, office-based steroid injections in 25 patients for mildmoderate vocal fold scar in combination with voice therapy was associated with improved patient-reported and functional voice measures. More specifically, the largest improvement in aerodynamic parameters occurred with a decreased phonation threshold pressure, most likely due to decreased vocal fold stiffness. Vocal fold steroid injections are procedures that can be performed in the office setting, are low risk, and do not preclude more invasive procedures later.[11] Treatment of fibrotic lesions in rat vocal folds using the potassium titanyl phosphate laser (KTP), as described by Sheu et al in 2013, induced an inflammatory response modulated by matrix metalloproteinases (MMPs) but resulted in little effect on the histologic appearance of the scar.[12]

Surgical Options to Restore Lamina Propria Depth

Various techniques and implant materials have been described to restore the bulk or depth of the lamina propria. Surgical manipulation of the lamina propria

through a subepithelial plane accessed through a window in the thyroid cartilage was first described by Steven Gray in 1999, specifically for the implantation of fat. This technique had two advantages over endolaryngeal approaches. First, the lamina propria was accessed without superior vocal fold surface dissection, thereby decreasing the risk of fat migration from the free edge to the superior surface. Second, there was no connection between the subepithelial space and the glottis, so the implant material could not extrude through the vocal fold surface. The use of fat implantation stems from the idea of improving tissue viscoelasticity, as fat has mechanical properties similar to those of the human vocal fold superficial lamina propria. Additionally, by separating the cover and body, this hopefully prevents fibroblast migration and resultant scar formation.[13] Mallur et al examined the outcome of 16 patients at a single institution undergoing a Gray's minithyrotomy procedure with fat (one patient with fat/fascia combination). All patients reported subjective improvement in their voice quality, while half showed an improvement in videostroboscopic parameters.[14] In an effort to improve the precision of Gray's minithyrotomy, microendoscopy of Reinke's space (MERS) was introduced to decrease the most commonly reported complication of mucosal perforation. The dissection of the lamina propria was performed with direct visualization of Reinke's space.[15]

Fascial implant into the vocal fold was first introduced by Rihkanen in 1998 to treat unilateral vocal fold paralysis.[16] Tsunoda adopted fascial implant to treat sulcus when autologous temporalis fascia was implanted superficially into the vocal fold.[17] Pitman et al retrospectively examined 19 vocal folds with scar or sulcus treated with temporalis fascia transplant with follow-up data after at least 1 year. Subjective improvements in voice handicap were noted in six of seven patients and 16 of 19 vocal folds demonstrated an improvement in mucosal wave.[18] In a prospective multi-arm evaluation comparing type I thyroplasty, injection laryngoplasty, and temporalis fascia implantation for vocal fold scar and sulcus, no single treatment modality demonstrated superiority overall. Type I thyroplasty and fascial implantation resulted only in improved VHI, while injection laryngoplasty resulted in no improvement on any vocal function index. Fascial implantation patients exhibited the slowest trajectory of improvement.[19] Pitman et al described a scaffold implant for the superficial lamina propria comprising small intestinal submucosa (SIS) that is porcine derived and contains key elements required for tissue regeneration. At 6 weeks post implantation into canine vocal folds, new, normal-appearing extracellular matrix components were diffusely dispersed throughout the implant. Future studies are necessary to evaluate functional outcomes.[20]

Dailey et al introduced a vascularized implant intended for Reinke's space.[21] This novel concept addressed the problem of eventual resorption of free grafts such as temporalis fascia. Two soft tissue rotational flaps were described: the thyroid ala perichondrium flap (TAP) and the composite thyroid ala perichondrium flap (CTAP).[21] These were raised and rotated into Reinke's space via a minithyrotomy. In 2015, the CTAP was further assessed using scarred canine vocal folds and revealed lower phonation threshold pressure and open quotient, as well as percent jitter and shimmer values.[22]

FUTURE TREATMENT OPTIONS

A variety of regenerative medicine and tissue engineering approaches have been proposed to address vocal fold scarring.[23] Growth factor therapy is predicated on the specific profile of the growth factor to direct the inflammatory response. As an example, the injection of hepatocyte growth factor (HGF) into scarred vocal folds has been shown to reduce collagen deposition, improve mucosal wave amplitude, and reduce glottal incompetence in animal models.[24,25]

Various tissue scaffolds have been proposed to restore the lamina propria. These can consist of decellularized biological tissue from sources such as liver, umbilical vein, or vocal fold that are rich with extracellular matrix (ECM), and the decellularized ECM can be seeded with cells with desired regenerative profile (see next paragraph). Other examples of biological scaffolds include hydrogels formed by collagen, cross-linked hyaluronic acid, or fibrin. Scaffolds can also be synthetic—for example, poly-(ethylene glycol)-diacrylate hydrogels. The purpose of any scaffold is not necessarily to persist and maintain structure in the target organ. Its function is to provide a microenvironment for native or transplanted cells to migrate into or populate an area of tissue deficiency so that over time new ECM can be established to restore the missing tissue.

Cell-based therapies have been proposed either alone or in combination with scaffolds.[26] Injections of autologous vocal fold fibroblasts into scarred vocal folds have shown benefit in animal models.[27,28] Similar benefits have been demonstrated for embryonic stem cells, bone marrow–derived mesenchymal stem cells (MSCs), adipose-derived stem cells (ASCs), and induced pluripotent stem cells, among others.[26]

A conceptually radical approach is to replace a diseased lamina propria altogether with a tissue engineered construct. This has been shown to be feasible in a rabbit model. ASCs embedded within a 3D fibrin scaffold comprised a total vocal fold mucosa replacement that was superior to a native free vocal fold mucosal graft in terms of histologic and functional outcomes.[29,30] This and other approaches that are successful in laboratories today will hopefully lead to clinical solutions in the future for vocal fold scarring.

SUMMARY

In summary, the myriad of treatment options for the severely dysphonic population who suffer with vocal fold scar and sulcus underscores the clinical challenge that is diseased lamina propria. Surgical treatment to address the resulting glottic insufficiency and/or injured lamina propria can be performed in addition to behavioral management in the form of voice therapy intervention. Indeed, working to prevent injury to the vocal fold mucosa is the most important intervention of all.

REFERENCES

1. Ford CN, Inagi K, Khidr A, Bless DM, Gilchrist KW. Sulcus vocalis: a rational analytical approach to diagnosis and management. *Ann Otol Rhinol Laryngol.* 1996;105:189–200.

2. Husain S, Sulica L. Familial sulcus vergeture: further evidence for congenital origin of type 2 sulcus. *J Voice.* 2015;30:761.e19–761.e.21.

3. Martins RH, Goncalves TM, Neves DS, Fracalossi TA, Tavares EL, Moretti-Ferreira D. Sulcus vocalis: evidence for autosomal dominant inheritance. *Genet Molec Res.* 2011;10(4): 3163–3168.

4. Hirano S, Minamiguchi S, Yamashita M. Ohno T, Kanemaru S, Kitamura M. Histologic characterization of human scarred vocal folds. *J Voice.* 2009;23(4):399–407.

5. Woo P, Casper J, Colton R, Brewer D. Diagnosis and treatment of persistent dysphonia after laryngeal surgery: a retrospective analysis of 62 patients. *Laryngoscope.* 1994;104:1084–1091.

6. Benninger MS, Alessi D, Archer S, Bastian R, Ford C, Koufman J, Sataloff RT. Vocal fold scarring: current concepts and management. *Otolaryngol Head Neck Surg.* November 1996;474–482.

7. Selleck AM, Moore JE, Rutt AL, Hu A, Sataloff RT. Sulcus vocalis (type III): prevalence and strobovideolaryngoscopy characteristics. *J Voice*. 2015;29(4):507–511.

8. Giovanni A, Chanteret C, Lagier A. Sulcus vocalis: a review. *Eur Arch Otorhinolaryngol*. 2007;264:337–344.

9. Yamauchi A, Yokonishi H, Imagawa H, Sakakibara KI, Nito T, Tayama N et al. Characterization of vocal fold vibration in sulcus vocalis using high-speed digital imaging. *J Speech Lang Hear Res*. 2017;60:24–37.

10. Pontes P, Behlau M. Sulcus mucosal slicing technique. *Curr Opin Otolaryngol Head Neck Surg*. 2010;18:512–520.

11. Young WG, Hoffman MR, Koszewski IJ, Whited CW, Ruel BN, Dailey SH. Voice outcomes following a single office-based steroid injection for vocal fold scar. *Otolaryngol Head Neck Surg*. 2016;155(5):820–828.

12. Sheu M, Sridharan S, Paul B, Mallur P, Gandonu S, Bing R, et al. The utility of the potassium titanyl phosphate laser in modulating vocal folds scar in a rat model. *Laryngoscope*. 2013;123:2189–2194.

13. Gray SD, Bielamowicz SA, Titze IR, Dove H, Ludlow C. Experimental approaches to vocal fold alteration: introduction to the minithyrotomy. *Ann Otol Rhinol Laryngol*. 1999;108(1):1–9.

14. Mallur PS, Gartner-Schmidt J, Rosen CA. Voice outcomes following the Gray minithyrotomy. *Ann Otol Rhinol Laryngol*. 2012;121(7):490–496.

15. Hoffman HT, Bock JM, Karnell LH, Ahlrichs-Hanson J. Microendoscopy of Reinke's space. *Ann Otol Rhinol Laryngol*. 2008;117(7):510–514.

16. Rihkanen H. Vocal fold augmentation by injection of autologous fascia. *Laryngoscope*. 1998;108:51–54.

17. Tsunoda K, Takanosawa M, Niimi S. Autologous transplantation of fascia into the vocal fold: a new phonosurgical technique for glottal incompetence. *Laryngoscope*. 1999;109:504–508.

18. Pitman MJ, Rubino SM, Cooper AL. Temporalis fascia transplant for vocal fold scar and sulcus vocalis. *Laryngoscope*. 2014;124:1653–1658.

19. Welham NV, Choi WH, Dailey SH, Ford CN, Jiang JJ, Bless DM. Prospective multi-arm evaluation of surgical treatment for vocal fold scar and pathologic sulcus vocalis. *Laryngoscope*. 2011;121:1252–1260.

20. Pitman MJ, Cabin JA, Iacob CE. Small intestinal submucosa implantation for the possible treatment of vocal fold scar, sulcus, and superficial lamina propria atrophy. *Ann Otol Rhinol Laryngol*. 2016;125(2):137–144.

21. Dailey SH, Gunderson M, Chan R, Torrealba J, Kimura M, Welham NV. Local vascularized flaps for augmentation of Reinke's space. *Laryngoscope*. 2011;121:S37–S60.

22. Hoffman MR, Glab R, Gunderson M, Maytag AL, Yang DT, Jiang JJ, Dailey SH. Functional and histological evaluation following canine vocal fold reconstruction using composite thyroid ala perichondrium flaps. *Otolaryngol Head Neck Surg*. 2015;153(1):79–87.

23. Long JL. Tissue engineering for treatment of vocal fold scar. *Curr Opin Otolaryngol Head Neck Surg*. 2010;18:521–525.

24. Hirano S, Bless DM, Rousseau B, et al. Prevention of vocal fold scarring by topical injection of hepatocyte growth factor in rabbit model. *Laryngoscope* 2004;114:548–556.

25. Hirano S, Bless DM, Nagai H, et al. Growth factor therapy for vocal fold scarring in canine model. *Ann Otol Rhinol Laryngol*. 2004;113:777–785.

26. Fishman JM, Long J, Gugatschka M, et al. Stem cell approaches for vocal fold regeneration. *Laryngoscope*. 2016;126(8):1865–1870.

27. Chhetri DK, Head C, Revazova E, Hart S, Bhuta S, Berke GS. Lamina propria replacement therapy with cultured autologous fibroblasts for vocal fold scars. *Otolaryngol Head Neck Surg*. 2004;131(6):864–870.

28. Thibeault SL, Klemuk SA, Smith ME, et al. In vivo comparison of biomimetic approaches for tissue regeneration of the scarred vocal fold. *Tissue Eng Part A*. 2009;15:1481–1487.

29. Shiba TL, Hardy J, Luegmair G, Zhang Z, Long JL. Tissue-engineered vocal fold mucosa implantation in rabbits. *Otolaryngol Head Neck Surg*. 2016;154(4):679–688.

30. Long JL. Repairing the vibratory vocal fold. *Laryngoscope*. 2018;128(1):153–159. doi: 10.1002/lary.26801.

CHAPTER 16

Chronic Laryngeal Inflammation

Andree-Anne Leclerc and Clark A. Rosen

CASE PRESENTATION

A 38-year-old woman presents with hoarseness. She has a 3 months history of progressive dypshonia, odynophonia, and odynophagia. With rest, her voice quality and pain improves but never returns to normal voice quality, nor does she become pain free. Drinking water helps temporarily for the dryness sensation and mentholated lozenges reduce the pain temporarily. She was recently treated with antibiotics and oral steroids by her primary care physician, but the slight improvement did not last (details of treatment, type, and duration not known).

Medical history: Gastroesophageal reflux disease (GERD), anemia, migraine, asthma.

Medication: Proton pump inhibitor (PPI) for more than 10 years.

Social: Stopped smoking 10 years ago, no alcohol, no drugs.

Work: Owns, manages, and works at a nail salon.

The term "laryngitis" is defined as an inflammation of the larynx, regardless of the etiology and can be subcategorized as acute or chronic. Acute laryngeal inflammation usually lasts less than 7 to 14 days[1–3] and is self-limiting.[4,5] Acute laryngeal inflammation is believed to result from viral infection most of the time, but a bacterial or fungal infection can also be the etiology.[4] The majority of those patients are never seen by an otolaryngologist. On the other hand, there is no specific definition of time for designation of "chronic" laryngeal inflammation. We propose that the term "chronic laryngitis" apply to any time frame after 30 days.[1,6] It is believed that as many as 21% of the population will suffer from chronic laryngeal inflammation at one point in their lives.[4] There is a multitude of causative agents that can be responsible for a chronic inflammatory process. Therefore, physicians should keep in mind that chronic laryngeal inflammation is only a clinical description and not a diagnosis. Thus practitioners should not use the terms laryngitis or chronic laryngitis as a diagnosis; a suspected etiology or etiologies should be attached to the clinical descriptor of all types of laryngitis even if the etiology is not confirmed yet.

INITIAL ASSESSMENT

History

During initial evaluation, the physician should allow the patient to explain his/her complaint(s) and related events as he/she experiences them. Sometimes, a precipitating event can be found: severe coughing, vomiting, laryngeal trauma, etc.[1] Inquiry should cover breathing, voice, and swallowing functions[2] and factors that increase or reduce symptoms. The most common complaint of a patient with chronic laryngeal inflammation is dysphonia (53%) that gets worse with use.[4,7] Pain and soreness, globus sensation, nonproductive cough, dysphagia, excessive throat clearing, post-nasal drip, scratchy throat, and laryngospasm are other common symptoms.[4,5,7,8] The intensity of those symptoms can be very different from one patient to another. History should also focus on trying to find the etiology and contributive factors of laryngeal inflammation with a detailed review of health habits, work exposure, allergies, immune deficiencies, infectious contact, travel history, systemic disease, etc.[2]

Examination

A comprehensive head and neck exam should be performed. The quality of the voice should also be noted including breathiness, roughness, asthenia.[9]

Endoscopy

Flexible or rigid (telescopic) laryngoscopy is an essential tool to diagnose and then follow the evolution of a patient with chronic laryngeal inflammation. The extent of the inflammation can be minimal and confined to the posterior glottis or can involve all laryngeal structures with edema, hypertrophic mucosa, or atrophic mucosa.[10] Edema, erythema, increased vascularity, nodularity, excessive and/or sticky mucus, pseudosulcus (infraglottic edema), and ulcerative changes are all possible findings.[5,7,11] Nevertheless, it is recognized that asymptomatic patients can have a certain degree of laryngeal inflammation, without having any medical problem. Hicks et al have reported finding signs of laryngeal irritation in 80% to 90% of asymptomatic volunteers.[12] Therefore, laryngoscopy should be used to document the extent of mucosal inflammation in symptomatic patients, to rule out other pathologies (including neoplasia) and to monitor disease longitudinally.

CASE: INITIAL EVALUATION

Her voice is rough, breathy, strained, and constricted. Her Voice Handicap Index 10 (VHI-10) score[13] is 40 and Reflux Symptom Index (RSI) score[14] is 42. Her head and neck examination is normal. Transnasal flexible laryngoscopy demonstrates significant laryngeal inflammation throughout her endolarynx, including bilateral vocal fold edema and erythema (moderate), and desiccated epithelium. Rigid telescopic examination with stroboscopy demonstrates bilateral reduced mucosal wave (severe on right, moderate on left side), irregular vocal fold edges, and incomplete glottic closure. See Figure 16–1.

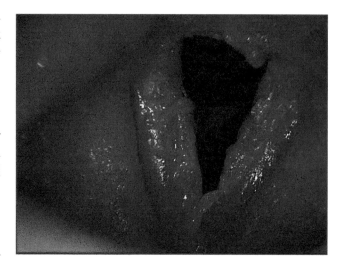

Figure 16–1. Laryngoscopic initial evaluation. See companion website for video.

Initial Diagnosis

Chronic laryngeal inflammation due to laryngopharyngeal reflux disease (LPRD) and severe dehydration.

Management

We recommend lifestyle and dietary modification (reflux counseling), proper hydration, and decreased intake of caffeine; omeprazole 40 mg p.o. b.i.d.; ranitidine 300 mg p.o. h.s. We emphasize proper timing of the acid suppression therapy.

Discussion

Given that the two most frequent etiologies associated with chronic laryngeal inflammation are tobacco and LPRD, they should be addressed first, if appropriate. Also, all obvious factors that can increase dehydration (caffeine, medications, etc.) and/or external caustic irritation components (smoke, fumes, etc) should be discontinued or reduced if possible. Proper hydration and vocal hygiene will help in management of chronic laryngeal inflammation due to dehydration and environmental irritants. For LPRD treatment, it is important to educate patients on the importance of lifestyle modifications because it can be sufficient to treat 50%

of patients with chronic laryngeal inflammation.[15] Empiric initial PPI is the most common treatment (79%) for chronic laryngeal inflammation.[4] An empiric trial with a PPI for a few months seems indeed reasonable when the history is supportive. PPI should be taken 30–60 minutes before a protein-based meal.

CHRONIC LARYNGEAL INFLAMMATION DUE TO LARYNGOPHARYNGEAL REFLUX DISEASE

LPRD is defined as a regurgitation of gastric content onto the superior aerodigestive tract, laryngeal mucosa, and pharyngeal mucosa.[16] It is one of the most frequent causes of chronic laryngeal inflammation.[4] It is often considered as an extraesophageal manifestation of GERD, with these patients demonstrating only 20–43% prevalence of classic GERD symptoms (heartburn, regurgitation).[17]

The RSI and the reflux finding scores (RFS) have both been investigated for their diagnostic role in chronic laryngeal inflammation due to LPRD. Park et al found a specificity of only 19% for RSI and 50% for RFS.[18] However, others have found that an improvement of those scores can mean that LPRD is the principal contributing factor to laryngeal inflammation.[19,20] With those results, it is hard to know to what extent we should rely on the RSI and RFS to diagnose LPRD in patients with chronic laryngeal inflammation. Diagnosis relies on a careful history and physical examination; however, the RSI and RFS can be useful to keep track of the progression of the patient. Even if not perfect, most will consider the double-probe 24 hour ambulatory pH and impedance monitoring to be the gold standard to diagnose LPRD. False negative results have been reported as high as 50% for this diagnostic test.[7]

CASE: THREE WEEKS FOLLOW-UP

Despite acid suppression therapy, lifestyle modification, and increased hydration, she feels that her voice is getting worse. Her voice is more strained than before. She has been compliant with the treatment plan. She is having a hard time at work because she is not able to talk with clients. Her VHI-10 and RSI scores are 40 and 42. There is only a mild improvement of the laryngeal edema and erythema on laryngeal endoscopy evaluation.

Diagnosis

Chronic laryngeal inflammation due to LPRD and severe dehydration and possible primary muscle tension dysphonia.

Management

She is scheduled for voice therapy. The goal is to: (1) help the patient not to strain her voice (direct voice therapy) and (2) address issues of vocal hygiene (indirect voice therapy).

Discussion

Persistence of chronic laryngeal inflammation, despite treatment of LPRD, can be caused by (1) inadequate compliance (not getting the treatment), (2) inadequate duration of treatment (too short treatment duration), and/or (3) other etiologies not recognized and treated (incomplete diagnosis). It is important to keep in mind that even if LPRD is the principal etiology, chronic laryngeal inflammation can be multifactorial and each problem needs to be addressed. Even when LPRD is not the principal factor, we know that an already traumatized laryngeal mucosa can be prevented from healing, even with only mild episodic reflux.[1] If the patient is not getting better with PPI treatment, some will argue that it is because of a non-acid reflux and/or intermittent reflux, and others that LPRD is not the etiology. In either of these situations, other investigations should be done to evaluate for other etiologies.[21] Furthermore, studies of the effect of PPI on LPRD are discordant. The effect of acid suppression treatment is shown to not be better than placebo to improve symptoms of LPRD in some studies,[22,23] to be better than placebo to improve only heartburn symptoms of LPRD,[24] or to work better than placebo for LPRD in others.[25–27] Lately, a meta-analysis by Yang et al in 2016 revealed that 2 to 3 months of PPI, two times a day, seems to be effective in treating chronic laryngeal inflammation due to LPRD.[28] This study also reveals that surgical treatment is probably more effective than PPI therapy. In patients with LPRD who do not respond or have a partial response to acid suppression treatment, a pH investigation should be done before doing more aggressive treatment (including surgery).[7] Among treatment options, alginates, traditionally used with PPI for treatment of GERD, has recently been studied to treat LPRD. In the presence of gastric acid, the alginate precipitate forms a gel, the bicarbonate releases carbon dioxide, and the combination will form a foam that floats at the surface of the gastric contents, thus blocking reflux. McGlashan et al studied the effect of Gaviscon Advance® QID compared with no treatment in patients with LPRD refractory to PPI treatment. The aim was to see if it can improve RSI and RFS scores.[29] They found that patients who took the alginate suspension solution had a better improvement in their RSI and RFS scores than those in the group with no treatment. Thus, alginates seem to be an effective complementary treatment for patients with LPRD.

CASE: FOUR WEEKS FOLLOW-UP

Upon follow-up, she is still compliant with her medications and treatments; however, she does not feel any better, even after voice therapy. Her VHI-10 score is still 40 and RSI score is increased to 45. The laryngoscopic exam is the same with moderate to severe erythema, edema, and desiccated mucosa.

Differential Diagnosis

Chronic laryngeal inflammation due to:

  LPRD and severe dehydration

  Idiopathic ulcerative laryngitis

  Inflammatory disease

  Autoimmune disease

  Vasculitis

  Infectious disease (fungal? bacterial?)

  Work exposure (nail salon)

Investigation

48 hour pH esophageal monitoring (Bravo™)

Erythrocyte sedimentation rate (ESR). C-reactive protein (CRP)

Rheumatoid factor (RF). Antinuclear antibodies (ANA). Cytoplasmic neutrophil antibodies (ANCA). Anti-Ro. Anti-La

Minor salivary gland biopsy

Lyme titers. Fluorescent treponemal antibody absorption test (FTA-ABS)

Rheumatology consultation

Management

While waiting for test results, the patient is instructed to wear a mask when she works with acrylic in her nail shop and maximize ventilation of her workplace.

Discussion

When initial treatment of LPRD and dehydration does not seem to work, proper LPRD investigation should be done and other diagnoses should be investigated. At this point, investigations should focus on the differential diagnosis and on tests that can evaluate for uncommon etiologies. Tests for vasculitis and systemic inflammatory and autoimmune diseases should be ordered, and a consultation in rheumatology can help to assess and eventually treat those conditions. Cultures will most of the time show multiple bacterial species that are part of the laryngeal biofilm.[6] This biofilm is a proposed contributing factor to chronic laryngeal inflammation and had been demonstrated on vocal folds of patients (62%) with chronic laryngeal inflammation by Kinnari et al.[30] Principal microbial species found were: *S. aureus, H. influenzae, C. albicans, Moraxella non-liquefaciens, P. acnes, N. meningitidis,* and *S. pneumoniae.* Given the possibility of a chronic bacterial laryngitis, one should consider 1–2 months of antibiotic treatment that will cover common bacterial pathogens such as methicillin-resistant *Staphylococcus aureus.* Biopsy can also be useful to eliminate neoplasia and some bacterial and fungal etiologies.

DIFFERENTIAL DIAGNOSIS (TABLE 16–1)

The most common etiologies are LPRD[44] and smoking.[31] Alcohol, coffee, pharmaceuticals, dehydration, and vocal abuse are other factors that can initiate or maintain

Table 16–1. Differential Diagnosis of Chronic Laryngeal Inflammation

Infectious	Viral	Herpes
	Bacterial	Actinomycosis
		Leprosy
		Tuberculosis
		Syphilis
	Fungal	Aspergillus
		Blastomycosis
		Candidiasis
		Coccidioidomycosis
		Histoplasmosis
	Parasite	Leishmaniasis
		Schistosomiasis
		Syngamosis
		Trichinosis
Neoplastic	Squamous cell carcinoma	
	MALT	
	Other laryngeal neoplasia	
Idiopathic	Idiopathic ulcerative laryngitis	
Irritants	Laryngopharyngeal reflux	
	Allergy	
	Chronic cough	
	Chemicals	
	Pollution	
	Smoking	
	Vocal misuse-abuse	
Autoimmune	Crohn's disease	
	Lupus erythematosus	
	Rheumatoid arthritis	
Vasculitis	Granulomatosis with polyangiitis (formerly known as Wegeners Granulomatosis)	
Inflammatory	Amyloidosis	
	Sarcoidosis	
Iatrogenic	Radiation therapy	
	Inhaled corticosteroids	
	Antihistamine	
	Anticholinergic	

inflammation.[4,5,32] Some studies had also shown that occupational and environmental exposure to irritants, pollutants, and allergens can also contribute to exacerbate laryngeal inflammation.[5,8,33] Even if chronic laryngeal inflammation is seldom considered of infectious origin,[6] bacterial and fungal organism can cause chronic symptoms, until treated.[4] Candidiasis,[2,34–36] tuberculosis,[37–42] and syphilis[2,43] are potential causative agent of chronic laryngeal inflammation. Less common organisms have also been reported: leprosy,[2] actinomycosis,[44] aspergillosis,[2,43] blastomycosis,[45,46] histoplasmosis,[43,47] coccidioidomycosis,[43] leishmaniasis,[48] trichinosis,[49] schistosomiasis,[50] and syngamosis.[51] In those rare cases, histopathological confirmation is essential to rule out neoplastic etiology and to confirm the diagnosis.[2] Chronic laryngeal inflammation can also be the result of systemic inflammatory diseases,[52–54] vasculitis,[40,55,56] or autoimmune diseases.[40,57] The laryngeal symptoms can be present with other manifestations of the disease or can be the first and only sign of it. In addition, the diagnosis of idiopathic ulcerative laryngitis should be considered.[3,58]

CHRONIC LARYNGEAL INFLAMMATION DUE TO ENVIRONMENTAL EXPOSURE

Nonspecific laryngeal inflammation can be caused or worsened by tobacco smoke, inhaled allergens, fumes, dust, or chemical substances.[10]

The majority of available studies on tobacco smoke have investigated the effect on the lower airway. However, laryngeal structures are anatomically positioned in a way that predisposes them to tobacco exposure and other airborne substances. Studies had shown that tobacco can increase the laryngeal mucin index (guinea pig study),[59] can induce prostaglandin E2 (via induction of COX-2 gene expression),[60] and can decrease laryngeal microbiome diversity.[61] Tobacco smoke is known to induce inflammatory responses in many different tissues, including laryngeal mucosa.

Inhaled allergens were first discussed as a potential cause of laryngeal inflammation in the early 1970s.[62] Since then, Simberg et al have shown that patients suffering from allergic rhinitis are at increased risk of voice complaints and reported vocal symptoms during allergy season compared with patients without allergies.[63] Lately the concept has arisen of the unified airway and the probability of viscous secretions, from the lungs and the nasal cavity, getting trapped near the larynx resulting in increased throat clearing, cough,

reactive edema, and hyperemia.[64] If inhaled allergens are suspected to be a contributing factor, an allergy workup can be useful. Allergic laryngitis can be hard to diagnose and there may be an overlap with LPRD diagnosis in many patients.[64]

Work-related exposure causing laryngeal inflammation is also hard to study. Most available literature are case reports or retrospective series of cases. Among health care workers, anesthetists' exposure to halothane[65] and dental personnel's exposition to acrylate compounds[66] and to surgical cement containing methyl methacrylate (MMA)[67] have been reported. MMA is also used in other materials: Plexiglass®, orthopedic bone cement and nail products.[67] MMA is a known respiratory tract irritant and skin sensitizer. Dyspnea and bronchospasms have been reported with this substance, as well as throat irritation to a lesser extent.[67] Workers in contact with asbestos, such as in an asbestos cement factory, have been studied by Kambic et al. They found a 22% incidence of chronic laryngeal inflammation, with hyperplastic chronic inflammation without laryngeal carcinoma.[68] Glassblowers have also been reported to have a six-fold increased risk of developing chronic laryngeal inflammation because of their chronic exposure to hot gases, dust particles, and metal oxides.[10] There are also case reports of formaldehyde exposure,[69] ammonium exposure,[70] and stainless steel welding fumes exposure[71] causing chronic laryngeal inflammation.

Patients will often complain of itching, cough, and globus sensation when exposed to the offensive substance(s). Some of these inhaled pollutants have water absorbent effect and will increase desiccation of the laryngeal mucosa and dehydration sensation.[5] The most effective treatment is to avoid the causative agent or, if not possible, to wear a mask. Increasing hydration may also result in symptomatic relief.

CHRONIC LARYNGEAL INFLAMMATION DUE TO IDIOPATHIC ULCERATIVE LARYNGITIS

Initially described in 2000,[72] idiopathic ulcerative laryngitis (IUL), or prolonged ulcerative laryngitis, is a chronic laryngeal inflammation of unknown etiology, characterized by unilateral or bilateral midmembranous ulcerative lesions of the vocal folds with a prolonged course of resolution. Based on the work of Rakel et al with a review of 14 patients,[73] Hsiao et al with 33 patients,[74] and Simpson et al with 15 patients,[3] IUL patients seem to be mostly nonsmokers (86–100%)

and nondrinkers (79–91%), female (66%), and with a mean age of presentation between 38 and 49 years old. The disease starts like a typical acute laryngitis but the symptoms will continue for several weeks.[3] Patients will present with severe cough and hoarseness,[73] and flexible laryngoscopy examination will show ulcer(s) on the vocal folds that may be coated with fibrinous exudate.[3] There is also a case report of bilateral mid-vocal fold granuloma instead of ulceration published by Sinclair et al.[58] Diagnostic criteria of IUL, presented by Simpson et al, included: preceding upper respiratory infection with cough; bilateral midmembranous ulcerative lesions of the vocal folds; prolonged course of ulcer resolution >6 weeks; and lack of response to pharmacologic management.[3]

Close follow-up with a laryngoscopic and stroboscopic exam is recommended. As IUL is a diagnosis of exclusion, obvious contributing factors to laryngeal inflammation (LPRD, alcohol, tobacco, dehydration) should be addressed first.[74] Specific infections and systemic diseases should be investigated with appropriate tests if risk factors or symptoms are present. Differential diagnosis of IUL include laryngeal malignancy. Even though one should try to avoid biopsy for IUL because of the risk of scar formation, patients with risk factors for malignancy, ulcers that do not heal, or any other factor that increases suspicion for a malignant process should have a biopsy.[3] Patients diagnosed with IUL should be counseled that their vocal symptoms will improve but the recovery process typically takes many months, patience is required, and often workplace voice demand modifications need to be implemented during the prolonged recovery period.

No specific etiology has been found for IUL. Few cases in literature present biopsy and culture results; biopsies had shown only inflammatory reaction without atypia, and cultures had not been able to isolate any viral, bacterial, or fungal organisms.[73] Furthermore, LPRD seems to be a contributing factor for persistence of symptoms.[3] Because we still do not know what causes IUL, there is no established effective treatment. Vocal rest or reduced voice use, because of the localization of ulcerations on vocal fold(s), and increased vocal hygiene are strongly encouraged in the latest published retrospective review.[3,73,74] Also, it seems prudent to treat those patients with PPI, even if midmembranous ulcers are not typical localization for LPRD and patients with IUL will usually not respond to PPI alone.[3,73] It makes sense that LPRD will exacerbate or prevent healing of laryngeal inflammation.

Voice symptoms get better when the ulceration heals and symptoms usually resolve in 4 to 20 weeks.[74]

There is a case report of a patient who suffered from IUL for 3 years,[75] but most of the cases resolved in less than 1 year.[73] In the review of Simpson et al, 60% of patients still have abnormal mucosal wave or vibration amplitude after resolution of the disease.[3] Recurrence occurs in 9 to 13% of cases and can be 6 months to 6 years later.

CASE: TEN MONTHS FOLLOW-UP

All tests ordered at the last visit were normal, except for the pH esophageal monitoring that showed an esophageal pH of less than 4 for 18.9% of the recording time (upright 24.4%, supine 11.9%) and a DeMeester score of 61.1. She underwent a Nissen fundoplication surgery 5 months ago. Postoperatively she feels that her voice is still a problem. Her VHI-10 is 40 and RSI 36. The laryngoscopic exam is slightly improved. See Figure 16–2.

Laryngoscopic exam, 5 months after Nissen fundoplication surgery.

Diagnosis

Chronic laryngeal inflammation due to LPRD, severe dehydration, and workplace environmental exposure.

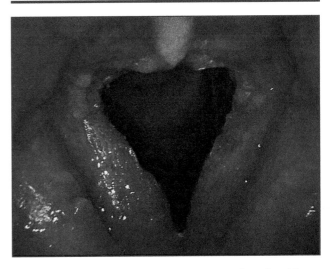

Figure 16–2. Laryngoscopic exam, 5 months after Nissen fundoplication surgery. See companion website for video.

Management

She is scheduled for surgery. The plan is to do a laryngoscopic exam under general anesthesia and depending on the findings, consider a limited resurfacing of the laryngeal mucosa with the KTP laser, steroids injection, and/or a biopsy.

Operating Room

Severe epithelial changes are seen on both vocal folds. There is also a subepithelial lesion on the right vocal fold. She underwent a microflap excision with excision of the right subepithelial fibrous mass lesion, a resurfacing of a small portion of the right vocal fold (posterior, superior surface approximately 3 mm × 3 mm) with KTP laser[76] and a bilateral superficial injection of dexamethasone, 0.2 mL each side.

One-Month Follow-up

She feels better about her voice even if her VHI-10 score is the same and there is still erythema, edema, and reduced mucosal wave on both side.

Three-Months Follow-up

She feels 70% better with reduced pain. Her VHI-10 score is now 20 and RSI score 16. See Figure 16–3.

Discussion

In this case, the presence of a subepithelial lesion on the right vocal fold could have been one of the reasons why symptoms were hard to improve. The previous Nissen fundoplication surgery, removal of workplace noxious exposure and the local injection of corticosteroids also potentially helped reduce laryngeal inflammation and assisted the healing process post-surgery. In chronic laryngeal inflammation, local steroids may have a healing modulation role. Local injection of corticosteroids for chronic laryngeal inflammation allows higher local tissue concentration with less sys-

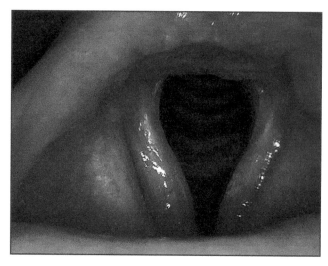

Figure 16–3. Laryngoscopic evaluation. See companion website for video.

temic effects.[77] Steroids can reduce granulation tissue formation and vocal fold fibrosis.[78] In counterpart, it has the theoretical potential to negatively impact wound healing. Multiple injections, with intervals of 6–12 weeks, have been suggested for inflammatory lesions.[78]

SUMMARY

Of otolaryngology consultations, 4% to 10% are for chronic laryngeal inflammation. Efforts should be undertaken to determine the etiology of the inflammation and the term "chronic laryngitis" should not be used as a stand-alone diagnosis.[79] Patients will complain mostly of dysphonia that can last several weeks to months. Detailed, high-quality laryngoscopic exam (often including stroboscopy) should be performed to assist with diagnosis and help follow the progression of the inflammation and to rule out other diagnoses. It is important to remember that chronic laryngeal inflammation is often multifactorial. An initiating event and an obvious etiology can sometimes be found, but a review of all possible causes and exacerbating factors is important to be able to address all of them and achieve treatment success. Failure to address all contributing factors can lead to disappointing results.

REFERENCES

1. Hanson DG, Jiang JJ. Diagnosis and management of chronic laryngitis associated with reflux. *American J Med.* 2000;108 Suppl 4a:112S–119S.
2. Tulunay OE. Laryngitis—diagnosis and management. *Otolaryngol Clin North Am.* 2008;41:437–451, ix.
3. Simpson CB, Sulica L, Postma GN, et al. Idiopathic ulcerative laryngitis. *Laryngoscope.* 2011;121:1023–1026.
4. Stein DJ, Noordzij JP. Incidence of chronic laryngitis. *Ann Otol Rhinol Laryngol.* 2013;122:771–774.
5. Dworkin JP. Laryngitis: types, causes, and treatments. *Otolaryngol Clin North Am.* 2008;41:419–436, ix.
6. Kinnari TJ. The role of biofilm in chronic laryngitis and in head and neck cancer. *Curr Opin Otolaryngol Head Neck Surg.* 2015;23:448–453.
7. Hanson DG, Conley D, Jiang J, Kahrilas P. Role of esophageal pH recording in management of chronic laryngitis: an overview. *Ann Otol Rhinol Laryngol Suppl.* 2000; 184:4–9.
8. Belafsky PC, Peake J, Smiley-Jewell SM, Verma SP, Dworkin-Valenti J, Pinkerton KE. Soot and house dust mite allergen cause eosinophilic laryngitis in an animal model. *Laryngoscope.* 2016;126:108–112.
9. Dejonckere PH, Lebacq J. Acoustic, perceptual, aerodynamic and anatomical correlations in voice pathology. *J Oto Rhino Laryngol.* 1996;58:326–332.
10. Baletic N, Jakovljevic B, Marmut Z, Petrovic Z, Paunovic K. Chronic laryngitis in glassblowers. *Industrial Health.* 2005; 43:302–307.
11. Kim CS, Lee SS, Han KD, Joo YH. Metabolic syndrome and chronic laryngitis: the Korean National Health and Nutrition Examination Survey 2008 to 2010. *Medicine.* 2015;94:e1890.
12. Hicks DM, Ours TM, Abelson TI, Vaezi MF, Richter JE. The prevalence of hypopharynx findings associated with gastroesophageal reflux in normal volunteers. *J Voice.* 2002;16:564–579.
13. Rosen CA, Lee AS, Osborne J, Zullo T, Murry T. Development and validation of the Voice Handicap Index-10. *Laryngoscope.* 2004;114:1549–1556.
14. Belafsky PC, Postma GN, Koufman JA. Validity and reliability of the Reflux Symptom Index (RSI). *J Voice.* 2002; 16:274–277.
15. Hanson DG, Kamel PL, Kahrilas PJ. Outcomes of antireflux therapy for the treatment of chronic laryngitis. *Ann Otol Rhinol Laryngol.* 1995;104:550–555.
16. Belafsky PC, Postma GN, Koufman JA. The validity and reliability of the reflux finding score (RFS). *Laryngoscope.* 2001;111:1313–1317.
17. Hopkins C, Yousaf U, Pedersen M. Acid reflux treatment for hoarseness. *Cochrane Database Syst Rev.* 2006:CD005054.
18. Park KH, Choi SM, Kwon SU, Yoon SW, Kim SU. Diagnosis of laryngopharyngeal reflux among globus patients. *Otolaryngol Head Neck Surg.* 2006;134:81–85.
19. Belafsky PC, Postma GN, Koufman JA. Laryngopharyngeal reflux symptoms improve before changes in physical findings. *Laryngoscope.* 2001;111:979–981.
20. Willems–Bloemer LH, Vreeburg GC, Brummer R. Treatment of reflux–related and non–reflux–related dysphonia with profound gastric acid inhibition. *Folia Phoniatr Logopaedica.* 2000;52:289–294.
21. Hammer HF. Reflux-associated laryngitis and laryngopharyngeal reflux: a gastroenterologist's point of view. *Dig Dis (Basel).* 2009;27:14–17.
22. Qadeer MA, Phillips CO, Lopez AR, et al. Proton pump inhibitor therapy for suspected GERD-related chronic laryngitis: a meta-analysis of randomized controlled trials. *American J Gastroenterol.* 2006;101:2646–2654.
23. Vaezi MF, Richter JE, Stasney CR, et al. Treatment of chronic posterior laryngitis with esomeprazole. *Laryngoscope.* 2006;116:254–260.
24. Ford C. Treatment of chronic posterior laryngitis with esomeprazole. *Laryngoscope.* 2006;116:1717–1718;author reply 1718.
25. Reichel O, Dressel H, Wiederanders K, Issing WJ. Double-blind, placebo-controlled trial with esomeprazole for symptoms and signs associated with laryngopharyngeal reflux. *Otolaryngol Head Neck Surg.* 2008;139:414–420.
26. Noordzij JP, Khidr A, Evans BA, et al. Evaluation of omeprazole in the treatment of reflux laryngitis: a prospective, placebo-controlled, randomized, double-blind study. *Laryngoscope.* 2001;111:2147–2151.
27. El-Serag HB, Lee P, Buchner A, Inadomi JM, Gavin M, McCarthy DM. Lansoprazole treatment of patients with chronic idiopathic laryngitis: a placebo-controlled trial. *Am J Gastroenterol.* 2001;96:979–983.
28. Yang Y, Wu H, Zhou J. Efficacy of acid suppression therapy in gastroesophageal reflux disease-related chronic laryngitis. *Medicine.* 2016;95:e4868.
29. McGlashan JA, Johnstone LM, Sykes J, Strugala V, Dettmar PW. The value of a liquid alginate suspension (Gaviscon Advance) in the management of laryngopharyngeal reflux. *Eur Arch Oto-Rhino-Laryngol.* 2009;266:243–251.
30. Kinnari TJ, Lampikoski H, Hyyrynen T, Aarnisalo AA. Bacterial biofilm associated with chronic laryngitis. *Arch Otolaryngol Head Neck Surg.* 2012;138:467–470.
31. Ward PH, Berci G. Observations on the pathogenesis of chronic non–specific pharyngitis and laryngitis. *Laryngoscope.* 1982;92:1377–1382.
32. Titze IR, Svec JG, Popolo PS. Vocal dose measures: quantifying accumulated vibration exposure in vocal fold tissues. *J Speech Lang Hear Res.* 2003;46:919–932.
33. de la Hoz RE, Shohet MR, Cohen JM. Occupational rhinosinusitis and upper airway disease: the World Trade Center experience. *Curr Allergy Asthma Rep.* 2010;10:77–83.
34. Chandran SK, Lyons KM, Divi V, Geyer M, Sataloff RT. Fungal laryngitis. *Ear Nose Throat J.* 2009;88:1026–1027.
35. Kobak S, Yilmaz H, Guclu O, Ogretmen Z. Severe candida laryngitis in a patient with rheumatoid arthritis treated with adalimumab. *Eur J Rheumatol.* 2014;1:167–169.

36. Nunes FP, Bishop T, Prasad ML, Madison JM, Kim DY. Laryngeal candidiasis mimicking malignancy. *Laryngoscope*. 2008;118:1957–1959.

37. Bhat VK, Latha P, Upadhya D, Hegde J. Clinicopathological review of tubercular laryngitis in 32 cases of pulmonary Kochs. *Am J Otolaryngol*. 2009;30:327–330.

38. Hemmaoui B, Bouayti B, Errami N, et al. [Laryngeal tuberculosis: a case report]. *Revue Laryngol Otol Rhinol*. 2007;128:93–96.

39. Kandiloros DC, Nikolopoulos TP, Ferekidis EA, et al. Laryngeal tuberculosis at the end of the 20th century. *J Laryngol Otol*. 1997;111:619–621.

40. Loehrl TA, Smith TL. Inflammatory and granulomatous lesions of the larynx and pharynx. *Am J Med*. 2001;111 Suppl 8A:113S–117S.

41. Porras Alonso E, Martin Mateos A, Perez-Requena J, Avalos Serrano E. Laryngeal tuberculosis. *Revue Laryngol Otol Rhinol*. 2002;123:47–48.

42. Sah SP, Raj GA, Bahadur T. Chronic ulceration of the tongue and laryngitis: first clinical sign of asymptomatic pulmonary tuberculosis. *J Infect*. 1999;39:163–164.

43. Silva L, Damrose E, Bairao F, Nina ML, Junior JC, Costa HO. Infectious granulomatous laryngitis: a retrospective study of 24 cases. *Eur Arch Oto-Rhino-Laryngol*. 2008;265:675–680.

44. Abed T, Ahmed J, O'Shea N, Payne S, Watters GW. Primary laryngeal actinomycosis in an immunosuppressed woman: a case report. *Ear Nose Throat J*. 2013;92:301–303.

45. Dumich PS, Neel HB, 3rd. Blastomycosis of the larynx. *Laryngoscope*. 1983;93:1266–1270.

46. Ebeo CT, Olive K, Byrd RP, Jr., Mirle G, Roy TM, Mehta JB. Blastomycosis of the vocal folds with life-threatening upper airway obstruction: a case report. *Ear Nose Throat J*. 2002;81:852–855.

47. Ferrari TC, Soares JM, Salles JM, et al. Laryngeal histoplasmosis in an immunocompetent patient from a non-endemic region: case report. *Mycoses*. 2009;52:539–540.

48. Moraes BT, Filho Fde S, Neto JC, Neto PS, Melo JEJ. Laryngeal leishmaniasis. *Int Arch Otorhinolargol*. 2012;16:523–526.

49. Nataro JD. Trichinosis of the vocal cords. Case report. *Eye Ear Nose Throat Monthly*. 1965;44:77.

50. Manni HJ, Lema PN, van Raalte JA, Westerbeek GF. Schistosomiasis in otorhinolaryngology: review of the literature and case report. *J Laryngol Otol*. 1983;97:1177–1181.

51. de Lara Tde A, Barbosa MA, de Oliveira MR, de Godoy I, Queluz TT. Human syngamosis. Two cases of chronic cough caused by Mammomonogamus laryngeus. *Chest*. 1993;103:264–265.

52. Baughman RP, Lower EE, Tami T. Upper airway. 4: Sarcoidosis of the upper respiratory tract (SURT). *Thorax*. 2010;65:181–186.

53. Butler CR, Nouraei SA, Mace AD, Khalil S, Sandhu SK, Sandhu GS. Endoscopic airway management of laryngeal sarcoidosis. *Arch Otolaryngol Head Neck Surg*. 2010;136:251–255.

54. Edriss H, Kelley J, Demke J. Sinonasal and laryngeal sarcoidosis. *Proceedings (Baylor University Medical Center)*. 2017;30:452–454.

55. Chiesa Estomba CM, Osorio Velazquez A, Perez-Carro Rios A. Wegener granulomatosis with supraglottic involvement. *Acta Otorhinolaryngol Espanola*. 2016;67:e24.

56. Gulati SP, Sachdeva OP, Sachdeva A, Singh U. Wegener's granulomatosis: a case with laryngeal involvement. *Indian J Chest Dis Allied Sci*. 1997;39:125–128.

57. Cheatum DE. Laryngeal involvement in systemic lupus erythematosus. *J Clin Rheumatol*. 2008;14:254.

58. Sinclair CF, Sulica L. Idiopathic ulcerative laryngitis causing midmembranous vocal fold granuloma. *Laryngoscope*. 2013;123:458–459.

59. Mouadeb DA, Belafsky PC, Birchall M, Hood C, Konia T, Pinkerton KE. The effects of allergens and tobacco smoke on the laryngeal mucosa of guinea pigs. *Otolaryngol Head Neck Surg*. 2009;140:493–497.

60. Branski RC, Zhou H, Kraus DH, Sivasankar M. The effects of cigarette smoke condensate on vocal fold trans-epithelial resistance and inflammatory signaling in vocal fold fibroblasts. *Laryngoscope*. 2011;121:601–605.

61. Jette ME, Dill-McFarland KA, Hanshew AS, Suen G, Thibeault SL. The human laryngeal microbiome: effects of cigarette smoke and reflux. *Scientific Reports*. 2016;6:35882.

62. Brodnitz FS. Allergy of the larynx. *Otolaryngol Clin North Am*. 1971;4:579–582.

63. Simberg S, Sala E, Tuomainen J, Ronnemaa AM. Vocal symptoms and allergy—a pilot study. *J Voice*. 2009;23:136–139.

64. Stachler RJ, Dworkin-Valenti JP. Allergic laryngitis: unraveling the myths. *Curr Opin Otolaryngol Head Neck Surg*. 2017;25:242–246.

65. Pitt EM. Halothane as a possible cause of laryngitis in an anaesthetist. *Anaesthesia*. 1974;29:579–580.

66. Piirila P, Kanerva L, Keskinen H, et al. Occupational respiratory hypersensitivity caused by preparations containing acrylates in dental personnel. *Clin Exp Allergy*. 1998;28:1404–1411.

67. Borak J, Fields C, Andrews LS, Pemberton MA. Methyl methacrylate and respiratory sensitization: a critical review. *Crit Rev Toxicol*. 2011;41:230–268.

68. Kambic V, Radsel Z, Gale N. Alterations in the laryngeal mucosa after exposure to asbestos. *Br J Industr Med*. 1989;46:717–723.

69. Roto P, Sala E. Occupational laryngitis caused by formaldehyde: a case report. *Am J Industr Med*. 1996;29:275–277.

70. Koleva M, Rangachev J, Boev M. Risk assessment of the occupational contact with ammonium. *Central Eur J Publ Health*. 2000;8:14–17.

71. Hannu T, Piipari R, Toskala E. Immediate hypersensitivity type of occupational laryngitis in a welder exposed to welding fumes of stainless steel. *Am J Industr Med*. 2006;49:402–405.

72. Spiegel JR, Sataloff RT, Hawkshaw M. Prolonged ulcerative laryngitis. *Ear Nose Throat J*. 2000;79:342.

73. Rakel B, Spiegel JR, Sataloff RT. Prolonged ulcerative laryngitis. *J Voice*. 2002;16:433–438.

74. Hsiao TY. Prolonged ulcerative laryngitis: a new disease entity. *J Voice*. 2011;25:230–235.

75. Toland BL, DeFatta RA, Sataloff RT. Prolonged ulcerative laryngitis in an 18-year-old voice major. *Ear Nose Throat J*. 2013;92:E24.

76. Zeitels SM, Burns JA. Office-based laryngeal laser surgery with the 532-nm pulsed-potassium-titanyl-phosphate laser. *Curr Opin Otolaryngol Head Neck Surg*. 2007;15:394–400.

77. Campagnolo AM, Tsuji DH, Sennes LU, Imamura R. Steroid injection in chronic inflammatory vocal fold disorders, literature review. *Braz J Otorhinolaryngol*. 2008;74:926–932.

78. Mortensen M, Woo P. Office steroid injections of the larynx. *Laryngoscope*. 2006;116:1735–1739.

79. Koufman JA. The otolaryngologic manifestations of gastroesophageal reflux disease (GERD): a clinical investigation of 225 patients using ambulatory 24-hour pH monitoring and an experimental investigation of the role of acid and pepsin in the development of laryngeal injury. *Laryngoscope*. 1991;101:1–78.

CHAPTER 17

Reinke's Edema

Ken Mackenzie

A 61-year-old woman presented with history of persistent hoarseness for over 3 years which had become worse in the last 6 months. In particular her voice had never been normal in the last 6 months and at no point had she had aphonia.

She complained that her voice was rough but the main characteristic which bothered her most was a reduction in the pitch of her voice, making her sound like a man.

She had no significant breathing or airway issues.

She had no associated dysphagia nor did she have any history of heartburn or upper gastrointestinal symptoms. She had not had any unintentional weight loss. She had no neck pain or referred otalgia.

She was an ex-smoker of 10 cigarettes per day and had stopped for approximately 6 months. She did not drink any alcohol.

Her job was as a packer in a noisy factory.

There was a family history of hypertension and she herself had been treated for hypertension for 10 years and had been type II diabetic, controlled by diet, for approximately 5 years.

At consultation she was audibly dysphonic with a reduced pitch to her voice. She appeared otherwise well and had a body mass index (BMI) of 32. Her ENT examination was unremarkable apart from the findings on nasolaryngoscopy. The nasolaryngoscopy revealed enlarged smooth surface and floppy vocal cords with the right slightly bigger than the left, both vocal cords being diffusely enlarged with possible bilobular changes on the right side. There were no areas of leukoplakia or irregularity of mucosa identified.

On quiet respiration the enlarged vocal cords prolapsed in and out of the glottic inlet; they were semi-translucent in appearance and almost appeared as a distinct swelling from the vocal ligament.

On phonation they were floppy with excessive vibration. The clinical appearances led to provisional diagnosis of Reinke's edema.

DISCUSSION POINTS

- Indications for surgery
- Type of surgery
- Management of smokers

CASE MANAGEMENT

Initial Evaluation

The clinical presentation of this patient is classical for the condition known as Reinke's edema. This condition originally was described by the German anatomist Friedrich B. Reinke in 1895. The definition of Reinke's edema is the accumulation of fluid deep to the mucosa, in the submucosal space known as a lamina propria (Figure 17–1). Within the fluid itself there may be gelatinous-type material but nil else of note. The mucosa is smooth and with it rare for there to be any findings in keeping with dysplastic changes and extremely rare for it to be associated with any in situ or malignant changes.

The standard examination of nasolaryngoscopy generally reveals smooth surfaced diffusely enlarged

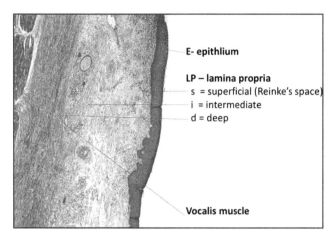

Figure 17–1. Histological coronal section through the membranous vocal cord showing its microstructure.

(almost semi-translucent on occasions) true vocal cords. In general an affected vocal cord will have changes throughout its length, in the majority of cases, in an almost uniform manner. The amount that the vocal cord will be enlarged can vary enormously from individual to individual. It should be noted that if the swelling is of a much smaller degree, in a smaller, more discreet lesion, then the lesion is more likely to be a polyp instead of classical Reinke's. A vocal cord polyp is a different distinct, histopathological process generally due to trauma or post inflammatory.

When comparing the right and left vocal cords it is frequently the case that both vocal cords are involved to a certain degree and may be symmetrical in their involvement, but it is equally common for them to be asymmetric in appearance.

Due to the semi-translucent appearance of the gelatinous material within the lamina propria, it is possible, on occasions, to see the vocal ligament quite clearly defined.

As the volume of the vocal cord increases there will be associated voice changes with dysphonia and masculinization. At consultation, as was the case here, the patient is audibly dysphonic, with a significant reduction in pitch. The reduction in pitch of voice, with her subsequently "sounding like a man," was her main complaint.

If the process continues, then not only will there be voice changes but there may also be obstruction of the proximal airway at the glottic inlet due to the bulk of the expanded vocal cords. If this is the case, then the patient may report stridor on mild exercise, or in extreme cases may be stridulous at rest or speaking.

On nasolaryngoscopy, on quiet respiration, the expanded smooth vocal cords tend to prolapse in and out of the glottic inlet passing into the subglottic space and back into the immediate supraglottic region on quiet respiration. This can be highlighted with the simple maneuver of asking the patient to take a deep breath in and out and forcing movement of the abnormal aspect of the vocal cords.

It is also possible to have separate multi-nodular areas of the affected vocal cords, as identified on the right side in this patient. This gives a slightly multi-lobulated type of appearance and may also appear as if it is a superimposed polyp, but in reality it is more than one lobule of Reinke's edema.

To assist with standardizing assessment of Reinke's edema, Tan et al suggested a grading system, assessing the involvement from grade 1 to grade 4, with a high inter- and intra-rater reliability.[1]

The suggested grading system relates to the residual airway as follows;

Grade 1: Lesions bilateral.

Grade 2: Bilateral lesions with expanded polypoid lesion affecting 25 to 50% of the glottic airway.

Grade 3: Bilateral lesions affecting at least 50% of the glottic airway, with no airway compromise.

Grade 4: Obstructed airway.

Previously, Yonekawa had suggested a clinical grading system, which was based on the extent of the polypoidal lesion at the glottic inlet.[2] The system is as follows:

Type I: Edematous swelling observed on the upper surface of the vocal folds, while patency of the glottis is adequately preserved.

Type II: Edematous swelling extends from the upper to lower surface beyond the margins of both vocal folds, which are partly in contact with each other.

Type III: Edematous swelling is further advanced so that an opening can be seen only at the posterior portion of the glottis, or the swelling is so bulged in sac-like shape that it hangs down to the subglottic space during inspiration.

While there may be a value in such grading systems if trying to correlate disease extent with patho-etiological factors, they are no substitute for high quality photo documentation in the assessment of disease progression. We do not routinely use a grading system in the recording of the disease process.

With respect to asymmetry of the features of Reinke's edema, given the underlying pathological processes involved, it would be anticipated that there would be some degree of change, similar in nature, affecting both true vocal cords. It is therefore extremely rare to have classical Reinke's edema affecting only one vocal cord. If, on examination, it is thought that one vocal cord is affected and the other is completely normal, then it must be strongly considered that on the side of the edematous changes of the vocal cord there may be an underlying malignancy. This could occur in subsites of the larynx, which might not be immediately obvious on nasolaryngoscopy, such as in the ipsilateral ventricle or subglottis. It is suggested therefore that "unilateral" Reinke's edema appearance should be considered as harboring a malignancy until proven otherwise.

In addition to the smooth mucosal expansion of the vocal cords and the expanded lamina propria, it is possible to have dysplastic changes of the mucosa. Although almost all of the patients with Reinke's edema are smokers, it might be anticipated that there would be a high prevalence rate of coexistent dysplastic changes. This does not appear to be the case. Although the reason is not known, the changes within the larynx as a result of smoking in women would appear to be either Reinke's edematous type of changes or dysplastic changes, rather than these two phenomena coexisting.

Some clinicians would consider the use of stroboscopic examination with a rigid endoscope also to be of value, and there is no reason why this should not be carried out. The most specific requirement for this, as the diagnosis can be made simply by nasolaryngoscopy, is for further detailed examination of the vocal cords. This is not mandatory in light of the risk of dysplastic or pre-malignant lesions being extremely low and if there is going to be progression to surgery for modification of the voice, then detailed examination will take place at the time of microlaryngoscopy.

In the UK population, it is our experience that Reinke's edema invariably occurs only in smokers with a very high female to male ratio. In our practice it is on the order of 9 to 1. The age of onset is from 40 to 50 years onward and there would not appear to be any marked associated socioeconomic preponderance reported. It also does not seem to be prevalent in the very old.

Reinke's space is the subepithelial space situated between the epithelium and the lamina propria, or vocal ligament (Figure 17–1).

In Reinke's edema there is an excess of matrix collecting in Reinke's space. The matrix contains collagen, elastin, and extracellular fluid. Sakae et al demonstrated that there is disarrangement of the collagen fibers in the fluid, resulting in loss of the flexible framework that maintains the uniformity of the lamina propria. The only significant correlation, however, in their series was between the extent of Reinke's edema and the age of the patient.[3] Volic et al reported in Reinke's edema that there was an excess of extracellular fluid and that this was due to phonotrauma and smoking.[4]

Why Reinke's edema occurs in certain individuals in the population is not known. Given the female preponderance, several theories have been proposed, such as hormonal; however, to date there is no clear cause for the patho-etiological process. What has been clearly identified is the almost exclusive association with smokers, the virtual exclusivity in females, and the lack of moderate to severe dysplastic changes and the virtual lack of invasive malignant changes.[5]

It is therefore clear, for whatever reasons, that some patients who are smokers may develop chronic laryngitic changes, with dysplasia extending into carcinoma in situ, and then invasive malignancy, whereas others will remain unaffected and still others will develop Reinke's edema. The reason for these different clinical paths is unknown.

COMORBIDITIES

Smoking and Laryngopharyngeal Reflux

Other than having type II diabetes, which was well controlled by diet for approximately 5 years, her only other significant comorbidity is that of hypertension, which was well controlled by losartan potassium 50 mg daily. There is no particular association with any of these medications and Reinke's edema.

She had smoked 10 cigarettes a day for approximately 40 years but had stopped smoking for the 6 months prior to consultation. She regularly attended her General Practitioner and to date had not any gross respiratory issues such as chronic obstructive airway disease or asthma noted.

Cessation of smoking is highly relevant in discussions on future management of this patient's Reinke's edema. Not only should it render her fitter for her surgical procedure, should that be deemed appropriate, but if management of her Reinke's edema has to have any significant degree of success, then it is imperative that smoking cessation occurs.

She is slightly overweight in that she has a BMI of 32. Although this is not a contraindication to general anesthesia, it should be considered when advising her of her relative fitness for general anesthesia. Her age and BMI raise the possibility of gastro-esophageal or laryngopharyngeal reflux disease.

From her symptoms there do not appear to be any that are in keeping with gross reflux disease, either gastro-esophageal or laryngopharyngeal; however, this should be borne in mind when considering future management.

It has been suggested, as in other laryngeal disorders such as laryngeal malignancy[6] and laryngotracheal stenosis,[7] that reflux disease has a significant role in Reinke's edema.[8] While theoretically reflux disorders may have an influence on Reinke's edema, not only as a co-patho-etiological factor but also to be considered during the healing phase following any surgical intervention, the exact role is unproven, as is the need for treatment. It would, however, be prudent, and indeed appropriate, to discuss with the patient prior to any surgical procedure the possible empirical treatment of reflux disorders by using agents such as regular antacids, H2 antagonists, or proton pump inhibitors over the period of treatment involving surgical intervention and voice therapy carried out by the speech and language therapists.

A further coexistent condition which should be considered, particularly in someone of this age, sex, and BMI, would be that of hypothyroidism.

PATIENT'S WISHES/EXPECTATIONS

The patient presented with increasing problems with her overall quality of life in relation to her voice quality. There were two main aspects of the quality of her voice which were problematic.

Firstly her voice was "never normal" in that it was persistently hoarse with an edge to it and lacked clarity. Secondly, the pitch of her voice was reduced and again persistently. Both of these features had been present for over 3 years and were significantly different from her previous "normal" voice.

These altered voice qualities had a significant impact on her quality of life both professionally and

socially. She worked as a packer in a very noisy factory where the environmental noise levels were such that the employees had to wear hearing protection when in the packing hall. To be effective at work she and her colleagues had to shout to be heard. She had been in this job for over 20 years and did not plan to retire for another 4 years.

Socially she and her husband liked to meet up with friends approximately once per week, at the local bowling club, and although she did not drink, she enjoyed conversation with her friends on a regular basis. For the last year or so, there had been several occasions when she was mistaken for being a man, notably on the telephone, and good friends had also commented on this issue to her on two occasions.

It is for these two key elements of her change in voice that she sought advice and wished her voice to be improved if at all possible.

She was well aware of the risk association between smoking and cancer development and although this was "at the back of her mind," the key reason for consultation was to achieve improvement in her voice, and return it to normal, if possible.

It is commonplace for referral of patients by general practitioners (GPs) for further assessment when they are hoarse for a period of 3 weeks or more to exclude malignancy. This practice has a low yield with respect to cancer diagnoses. This is generally recognized as being as low as 8%,[9] and as such there may be a mismatch between GP referral for excluding a cancer and patient expectation of ENT consultation. To try to clarify patients' wishes and expectations from the consultation, the use of questionnaires in relation to hoarseness has been reported.

Crosbie et al reported ACAPELA, a patient report questionnaire which aims to establish, with some form of rank order, patients' expectations from the ENT clinician's consultation with respect to their dysphonia.[10]

In clinical practice this is useful in confirming patients' expectations, as frequently the GP has a different aim, and indeed the ENT clinician may have made several presumptions of the reason for referral. This is important in dysphonic patients in general but is of particular importance in patients with Reinke's edema.

For many years the role of microlaryngeal surgery in Reinke's edema has been based on two key aims, firstly that of trying to improve the voice but secondly to exclude a malignancy. This has been based on the very high prevalence of smokers within the Reinke's edema group and the theoretical exclusion of malignancy in relation to this. However, it is clear from pathological studies of substantive cohorts of patients that the coexistence of moderate or severe dysplasia or carcinoma in situ and invasive malignancy is extremely rare.[5] On this basis it is recommended that when agreeing on the aims of any treatment, particularly surgical intervention, the principal aims should be improvement of voice and that there is no realistic need to have exclusion of malignancy as an aim of the surgical procedure.

Clearly any excised tissue from the microlaryngeal procedure will be examined in detail histopathologically; however, this is for completion purposes and is not a principal surgical aim.

Having agreed that the treatment aim is for improvement in the voice, then an indication must be given as to the relative chances of success, or otherwise, of the surgical procedure. Such indications ideally should be based on personal or team figures, rather than those quoted in the literature. In previous reports, however, it is generally recognized, by patient report measures, that surgical treatment for Reinke's edema can be of benefit to the patient.[11,12] So any improvement or modification in voice has to be taken in the context of the patient's requirements not only in the professional setting, as in this patient's case as a packer in a factory, but also in social circumstances. If it is not necessary to improve the voice, then there is little indication to carry out the surgical intervention.

Potential complications of the surgical interventions for voice will be discussed within the treatment outcomes section.

When discussing patient expectations from management of Reinke's edema, integral to the success of the treatment is the combination of supportive measures in the form of voice therapy, by speech and language therapists, and cessation of smoking. These are of equal importance; however, it is mandatory that the patient commit to cessation of smoking in conjunction with the other treatments. Given that the condition essentially only occurs in smokers, then clinical experience is such that if patients do not stop smoking there is a very high likelihood that, irrespective of surgical resection and voice therapy, there will be a high recurrence rate of the condition.

Given the large choice of methods which may be used to assist cessation of smoking, this key element for success cannot be emphasized too strongly.

Voice therapy is also integral to the success of the treatment of Reinke's edema. Voice therapy delivered by the speech and language therapy team needs to be comprehensive, individualized, and dependent on the patient's needs and professional and social lifestyle conditions.

Voice therapy can be a significant consideration for those in certain employments, not only in having time to access speech and language therapy but also in how they may or may not be able to modify their voice use in occupational situations. This is particularly the case with this patient in having to speak when there is challenging background noise.

PROCEDURE

Indications

The patient's laryngeal findings were considered clinically to be in keeping with classical Reinke's edema and because of no other medical conditions (such as hypothyroidism) needing treatment, microlaryngeal surgery was considered appropriate as part of the combined treatment process.

Given that she had stopped smoking 6 months prior to her presentation, it was considered extremely likely that this status could be maintained during and following microlaryngeal surgery.

All studies involving the successful treatment of Reinke's edema report the cessation of smoking as being essentially mandatory in case management. Although working in a challenging environment with respect to her voice use, she recognized that it would be possible to modify certain aspects of her voice use in relation to her work and in addition participate in a full course of voice therapy.

So in summary, given her wish to have her voice improved, her willingness to take part in voice therapy, and her smoking being stopped, then it was agreed that microlaryngoscopy surgical management of her Reinke's edema was indicated.

Contraindications

There are no absolute contraindications to microlaryngeal surgical technique. Her type II diabetes was well controlled, as was her hypertension. Her respiratory function was reasonable given both her BMI and her having stopped smoking 6 months earlier. It was considered that she would be fit for surgical technique under general anesthesia with all forms of perioperative ventilation feasible.

Expected Results Including Team Experience

This is a key element in the management of Reinke's edema. Given that this is the classical form of Reinke's edema, with no suspicious areas within the larynx, and that the patient is fit for all forms of general anesthesia, she is able to have all aspects of microlaryngeal surgery and anesthesia considered.

Previously reported experience with Reinke's edema is that in general it can be regarded as being of benefit to the patient, with an improvement in the quality of voice.[11]

The quantification of any such improvement tends to be reported in relation to certain specific surgical techniques, such as micro-suturing after vocal fold lesion removal,[13] or using a modified "M" shaped flap,[14] or other techniques such as the microdebrider.[15] In addition to the reporting of these novel and innovative approaches, the results of microlaryngeal surgical intervention are generally within heterogeneous laryngeal pathology cohorts, with Reinke's edema being a subgroup.[16] In general, therefore, the results of microsurgical intervention in these observational cohorts is that there is overall an improvement in the voice. Exactly what aspects of the voice and by how much it has improved are difficult to derive from the reported data.

Each individual team should be able to report the results of the surgical intervention and supportive measures used in their management of Reinke's edema.

Over a 5-year period, Ansari et al reported our team experience in a prospective evaluation of a heterogeneous cohort of patients undergoing endolaryngeal surgery. The assessment technique reported was a change of state assessment using a patient report voice questionnaire.[12]

There are several well-recognized patient-report voice questionnaires, namely the VoiSS (Voice Symptom Scale), the VHI (Vocal Handicap Index), and the VPQ (Voice Performance Questionnaire), which have been demonstrated to be applicable and sensitive to change.[17–20]

Although perceptual analysis may have a greater degree of accuracy, it is difficult to apply in a routine clinical situation. It is therefore strongly recommended that routinely a patient-reported voice questionnaire be used to assess the outcomes of any form of microlaryngeal surgery but particularly in the case of Reinke's edema, where the aim of the microlaryngeal procedure is improvement in voice.[20]

In the heterogeneous cohort reported by Ansari et al, when the group whose aim was "improvement in voice" was assessed, there was a statistically significant improvement in the VoiSS scores post surgical intervention compared with the preoperative levels.[12]

When the Reinke's edema group from this subgroup was reported specifically, then this was also shown to be statistically significant improvement using the team's surgical technique.[11]

Of relevance within this observational cohort is that the surgery carried out was by supervised trainees and by the lead consultant and is therefore regarded as being representative of the surgical intervention and able to be quoted to the patient when considering the microlaryngeal procedure. The patient can therefore be advised that the results of intervention using a similar microsurgical technique should, on the balance of probabilities, result in a reported improvement in voice.

Risk Benefit

In this patient's case, it was considered that it was likely that the patient was going to benefit from the microsurgical procedure given her favorable status with respect to cessation of smoking and general health prior to the surgical procedure. The risks involved are that during the surgical procedure it may be considered that, given the extent of the Reinke's edema, only one vocal cord could and should be addressed at the time and so there is potential risk that the patient might have to return for a second procedure for the contralateral vocal cord. A further risk is that there is not an improvement in voice and that her voice may deteriorate. While this may be the outcome, it would be anticipated that she would have voice improvement. If it was not significantly noticeable, then as the quality of voice for professional reasons is not absolutely critical, she still considered it was appropriate to proceed with the microlaryngeal surgical procedure.

Therapeutic Alternative

If a substantial improvement in the quality of the voice is required, then there is no real therapeutic alternative to microsurgical intervention. Smoking cession and voice therapy themselves can be instituted; however, the Reinke's edematous changes within the larynx are essentially irreversible to any significant extent. A change in voice will only be noticed if the bulk of the vocal cord is modified by reducing the fluid in the lamina propria and excising the excess mucosa.

TECHNIQUES AND RESULTS

Anesthesia/Perioperative Care

Close collaboration between the anesthetist and the surgical team is necessary when planning, and subsequently carrying out, the microlaryngeal procedure. The key elements to consider are being able to guarantee optimal ventilation of the patient during the procedure while at the same time allowing access to all aspects of the larynx, and the vocal cords in particular, without any significant distortion of these tissues. If, as in most cases, the aim is to access the vocal cords in the most natural position, with Reinke's edema causing change to only voice and not causing airway obstruction, then consideration can be given to ventilation of the patient by supraglottic jet insufflation, microlaryngeal tube insertion, or infraglottic or subglottic ventilation.

If there is any degree of obstruction which is apparent preoperatively or there is significant comorbidity, such as chronic obstructive airway disease which necessitates intubation, then a microlaryngeal endotracheal tube should be used. Use of such a tube can be regarded as being standard in some teams; however, we tend to use subglottic jet ventilation, as it allows minimal distortion of the Reinke's edema, and in particular the vocal ligament and lamina propria which are going to be addressed by the microlaryngeal surgery.

Once the form of ventilation has been agreed upon, the patient is anesthetized. In our practice if subglottic jetting is to be used, total intravenous anesthesia (TIVA) with propofol, using target controlled infusion (TCI) rocuronium as the muscle relaxant of choice, allows adequate dose administration to ensure appropriate degree of relaxation for surgery with reversal, if required, with sugammadex. The anesthetist places the microlaryngeal tube or a subglottic jet in place with the surgical team taking over thereafter. If it is going to be supraglottic jet ventilation, then the ventilation is through the rigid endoscope and a jet insufflation Venturi system.

Surgical Technique

Our method of choice is the standard microlaryngeal "cold" surgical technique using the Dedo laryngoscope

with the suspension apparatus, and the microlaryngeal technique using MicroFrance instruments, principally the "heart" forceps and straight and curved scissors as appropriate. Once the microlaryngeal tube or the subglottic jetting catheter is in place and the patient ventilated, topical 1:1000 adrenaline is applied to the vocal cord to be addressed by using neurosurgical neuropatties soaked in 1:1000 adrenaline. This allows some local vasoconstriction of the overlying mucosa prior to the incision.

A cordotomy is made in the superior aspect of the true cord, through the mucosa longitudinally into Reinke's space and extended throughout its length but leaving the antero-superior aspect of the cord and preserving the anterior commissure mucosa.

The submucosal space is entered and gently opened and Reinke's space decompressed carefully by aspiration of fluid from Reinke's space without trauma to the underlying vocal ligament. Once a subjective assessment that Reinke's space has been decompressed sufficiently, then the excess mucosa which will be lying supralateral to the free edge of the vocal cord is excised, and this is carried out judiciously preserving and not traumatizing the free edge of the vocal cord. Once this has been achieved once again, hemostasis is secured with a neuropattie and the final position of the mucosa and the two edges of the cordotomy assessed. Providing there has been no trauma to the free edge of the vocal cord, then the process can be repeated on the contralateral vocal cord, again taking care through each stage of the procedure but particularly at the anterior commissure and at the free edge of the vocal cord.

Once the position of the overlying mucosa has been deemed satisfactory, the patient's anesthesia is reversed and the patient extubated with care to avoid injudicious suction in the laryngopharyngeal region by the anesthetist on extubation.

As a standard form of examination prior to all microlaryngeal techniques, it is our practice to examine the vocal cords using Hopkins rods 0, 30, and 70 degrees to ensure that all aspects of the overlying mucosa, as would be expected, had no areas of abnormality such as mild dysplasia. Photo documentation as appropriate.

In cases of marked asymmetry of Reinke's edema and in particular the unilateral Reinke's type of edema, then underlying malignancy needs to be excluded, and so use of the telescopes 0, 30, and 70 degrees is invaluable in such situations.

All resected specimens from the vocal cords are sent to histopathology for definitive histopathological assessment. This is not only to ensure that there is no dysplasia associated with the condition but to confirm that the diagnosis is in keeping with Reinke's edema.

Immediately postoperatively we are keen that any excess coughing is avoided if possible. With respect to voice rest, we ask our patients to avoid excessive voice use, particularly in the first 48 hours, but if they have to speak, then to speak normally without any excessive shouting, straining, or whispering. We also encourage optimal fluid intake of at least 3 liters daily during this period.

There is considerable debate about the optimal amount of voice rest following microsurgery to the larynx. Kaneko et al reported that following microlaryngeal surgery for a heterogeneous group of conditions, including Reinke's edema, a range of measures, including patient report and perceptual assessments, were significantly better after 3 days of voice rest rather than 7 days.[21]

Returning to work is almost exclusively dependent upon the individuals, their need to work, and the type of work they undertake. If they have minimal voice use at work and can avoid a lot of conversation, then they can return to work within a few days once they have recovered from the effects of the general anesthesia. If, as in our patient's case, there is considerable challenge when at work—either in having to shout when there is excessive background noise, having to speak in an environment which might have certain irritating fumes such as a hairdresser, or having to speak to customers regularly such as in a call center—patients may be advised to take a longer period off work, such as 1 to 2 weeks.

There are modifications of the above techniques which have been suggested by various groups.

We have used the carbon dioxide laser to create the cordotomy and subsequent excision of the redundant glottic mucosa. I would suggest that this is an individual surgeon's preference, but clearly the only disadvantage would be that you either have to have the patient ventilated through a laser-resistant tube or by tubeless anesthesia with a supraglottic jetting technique. If that is found to be acceptable, then the CO_2 laser works well; and in this situation there are no concerns about the dissipation of the thermal effect of the CO_2 laser, as the fluid in Reinke's space will act as an absorber of any dissipated heat.

A further suggestion has been the use of the microdebrider for removal of the mucosa and aspiration of the fluid.[15] Although there have been positive reports of its use, we do not use it in our group, principally because it was felt that we could have more accurate resection and preservation of the medial glottic

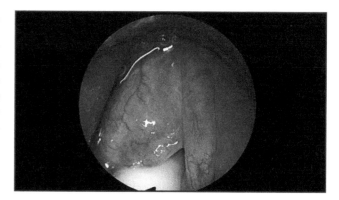
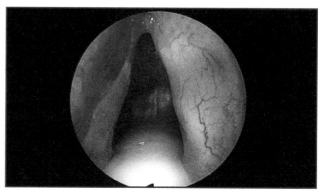

Figure 17–2. Reinke's edema seen through the operating microscope, before and after treatment.

mucosa with cold techniques using the MicroFrance instrumentation.

Adjuncts to improving the healing process have been suggested.

The micro-suturing of the flap on completion of mucosal resection and aspiration of the fluid has been advocated with good result.[13] Furthermore, to try to improve the design of the micro-flap, an "M" shaped flap has been advocated.[14] We do not use either of these techniques, as we have not found it to be necessary in the production of a good voice outcome. See Figure 17–2.

Results and Procedure–Related Complications

With all rigid endoscopic procedures of the proximal aerodigestive tract, there is risk to the dentition, particularly the upper dentition. This may be particularly problematic in the age group who may be suffering from Reinke's in that they may have had previous dental extractions, needing the use of a partial upper denture, or alternatively they may be edentulous with respect to the upper dentition.

Although being completely edentulous renders access easier to the proximal aerodigestive tract with a rigid endoscope, there is still the possibility of irritation of the upper alveolar mucosa by abrasion of it—for example, when protecting the upper gum with a wet gauze swab. To avoid this, we would use another material, a dental dam, and have found this to be effective in reducing the rate of upper gum abrasion.[22]

Furthermore on those where there is retained dentition, particularly if it is complete or in poor state, then we use a personalized upper mouth guard, particularly if there is going to be repeated endoscopic procedures—for example, in a two-stage procedure for the Reinke's procedure or in those patients with dysplasia or low volume laryngeal cancer needing repeated endoscopic procedures.

If either a microlaryngeal tube or a subglottic jet catheter is going to be inserted, then the anesthetic team must be aware of the potential risk to the dentition as mentioned but also to the potential risk of causing trauma within the laryngotracheal tract. This is of particular relevance in Reinke's edema, where the increased volume of the vocal cords may temporarily obstruct the passage on insertion of the microlaryngeal tube or the subglottic catheter with subsequent either hematoma creation or possibly even removal of the mucosa.

The key element in the resultant improvement in voice is to ensure that the anterior commissure mucosa is left with minimal disruption and that the medial aspect of the vocal cord mucosa is left in a good position following the mucosal resection. If the latter does not take place, then it is likely that the voice outcome result will not be optimized. It is imperative that the anterior commissure mucosa be left undisturbed and preserved, otherwise the risk of web formation becomes high. This is essentially the worst outcome conceivable, as the patient will inevitably become grossly dysphonic, and is completely unacceptable in a procedure where the aim is to improve the quality of the voice.

In this case, the cordotomy was performed, with the excision of the excess mucosa micro-flaps positioned well. At 6 weeks postoperatively, her voice was significantly improved, with increased quality of her voice and overall increase in pitch.

In our practice the patient-report voice questionnaire, the VoiSS, is used. We reported the results of the cold technique described.[11]

In this observational cohort, 95% of the patients were female, 100% were smokers. Of the 33 patients who had pre- and postop impaired voice outcome data,

using the VoiSS questionnaire revealed there was a significant improvement in the patient-reported VoiSS scores ($p = 0.008$). It is therefore concluded that in this practice using cold surgical techniques in the routine clinical setting, patients have a significant improvement in the quality of voice.

It can therefore be concluded that improvement in voice, as reported by patient-report questionnaire, can be demonstrated following treatment of Reinke's edema.

LONG-TERM MANAGEMENT

Referral

It is strongly advocated that, not only to optimize the outcome in relation to voice following the microlaryngeal surgical procedure, but also to ensure that this is maintained with time, referral to speech and language therapy for appropriate individualized voice therapy is made.

Attendance at this is to be strongly encouraged. In this patient's case this was extremely important, as she was in a challenging occupational environment for her voice use, with competing background noise present while she was in the packing hall and trying to communicate with her colleagues.

Simple supportive measures such as maintaining adequate fluid intake, communicating only when necessary with her colleagues, and trying to optimize lip reading techniques were recommended.

Follow-Up Test and Procedures

It is advisable to carry out review in the outpatient setting with flexible nasendoscopy or the instrument with which the patient was initially assessed. On this occasion there was a very good result, with no apparent residual edematous changes at 6 weeks review following the surgical procedure. Both vocal cords were healthy and well healed, with a good quality of voice on phonation.

On review, she was advised that the excision of the mucosa from both vocal cords had a histopathological report in keeping with Reinke's edema and there was no evidence of dysplasia or any other significant mucosal change. At the 6-week review, she had had her first appointment for voice therapy and she had continued to stop smoking.

Consulting with the patient to advise her of this histopathological result and reinforcing each of these supportive aspects were imperative, hopefully ensuring long-term success.

Long-term improved voice results should be maintained so long as each key aspect of the patient's management is maintained, in particular smoking cessation and modification of voice use.

DISCUSSION POINTS

Indications for Surgery

The indications for surgery, in this case microlaryngeal surgery consisting of aspiration of fluid from Reinke's space followed by excision of excess glottic mucosa, have to be considered carefully before advising the patient. This is the case with all forms of surgery but is of particular relevance in those patients in whom surgery is being considered to improve what is essentially a quality of life issue. This arises frequently in otorhinolaryngological practice—for example, when considering middle ear surgery to address a hearing impairment, and for this as well as to assess other otorhinolaryngological interventions, the Glasgow Benefit Inventory was derived. Recent systematic review of this outcome measure reports its generic value.[23]

So in the case of a patient presenting with Reinke's edema in the outpatient setting, the first decision to be made is whether the patient needs formal sampling of the laryngeal mucosa for histopathological assessment. If the patient presents with "classical" Reinke's, with smooth, diffusely expanded, glottic mucosa, affecting both true vocal cords and with mobile vocal cords, then there is no need to sample the mucosa. This is because it has been clearly demonstrated that there is an extremely low prevalence of dysplastic changes, and a virtual nonexistence of malignant changes, in patients with this clinical presentation. Conversely, however, if there are any areas of suspicion in the mucosal lining, with altered color or texture, then those areas should be sampled, or excised, for definitive histopathological assessment. Furthermore, if the edematous changes are primarily unilateral, then microlaryngoscopy is mandatory to exclude any underlying malignancy which might have resulted in the unilateral changes.

In the case of classical Reinke's edema, with no suspicious characteristics, the principal indication for surgery is for alteration of voice. The desired alterations to the voice must be clarified, and documented, with the patient and are almost certainly to raise the pitch of the voice and make it less rough. Once the chances of this occurring have been discussed and agreed with the patient, then the planned surgery can proceed.

Type of Surgery Employed

From the literature and clinical experience, it would appear that the exact method used to incise the laryngeal glottic mucosa, aspirate the fluid from Reinke's space, and excise the residual excess mucosa is of little difference from one method to another. The most important aspect is that the surgery should be carried out judiciously, with all of the usual considerations of microlaryngeal surgery, such as not encroaching upon the anterior commissure when excising the mucosa.

The type of surgery employed should therefore be that normally used by the surgeon and is able to be demonstrated as being effective by using voice outcomes.

Furthermore, the adjuncts to microlaryngeal surgery, such as suturing of the micro-flap, would appear to be a matter of an individual surgeon's preference.

Management of Smoking

In this case there was not an issue, as she had stopped smoking approximately 6 months prior to the consultation. In most patients it is a significant issue and some clinicians may propose that patients should have stopped smoking prior to definitive microlaryngeal surgery. This approach is subject to debate, but the protagonists would justify it, as this is primarily a quality of life issue and will almost certainly recur if smoking persists. We do not make stopping smoking a prerequisite of performing microlaryngeal surgery.

In general what method is used to stop smoking is of little significance. What is not known is if the use of methods such as e-cigarettes has any adverse effects on the larynx and in particular the association with recurrence of Reinke's edema.

REFERENCES

1. Tan M, Bryson PC, Pitts C, Woo P, Benninger MS. Clinical grading of Reinke's oedema. *Laryngoscope*. 2017;127: 2310–2313.

2. Yonekawa H. A clinical study of Reinke's oedema. *Auris Naris Larynx (Tokyo)*. 1988;15:57–78.

3. Sakae FA, Imamura R, Sennes LU, Mauad T, Saldiva PH, Tsuji DH. Disarrangement of collagen fibres in Reinke's edema. *Laryngoscope*. 2008;118(8:1500–1503.

4. Volic SV, Kaplan I, Seiwerth S, Ibrahimpasic T. Extracellular matrix of Reinke's space in some pathological conditions. *Acta-Otolaryngologica*. 2004;24(4):505–508.

5. Lim S, Sau P, Cooper L, McPhaden A, MacKenzie K. The incidence of pre-malignant and maligant disease in Reinke's oedema. *Otolaryngol Head Neck Surg*. 2014; 150(3):435–437.

6. Zhang D, Zhou J, Chen B, Zhou L, Tao. Gastro-oesophageal reflux and cancer of the larynx and pharynx: a meta-analysis. *Acta Otolaryngol*. 2014;134(10) 982–989.

7. Maronian NC, Azadeh H, Waugh P, Hillel A. Association of laryngopharyngeal reflux disease and subglottic stenosis. *Ann Oto Rhinol Laryngol*. 2001;110:606–612.

8. Kamargiannis N, Gouveris H, Katsineelos P, Katotomichelakis M, Riga M, Beltsis A, Danielides V. Chronic pharyngitis is associated with laryngopharyngeal reflux in patients with Reinke's oedema. *Ann Otol Laryngol*. 2011;120(11):722–726.

9. Langton S, Siau D, Bankhead C. Two week rule in head and neck cancer 200-2014: a systematic review. *Br J Oral Maxillofac Surg*. 2016;54(2):120–131.

10. Crosbie R, McKendrick M, Corson S, Lowit A, MacKenzie K. Patient expectation of a voice consultation: development of the ACaPELa questionnaire by assessment of four hundred and fifty-five patients. *Clin Otolaryngol*. 2017;42:182–185. doi:10.1111/coa.12593.

11. Ansari S, MacKenzie K. Why should we operate on Reinke's oedema? The 3rd International Conference and Exhibition in Rhinology and Otology, April 25–27, 2016, Dubai UAE. *Scientific Tracks Abstracts: Otolaryngology*. doi:10.4172/2161–119X.C1.013

12. Ansari S, MacKenzie K. Voice outcomes following endolaryngeal surgery: are we achieving our aims? *Clin Otolaryngol*. 2015;40(6):580–586.

13. Yilmaz T, Sozen T. Microsuture after benign vocal fold lesion removal: a randomised trial. *Am J Otolaryngol*. 2012;33(6):702–707.

14. Tan NC, Pittore B, Puxeddu R. M shaped microflap for treatment of complex Reinke's space oedema of the vocal cords. *Acta Otorhinolaryngol Ital*. 2010;30(5):259–263.

15. Honda K, Haji T, Maruyama H. Functional results of Reinke's oedema surgery using a microdebrider. *Ann Otol Rhinol Laryngol*. 2010;119(1):32–36.

16. Geyer M, Ledda GP, Tan N, Brennan PA, Puxeddu R. Carbon dioxide laser assisted phonosurgery for benign glottic lesions. *Eur Arch of Otorhinolaryngol*. 2010;267(1):87–93.

17. Deary IJ, Wilson JA, Carding PN, MacKenzie K. VoiSS: a patient derived voice symptom scale *J Psychosom Res*. 2003:54(5):483–489.

18. Wilson JA, Webb A, Carding PN, Steen IN, MacKenzie K, Deary IJ. Optimising outcome assessment of voice interventions I: the reliability and validity of three self report scales. *J Laryngol Otol*. 2007;121:763–767.

19. Steen IN, MacKenzie K, Carding PN, Webb A, Deary IJ, Wilson JA. Optimising outcome assessment of voice interventions II: the sensitivity to change of self report and observer rated measures. *J Laryngol Otol*. 2008;122:46–51.

20. Carding PN, Wilson JA, MacKenzie K, Deary IJ. Measuring voice outcomes: state of the science review. *J Laryngol Otol*. 2009;129:823–829.

21. Kaneko M, Shiromoto O, Fujiu-Kurachi M, Kishimoto Y, Tateya I, Hirano S. Optimal duration for voice rest after vocal fold surgery: randomised controlled clinical study. *J Voice*. 2017;31(1):97–103.

22. Hey SY, Harrison A, MacKenzie K. Oral trauma following rigid endoscopy and a novel approach to its prevention—prospective study of one hundred and thirteen patients. *Clin Otolaryngol*. 2014;39(6):389–392.

23. Hendry J, Chin A, Swan I, Akeroyd M, Browning G. The Glasgow Benefit Inventory: a systematic review of the use and value of an otorhinolaryngological generic patient-recorded outcome measure. *Clin Otolaryngol*. 2016; 41(3):259–275.

CHAPTER 18

External Laryngeal Trauma

S. A. Reza Nouraei and Natasha Quraishi

KEY POINTS

- Laryngeal trauma is rare but includes life-threatening injuries which if not rapidly recognized and treated can cause major long-term morbidity.
- Laryngeal trauma may be due to blunt or penetrating trauma, and the latter may be due to knife or projectile injury. Over the past decades, the incidence of penetrating laryngeal trauma has increased.
- The principal objective of early management of laryngeal trauma is securing the airway while protecting the cervical spine. In the majority of cases this requires computed tomography (CT) scanning of the neck and the cervical spine.
- Approximately 40% of patients can be managed conservatively.
- With increasing use of advanced endoscopic techniques, an increasing number of patients with laryngeal trauma may be managed endoscopically.
- All cases of laryngeal trauma require careful laryngological follow-up to identify and rehabilitate post-injury sequelae, including vocal decrement, swallow impairment, and aspiration.

INTRODUCTION

The larynx is the narrowest part of the adult airway.[1] It houses the organ of phonation, controls the respiratory time constant, and most importantly, acts to prevent ingress of swallowed material into the airway. It is connected, via the hyoid bone and the supra- and infrahyoid musculature, to the facial skeleton,[2] and its displacement during swallowing acts to protect the airway and distract and open the upper esophageal sphincter. External laryngeal trauma is rare but can be acutely life-threatening.[3–5] If not promptly recognized and treated, laryngeal trauma can cause significant long-term morbidity in as many as a quarter of patients due to any combination of persistent disruption of phonation, swallowing, or airway architecture.[5–7] Laryngeal trauma is often associated with concomitant cervical and intracranial injuries, and frequently occurs in the context of poly-trauma.[5] It is vital therefore that all patients with suspected laryngeal injury be managed by a multidisciplinary trauma team according to Advanced Trauma Life Support® guidelines.

CASE PRESENTATIONS

A Case of Cricoarytenoid Joint Injury

A previously fit and well 28-year-old male presented with sudden-onset dyspnea, loss of voice, and stridor. While playing rugby, he collided with another player and received a direct blow to his cricoid from the other player's elbow. He did not suffer any head injuries or loss of consciousness. There was no medical history of note. He was initially treated with steroids and nebulized adrenaline. After 3 hours, the patient's stridor improved and his voice returned; however, he had severe dysphonia, only managing to whisper. He also complained of odynophagia.

On inspection of the neck there was localized erythema and edema at the level of the larynx. His oropharynx appeared normal. A chest radiograph ruled out pneumothorax or rib fractures. The initial flexible nasal endoscopy (FNE) showed edema of the supraglottis, bowing of the right vocal fold, and possible restriction in vocal fold mobility. The airway was judged safe and the patient underwent a CT examination of the neck to clear the cervical spine of injury and to further assess the larynx. Initially this was considered to show no fracture or dislocation of the larynx and so he was treated with intravenous antibiotics (co-amoxiclav) and steroids, nebulized saline and adrenaline, and analgesia. He was allowed sips of water only.

The next day the patient's symptoms appeared to be improving. On examination with FNE, his left arytenoid was swollen and bruised, overlapping the posterior commissure. There was restricted mobility of both arytenoids. No pooling of secretions was seen in the piriform fossa (Figure 18–1).

Review of the CT images by a specialist radiologist identified a vertical fracture of the left side of the posterior arch of the cricoid cartilage with a 4 mm fracture diastasis causing displacement and possible impaction of the left arytenoid cartilage into the fracture line. There was associated diffuse edema in the anterior neck but no subcutaneous air (Figure 18–2).

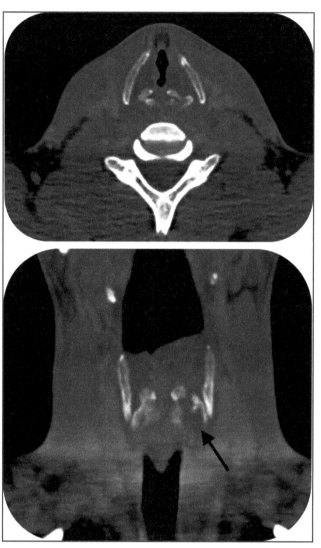

Figure 18–2. The top image is an axial CT scan which shows a fracture of the left posterior cricoid cartilage with associated lateral displacement of left arytenoid cartilage into the fracture line. The bottom image is a coronal Maximum Intensity Projection (MIP) CT reconstructed image which shows a widely separated fracture of the left posterior cricoid cartilage (black arrow) resulting in disruption of the cricoarytenoid joint. The right cricoarytenoid joint demonstrates the normal relationship between the two cartilages at this level. This figure is provided courtesy of Dr Paul F Castellanos MD.

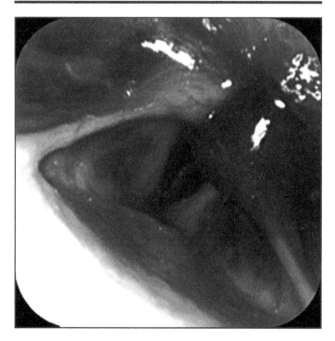

Figure 18–1. Widespread pharyngo-laryngeal swelling and hematoma which is centered on the left arytenoid area. This figure is provided courtesy of Dr Guri Sandhu.

The patient was commenced on antacid medication (omeprazole 20 mg twice a day and Gaviscon Advance after every meal). Counseling was provided regarding the possibility that there may be impairment of voice and reduction in maximal air flow through the larynx. A flexible endoscopic evaluation of swallowing

(FEES) on day 2 showed reduced laryngeal excursion but adequate airway protection during swallowing. Post-swallow residue, present on swallowing of fluids, was seen to cross the laryngeal vestibule (penetrate) and was not immediately cleared (Penetration Aspiration Score [PAS] = 5). There was trace to mild diffuse residue throughout the pharynx secondary to structural changes and swelling.

The patient's vocal folds appeared erythematous and hemorrhagic with altered closure. He showed signs of increased effort to voice and maintain vocal fold contact. He was advised to continue eating and drinking a normal diet and avoid further trauma to his vocal cords.

Four days after the injury the patient was discharged with antibiotics, steroids, anti-reflux medication, and follow-up with an ear-nose-throat specialist and a speech-language therapist. At 3 months following injury his voice had returned to normal and while he had residual reduction in the range of left vocal fold mobility, the two vocal folds were at the same vertical height. The patient had no airway restriction and was able to resume professional rugby.

A Case of Vocal Fold Avulsion

A previously fit and well 17-year-old male sustained a strangulation injury (Figure 18–3) while water-skiing. He became acutely aphonic and stridulous and expe-

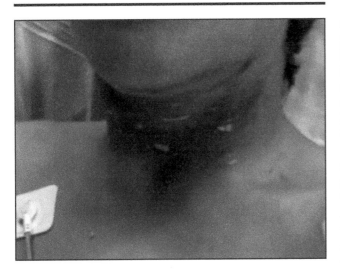

Figure 18–3. Clinical photograph of a patient with external laryngeal trauma secondary to strangulation. This figure is provided courtesy of Dr Paul F Castellanos MD.

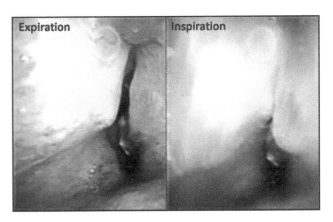

Figure 18–4. Flexible laryngoscopy performed in the resuscitation room showing significant laryngeal injury and a flail segment with inspiratory in-drawing causing stridor. This figure is provided courtesy of Dr Paul F Castellanos MD.

rienced large-volume hemoptysis. He was air-lifted to a trauma center and was received to the resuscitation area. On arrival he was breathing spontaneously, was awake and alert, but was aphonic and had predominantly inspiratory stridor. Flexible laryngoscopy showed a significant glottic injury with a flail segment with inspiratory in-drawing causing stridor (Figure 18–4). The patient was transferred to radiology with full medical escort, including a laryngologist poised to perform a front-of-neck access, and after the cervical spine had been cleared, was taken directly to the operating room. The imaging demonstrated no major bony or cartilaginous hyolaryngeal framework injuries.

The patient received induction of anesthesia and a small endotracheal tube was initially and uneventfully placed. Suspension laryngoscopy using a Benjamin–Lindholm laryngoscope was established and the endotracheal tube was carefully removed and replaced by subglottic jet ventilation. Examination of the larynx under anesthesia revealed avulsion and shearing of the left vocal fold from the body of the arytenoid cartilage (Figure 18–5).

The injury was repaired using reconstructive transoral laser microsurgical techniques. Three P-3 cutting needles and a 4-0 absorbable monofilament suture were used in figure-of-eight configuration to anchor and reapproximate the avulsed tissues back into anatomical configuration (Figure 18–6). Following the procedure, the patient was reintubated and transferred to the intensive care unit. Successful extubation occurred within 24 hours. Three months after the surgery the patient had a near-normal voice, no dysphagia, and no airway restriction.

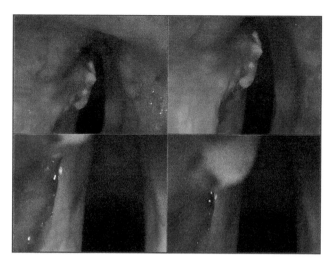

Figure 18–5. Shearing and subligamentous avulsion of the left vocal fold from the arytenoid cartilage. This figure is provided courtesy of Dr Paul F Castellanos MD.

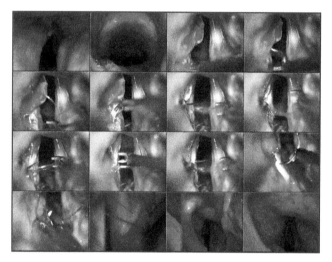

Figure 18–6. Steps of reconstructive transoral laryngeal microsurgery. No cricotracheal injuries were seen and subligamentous avulsion of the left vocal fold was repaired and tissues were re-approximated back into their anatomical positions using absorbable monofilament sutures. This figure is provided courtesy of Dr Paul F Castellanos MD.

A Case of Thyroid Cartilage Fracture

A 36-year-old previously fit and well construction worker was involved in a crush injury involving a pedestrian versus a heavy-goods vehicle during which he received crush injuries to his legs, his chest, and bluntly, to his neck. He was immediately stridulous and received intubation at the scene of the accident, following which he was air-lifted to the regional trauma center. He had bilateral chest drains placed for pneumothoraces and underwent open reduction and internal fixation with flap coverage of a compound tibia and fibula fracture. Note was made by the trauma team of the presence of anterior neck bruising and subcutaneous emphysema was documented.

Initial laryngoscopy was performed on the first day of the patient's admission and note was made of significant swelling in the supraglottis and circumferential ecchymosis of the supraglottic, post-cricoid, and piriform mucosal surfaces. There were no obvious lacerations. Glottic assessment was confounded by swelling, presence of an endotracheal tube, and an intubated and ventilated patient.

Given that the patient's airway was secure, he underwent open reduction and internal fixation with free flap coverage of his compound open tibia and fibula fractures, and then underwent a separate procedure for repair of laryngeal fracture. A cervical collar incision was used, with elevation of superior and inferior subplatysmal flaps. A separate small incision was made in the inferior flap, a tracheostomy window was established, and a soft endotracheal tube was placed. Following this, suspension laryngoscopy was performed. Given the presence of pneumothoraces and subcutaneous emphysema, use of jet ventilation was avoided.

Endoscopic examination revealed the presence of vocal fold granulation tissue, either an avulsion injury or contact ulceration (secondary to endotracheal intubation) of the left arytenoid cartilage, shortening of the anteroposterior laryngeal diameter, general vocal fold swelling, but no evidence of cricotracheal separation. Flexible esophagoscopy was performed on the table ruling out esophageal injury (Figure 18–7).

A single displaced thyroid cartilage fracture line was identified, reduced, and held in place with laryngeal mini-plates and screws (Figure 18–8). The endotracheal tube was replaced with a tracheostomy at the end of the procedure. The patient was returned to the intensive care unit, from where he was successfully discharged to the care of the ward trauma team 2 days later. The tracheostomy was removed after 7 days and at the time of discharge on day 19 the patient had mild rough (G1) dysphonia but no dysphagia, odynophagia, aspiration, or airway obstruction. Both vocal folds were mobile. Following discharge from the hospital the patient returned to Australia, no further contact could be made, and as such, longer-term outcomes could not be ascertained.

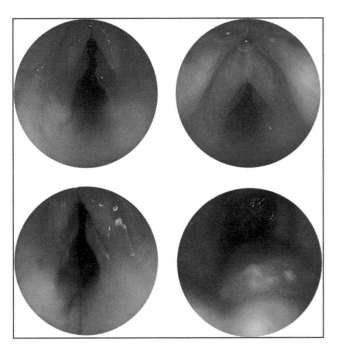

Figure 18–7. Endoscopic assessment of a case of blunt anterior laryngeal trauma causing displaced fracture of the thyroid cartilage with reduction in the anteroposterior laryngeal dimensions, laryngeal granulation tissue, and partial avulsion of the soft tissues overlying the left arytenoid cartilage. This figure is provided courtesy of Professor Reza Nouraei and Dr Edwin B Dorman.

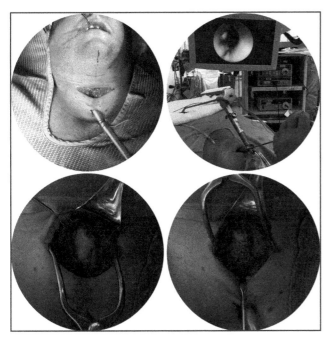

Figure 18–8. Open reduction and plate fixation of a displaced thyroid cartilage.

DISCUSSION

Incidence of Laryngeal Trauma

External laryngeal trauma occurs in 1 in 137,000 adults.[5]

Etiology of Laryngeal Trauma

The principal susceptibility of the larynx to blunt trauma is due to exposure in the neck, and the most frequent injury mechanism is through a compression injury whereby the larynx is crushed against the spinal column. This may lead to comminuted fractures particularly in the presence of laryngeal calcification in older adults.[8] Road traffic accidents (particularly dashboard or steering-wheel injuries),[9] clothesline injury,[10] sports injuries, and hanging/strangulation are the main causes of blunt laryngeal trauma.[11–14] The incidence of penetrating laryngeal trauma both in civilian life and in theaters of war has been increasing (Figure 18–9).[15]

Diagnosing Laryngeal Trauma

Pertinent History

The mechanism of injury has a significant influence on the likely pattern and severity of injury. In the case of road traffic accident, the use of seatbelt or lap belts, and the speed and configuration of collisions should be ascertained. There are differences between suicidal and homicidal strangulation,[16] with the latter more likely to cause laryngotracheal separation and neurovascular injuries. In the case of penetrating trauma, information about the nature and trajectory of a knife used, and in the case of projectile injuries, the type of weapon and the distance from which it was fired should be inquired about.

Symptoms

The most common symptom of laryngeal trauma is hoarseness (82%), followed by dysphagia (52%), odynophagia (42%), dyspnea (21%), and hemoptysis (18%).[6]

Clinical Examination

Assessment of laryngeal trauma must be conducted as part of primary and secondary surveys according to

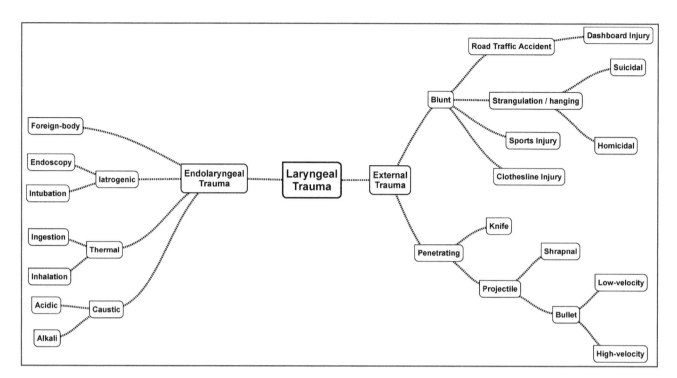

Figure 18–9. Etiology of laryngeal trauma.

Advanced Trauma Life Support (ATLS)® guidelines. As many as 20% of patients with laryngeal injury also have neck, maxillofacial, or intracranial injuries and over 10% of patients have associated chest injuries.[5] The primary objectives in managing laryngeal trauma are establishing a safe airway and protecting the cervical spine. For approximately 3% of patients this entails an emergency room intubation or tracheotomy tube placement.[17] The neck must be managed with in-line immobilization until a cervical spine injury has been excluded with CT. In the presence of significant endolaryngeal trauma, an endotracheal tube should be converted to a tracheostomy at the earliest opportunity to prevent long-term morbidity.

Inspection. Evidence of injury such as skin abrasions, bruising (see Figure 18–3), and entry and exit puncture wounds should be sought in penetrating trauma incidents. Open wounds must not be explored until the airway has been secured.

Palpation. This aims to identify subcutaneous emphysema, localized pain, and evidence of loss of normal laryngeal framework anatomy. Loss of laryngeal crepitus may indicate swelling and hematoma in the posterior cricoid or prevertebral region.

Flexible Laryngoscopy. Endoscopic examination should be performed to assess the oropharynx and hypopharynx for evidence of edema, contusions, hematoma, and lacerations. Evolving supraglottic edema and supraglottic airway obstruction is a particular concern in strangulation cases and in younger patients, and its surveillance necessitates regular serial endoscopy. The laryngeal mucosa is assessed for lacerations and hematomas (see Figure 18–1). It is not always possible to adequately examine the vibratory surface during the initial assessment or in the presence of significant swelling but it must be documented at the earliest feasible opportunity over the course of the patient's admission. Gross vocal movements are assessed through phonation and sniffing, and when possible, a stroboscopy is performed looking in particular for evidence of phase asymmetry.[18] Presence or absence of vertical height difference between the vocal folds is specifically sought and documented (Figure 18–10).

Computed Tomography

Radiological assessment of trauma patients is determined by ATLS guidelines, which in many cases mandate assessing the cervical spine. We consider CT of the cervical spine a minimum standard of care in all but the most minor of laryngeal injuries. In our practice CT is performed as soon as the airway is deemed stable, either following a tracheostomy or endotracheal intubation or following the initial laryngoscopy which judges the patient safe for transfer to a CT scanner. Laryngeal trauma is associated with cervical spine fracture in approximately 10% of patients.[5] At the same time, National Emergency X-Radiography Utilization Study (NEXUS) criteria[19] state that for a patient to be deemed low-risk for cervical spine injury, he or she should have no posterior midline cervical tenderness, no evidence of intoxication, normal level of alertness, no focal neurological deficit, and no painful distracting injuries. Any patient with laryngeal trauma should be considered to have a distracting injury,[20] and in fact one that is both close to the site of a possible cervical spine injury, and one that is known to be associated with a cervical spine injury in a significant minority of cases.[5] Using these criteria, every laryngeal trauma case requires cervical spine imaging; a CT scan has higher sensitivity and specificity for identifying cervical spine injury compared with plain radiography,[21,22] and at the same time provides vital information about the status of the larynx and hyoid bone. It is, in our practice, the investigation of choice in all but the most minor of laryngeal trauma cases.

Classifying Laryngeal Trauma

External laryngeal trauma can be classified according to the Schaefer–Fuhrman (Figure 18–10)[23,24] or the Lee–Eliashar classifications.[25] For the purposes of clinical

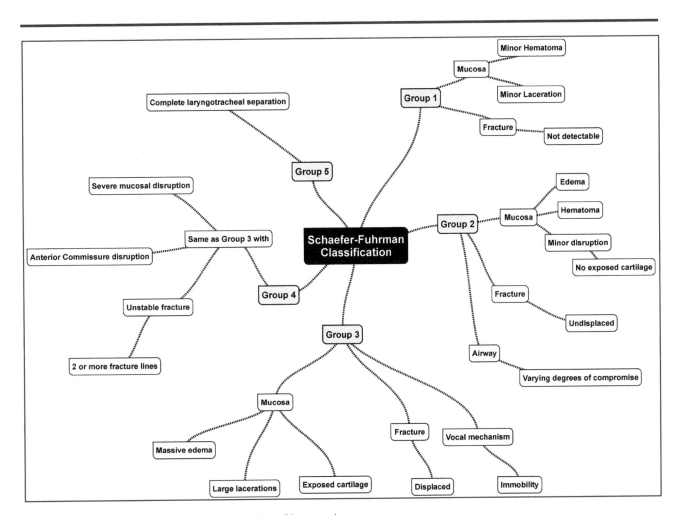

Figure 18–10. Schaefer–Fuhrman classification of laryngeal trauma.

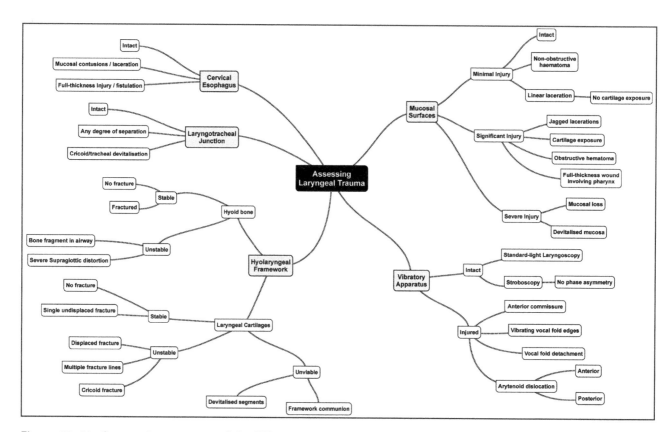

Figure 18–11. Systematic assessment of the different components of laryngeal trauma.

management, we classify and document each component of the injury separately (Figure 18–11).

MANAGING LARYNGEAL TRAUMA

Managing the Airway

Securing the airway while protecting the cervical spine is the principal priority in the early management of laryngeal trauma. Just under 40% of patients with laryngeal trauma do not require major airway intervention.[5] In cases of impending airway obstruction, a tracheostomy under local anesthesia is the preferred option, but in real life, the majority of patients who require emergency room airway intervention do in fact get intubated.[17] Once the airway has been secured, a CT scan should be performed to clear the cervical spine and at the same time obtain laryngeal imaging. Endotracheal intubation should be converted to tracheostomy at the earliest possible opportunity, which in our practice is no later than 24 hours.

Conservative Management

The decision whether to manage a laryngeal trauma patient conservatively or surgically depends on the pattern and severity of injury to the different structures (see Figure 18–11). Conservative management should be performed in a high-dependency unit with a minimum of 24 hours of observations, serial flexible laryngoscopy, and use of humidified oxygen. High-flow warmed and humidified nasal air reduces the work of breathing[26] and its use may be considered. A mixture of oxygen and helium should be on standby. The patient's head is elevated to reduce venous congestion, and corticosteroids are administered. All patients are given proton pump inhibitor and, in the case of open injuries, prophylactic broad-spectrum antibiotics.

Operative Management

Patients with significant injuries require surgical intervention. In patients who have suffered poly-trauma, the optimal timing of surgery should be coordinated with other specialties. We aim to repair injuries that require surgery within 12 hours of presentation, and no later than 24 hours. Delays in treatment can lead to granulation (Figure 18–7) and scar tissue formation, which can progress to laryngeal stenosis. In practice, however, some patients cannot be operated on acutely and in these individuals it is important to reduce further laryngeal trauma caused by trans-laryngeal intubation through performing an early tracheostomy.

Endoscopic Surgery

All surgical interventions must involve a microlaryngoscopy and tracheoscopy, direct pharyngoscopy, and direct esophagoscopy. With increasing deployment of advanced endoscopic instrumentation and techniques, an increasing range of conditions that would historically have required open repair, principally a laryngofissure for access, are now amenable to endoscopic treatment (see Figure 18–6). If there have been extensive injuries to opposing laryngeal mucosal surfaces, stents may be deployed endoscopically.[27]

Open Surgery

The main indications for open repair are unstable or comminuted laryngeal fractures, cricotracheal separation, detachment of the anterior commissure, or extensive mucosal disruption. The most common approach utilizes a cervical collar incision situated over the cricoid (see Figure 18–8). Mucosal loss can often be reconstructed with local mucosal flaps, and in particular, posterior commissure injuries should be reconstructed with posterior cricoid mucosal advancement flaps to prevent laryngeal stenosis. In selected cases this may still be performed endoscopically.[28] The anterior margins of the vocal folds are attached to the anterior thyroid cartilage or its outer perichondrium using a slow-absorbing monofilament suture. It is important to reestablish the appropriate height of the vocal folds. Thyroid cartilage fractures are repaired using permanent or resorbable miniplates (see Figure 18–8). Most cases of cricoid fractures can be treated with sutures, but in the case of posterior fractures, a nuanced judgment needs to be made about the likelihood of benefit in terms of fracture reduction (see Figure 18–2) and the morbidity associated with surgical access. Figure 18–12 provides some of the surgical

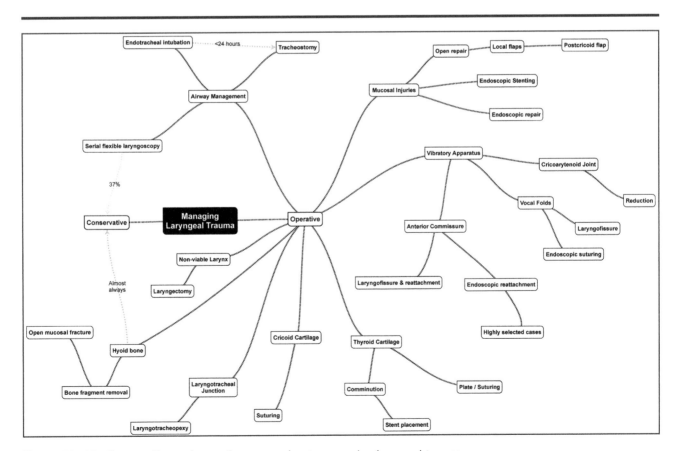

Figure 18–12. Conservative and operative approaches to managing laryngeal trauma.

approaches used to treat different components of laryngeal trauma.

POSTOPERATIVE MANAGEMENT

Strict voice rest of 48 to 72 hours duration should follow any surgery to the vibratory mechanism. A nasogastric tube should be inserted after surgery and should remain in place until the safety of swallowing is confirmed using either videofluoroscopy or fiberoptic endoscopic evaluation of swallowing. However, care must be exercised in individuals who may have sustained a burst perforation of the pharynx or esophagus, as can occur with the contact force of the larynx meeting the vertebral column. Free air in the neck or mediastinum indicates a communication between the pharyngo-esophagus and soft tissues. Nasogastric tube placement may then need to be radiologically guided or alternative options such as gastrostomy tube considered. All patients with laryngeal mucosal tears should be placed on antireflux therapy and prophylactic antibiotics. The patient is nursed in head-up position to reduce edema and standard tracheotomy care should be provided. Stents are removed at 10 to 14 days. Most patients are decannulated in 7 to 10 days. Regular assessments and intralesional steroid injection either in the operating room or in an interventional clinic is used to manage postoperative granulation tissue. In patients with cricotracheal separation, the neck is kept in flexion using a reverse soft collar 7 days to reduce anastomosis tension. Injury to the hyoid bone or esophageal contusions significantly predispose the patient to postoperative oropharyngeal dysphagia, and this should be carefully evaluated and managed to prevent aspiration and pneumonia.

FOLLOW-UP OF LARYNGEAL TRAUMA

All patients should be regularly followed up for a minimum of 12 months. Long-term morbidity results from any combination of laryngeal stenosis, glottal scar, and glottal incompetence as a consequence of both structural and neurovascular injuries. Patients with vocal fold paralysis should be carefully monitored for recovery with a low threshold for use of electromyography. An injection laryngoplasty should be considered early in the course of rehabilitation, but a definitive medialization thyroplasty should only be performed when there is minimal evidence of recovery after a sufficient time period has elapsed (minimum 9–12 months). In cases of recurrent laryngeal nerve injury, a laryngeal reinnervation procedure should be considered depending on patient characteristics and comorbidities.

In cases of bilateral vocal fold palsy, consideration should be given to retaining the tracheotomy over performing an early laser arytenoidectomy. Patients with injury to the hyoid should be carefully followed up and evaluated early with videofluoroscopy for evidence of aspiration. Active steps should be taken to reduce the risk of aspiration pneumonia through eating strategies, oral cares, pulmonary cleansing techniques, and mobilization. Laryngeal stenosis due to posterior commissure or tracheal granulation tissue should be promptly treated with intralesional steroid injections and granulation tissue reduction.[29]

OUTCOME

Outcome is dependent both on the nature and the severity of the original injury, and on whether the injury was promptly recognized and adequately treated. Schaefer and, more recently, Luutilainen et al found that the voice, but not the airway outcome related to the severity of the initial injury,[6,30] but Bent and colleagues found that intervention within 48 hours was associated with an improved outcome.[31]

SUMMARY

Laryngeal trauma is a rare but potentially acutely life-threatening injury, which if not promptly recognized and appropriately treated, can be associated with significant long-term morbidity due to permanent injury to the phonatory mechanism, airway dimensions, and interference with the respiratory control of the larynx. The greatest risk is glottal incompetence leading to airway violation. Management should be according to ATLS guidelines, and a CT scan of the neck and the cervical spine should be considered mandatory in all but the most minor cases. Some injuries, e.g., hyoid bone fractures, can almost always be managed conservatively, whereas other injuries such as anterior commissure detachment or laryngotracheal separation almost always require operative intervention. The outcome of treating this condition is dependent on the nature of the injury, speed of recognition of the injury, and administration of prompt and appropriate treatment.

REFERENCES

1. Lumb AB. *Nunn's Applied Respiratory Physiology.* 6th ed. Oxford, UK: Elsevier Butterworth-Heinemann; 2005.
2. Brates D, Molfenter SM, Thibeault SL. Assessing hyolaryngeal excursion: comparing quantitative methods to palpation at the bedside and visualization during videofluoroscopy. *Dysphagia.* 2019;34:298-307.
3. Bhojani RA, Rosenbaum DH, Dikmen E, Paul M, Atkins BZ, Zonies D, et al. Contemporary assessment of laryngotracheal trauma. *J Thorac Cardiovasc Surg.* 2005; 130:426-432.
4. Gussack GS, Jurkovich GJ, Luterman A. Laryngotracheal trauma: a protocol approach to a rare injury. *Laryngoscope.* 1986;96:660-665.
5. Jewett BS, Shockley WW, Rutledge R. External laryngeal trauma analysis of 392 patients. *Arch Otolaryngol Head Neck Surg.* 1999;125:877-880.
6. Luutilainen M, Vintturi J, Robinson S, Back L, Lehtonen H, Makitie AA. Laryngeal fractures: clinical findings and considerations on suboptimal outcome. *Acta Oto-Laryngologica.* 2007. doi 10.1080/00016480701477636.
7. Minrad G, Kudsk KA, Croce MA, Butts JA, Cicala RS. Laryngotracheal trauma. *Am Surg.* 1992;58:181-187.
8. Mupparapu M, Vuppalapati A. Ossification of laryngeal cartilages on lateral cephalometric radiographs. *Angle Orthod.* 2005;75:196-201.
9. Pennington CL. External trauma of the larynx and trachea. Immediate treatment and management. *Ann Otol Rhinol Laryngol.* 1972;81:546-554.
10. Rejali SD, Bennett JD, Upile T, Rothera MP. Diagnostic pitfalls in sports related laryngeal injury. *Br J Sports Med.* 1998;32:180-181.
11. Zatopkova L, Janik M, Urbanova P, Mottlova J, Hejna P. Laryngohyoid fractures in suicidal hanging: a prospective autopsy study with an updated review and critical appraisal. *Forens Sci Int.* 2018;290:70-84.
12. Knapik DM, Royan SJ, Salata MJ, Voos JE. Hyoid dislocation following subacute fracture in an american high school football athlete. *Orthop J Sports Med.* 2018; 6(2):2325967117753594.

13. Es H, Sahin MF, Ozdemir E. Laryngohyoid fractures in fatal nonhomicidal falls from a height. *Am J Forens Med Pathol.* 2017;38(4):289-293.
14. Hlavaty L, Sung L. Strangulation and its role in multiple causes of death. *Am J Forens Med Pathol.* 2017; 38(4):283-288.
15. Danic D, Prgomet D, Sekelj A, Jakovina K, Danic A. External laryngotracheal trauma. *Eur Arch Otorhinolaryngol.* 2006;263:228-232.
16. Maxeiner H, Bockholdt B. Homicidal and suicidal ligature strangulation—a comparison of the post-mortem findings. *Forens Sci Int.* 2003;14:60-66.
17. Sethi RKV, Khatib D, Kligerman M, Kozin ED, Gray ST, Naunheim MR. Laryngeal fracture presentation and management in United States emergency rooms. *Laryngoscope.* 2019, doi:10.1002/laryn.27790. [Epub ahead of print].
18. Sielska-Badurek EM, Jedra K, Sobol M, Niemczyk K, Osuch-Wojcikiewicz E. Laryngeal stroboscopy—normative values for amplitude, open quotient, asymmetry and phase difference in young adults. *Clin Otolaryngol.* 2019; 44:158-165.
19. Hoffman JR, R MW, Wolfson AB, Todd KH, Zucker MI. Validity of a set of clinical criteria to rule out injury to the cervical spine in patients with blunt trauma. National Emergency X-Radiography Utilization Study Group. *N Engl J Med.* 2000;343:94-99.
20. Heffernan DS, Schermer CR, Lu SW. What defines a distracting injury in cervical spine assessment? *J Trauma.* 2005;59:1396-1399.
21. Griffen MM, Frykberg ER, Kerwin AJ, Schinco MA, Tepas JJ, Rowe K, et al. Radiographic clearance of blunt cervical spine injury: plain radiograph or computed tomography scan? *J Trauma.* 2003;55:222-226.
22. Mathen R, Inaba K, Munera F, Teixeira PG, Rivas L, McKenney M, et al. Prospective evaluation of multislice computed tomography versus plain radiographic cervical spine clearance in trauma patients. *J Trauma.* 2007;62:1427-1431.
23. Fuhrman GM, Stieg FH, Buerk CA. Blunt laryngeal trauma: classification and management protocol. *J Trauma.* 1990;30:87-92.
24. Schaefer S. Primary management of laryngeal trauma. *Ann Otol Rhinol Laryngol.* 1982;91:399-402.
25. Lee WT, Eliashar R, Eliashar I. Acute external laryngotracheal trauma: Diagnosis and management. *Ear Nose Throat J.* 2006;85:184.
26. Adams CF, Geoghegan PH, Spence CJ, Jermy MC. Modelling nasal high flow therapy effects on upper airway resistance and resistive work of breathing. *Respir Physiol Neurobiol.* 2018;254:23-29.
27. Mace A, Sandhu GS, Howard DJ. Securing tracheal stents: a new and simple method. *J Laryngol Otol.* 2005; 119:207-208.
28. Atallah I, Manjunath MK, Omari AA, Righini CA, Castellanos PF. Reconstructive transoral laser microsurgery

for posterior glottic web with stenosis. *Laryngoscope.* 2017;127(3):685–690.

29. Nouraei SAR, Singh A, Patel A, Ferguson C, Howard DJ, Sandhu GS. Early endoscopic treatment of acute inflammatory airway lesions improves the outcome postintubation airway stenosis. *Laryngoscope.* 2006;116:1417–1421.

30. Schaefer SD. The acute management of external laryngeal trauma. A 27-year experience. *Arch Otolaryngol Head Neck Surg.* 1992;118:598–604.

31. Bent JP, Silver JR, Porubsky ES. Acute laryngeal trauma: a review of 77 patients. *Arch Otolaryngol Head Neck Surg.* 1993;109:441–449.

CHAPTER 19

Laryngitis

Aaron J. Jaworek, Kranthi Earasi, and Robert T. Sataloff

INTRODUCTION

Acute infectious laryngitis is one of the most common disorders of the larynx and is often associated with upper respiratory tract infection (URI).[1] The resulting laryngeal inflammation can cause hoarseness, sore throat, and difficulty swallowing, which can be particularly troublesome for singers and other professional voice users. These symptoms usually subside within 3 weeks, but chronic forms may persist for much longer (months). Clinically, it can be difficult to distinguish between bacterial and viral origins.[1] Viral laryngitis can be caused by many organisms, including, but not limited to, influenza virus, adenovirus, and even varicella zoster virus. Acute bacterial laryngitis presents similarly; however, purulent secretions are observed more commonly in these patients.[2] Treatment for viral causes remains supportive with adequate hydration and at least relative voice rest, while the bacterial form may benefit from the addition of an antibiotic. Most patients with URI symptoms are evaluated and treated by a primary care physician. It is much less common for an otolaryngologist to treat an acute episode unless there is a complicating feature (a protracted course, persistent symptoms following the URI, recurrent episodes, etc.). For this reason, high quality images of the larynx during an acute infection often are not available. Jaworek et al presented a series of patients with acute infectious laryngitis and their coinciding laryngoscopic images to highlight salient features,[3] and much of this chapter is derived from that article.

PATIENT 1

A 17-year-old female singer had a history of vocal fold nodules and reflux laryngitis. She reported a productive cough for the past 24 hours. Strobovideolaryngoscopy (SVL) revealed edema of the true vocal folds and erythema of the larynx, and thick yellow mucus was observed from within the trachea (Figure 19–1). A diagnosis of acute laryngotracheitis was made, and the patient was started on amoxicillin-clavulanate for

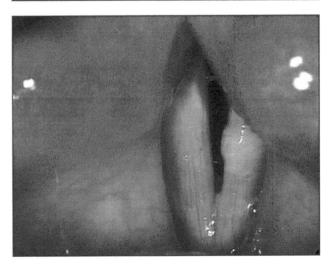

Figure 19–1. Patient 1 during acute infectious laryngitis episode.

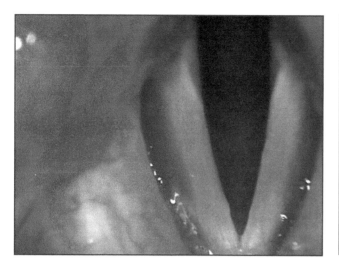

Figure 19–2. Patient 1 following resolution of acute infectious laryngitis.

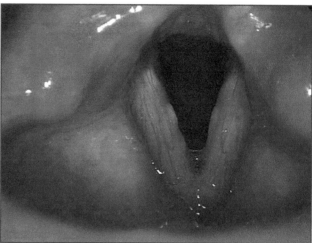

Figure 19–3. Patient 2 during acute infectious laryngitis episode.

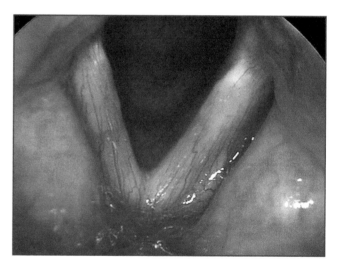

Figures 19–4. Patient 2 following resolution of acute laryngitis episode.

10 days. The patient did not follow up until 15 weeks later, at which time SVL confirmed resolution of the infection (Figure 19–2).

PATIENT 2

A 29-year-old woman presented with an acute episode of hoarseness progressing to aphonia, which she experienced 3 days before her appointment. She also reported a sore throat, odynophagia, and cough for 5 days. She had been taking a cough suppressant, antihistamine, decongestant, and acetaminophen to relieve her symptoms, and she had increased oral hydration. SVL revealed Reinke's edema and new bilateral midmembranous vocal fold masses (Figure 19–3). The amplitude and wave form of the vocal folds were decreased. She was diagnosed with acute laryngitis and treated with amoxicillin-clavulanate for 10 days and a methylprednisolone taper. At follow-up 1 week later, her voice had improved markedly. She reported that she had been able to speak "normally" after 5 days of treatment. SVL revealed resolution of the inflammatory vocal fold masses and return to baseline of laryngeal erythema and edema, and the vibratory characteristics of the vocal folds had improved (Figure 19–4).

DISCUSSION

Acute infectious laryngitis is characterized by inflammation of the larynx that usually resolves within 3 weeks. The condition often accompanies URI, with symptoms that may include hoarseness, sore throat, odynophonia, odynophagia, dysphagia, dyspnea, cough, congestion, post nasal drip, and mucous. The hoarseness often is accompanied by lowering of pitch that persists for 3 to 8 days in most cases.[1] The voice may sound breathy and/or raspy, and compensatory muscle tension dysphonia often is present. SVL frequently reveals erythema and edema of the larynx involving the true vocal folds, resulting in alteration of the mucosal wave and vibratory characteristics. Inflammatory masses also can develop on the true vocal folds, further exacerbating the dysphonia and altered pitch.[1] Jaworek et al published an interesting small series that includes seven professional voice users who had undergone baseline SVL previously and who returned with acute laryngitis.[3] Sequential SVL showed not only the expected erythema, edema, cough, and dysphonia, but also new masses in five of the seven subjects. All the signs including the masses returned to baseline. This series highlighted the reversible structural changes that can be expected in patients with acute laryngitis and the value of conservative management of the masses, all of which resolved following routine treatment for laryngitis.

Acute infectious laryngitis is caused by numerous pathogens. Among these, viral pathogens are believed to be most prevalent following patterns similar to those for URI. They include para-influenza, rhinovirus, influenza virus, and adenovirus. Bacterial pathogens that have been associated with acute laryngitis include *Moraxella catarrhalis*, *Haemophilus influenzae*, and *Streptococcus pneumoniae*, with *M. catarrhalis* being the most common.[2] Both acute viral and bacterial laryngitis are transmitted from infected individuals through inhalation or direct contact of the pathogen within aerosolized droplets from a sneeze or cough. Extension to the larynx of an infection involving the upper aerodigestive tract can occur as well. Although these bacterial and viral etiologies of acute laryngitis can be difficult to differentiate clinically, the presence of purulent secretions may favor a diagnosis of bacterial laryngitis.[2] In some cases, a sputum culture may be helpful to direct therapy.

The treatment for viral and bacterial laryngitis includes supportive measures. At least relative voice rest, humidification, analgesics, and hydration should be considered along with mucolytics, decongestants, and glucocorticoid steroids. In addition, antibiotics may be prescribed in cases in which a bacterial infection is suspected (eg, tracheitis, purulent secretions, immunocompromised state, protracted course). They may also be used when the etiology is uncertain but pressing voice commitments are imminent. A *Cochrane Review* study was completed in 2013 investigating the benefits of antibiotic usage for acute laryngitis. After reviewing the only two placebo-controlled, randomized trials that met their inclusion criteria, the authors concluded that antibiotics appeared to have no benefit; however, they acknowledged that one of the studies demonstrated a significant reduction in severity of reported vocal symptoms after 1 week on erythromycin (vs placebo) and a significant reduction in cough after 2 weeks with antibiotics.[1] Since the patients in our series were professional voice users, expeditious return to baseline vocal function was a primary concern. Therefore, prescribing an antibiotic was justified based on the conclusions of the study included in the *Cochrane Review*, as well as on the uncertainty of the etiology and the need for rapid return to safe phonation.

Laryngopharyngeal reflux (LPR), a chronic form of laryngitis, can have signs and symptoms that overlap with those of acute infectious laryngitis. The distinguishing features of reflux laryngitis include a longer duration of symptoms (usually over many weeks, months, or even years), exacerbating factors (symptoms with meals or certain foods and during specific activities), response to proton pump inhibitor/H2 blocker, and erythema/edema commonly most prominent on or isolated to the region of the arytenoids.[4] When the two pathologies coexist, it is prudent to allow the acute laryngitis episode to resolve before making any assessment on the need for long-term treatment for the reflux, but acute treatment of LPR reduces inflammation caused by both LPR and infection. When any uncertainty in the diagnosis remains, a 24-hour dual sensor pH impedance test can be completed.

Another form of chronic laryngitis, prolonged ulcerative laryngitis (PUL), also has been reported by the senior author, among others.[5] Symptoms and abnormal SVL may persist for many weeks (up to 5 months or longer in some cases). Antibiotics and corticosteroids are ineffective, and the etiology remains unknown, although the senior author suspects that biofilms may play a role.

CONCLUSION

Acute infectious laryngitis presents commonly during URI. Through SVL images, the changes along the musculomembranous vocal folds have been defined clearly and documented in this case series. Further investigation with prospective, randomized, controlled trials is needed to improve our understanding of ways to differentiate viral from bacterial causes, to determine whether the structural changes seen in this series of voice professionals also occur routinely in other patients, to help guide appropriate use or non-use of antibiotics without delays awaiting culture results, and to identify the most effective treatment strategies in various patient populations.

REFERENCES

1. Reveiz L, Cardona AF, Ospina EG. Antibiotics for acute laryngitis in adults. *Cochrane Database Syst Rev.* 2007; 18;(2):CD004783.

2. Dworkin JP. Laryngitis: types, causes, and treatments. *Otolaryngol Clin North Am.* 2008;41(2):419–436.

3. Jaworek AJ, Hu A, Lyons KM, Earasi K, Dagumatti BS, Sataloff RT. Acute infectious laryngitis. *Ear Nose Throat J.* 2018;97(9):306–313.

4. Sataloff RT, Castell DO, Katy PO, Sataloff DM, Hawkshaw MJ. Reflux and other gastroenterologic conditions that may affect the voice. In: Sataloff RT, ed, *Professional Voice: The Science and Art of Clinical Care.* 4th ed. San Diego, CA: Plural Publications; 2017:907–997.

5. Sataloff RT. Structural abnormalities of the larynx. In: Sataloff RT, ed, *Professional Voice: The Science and Art of Clinical Care.* 4th ed. San Diego, CA: Plural Publications; 2017:1564–1566.

CHAPTER 20

Tuberculosis of the Larynx

Nick Gibbons

PRESENTING HISTORY

This chapter is based on the presentation of a previously fit and well 76-year-old man originally from India who had emigrated to the UK 2 years previously. He was married with two children, both of whom lived in the UK and were fit, practicing yoga regularly. He was a non-smoker and non-drinker and his wife lived independently. However, his past medical history included pulmonary sarcoidosis that was being monitored by the respiratory physicians and kept quiescent. He also had B-thalassemia trait and well-controlled hypertension.

For approximately 4 weeks prior to presentation, he had become increasingly hoarse with concurrent dysphagia. He presented to the ENT department, and indirect laryngoscopy by means of flexible nasendoscopy (FNE) had shown a mass affecting the supraglottis bilaterally with decreased movements of both vocal folds (Figure 20–1). Further examination revealed no other mucosal abnormalities of the head and neck and no cervical lymph nodes.

He was taken urgently to theater for microlaryngoscopy and biopsy with the concern being that this represented a laryngeal malignancy. Multiple biopsies of the false vocal folds were taken and sent for histological analysis. The airway was not threatened at this point (no stridor, increased work of breathing, tachypnea) and no debulking of the laryngeal tissues was needed. He recovered uneventfully and was discharged as a day case procedure with an appointment for the following week to be seen with the results.

Over the following 4 days he became increasingly lethargic, with reduced mobility. According to his wife, his appetite decreased and he was passing urine with

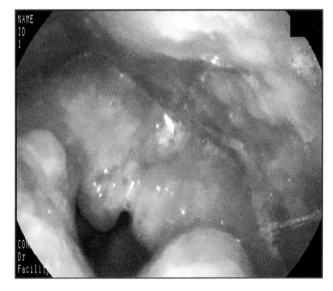

Figure 20–1. Initial FNE appearance of the patient's larynx (note very bulky arytenoids).

increased frequency. Once he started becoming confused, his family brought him to the Emergency Department for urgent review.

Examination at this time concurred that he was moderately confused with a Mini-Mental State Exam score of 7/10. His thorax and abdomen were clear, his respiratory rate was 17, his O_2 saturations were 97% on room air, and he was cardiovascularly stable.

Blood tests revealed a hyponatremia with his Na+ measured at 125 mmol/L, HIV screen was negative, C-reactive protein and erythrocyte sedimentation rate were raised and a CT showed thickening of the soft sites of the larynx and mid-esophagus, so an initial diagnosis of syndrome of inappropriate antidiuretic hormone secretion secondary to either a laryngeal or esophageal malignancy was made.

The hyponatremia responded to fluid management but his confusion remained, so a lumbar puncture was undertaken. The tap was clear and colorless and showed a white cell count of 732, no Gram stain, and no acid fast bacilli (AFBs) seen. At this point the biopsy from the larynx was confirmed as laryngeal tuberculosis (TB). The combination of the lumbar puncture and confusion in combination with the laryngeal TB led to a diagnosis of disseminated TB with laryngeal and meningeal involvement.[1] The patient was started on 12 months of anti-tuberculous treatment with quadruple therapy under the care of the respiratory and TB teams, with the current guidelines suggesting that a minimum of 10 months is needed for eradication of the bacterium.[2]

Unfortunately, within a few days he had developed an acute kidney injury and a week after diagnosis he had developed a lower respiratory tract infection. This was the first of a series of minor lower respiratory tract issues that became a pattern indicating gradual possible deterioration in laryngeal sensation and overall function. His voice and swallow continued to deteriorate and repeat examinations over a few weeks with FNE demonstrated the following (Figure 20–2):

1. Decreasing sensation of the larynx over the following few weeks

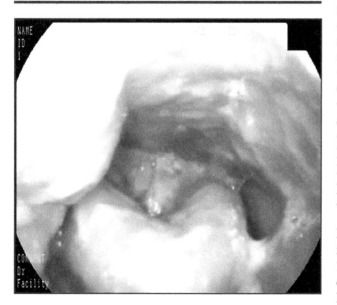

Figure 20–2. Increasing swelling with epiglottic involvement on FNE.

2. Continued movement and reasonably normal function of the vocal folds
3. Increasing bulk of the false vocal folds and epiglottis
4. Mild biphasic stridor

A multidisciplinary meeting was formed to discuss the onward management of the patient, where a discussion regarding the safety of his airway was of paramount importance. The debate was whether to remove some bulk of the false vocal folds, hopefully resolving the stridor, and leave the vocal folds fully functioning, allowing time for the anti-tuberculous treatment to reduce the size of the affected tissues, or to perform a tracheostomy.

INTRODUCTION TO TUBERCULOSIS

TB is an infectious disease caused by the bacterium mycobacterium tuberculosis and is treatable and preventable. In 2016, 10.4 million people fell ill with TB and 1.7 million died from it. It can affect any part of the body but is most commonly seen in the lungs.[3] Approximately 20% of infections are in extrapulmonary sites[4] and occur more frequently in immunocompromised patients. The most common extrapulmonary sites for TB are the lymphatic system, the central nervous system (CNS), the pleura, and the bones in the form of osteomyelitis or osseous TB. Those clinicians working in head and neck units, and especially those in city centers, will be familiar with patients presenting with an isolated neck lump[5] that ultrasound and fine-needle aspiration cytology confirm as mycobacterial infection. TB is a worldwide disease, with the World Health Organization suggesting that up to one quarter of the world population is infected,[3] but in the UK with its childhood vaccination program, most presenting patients are now from first-generation immigrant families originally from Africa or the Indian subcontinent. It can be seen in any race or background and has a propensity for low socioeconomic status, overcrowding, and poor hygiene areas.

Mycobacterium tuberculosis is an aerobic bacillus (Figure 20–3). It is an interesting pathogen, as it is the tortoise of the bacterial world; it divides every 16 to 20 hours,[6] which is very slow for bacteria (most divide every hour or less) but has a tough bilipid outer layer.[7] It is this outer layer that allows it to survive disinfectants or in a dry state for weeks. Although it can "hibernate" for a while outside the body, it can

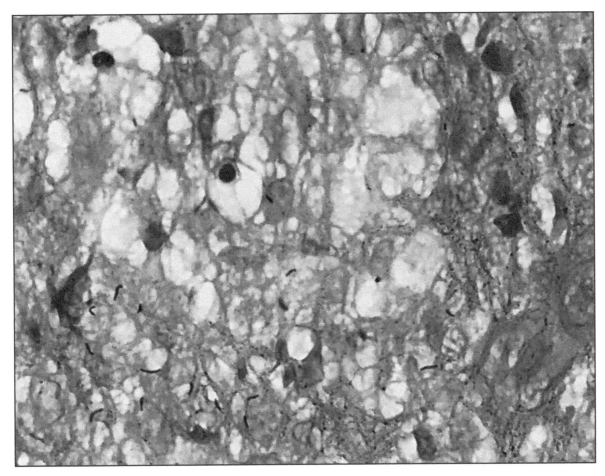

Figure 20–3. Histopathological specimen showing AFBs and granuloma formation (courtesy of Dr Andrew Giles, Pathologist University Hospital, Lewisham).

only replicate within the confines of a living organism. It is this resilience that has accounted for its presence and description throughout human history—the earliest known presence of TB infection is from 9000 years ago, found in human remains from Atlit Yam, in the eastern Mediterranean.[8] Accounts suggest that TB did not change very much over 9 millennia until the start of the antibiotic era. Since then, resistant strains have evolved, mainly to the two most powerful first-line anti-TB drugs, isoniazid and rifampicin; but more recently some strains have been found to also be resistant to second-line drugs. These strains are known as extensively drug-resistant TB (XDR-TB).[9]

Laryngeal TB is rare, accounting for less than 1% of all TB cases,[10] and its incidence has remained stable.[11]

Juxtaposed to this is the fact that TB is the most common granulomatous disease of the larynx.[12] When seen, it is usually secondary to a tuberculous lesion elsewhere in the body; however, case reports of primary laryngeal TB have been described.[13] It can often be difficult to diagnose as there are no pathognomic features of laryngeal TB and it can mimic laryngeal cancer in both its appearance and occasionally rapid growth.[14] Diagnosis, therefore, must rely on a good history, appropriate investigations and laryngeal biopsy. Due to the wide variation in clinical presentation, a high degree of suspicion must be maintained in high risk individuals, such as those from geographical areas where TB is endemic, and the immunocompromised individuals (diabetes, HIV, or transplant patients).

EFFECTS OF TUBERCULOSIS ON THE LARYNX

Laryngeal TB can affect any part of the larynx due to both hematological and lymphatic spread, so presentation may include any symptoms associated with the larynx: dysphonia, dysphagia, dyspnea, and odynophagia (Figure 20–4A and B). TB infection of the larynx begins

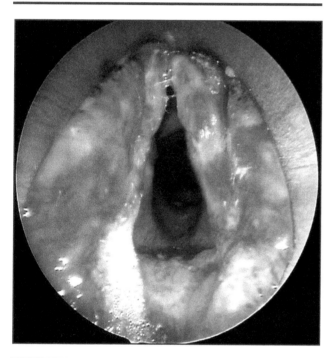

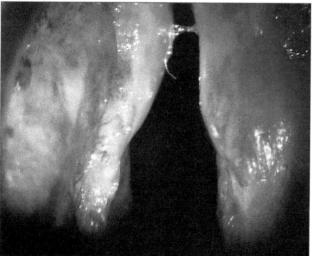

Figure 20–4. Laryngeal TB with true and false vocal fold involvement at microlaryngoscopy (courtesy of G. Sandhu).

with an inflammatory response in the subepithelial space, followed by round cell infiltration and fibrotic healing.[15] If this occurs in the superficial lamina propria, the resulting fibrosis can permanently alter the epithelial vibration and subsequently the voice. Vocal fold scarring is one of the most difficult epithelial defects to treat within the larynx, and the search for a treatment with good and repeatable outcomes has and continues to generate volumes of research. So far, a lamina propria replacement or injectable material have yet to be found, so protecting and maintaining the vocal fold vibration is particularly important.

As well as the soft tissues of the larynx, TB can involve the underlying skeleton of the larynx; the arytenoid, corniculate, and cuneiform cartilages especially. Infiltration of cartilage by TB is caused by hematogenous spread. It can cause fibrosis and thickening of the cartilage that can cause sluggish movements of the crico-arytenoid joint (CAJ).[16] Hematogenous spread into the joint synovium causes an inflammatory reaction followed by granulation tissue formation that can erode the cartilage itself. TB is not a pyogenic infection and does not produce proteolytic enzymes. These proteolytic enzymes destroy peripheral cartilage and so without them the joint space is preserved for much longer than might be expected.[17] However, if the infection progresses unchecked or with inadequate levels of treatment, abscesses may form in the tissues surrounding the joint and destroy the synovium, rendering the CAJ immobile. If immobile, the larynx is at risk of becoming incompetent and exposing the patient either to the risks of aspiration due to an inability to close the glottis or to airway compromise due to bilateral vocal fold palsy secondary to bilateral CAJ fixation.

There is no evidence to suggest the most common areas of the larynx affected by TB, but case reports suggest that the interarytenoid region, the arytenoid cartilages, the superior surface of the vocal folds, and the laryngeal surface of the epiglottis are most likely to be affected.[12,18,19] In the past, pulmonary TB was managed with bed rest, and the hypothesis was that as patients were on their backs for extended periods of time, the AFBs present in lung cavities, when expelled, would more likely come to rest in the posterior larynx. However, with prolonged bed rest no longer used, the incidence of TB in different parts of the larynx is much more even.[20]

The knowledge that the cartilage, the lamina propria, and the synovium can be affected, all of which can cause long-term problems with the competency of the larynx and with the voice, suggests that aggressive treatment with anti-tuberculous treatments should be employed to try to prevent these problems. If medical treatment is successful, the function of the larynx should return to normal, but if not successful, or if the diagnosis or treatment is delayed, or if the TB is a particularly aggressive or resistant strain, both voice outcomes and overall competency of larynx can be compromised.

DECISION MAKING

When deciding a management plan for patients with TB of the larynx, a multidisciplinary approach should always be employed, as it is rare that the larynx is affected in isolation. It is likely that the larynx will not be affected to a degree where the airway is at risk, and so medical treatment of the systemic condition is of paramount importance. Likewise, in this case, the patient had two rare complications of TB: tuberculous meningitis and tuberculous laryngitis. The patient's tuberculous meningitis had been confirmed on lumbar puncture and was being treated aggressively with quadruple antibiotic therapy, but he still had a hugely engorged supraglottis that was compromising his airway.

A decision had to be made as to whether trying to improve his normal airway by means of debulking the tumor would be better or worse than inserting a (hopefully temporary) tracheostomy during the medical treatment of his meningeal TB, with the hope that resolution of his meningeal disease would concurrently lead to regression of the laryngeal portion of his condition.

The arguments for debulking included:

- The arytenoids were moving and his cough was good, indicating a competent larynx.
- His meningeal TB appeared to be slowly improving.
- The family did not want a tracheostomy if possible (important as they would be the people looking after it in the community, when patient is discharged from hospital).
- There was no guarantee that the tracheostomy would be temporary.

Arguments against debulking and for tracheostomy were:

- Definitive, safe airway would be immediately obtained.

- Once the TB had been treated, the tracheostomy would be removed, leaving a normal larynx.

After prolonged discussions with the medical respiratory team looking after the patient and the family, a debulking procedure was opted for as first-line surgical management. If the false vocal folds could be debulked, it was hoped that patient would be able to maintain his own airway, and tracheostomy would be avoided. The family, as advocates for the patient, who was unable to consent for himself due to altered mental state from the meningeal TB, were keen to avoid a tracheostomy if possible. This did not remove the possibility of proceeding to tracheostomy at a future time if the situation deteriorated.

The patient underwent a microlaryngoscopy examination under anesthesia and debulking of the false vocal folds using coblation—a minimally invasive technology that removes tissue using a controlled, stable plasma field at low temperatures. Only the false vocal folds were debulked, with the true vocal folds and arytenoids left untouched. Although there was significant tissue swelling on and around the arytenoids, any iatrogenic trauma ran the risk of causing scarring of the cartilage and synovial joints. Tissue was sent for histology, which confirmed the continued presence of tuberculous granulomata.

The patient made an uneventful recovery over the following few days and continued his treatment. Unfortunately his airway deteriorated and the decision to obtain a definitive airway in the form of a tracheostomy was made in collaboration with the medical team and the patient's family. At the time of tracheostomy insertion, a repeat examination of the larynx was performed that showed increased size of the false vocal folds since the debulking procedure a few days previously. In addition, palpation of the arytenoid cartilages revealed reduced movements in both arytenoid joints. Although not completely fixed, movements were minimal. It was therefore likely that unless there was fairly rapid resolution of the patient's overall TB load and disease burden, then his arytenoids would become fixed.

There are no data in the literature regarding the fate of fixed arytenoid due to TB, when the patient's systemic TB is subsequently treated. However, extrapolating from the basic science, it is likely that direct effect on the cartilage by hematogenous spread and infiltration of the synovial by granuloma formation would lead to irreversible fibrosis and CAJ fixation.

The patient continued to be treated with high dose anti-tuberculous medication and his overall picture slowly improved. Interval examinations under anesthesia (EUA), every 4 to 6 weeks showed gradual improvement in the overall state of the larynx; the bulk of the false vocal folds and overlying of the arytenoid cartilages receded until the larynx looked almost normal. Unfortunately, further EUAs confirmed CAJ fixation, so although the soft tissues of the larynx appeared almost normal, the patient was left with bilateral vocal fold fixation (not to be confused with bilateral vocal fold palsy, as the neurology was intact, although the final effect is much the same).

LIVING WITH THE CONSEQUENCES

The patient was an in-patient for over 14 months. He had prolonged anti-tuberculous treatment and because the primary site was meningeal, he had had severe global neurological deficit. His airway had become critical and a tracheostomy was inserted. This gave the larynx time to recover, with the huge glottic and arytenoid swelling reducing over the course of a couple of months to the point where the larynx looked normal to outward appearances.

However, a consequence of the severe nature of the TB infection of the larynx was to cause CAJ fixation. On examination while the patient was awake using FNE it was noted that the glottis now appeared insensate. One was able to touch the glottis, including the vocal folds with the endoscope without any reaction from the patient. During these examinations, it was possible to watch secretions flow into the glottis with no effort from the patient to clear his throat or cough.

In the case of other, isolated non-iatrogenic neurological deficits—for example, an idiopathic recurrent laryngeal nerve palsy, the consensus has varied as to how long to wait before offering the patient a permanent surgical procedure to restore the voice. Length of time has been variously reported but most guidelines have traditionally suggested between 6 and 12 months. However, Gayle Woodson and Robert Miller published the definitive review on this topic in 1981,[21] which suggested there was little evidence for these time frames, and there has been no published evidence to counter this conclusion in the intervening 35 years.

However, what has improved in the last two decades in this regard has been the role of injection media-

lization thyroplasty as an early intervention to maintain the competence of the larynx in the case of unilateral vocal fold palsy. This allows a temporary fix for a problem that may resolve over the next few months. Anecdotally, in the author's practice, there have been a handful of cases in which idiopathic laryngeal nerve palsy has resolved between 12 and 18 months post-onset, but this is a subject for another book. In short, the length of time one should wait until performing permanent surgical intervention on the larynx for neurological deficit is currently a matter of clinical judgment.

With this in mind, the treatment options for this patient were influenced by the following factors:

1. 70-year-old gentleman.
2. He had physically but not mentally recovered from meningeal TB after a year of anti-tuberculous treatment.
3. Had spent 15 months in hospital almost bed bound (with transfers to chair occasionally possible).
4. He had suffered, among other things, three separate episodes of aspiration pneumonia despite an inflated, non-fenestrated tracheostomy tube in situ.
5. He was being fed via a gastrostomy tube due to his unsafe swallow.
6. He needed round the clock nursing care.

The treatment options were now on the basis that there would be no resolution of laryngeal nerve function, leaving the patient with bilateral vocal fold fixation by means of arytenoid cartilage sclerosis (minimal airway) and an insensate larynx by soft tissue and possibly neural involvement of the supraglottic tissues. The treatment options were therefore limited to a permanent tracheostomy or a laryngectomy.

In a case of bilateral vocal fold palsy with airway compromise, an option often employed is a posterior partial arytenoidectomy.[22] Ninety percent of the airflow in the larynx is through the posterior glottis, so increasing the diameter in this area should improve the airway. Pouseille's law regarding the fluid dynamics in laminar flow through a cylinder shows that, all other things being equal, flow is proportional to the radius to the fourth power: In other words a small increase in radius leads to a large increase in flow. The voice is mostly maintained, as the anterior half of the vocal folds is the main area of contact during phonation, although there is always an inevitable balance that must be struck between airway and voice. However, in this patient's case, arytenoidectomy was immediately ruled out as an option. The patient was aspirating secretions due to his insensate larynx and any further widening of the glottis to improve the airway would inevitably lead to increased aspiration.

The idea of a laryngectomy initially dismayed the relatives of the patient, as it was a difficult psychological jump from meningeal TB that had mostly resolved to a laryngectomy. However, the patient had already had three bouts of aspiration pneumonia, with secretions having managed to pass the cuff on the tracheostomy tube. This was while the patient was on a monitored ward in the hospital. The risk of aspiration would most likely be higher in the community unless specialist tracheostomy care could be sourced and paid for. Having had a year in hospital, it was inevitable that the patient's physiological reserves would be depleted and so there would only be a certain number of lower respiratory infections that he would be able to recover from. In addition, due to the patient's reduced mental faculties, it would be impossible for him to look after the tracheostomy himself, so specialist nursing would have to be sourced.

A laryngectomy, on the other hand, would create a definitive and relatively safe airway and avoid the risk of overspill aspiration. It would involve a large operation and physiological insult, but unlike a laryngectomy for cancer, it would not involve neck dissections and the morbidity from it would potentially be lower. Now that the larynx looked normal on indirect laryngoscopy, it was assumed that the surrounding subepithelial tissues would also have returned to normal.

It should be noted that if the larynx had preserved neurological function and the patient had been protecting his own airway, a supraglottic hemilaryngectomy could have been considered, preserving the vocal folds—but the tissue of the false vocal folds had been large and was compromising the airway.

FINAL OPTIONS

The decision was made to persist with a tracheostomy, as the family wanted to wait and see if there would be some return of function of the larynx. If the patient were able to protect his own airway, then this might negate the need for a laryngectomy. The patient was transferred into the community to the family home after 15 months as an in-patient with 24-hour tracheostomy specialist nursing care. There was no provision for changing the tracheostomy tube in the community, so he was brought into hospital on a monthly basis to do this and to check both the stoma site and the larynx via FNE. For 6 months the patient continued to attend appointments for tube changes but in this time no recovery of laryngeal function was detected. During these 6 months he had had two episodes of lower respiratory tract infection, during one of which he had expectorated some of his gastrostomy feed. This led to the conclusions that he was suffering from reflux, regurgitating his feed, and that the regurgitated substance had then been aspirated and found a way inferiorly past the cuffed tracheostomy tube.

The reflux of feed was visible on FNE and was treated with pro-motility agents with some, but not complete, success. However, the family agreed that the patient's airway was still precarious and now that he was 21 months post admission to hospital it was very likely that no recovery of the laryngeal function was likely.

It was agreed with the family to explore the possibility of a laryngectomy. A laryngectomy for persistent aspiration is a recognized procedure but for a larynx that had been infiltrated by TB had not previously been described in the literature. It was assumed that the granulomatous inflammation would have caused significant scarring of the paralaryngeal tissues and would make the dissection more difficult, even though the FNE appearance was now normal. Whether or not the surgical site and neck wounds would heal was also a consideration while deciding on whether the operation would be feasible. It is well known that the incision of active TB in the neck can produce a non-healing discharging sinus (when spontaneously discharging, this is known as scrofula—Figure 20–5), so any active residual TB in the larynx could potentially lead to breakdown of the post-op wound and a pharyngocutaneous fistula. Therefore, repeat microlaryngoscopy and biopsy were performed to exclude any obvious infection, and a repeat of a CT scan of the neck was performed to exclude any obvious cartilaginous involvement. Both were negative for signs, and so laryngectomy was deemed technically possible.

Further consideration was taken of the patient's overall health status. At the time of writing, he is still bed bound and needing 24-hour specialist care. His physical reserves are low and it is currently the determination that a 2 to 3-hour operation may be too much physiological stress and is currently too high an anesthetic and surgical risk for him to undertake. The operation is currently not being pursued.

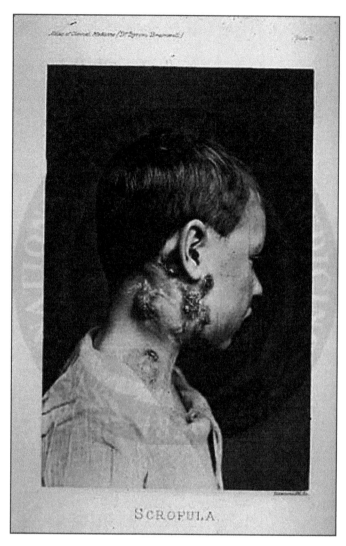

Figure 20–5. Historical picture of scrofula of the neck. From: Bramwell, Byron Edinburgh, Constable, 1893 Atlas of Clinical Medicine. Source: National Library of Medicine, National Institutes of Health, USA.

DISCUSSION

This gentleman's case highlights a number of areas that must be addressed when managing and treating a patient with laryngeal TB:

1. Isolated TB of the larynx is rare and it is more likely that other systems would be affected, so look for other signs and symptoms (in this case, disseminated disease with pulmonary and meningeal involvement).

2. Although this gentleman was a recent arrival from the Indian subcontinent and so TB was considered as a diagnosis early on in the investigative process, TB in the Western world is on the increase and must be considered when assessing laryngeal masses in patients of any ethnic background.

3. TB of the larynx can affect any part of the larynx, including the soft tissue, cartilage, and synovium.

Each affected area can cause different signs and symptoms.

4. TB of the larynx presents as, and can easily be mistaken for, laryngeal carcinoma. Diagnosis is from biopsy.

5. Early anti-tuberculous treatment may remove the need for surgical treatment to the larynx.

6. Late diagnosis and treatment or aggressive or drug-resistant TB may cause vocal fold fixation.

7. Surgical treatment options depend on the ability of the patient to protect his/her airway.

8. The patient's larynx should be treated holistically in conjunction with family rather than in isolation.

9. Laryngectomy for TB of the larynx is a feasible option once active disease has been proven to be eradicated.

Early and accurate diagnosis is of the utmost importance to give your patient the best chance of a full recovery. An accurate and detailed description of any surgical procedure concentrating on the after-effects and what the patient will need to deal with postoperatively is important. One may aim for short-term improvement of symptoms, but it should be balanced with the patient's potential long-term outcome.

TB is a prevalent disease in the developing world, and—thanks to the rise of HIV, immunosuppression from chronic disease treatments or post-transplant surgery, and the appearance of drug-resistant strains—laryngeal TB may again become a common sight in our future practice.

REFERENCES

1. https://www.nice.org.uk/guidance/ng33/chapter/recommendations#active-tb
2. Thwaites G, Fisher M, Hemingway C, Scott G, Solomon T, Innes J. British Infection Society guidelines for the diagnosis and treatment of tuberculosis of the central nervous system in adults and children. *J Infect*. 2009; 59:167–187.
3. Tuberculosis fact sheet No. 104. WHO. Updated Oct 2017.
4. Golden MP, Vikram HR. Extrapulmonary TB: an overview. *Am Fam Phys*. 72(9):1761–1768.
5. Rockwood RR. Extrapulmonary TB: what you need to know. *Nurse Pract*. 32(8):44–49.
6. Latawa R, Verma I. Mycobacteria: an overview. In: Jindal S, ed, *Textbook of Pulmonary and Critical Care Medicine Vols 1 and 2*. Jaypee Brothers Medical Publishers; New Delhi, IN, 2015:525–527.
7. Niederweis m, Danilchanka O, Huff J, Hoffmann C, Engelhaft H. Mycobacterial outer membranes: in search of proteins. *Trends in Microbiology*. 2010;18(3):109–116.
8. Hershkovitz I, Donoghue HD, Minnikin DE, et al. Detection and molecular characterisation of 9000-year-old Mycobacterium tuberculosis from a neolithic settlement in the eastern Mediterranean. *Plos One* 2008; 3(10): e3426. https://doi.org/10.1371/journal.pone.0003426
9. Velayati AA, Masjedi MR, Farnia P, et al. Emergence of new forms of totally drug-resistant tuberculosis bacilli: super extensively drug-resistant tuberculosis or totally drug-resistant strains in Iran. *Chest*. 2009;136(2):420–425.
10. Egeli E, Oghan F, Alper M, Marputluoglu U, Bulut I. Epiglottic tuberculosis in patient treated with steroids for Addison's disease. *Tohoku J Exp Med*. 2003;201:119–125.
11. Yencha MW, Linfesty R, Blackman A. Laryngeal tuberculosis. *Am J Otolaryngol*. 2000;21(2):122–126.
12. Özüdogru E, Çakli H, Altunas EE, Gürbüz MK. Effects of laryngeal tuberculosis on vocal fold functions: case report. *Acta Otorhinolaryngol Ital*. 2005;25:374–377.
13. El Ayoubi F, Chariba I, El Ayoubi A, CHariba S, Essakalli L. Primary tuberculosis of the larynx. *Eur Ann Otorhinolaryngol Head Neck Dis*. 2014;131(6):361–364.
14. Verma SK. Laryngeal tuberculosis clinically similar to laryngeal cancer. *Lung India*. 2007;24(3):87–89.
15. Broek PV. Acute and chronic laryngitis. In: Kerr AG, ed, *Scott Brown's Otolaryngology*. 6th ed. Oxford, UK: Butterfield-Heinemann Reed Educational and Professional Publishing; 1997:1–20.
16. Travis LW, Hybels RL, Newman MH. Tuberculosis of the larynx. *Laryngoscope*. 1976;86:549–558.
17. Mousa AM. Bones and joints tuberculosis. *Bahrain Medical Bulletin*. 2007;29(1):17–21.
18. Kandiloros DC, Nikolopoulos TP, Ferekidis EA, et al. Laryngeal tuberculosis at the end of the 20th century. *J Laryngol Otol*. 1997;111(7):619–621.
19. Rizzo PB, Da Mosto MC, Claro M, Scotton PG, Vaglia A, Marchiori C. Laryngeal tuberculosis: an often forgotten diagnosis. *Int J Infect Dis*. 2003;7(2):129–131.
20. Travis LW, Hybels RL, Newman MH. Tuberculosis of the larynx. *Laryngoscope*. 1976;86:549–558.
21. Woodson GE, Miller RH. The timing of surgical intervention in vocal cord paralysis. *Otolaryngol Head Neck Surg*. 1981;89(2):264–267.
22. Li Y, Garrett G, Zealear D. Current treatment options for bilateral vocal fold paralysis: a state-of-the-art review. *Clin Exp Otorhinolaryngol*. 2017;10(3):203–212.

CHAPTER 21

Recurrent Respiratory Papillomatosis Disease Progression in Pregnancy

Paul C. Bryson and Faez H. Syed

A 30-year-old woman (Jane Doe) presented with adult-onset recurrent respiratory papillomatosis (AORRP) involving the larynx beginning at age 20 for which she has received periodic debulking procedures every 1–3 years. She has recently become pregnant and lesions have spread to her trachea with symptoms of both hoarseness and shortness of breath. She has a 15-pack-year smoking history and denies alcohol consumption since becoming pregnant. The patient is single but lives with her mother and father in the inner city and works as a convenience store manager as the family breadwinner.

What are her options for management during pregnancy?

BACKGROUND

RRP is a chronic viral disease in both children and adults that is caused most commonly by human papillomavirus (HPV) types 6 and 11. It is typically characterized by exophytic benign papillary condylomatous neoplasms of the upper airway[1-3] that can result in hoarseness and in extreme cases obstruct the airway.[4] RRP tends to recur despite repeated surgical and adjuvant medical treatment[5] and can, rarely, undergo malignant transformation and spread throughout the airway.[6] Patients with RRP may require numerous surgical procedures throughout their lives to maintain airway patency, limit tracheal and pulmonary spread

of the virus, and maintain vocal function, thus placing significant physical, emotional, and financial burden on patients and their families.[7]

RRP is a rare disease, with an incidence of 3.5 per million person-years and a prevalence of 4 in 100,000 children[8] and 1.8 in 100,000 adults.[9] The age of onset for AORRP has a bimodal distribution with a peak at 35 years, and an additional peak in prevalence at 64 years.[10] While cases have been diagnosed as early as 1 day,[9] the average age of diagnosis in children is 3.8 years.[10] According to results from the National Registry of Juvenile Onset Recurrent Respiratory Papillomatosis (JORRP), 62.7% of children with RRP were white, 28.3% were black, and 2.3% were Asian or Native American.[11]

VIROLOGY/HISTOLOGY

The most common HPV subtypes in RRP are types 6, 11, 16, 18, 31, and 33.[12] Types 6 and 11 are less likely to become malignant, but compared with type 6, type 11 is more locally aggressive and carries a higher risk of malignant transformation.[13] On the other hand, HPV types 16 and 18 are more rare and more commonly associated with malignant transformation.[12] It has been thought that differential interaction between early viral proteins E6 and E7, with tumor suppressors protein 53 (p53) and retinoblastoma protein (pRB), respectively, determines the risk of progression to malignancy. This correlates with the fact that in type 6 and type 11 HPV, E6/E7 possess lower biological activity compared with E6/E7 in types 16 and 18, which more commonly lead to cell immortalization.[14] However, there have also been cases where expression of p53 and pRB was un-altered in tumor progression.[15] While malignant transformation is still not completely understood, risk factors include cigarette smoking and radiation therapy.[16]

On gross examination, RRP lesions are exophytic, and may be either pedunculated or sessile. Their coloration is usually pinker compared with normal larynx and they may have a lobulated surface with a spotted, angiogenic pattern (due to vasculature at the center of each individual papilla) (Figure 21–1). As described by Kashima et al, lesions typically occur at junctions of the respiratory and squamous epithelia such as the vestibule, nasopharyngeal soft palate, laryngeal aspect of the epiglottis, margins of the ventricle, inferior surface of the vocal folds, carina, and bronchial spurs.[17]

Microscopically, lesions are characterized by squamous epithelium in finger-like projections with thin fibrovascular cores, hyperplastic basilar and parabasilar cells, and koilocytes (Figure 21–2). The epithelial cells of the lesion have been characterized with an increased nuclear-to-cytoplasmic ratio and perinuclear halo with irregular membranes and hyperchromasia.[18] While the most common serotypes of HPV cause benign lesions, all grades of dysplasia and carcinoma have been diagnosed from biopsy specimens of even non-malignant lesions, with rare instances of mild or even severe dysplasia progressing to squamous cell carcinoma.[19] It has also been observed that squamous metaplasia of normally ciliated pseudo-columnar epithelium in the larynx as a result of uncontrolled gastroesophageal

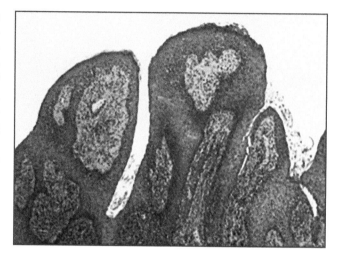

Figure 21–2. Histological section of laryngeal papilloma with polypoid growth and fibrovascular core (H&E; magnification, x33) (from Derkay and Wiatrak, 2008[30]).

reflux disease (GERD) is potentially a conducive environment for RRP.[20]

MODE OF TRANSMISSION

Transmission in adults is primarily horizontal through sexual contact, though cases of latent juvenile infection activated by changes in host environment should be considered.[12] In children, transmission may be perinatal, via auto/hetero inoculation, and possibly via fomites or sexual abuse.[21]

PRESENTATION AND COURSE

RRP is the most prevalent benign laryngeal neoplasm in children.[22,23] The vocal fold is the earliest and most common site of involvement, and hoarseness is the main presenting symptom in adults, while airway signs such as stridor are more common in children.[17] Less typically children present with cough, pneumonia, failure to thrive, or acute respiratory distress secondary to upper respiratory tract infection. The natural history is variable, with periods of more frequent regrowth or periods of remission.[24] Regardless, recurrence is the rule.

Younger age of onset (and therefore smaller airways) and lower airway lesions are associated with

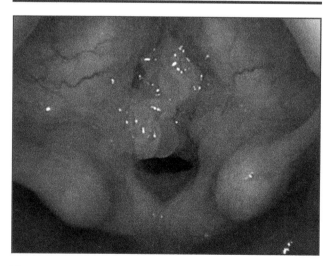

Figure 21–1. Gross papilloma lesions as seen on direct laryngoscopy (from Derkay and Wiatrak, 2008[30]).

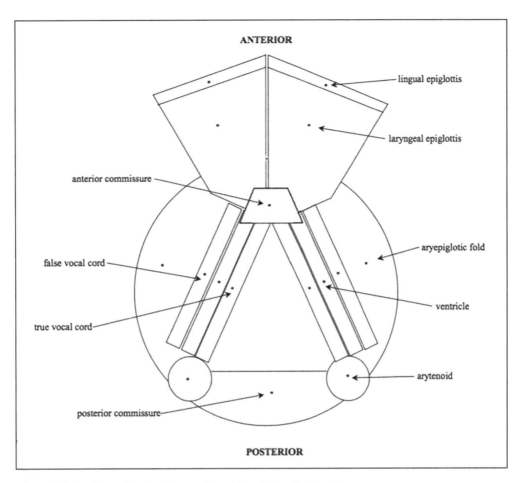

Figure 21–3. Map of lesional spread for determining Derkay stage.

tracheal obstruction, which may require tracheotomy to preserve the airway; however, it is felt that this can increase the risk of seeding at the tracheostomy and is thus avoided if possible.[25] Studies indicate that 30% of children have extralaryngeal spread, with the most common sites in children in order of frequency being oral cavity, trachea, bronchi, and esophagus.[9,17,26] In one study, children with HPV 11 had a higher risk of airway obstruction and a greater likelihood of needing a tracheotomy.[27]

In fewer than 1% of cases, JORRP can spread to affect the lungs in children, which is associated with a poor prognosis. Lesions begin as non-calcified nodules that do not present with symptoms[28]; eventually they enlarge, cavitate centrally, and undergo necrosis. This rare patient population may then present with recurrent bronchiectasis or pneumonia, or simply declining pulmonary function due to destruction of lung parenchyma.[29]

Studies report that a minority of adults have extralaryngeal spread.[27] The most common laryngeal signs and symptoms include first hoarseness, then dyspnea, cough, recurrent pneumonia, dysphagia, and respiratory distress.[30] Tracheal and pulmonary spread and course in adults will be discussed in subsequent sections of the chapter.

STAGING

The staging system proposed initially in 1998 by Derkay has achieved wide acceptance among otolaryngologists[31] and has shown to be reliable.[32] Furthermore, the anatomic burden of disease from Derkay staging has been shown to correlate positively with voice-related quality of life in adults as designated by the Voice Handicap Index 10 (VHI-10), though results cannot be extended to children due to sample size.[33] The Derkay staging system (Figure 21–3) consists of functional parameters (voice quality, urgency of intervention, stridor) and anatomic parameters (25 sites of respiratory and upper gastrointestinal tracts with lesions at each site being further characterized as absent, surface, raised, or bulky). In pediatric patients, the Derkay staging system has shown to effectively predict surgical interval for anatomic score, stridor with activity compared with lack of stridor, and urgency of intervention.[34]

> **Case Consideration 1:** Is caesarian section indicated for pregnant women with RRP?

It used to be thought that perinatal transmission occurred only through contact with the birth canal, but it has been demonstrated that vertical transmission from mother to baby has also occurred during caesarian birth.[35] Other possible routes include an ascending infection after rupture of membranes, infection from spermatozoa during fertilization, and hematogenous transmission.[21] Overt maternal condyloma are found in over 50% of mothers who deliver children with RRP; however, a child's risk of getting RRP from a mother with active genital condyloma is only 1 in 231 to 400.[7,36–38] Kashima et al[35] have demonstrated that caesarean delivery does not significantly reduce the risk of developing JORRP in high risk neonates (first-born, vaginal delivery, and teenage mother). As a result, caesarean delivery is not mandated in high risk mothers (primigravida, teenage, HPV history).[36]

SURGICAL MANAGEMENT AND CONSIDERATIONS

The primary modality of treatment for RRP is surgical debridement and removal of lesions with or without adjuvant medical therapy. The approach should begin with direct laryngoscopy or bronchoscopy to characterize the extent of lesional spread and procurement of a biopsy sample for histology and for viral subtype analysis, followed by debulking and removal via a number of different modalities available to the surgeon.[12] Preferences vary depending on the surgeon and his/her experience and level of comfort using various modalities, including cold steel removal, microdebridement, and laser ablation. To date there have been few to no studies that directly compare surgical modalities.

CLASSICAL MODALITIES OF SURGICAL MANAGEMENT

Phonomicrosurgery with Cold Steel Instrumentation

Cold steel instruments are the traditional modality for debulking and removal of papillomata in the aerodigestive tract and was the dominant technique utilized before the advent of the CO_2 laser and other powered instrumentation. Cold steel has also been used successfully for treatment of early glottic cancer and premalignant lesions.[39] One possible advantage of cold steel instruments compared with other modalities is that they can make use of micro-flap surgery techniques for the potentially complete removal of epithelial lesions in RRP. However, this is mitigated by the fact that virus is likely present in normal epithelium. Sataloff et al conducted a study of 22 patients treated with cold steel phonomicrosurgical techniques and documented a 38% rate of relapse after lesion removal.[40] They did not record voice outcomes. Uloza et al examined 89 patients treated with cold steel with a 2-year follow-up period and documented a 71.9% recurrence rate in cases of JORRP and 22.8% in AORRP; they also did not record voice outcomes.[41] A more recent study by Kim et al examined 29 subjects receiving en bloc resection of lesions (including submucosal glands) with cold instruments followed by treatment with 585 nm pulse-dye laser (PDL) to try to prevent vocal fold scarring as well as intralesional anti-viral injection of cidofovir. They found significantly decreased rate of recurrence, restoration of mucosal wave, and improved voice quality according to patient-reported VHI scores. While their study did not directly compare treatment modalities, they did document a correlation between site of recurrence and high density submucosal gland sites, removal of which could present a possible future surgical goal of treatment particularly amenable to cold instruments.[42] The concern with deeper surgical resection will continue to be loss of vocal fold pliability with permanent hoarseness in the setting of a benign and recurrent disease.

Carbon Dioxide Laser

The carbon dioxide laser, first described in 1976, is characterized by a 10,640 nm wavelength that is absorbed primarily by water. Its use allows for either total or subtotal removal of lesions with less bleeding and decreased surgical time. Furthermore, the CO_2 laser offers the surgeon a less obstructed view of the operative field.[43] Post-surgical scarring in the initial studies has been a concern. In Strong's original article, total removal led to increased rates of anterior glottic web formation, likely as a result of thermal energy damage to normal epithelium.[44] Wetmore et al have also documented delayed complications of anterior and posterior glottic web, dysphagia, and edema in 11/12 patients in their study who had more than 5 procedures with the CO_2 laser.[45] Crockett et al describe the added complications of glottic stenosis and vocal fold scarring with total removal.[46] On the other hand, Benjamin and Parsons document a 10-year study of 60 patients having undergone a total of 1518 procedures with CO_2 laser in combination with forceps for greater intraoperative control. While 12 patients developed post-surgical glottic webbing, the webs were visible only under image magnification while patients were under general anesthesia.[47] This may have been due to their deliberate focus on unilateral treatment of the anterior commissure as opposed to total resection pursued by both Wetmore and Crockett.[48(p1165)] Ossoff et al describe only 3 of their 22 patients as having laser-related soft-tissue complications. They utilized a microspot manipulator to minimize thermal damage to lateral tissue and took care to avoid total resection when it risked damaging underlying soft tissue.[48]

Cold Steel Versus Carbon Dioxide Laser

The literature includes conflicting reports on this issue.[49] Cold steel instrumentation has been associated with increased rates of surgical complications such as tracheotomy-requiring airway compromise, glottic web, and glottic scarring compared with CO_2 laser ablation, with no significant difference in recurrence rates.[50] However, it is unclear which specific surgical technique was employed with the cold steel in this study (micro-flap, etc). There are also examples of the CO_2 laser approach producing fewer instances of anterior glottic web, posterior synechia, and stenosis of the larynx.[50] On the other hand, another study of 50 patients with JORRP showed significantly increased rates of glottic stenosis as a post-op complication in patients treated with CO_2 laser compared with cold steel.[51] Dedo et al conducted a study of 244 patients treated with CO_2 laser that indicated a 27% rate of anterior commissure synechia.[52] A retrospective analysis of patients treated for laryngeal papillomatosis from 1983 to 2014 at Magdeburg University Hospital attempted to compare cold steel with CO_2 laser and their

combination in terms of treatment safety and efficacy. The study consisted of 79 patients with AORRP and 27 with JORRP with a total of 62 procedures with cold instruments only, 28 with CO_2 laser only, and 16 with a combination of the two modalities. The authors of the study found no statistically significant difference in terms of the number of procedures required per year or the mean relapse interval across the modes of treatment. Postoperative complications were present in 37 cases, with the most common complication among all techniques being synechia of the anterior commissure, but there was no significant difference in the rate of complication across modes of treatment.[49] Overall, regardless of technique, care should be taken in the anterior commissure region.

Microdebrider

The laryngeal microdebrider was first described by Myer et al in 1999 and consists of a single device with a rotating blade that physically debulks the lesion as well as incorporated suction which allows greater freedom of the surgeon's contralateral hand.[53] The aim of microdebrider use is to preserve as much normal epithelium as possible while removing bulky, exophytic lesions. While the microdebrider has an advantage over lasers in the sense that there is no thermal radiation to normal tissue, the lack of tactile feedback and the suction makes this modality potentially riskier in regard to deep lesion resection and vocal cord scarring.[54] Studies have shown that use of the microdebrider compares favorably with other modalities in terms of operating time.[55] Pasquale et al examined 19 patient outcomes to compare microdebrider with CO_2 laser and found the same postoperative pain scores, but better voice quality outcomes with the microdebrider, confirmed shorter operating times, and less cost as well.[56] Another retrospective study comparing microdebrider vs. CO_2 laser for JORRP treatment further confirmed decreased operating times and demonstrated lack of soft tissue complications.[57]

PHOTOANGIOLYTIC LASERS AND THE EVOLUTION OF OFFICE-BASED LESION ABLATION

The advent of photoangiolytic lasers and their use in the larynx for RRP has been a major advance in treatment of the disease. The wavelengths of these lasers are close to that of oxyhemoglobin and therefore target the vascularity of the lesions as opposed to the CO_2 laser. The pulsed nature of these lasers allowed for more thermal relaxation, less heat dispersion to surrounding tissue, and shallower depth of penetration into the vocal fold. These lasers also employ a fiber-based delivery system that allows for more precision and freedom of motion under the microscope. The fiber-based delivery system also allows for the laser to be used through the operating port of a flexible laryngoscope, thus allowing surgeons to treat patients in the office setting without general anesthesia.

PULSE-DYE LASER

The pulse-dye laser is characterized by a wavelength of 585 nm that is absorbed by oxyhemoglobin within the vasculature of the lesion. This has the distinct advantage of preservation of the surface epithelium and superficial lamina propria with less heat being dispersed to healthy tissue compared with CO_2 laser. Its action results in intravascular coagulation, intralesional ischemia, and subsequent necrosis of papillomata.[12] The PDL was first used to treat RRP in 1998 by McMillan et al and showed significant remission rates in patients.[58] Franco et al supported these results in their study with a 70% rate of remission in patients with no anterior commissure webbing.[59] Other studies have shown similar results in children as well.[60] One of the greatest advantages of the PDL is that it can be used in-office, with topical as opposed to general anesthesia, and does not require direct laryngoscopy.[12] Other studies have suggested that the PDL as a modality is particularly suited to scar suppression.[61] A study of in-office treatment of vascular polyps showed effective complete clearance of small lesions (defined as constituting less than 1/3 of the vocal fold) in patients who had declined further operative procedures.[62] Another study of 59 RRP patients having undergone a total of 212 in-office procedures was conducted. These patients received either topical anesthesia (lidocaine), nebulized lidocaine, or local nerve blocks. Of these patients, 15% required operating room (OR) procedures because the bulkiness of their lesions limited laser access. There were no complications reported in this population in this study.[63] A retrospective chart review carried out by Centric et al found 32 of 33 patients treated for RRP with PDL had no complications, with 6 having complete resolution and 26 requiring further surgery in the OR.[64]

While the PDL was the first photoangiolytic laser to be used in the larynx, there were several technical limitations. These included the disposable dye packs that required refills, a laser with set parameters that did not permit changes to pulse width or pulses per second, and finally a large fiber that was at times difficult to insert and advance through the channeled laryngoscope.

POTASSIUM TITANYL PHOSPHATE LASER

The potassium titanyl phosphate (KTP) laser was first described as effective for in-office use in treating RRP in 2006 by Zeitels et al,[65] with a more recent study by Kuet and Pitman showing improvement in objective measures such as Derkay score and VHI-10.[66] In addition to in-office use, the KTP laser has also been shown to be effective in treating RRP for patients under general anesthesia.[67] Its increased pulse width allows for less vessel rupture and greater stability.[68] Zeitels et al have also shown using a retrospective analysis of 10 patients that adjuvant bevacizumab may enhance 532-nm KTP photoangiolysis and result in a decreased rate of recurrence compared with laser photoangiolysis alone.[69] This study was followed up with a prospective open-label study in which 20 adults with bilateral RRP received KTP photoangiolysis with either bevacizumab or sham saline injections (control) in each vocal fold with similar results.[70] KTP laser is the now preferred option compared with PDL because of improvements on the technical limitations listed above. It is a steady-state laser with no dye packs and less frequent maintenance, smaller fibers that can be used in both the OR and the office setting with better fit through the flexible laryngoscope, and more adjustability in regard to pulse width and pulses per second.

NARROW BAND IMAGING

Narrow band imaging (NBI) is a type of endoscopy that allows for enhanced visualization of mucosal and submucosal microvascular patterns associated with neoplastic angiogenesis that would otherwise be undetectable under white light. It utilizes the principle of differential absorption of light wavelengths (415 nm and 540 nm, for blue and green light, respectively) by hemoglobin compared with mucosal tissue. When endoscopic light is filtered for these wavelengths only, superficial vasculature can be visualized in contrast to surrounding tissue.[71(p473)] Tjon Pian Gi et al performed 24 microlaryngoscopies on 14 patients with RRP using both white light (WL) and NBI. They then took a total of 86 biopsies, 13 of which were based on NBI findings suspicious for papillomata. Eleven of those 13 additional biopsies were confirmed as papillomatous lesions. Their study found that using NBI significantly increased sensitivity from 80% to 97% compared with solely using WL, while specificity remained low for both techniques (32% for WL, 28% for WL with NBI).[72] In a study carried out by Ochsner and Klein in which both WL and NBI photos from 10 patients treated for RRP were sent for evaluation to fellowship-trained laryngologists, it was found that NBI both revealed previously unappreciated lesions as well as enhanced visualization of diseased areas. Respondents also felt that NBI helped to more clearly demarcate the borders of diseased versus normal tissue. A significant minority found that it was more difficult to visualize lesions using NBI.[73] Narrow band imaging has also been demonstrated to successfully help demarcate lesions otherwise missed by conventional laryngoscopy in two case reports by Adachi et al.[74] An additional case report by Imaizumi et al demonstrated its use for patients with common RRP recurrences and how it helped improve visualization of the margins, which allowed for a decrease in recurrence upon removal.[75]

TRACHEAL AND LOWER RESPIRATORY TRACT SPREAD

Tracheal spread is defined as extension of disease distal to the lower border of the cricoid cartilage. Cited frequencies of RRP with tracheal spread range from 2 to 17%.[76–80] Tracheal spread may initially be asymptomatic, but in children there is the potential for airway obstruction.

A study done by Weiss and Kashima reviewed 39 RRP patients and found a higher risk of tracheal spread in patients who have had tracheotomies. They also found tracheal papillomata isolated to the tracheotomy site in these patients, which supports a hypothesis in which damage to epithelium from tracheotomy procedures can provide fertile ground for viral particles to seed and grow.[81] However, the presence of more aggressive disease in patients that go on to require tracheotomy raises the question of whether tracheal spread is a consequence of iatrogenic trauma or simply part of an aggressive disease course.[25]

Other potential risk factors are believed to include multiple intubations, aggressive bronchoscopy, and Venturi ventilation. Silver et al cite that in their experience PS is associated with HPV type 11. The development of pulmonary spread (PS) is almost always fatal, with mortality most likely within 4 to 10 years after the PS diagnosis. It is recommended to follow patients with distal tracheal spread very closely for PS (seen on CT scan) and to maintain a high index of suspicion for malignancy. Possible sequelae of distal tracheal or pulmonary spread include alveolar destruction, restrictive lung disease, abscess formation, malignant transformation to squamous cell carcinoma (SSC), and death.[29]

Lower respiratory tract papillomata have a poor prognosis, worsening with bronchial or pulmonary spread. Such patients require more surgical procedures and have a decreased mean surgical interval and an increased likelihood of tracheotomy (and likely of further seeding of viral particles).[82] Their treatment is often challenging and requires multiple endoscopic interventions[83] and possibly a multidisciplinary approach with interventional pulmonology or thoracic surgery. As long as symptoms are mild or controlled via medication, observation is preferred. Once symptoms manifest and if there is any sign of airway compromise, treatment is expected. Various surgical modalities have been attempted to treat RRP that has spread to the trachea, though lasers are most popular. Radiofrequency coblation has been used with favorable results compared with CO_2 laser.[84] Photodynamic therapy with dihematoporphyrin has been used,[85] as well as microdebrider.[86] Cryotherapy has also been used.[87] In these severe circumstances, systemic adjuvant therapy likely plays a role. Adjuvant medical therapy may involve long-term chemotherapy with methotrexate, interferon therapy, and isotretinoin with the aim of slowing progression.[29] Zur and Fox administered systemic bevacizumab to a 12 year-old female with PS upon deterioration of pulmonary status and found significant improvement of laryngotracheal disease at 6 weeks, with complete resolution at the larynx and near-complete resolution at the trachea after 3 months of therapy. At 5 months, CT scan indicated complete resolution of pulmonary nodules without complications.[88]

Case Consideration 2: What Is Appropriate Surgical Management for Jane Doe?

Upon direct laryngoscopy, it is ascertained that Ms. Doe has the presence of warty growths from the inferior larynx and throughout and into the distal trachea but without bronchial spread.

Anesthesia Considerations for Pregnant Women

General anesthesia is usually recommended for pregnant women only when it is absolutely necessary, as the requirement of balancing the needs of the fetus with those of the mother severely complicate anesthetic management in the pregnant patient. While there have not yet been conclusive studies indicating fetal toxicity of general anesthetic drugs, they generally do cross the placenta and have been shown to have toxic effects in animal studies that manifest as behavioral deficits and neuronal apoptosis in later development. Furthermore, pregnant women have a particularly vulnerable airway. Airway changes in pregnancy include swelling and friability that effectively decrease the size of the glottal opening. These physiological changes, which manifest more toward the end of the pregnancy but as early as the mid-second trimester, make ventilation and intubation difficult in an unconscious pregnant patient.[89] The leading cause of anesthesia-associated maternal death is loss of airway control.[90] Furthermore, while short periods of maternal hypoxia are well tolerated by the fetus, prolonged periods of hypoxia can cause placental vasoconstriction resulting in fetal hypoxia, acidosis, and death.[91,92] The two primary concerns in this case would be unnecessary exposure of the fetus to medication, and protection of the vulnerable maternal airway. As such, it would be recommended to avoid general anesthesia if possible in favor of office procedures that make use of local anesthesia.

Treatment under local anesthesia could be considered if the disease is not bulky and airway obstructive. What would likely be necessary would be consideration of treatment in the bronchoscopy suite under sedation and topical anesthesia. The laser might be able to be used. Usually if they require treatment the lesions are causing airway compromise or growing rapidly. OB/GYN consult would be required. The patient may have to give serious consideration to aborting the pregnancy if the mother's life is endangered by the lower airway papilloma. Systemic chemotherapy may be considered in life-threatening disease with this degree of lower airway involvement.

ADJUVANT MEDICAL TREATMENT

Adjuvant medical therapy for RRP has a long history. Unfortunately, no one treatment has definitively been found to limit recurrence, as the natural history of the disease is one of relapses and recurrences. Adjuvant therapy is typically recommended in patients with rapid regrowth or in those with airway compromising disease. The threshold for offering these therapies will vary between surgeons.

Cidofovir

Cidofovir is a nucleotide analog of cytosine and a prodrug that must be de-phosphorylated to its diphosphate form, which is then incorporated into newly synthesized DNA and terminates synthesis upon addition.[12(p746)] Currently it is only approved by the FDA for cytomegalovirus retinitis in AIDS patients, but is the most commonly used adjuvant (off-label) to treat RRP.[12(p747)] Despite enjoying widespread usage, cidofovir has produced mixed therapeutic results. Several studies have shown therapeutic effect. Pransky et al have demonstrated increasing time between procedures after cidofovir injection and decreased disease severity.[93,94] Bielamowicz et al treated 15 patients solely with cidofovir injection and achieved remission, but only temporarily.[95] Akst et al have utilized stepped dosing with better results.[96] Chhetri and Shapiro demonstrated a decrease in papilloma stage in 4 out of 5 patients, as well as a decrease in need for laser ablation of bulky lesions upon intralesional administration of cidofovir.[97] Tanna et al looked at adults over a 10-year retrospective and out of 13 patients were able to achieve long-term remission in only 3 of them, with a mean of six injections.[98] Wierzbicka examined 32 patients treated with cidofovir as adjuvant to surgery and found that 18 had complete remission, 13 had local remission only at the injection site, and 1 was a non-responder.[99] Two studies have demonstrated the efficacy of cidofovir in very young children. One has shown good response in an infant,[100] while another has shown the possibility of administering a nebulized formulation to a 4-month–old, which improved disease burden.[101] Studies have also shown that whether cidofovir is given in-office or in the OR does not affect its efficacy.[102,103]

While these studies demonstrate efficacy in reducing lesional burden, lack of permanent remission and other evidence disputes their generalizability. For example, El Hakim et al showed no benefit to cidofovir use,[104] and Milczuk demonstrated a rebound effect in 2 of 4 patients and a non-responder in their study,[105] though these results may have been due to the long interval between injection (similar responses were seen in a study by Peyton and Wiatrak).[106] Additionally, Shi et al saw short-term remission but eventual relapse in all 5 of the patients in their study and concluded that while cidofovir might be valuable in reducing severity of course, it did not appear to provide any long-term benefit in their study.[107] The only as yet double-blind randomized control trial carried out to determine the efficacy of cidofovir yielded the result that there was no significant difference between cidofovir use compared with placebo saline. Unusually, both treatment and control groups in this study showed significant improvement in Derkay score and VHI at 2- and 12-month follow-up, but no significant difference in response relative to each other. However, 7 of 10 of these patients received doses far lower than standard therapeutic range and this may have influenced the lack of response.[108]

Side effects of cidofovir usage are mostly local and tend to resolve with discontinuation. Non-local side effects include elevated serum creatinine within normal limits[109] and acute kidney inflammation (AKI) that resolved with discontinuation of therapy.[110]

> Is Cidofovir Associated with Progression to Squamous Cell Carcinoma?

One of the major concerns of using cidofovir has been the fear of progression to malignancy in injected lesions. A dysplasia to squamous cell carcinoma transition was reported in rats,[115] and there has been a report of a patient going on to develop squamous cell carcinoma, but this was after receiving 13 injections of intralesional cidofovir.[116] One study examined 13 patients' dysplasia grades before and after injection and found that 2 had gotten worse, 4 were better, and 7 were the same.[117] A more powerful study reviewed 96 patient samples and showed no dysplastic changes associated with cidofovir injection.[118] Fusconi et al's 2014 study also indicated that cidofovir is not associated with dysplasia and when combined with surgical removal of lesions produces a favorable treatment response.[119] Supporting this latter result, a 10-year retrospective chart review found that cidofovir was not associated as a risk factor of progression to dysplasia or carcinoma-ex-papilloma in JORRP or AORRP.[120] Broekema et al found that the rate of malignant transformation after receiving intralesional cidofovir was the same as the rate of spontaneous transformation (2–3%). They conclude that intralesional cidofovir

appears safe as long as the injected dose is less than 3 mg/kg body weight.[121]

One incident of vocal fold necrosis has been documented in a patient who received five injections which totaled an unusually high dosage.[111] Derkay et al conducted a study reporting a survey of 82 surgeons and concluded that cidofovir is indicated if more than one of the following criteria are met: the patient requires more than four procedures per year, has continued anterior and posterior commissure lesions, or has had no response to surgery alone. They report dosing cidofovir at 2.5 to 7.5 mg/mL and total injected volumes of <4 and <2 mL (for adults and children, respectively) with five total treatments spread out every 2 to 6 weeks.[110] Intravenous cidofovir was administered in several cases of pulmonary spread[112–114] and was well tolerated in all cases except the case study conducted by Dancey, in which there were side effects of partial alopecia and leukopenia.[112]

Bevacizumab

Bevacizumab is a monoclonal antibody of vascular endothelial growth factor (VEGF) and thus has an anti-angiogenic mechanism of action that prevents the growth of new blood vessels within the papilloma. Studies have found injected bevacizumab to be effective for decreasing lesional burden as well as treating areas requiring less KTP photoangiolysis during treatment compared with sham saline injections.[122] Mohr et al demonstrated immediate response in five patients receiving bevacizumab.[123] A limited case series was carried out recently in which eight patients with aggressive disease refractory to surgical and adjuvant therapy with pulmonary spread (in seven out of eight) were treated with systemic bevacizumab. Seven out of eight achieved partial response, and one achieved complete response. All patients exhibited an increased treatment interval. This response was maintained in seven out of eight patients long term, with the only complications being hemoptysis and proteinuria.[124] Injected bevacizumab also appears to be safe, with a review of 100 injections with a mean dosage of 30 mg showing no significant adverse effects.[125]

Indole-3-Carbinol

Indole-3-carbinol is a molecule found naturally in cruciferous vegetables like cabbage, broccoli, Brussels sprouts, and cauliflower. It acts to increase cytochrome p450 (CYP) 2-hydroxylation of estradiol while decreasing its 16-hydroxylation, in sum leading to decreased proliferative effect of estradiol in laryngeal papilloma due to HPV-11 infection. In a prospective study of children and adults treated with indole-3-carbinol, at a mean follow-up of 14.6 months, one-third had resolution of lesions, one third had reduced regrowth, and one third had no response.[126] A similar study was conducted with a longer mean follow-up time of 4.8 years and had similar findings. No side effects were noted.[127]

Interferon–Alpha

Interferon (IFN)-alpha is a pro-inflammatory cytokine released by monocytes and macrophages to induce helper T-cell response as part of normal anti-viral immune defense. It was first used in a study in 1981 where 7 patients were treated with IFN-alpha as an adjuvant to surgery. All of them exhibited response to therapy, but 5 recurred after termination of treatment.[128] In another study, 14 patients received initial doses of 2 million units (MU), which were then modified per favorable response or adverse effect, and half had sustained favorable responses even after termination of therapy.[129] In another study, 19 patients were given three injections per week and had their doses adjusted every 3 months. Six out of 19 had remission, but 2 of these had papilloma regrowth after termination of treatment and 1 could not tolerate side effects. There was significant benefit to tracheal and pulmonary lesions found in this study.[130] Similar results have been reported elsewhere.[131,132] A larger-scale study of 125 patients (92 children and 33 adults) examined the effect of surgical removal of lesions followed by an IFN schedule that was adjusted based on response and found 71% of patients in remission after 3 years. In those who had relapses, the frequency of recurrence was decreased in all but 4. In this study 14 patients had relapses that persisted despite several cycles of IFN treatment and were hence considered resistant. Only mild side effects were reported in this study.[133] In a separate 20-year follow-up of 42 patients given 3 MU/cubic meter of body surface area of IFN, an event-free survival of 42.8% was found, with those who had HPV 11 being more resistant to treatment.[134] Kashima et al conducted a multi-institutional randomized trial of surgery versus IFN-alpha-n1 (across various age groups) in which they administered 5 MU/m³ body surface area to patients for 28 days, then three times a week for 5 months and found the following: a decreased papilloma score that was significantly lower in the IFN-alpha treatment group. Patients reported minimal adverse effects.[135] Leventhal et al followed up Kashima et al's multi-institution randomized trial and showed patients given IFN therapy were in complete or partial remission.[136] Suter-Montano et al combined IFN-alpha treatment with granulocyte monocyte colony stimulating factor (GM-CSF) and administered the combination via weekly subcutaneous injections and at 18 months follow-up found all patients to have improved voice quality, less disease burden, and a lower surgical intervention frequency.[137]

However, in contrast, another randomized trial compared surgery alone with surgery plus IFN-alpha-n3 administered at a dose of 2 MU per meter body surface area 1×/day for 1 week, then 3×/week for 12 months. This study found that IFN therapy showed a significant decrease in papilloma growth rate through the first 6 months, but then approached the control growth rate for the next 6 months. This is the only major study to the author's knowledge showing that IFN therapy does not have a significant effect on outcome.[138]

Unfortunately, while injected forms seem to be well tolerated, systemic interferon therapy has significant side effects, including elevated aspartate aminotransferase, fever, leukopenia, myalgias, anorexia, and fatigue—so much so that patients will often demand discontinuation of therapy.[12]

Cimetidine

Cimetidine is a histamine-2 receptor antagonist (H2RA) that is normally used to treat GERD. However, it has been found that higher doses of cimetidine inhibit suppressor T cells, thus increasing the body's normal antibody response.[139–141] At least one case report exists in the literature in which a patient was given 40 mg/kg body weight of cimetidine for 4 months and experienced significant improvement in tracheo-bronchial pulmonary disease.[142]

Photodynamic Therapy (PDT)

PDT involves administration of a photosensitizing drug that is taken up preferentially by lesions and has a chemical that is activated by light and causes cell death through creating a singlet (high energy quantum state) of oxygen.[12] Shikowitz et al have demonstrated use of hematoporphyrin in a rabbit model for RRP and showed regression of lesions upon light activation.[143] In one study, 33 patients were administered 2.5 mg/kg body weight of IV dihematoporphyrin ether (DHE) 48 to 72 hours before argon pump dye laser treatment. Fifty percent of the patients in the study showed a decrease in lesion growth and without side effects.[144] Another study found that in PDT, increasing light dosage had no benefit,[145] while increasing DHE to 4.25 mg/kg body weight inhibited papilloma growth further and was maintained at 3-year follow-up.[146] A major concern for PDT is the post-treatment inflammatory response that could cause airway obstruction, long-term airway stenosis or vocal cord scarring.

MMR Vaccine

A randomized control trial consisting of 26 children with JORRP showed no statistically significant difference in giving topical measles, mumps, and rubella (MMR) vaccine after surgical removal of lesions.[147] A more recent study of 15 children ages 1 to 16 years with confirmed RRP actually showed no significant difference in terms of number or frequency of adjuvant treatments or in remission rate when comparing MMR vaccine with cidofovir.[148]

HspE7

HspE7 is a recombinant protein combining Mycobacterium bovis bacillus Calmette-Guerin Hsp 65 with part of the HPV E7 protein's C terminal end.[12] In a study it was given as an injection within 7 days postop and again at 4 weeks and 8 weeks and was found to result in a significantly increased surgical interval as well as improvement in Derkay score.[149]

HPV Vaccination

Therapeutic vaccine research has failed to show any benefit in anogenital papilloma.[150] However, several retrospective studies as well as case reports have presented provisional data that support the HPV vaccine's efficacy in altering RRP disease course. A retrospective study comprising 10 patients ranging in age from 13 to 46 with follow-up times from 12 to 52 months who received the quadrivalent HPV vaccine (also known

as Gardasil, which covers HPV types 6, 11, 16, and 18) found a significant increase in intersurgical interval (ISI) as well as a significant decrease in total number of procedures—however, without any difference in Derkay score, relative to prior surgical treatment.[151] In a retrospective observational study of 6 patients with RRP, Tjon Pian Gi et al also showed a decreased rate of surgical intervention at median follow-up of 4 years when patients were given the quadrivalent HPV vaccine. This was also correlated with a significant increase in anti-HPV antibodies.[152] Another retrospective study of 20 patients having received Gardasil as part of their treatment for RRP demonstrated an increase in ISI isolated to male patients, and complete or partial remission in 13/20 patients (9 male, 4 female).[153] Interestingly, 1-year follow-up in another study comprising pediatric patients did not show any significant change in disease course.[154] Case reports have shown increases in ISI in pediatric patients with RRP treated with both the quadrivalent HPV vaccine[155] as well as the 9-valent vaccine (which additionally covers HPV types 31, 33, 45, 52, and 58).[156] In the case of a 2-year-old boy with JORRP with esophageal involvement and the presence of both HPV types 6 and 11, Gardasil led to complete remission of laryngeal and esophageal lesions at 2-year follow-up.[157] In another case study of a 2-year-old boy, who received three therapeutic immunizations with Gardasil, aggressive JORRP was found to stabilize.[158] Overall, the possibility of HPV vaccination as a safe and effective therapy for RRP is promising, but current studies seem to be limited by their retrospective design and small sample sizes.

COX-2 Inhibitors

Cyclooxygenase 2 (COX-2) inhibitors are a new area of therapeutic research in RRP. COX-2 leads to increased downstream prostaglandin E2 expression (PG-E2), which is implicated in many cancers, including those of the head and neck.[159,160] Lucs et al, in a 2012 paper, demonstrated that Rac1 expression was increased throughout the aerodigestive tract of RRP patients, even where there was no active lesion indicating viral activation. This led to the hypothesis that Rac1 expression, which induces COX-2 expression, might be a susceptibility factor in the minority of people who end up developing lesions upon infection with HPV.[161]

In a subsequent experiment they administered the COX-2 inhibitor celecoxib to three patients with AORRP and found that two of them went into extended remission and that the final patient, while not going into remission, had significant improvement of tracheal disease.[161] In another study, Limsukon et al treated a patient with extensive bronchial disease who was refractory to cidofovir, with a combination of celecoxib and erlotinib (a small-molecule inhibitor of the tyrosine kinase epidermal growth factor receptor [EGFR]) and found a favorable response.[162] The rationale for including erlotinib as part of the treatment was the overexpression of EGFR in papillomata (demonstrated by Vambutas et al)[163] and the fact that EGFR blockade can indirectly suppress COX-2 and PG-E2.[164]

Another indirect inhibitor of COX-2 and direct inhibitor of EGFR is the drug gefitinib, which has been approved for refractory lung cancer.[165] Gefitinib was used to treat a 42-year-old with JORRP diagnosed within his first year of life who subsequently experienced complete regression of disease from the vocal cord and trachea.[166] There is also a case study of a 14-year-old patient with tracheal spread who received gefitinib and subsequently had increased time between debulking procedures and minimal recurrence in the trachea and carina.[167]

Checkpoint Inhibitors

Checkpoint inhibitors are another rapidly developing area of therapeutic research within cancer immunotherapy. Recent research in immunology has demonstrated that programmed cell death ligand 1 (PD-L1) is a ligand for programmed cell death protein 1 (PD-1), the immune-inhibitory receptor on T cells, B cells, monocytes, and tumor-infiltrating lymphocytes (TILs).[168] Binding of PD-L1 to PD-1 suppresses T-cell function by inducing apoptosis, anergy, and exhaustion.[169] When Lieu et al stained and analyzed lesions from seven children with a mean age of 7.43 years with RRP for expression of PD-L1 they found that it was present in both TIL+ lesions and those without TILs.[170] Furthermore, in another study, PD-L1 expression was correlated with HPV positivity and chromosomal instability (CIN) grade[171] and immune suppression mediated by PD-L1/PD-1 was found in HPV-related head and neck cancer.[172] This led to the rationale for a potential therapy: If the RRP lesional microenvironment has increased PD-L1 expression that is leading to immune blockade of T cells, then an inhibitor of the PD-L1/PD-1 interaction should help boost the host immune response against the lesions. Indeed, in vitro blockade of PD-L1/PD-1 signaling restored function of TILs. Such an approach

has shown efficacy in activating immune response to melanoma[173] and colorectal cancer,[174] as well as head and neck cancer when anti–PD-1 antibody is given with HPV vaccine.[172] There are several clinical trials under way seeking to evaluate the in vivo efficacy of inhibiting PD-L1/PD-1 mediated immuno-blockade in RRP.

> **Case Consideration 3:** What Is Appropriate Adjuvant Treatment for Jane Doe?

Options include cidofovir, bevacizumab, indole-3-carbinol, and IFN-alpha. The patient is pregnant and has lesional spread to the lower respiratory tract but not the lungs. Cidofovir and Avastin (bevacizumab) can be given in the office as intralesional injections or intravenously, hence no general anesthesia will be required. If intralesional injections are utilized, cidofovir appears to have the greatest data supporting its efficacy, but Avastin appears to have a higher safety profile and no reported cases of potential carcinogenicity in adults or children. With cidofovir, care should be taken to maintain the injected dose below 3 mg/kg body weight in adults and one should be reserved with its use in pregnant women. In the present case, while there is no pulmonary spread, judicious prophylactic use of cidofovir or Avastin may be helpful. Systemic cidofovir is contraindicated, as it is a class C drug and has shown teratogenic and embryotoxic potential in animal studies (Gilead Sciences, Vistide package insert; 2000). Systemic bevacizumab and IFN-alpha appear well tolerated in pregnancy, and are also options, though there are fewer studies on their efficacy compared with cidofovir, and the latter usually has serious side effects. (For further specific recommendations and guidelines, see Derkay, 2005, RRP Task-force.) Given the alleged carcinogenicity of cidofovir, intralesional Avastin may be a safer choice. Regardless, the patient should be counseled about the potential risks to the fetus including miscarriage. Further, in patients with airway obstructive disease, general anesthesia may be unavoidable and pregnancy termination is a possibility.

REFERENCES

1. Bennett RS, Powell KR. Human papillomaviruses: associations between laryngeal papillomas and genital warts. *Pediatr Infect Dis J*. 1987;6:229–232.

2. Mounts P, Shah KV, Kashima H. Viral etiology of juvenile- and adult-onset squamous papilloma of the larynx. *Proc Natl Acad Sci U S A*. 1982;79:5425–5429.

3. Silverberg MJ, Thorsen P, Lindeberg H, et al. Clinical course of recurrent respiratory papillomatosis in Danish children. *Arch Otolaryngol Head Neck Surg*. 2004;130: 711–716.

4. Verma H, Solanki P, James M. Acoustical and perceptual voice profiling of children with recurrent respiratory papillomatosis. *J Voice*. 2016;30(5):600–605.

5. Lindman JP, Lewis LS, Accortt N, Wiatrak BJ. Use of the Pediatric Quality of Life Inventory to assess the health-related quality of life in children with recurrent respiratory papillomatosis. *Ann Otol Rhinol Laryngol*. 2005; 114:499–503.

6. Steinberg BM, DiLorenzo TP. A possible role for human papillomaviruses in head and neck cancer. *Cancer Metastasis Rev*. 1996;15:91–112.

7. Bishai D, Kashima H, Shah K. The cost of juvenile-onset recurrent respiratory papillomatosis. *Arch Otolaryngol Head Neck Surg*. 2000;126(8):935–939.

8. Tasca RA, Clarke RW. Recurrent respiratory papillomatosis. *Arch Dis Child*. 2006;91(8):689.

9. Derkay CS. Task force on recurrent respiratory papillomas. *Arch Otolaryngol Head Neck Surg*. 1995;121:1386.

10. San Giorgi M, van den Heuvel ER, Tjon Pian Gi RE, et al. Age of onset of recurrent respiratory papillomatosis: a distribution analysis. *Clin Otolaryngol*. 2016;41(5): 448–453.

11. Armstrong LR, Derkay CS, Reeves WC. Initial results from the National Registry for Juvenile-Onset Recurrent Respiratory Papillomatosis. RRP Task Force. *Arch Otolaryngol Head Neck Surg*. 1999;125(7):743–748.

12. Berzofsky C, Pitman MJ. Laryngeal papilloma. In: Benninger MS, ed. *Sataloff's Comprehensive Textbook of Otolaryngology Head and Neck Surgery: Laryngology*. Philadelphia, PA: Jaypee Medical Inc; 2016:739.

13. Reidy PM, Dedo HH, Rabah R, et al. Integration of human papillomavirus type 11 in recurrent respiratory papilloma-associated cancer. *Laryngoscope*. 2004;114: 1906–1909.

14. Barbosa MS, Vass WC, Lowy DR, et al. In vitro biological activities of the E6 and E7 genes vary among human papillomaviruses of different oncogenic potential. *J Virol*. 1991;65:292–298.

15. Xu H, Lu DW, El-Mofty SK, Wang HL. Metachronous squamous cell carcinomas evolving from independent oropharyngeal and pulmonary squamous papillomas: association with human papillomavirus 11 and lack of aberrant p53, Rb, and p16 protein expression. *Hum Pathol*. 2004;35(11):1419–1422.

16. Bauman NM, Smith RJ. Recurrent respiratory papillomatosis. *Pediatr Clin North Am*. 1996;43:1385–1401.

17. Kashima H, Mounts P, Leventhal B, et al. Sites of predilection in recurrent respiratory papillomatosis. *Ann Otol Rhinol Laryngol*. 1993;102:580–583.

18. Gale N, Zidar N. Benign and potentially malignant lesions of the squamous epithelium and squamous cell carcinoma. In: Wenig BM, Bordin GM, eds, *Atlas of Head and Neck Pathology*. Philadelphia, PA: Elsevier; 1993.

19. Hall JE, Chen K, Yoo MJ, et al. Natural progression of dysplasia in adult recurrent respiratory papillomatosis. *Otolaryngol Head Neck Surg*. 2011;144:252–256.

20. Borkowski G, Sommer P, Stark T, Sudhoff H, Luckhaupt H. Recurrent respiratory papillomatosis associated with gastroesophageal reflux disease in children. *Eur Arch Otorhinolaryngol*. 1999;256(7):370–372.

21. Syrjanen S, Puranen M. Human papillomavirus infections in children: the potential role of maternal transmission. *Crit Rev Oral Biol Med*. 2000;11(2):258–274.

22. Tasca RA, Clarke RW. Recurrent respiratory papillomatosis. *Arch Dis Child*. 2006;91(8):689.

23. Armstrong LR, Derkay CS, Reeves WC. Initial results from the National Registry for Juvenile-Onset Recurrent Respiratory Papillomatosis. RRP Task Force. *Arch Otolaryngol Head Neck Surg*. 1999;125(7):743.

24. Derkay CS, Faust RA. Recurrent respiratory papillomatosis. In: Lesperance MM, Flint PW, eds. *Cummings Pediatric Otolaryngology*. Philadelphia, PA: Saunders; 2015:336.

25. Shapiro AM, Rimell FL, Shoemaker D, Pou A, Stool SE. Tracheotomy in children with juvenile-onset recurrent respiratory papillomatosis: the Children's Hospital of Pittsburgh experience. *Ann Otol Rhinol Laryngol*. 1996; 105(1):1–5.

26. Schraff S, Derkay CS, Burke B, Lawson L. American Society of Pediatric Otolaryngology members' experience with recurrent respiratory papillomatosis and the use of adjuvant therapy. *Arch Otolaryngol Head Neck Surg*. 2004; 130:1039–1042.

27. Rimell FL, Shoemaker DL, Pou AM, Jordan JA, Post JC, Ehrlich GD. Pediatric respiratory papillomatosis: prognostic role of viral typing and cofactors. *Laryngoscope*. 1997;107(7):915–918.

28. Kramer SS, Wehunt WD, Stocker JT, Kashima H. Pulmonary manifestations of juvenile laryngotracheal papillomatosis. *AJR*. 1985;144:687–694.

29. Silver RD, Rimmel FL, Adams GL, et al. Diagnosis and management of pulmonary metastasis for recurrent respiratory papillomatosis. *Otol Head Neck Surg*. 2003; 129:622–629.

30. Derkay CS, Wiatrak B. Recurrent respiratory papilloma: a review. *Laryngoscope*. 2008;118:1236–1247.

31. Derkay C, Malis D, Zalzal G, Wiatrak B, Kashima H, Coltrera M. A staging system for assessing severity of disease and response to therapy in recurrent respiratory papillomatosis. *Laryngoscope*. 1998;108:935–937.

32. Hester RP, Derkay CS, Burke BL, Lawson ML. Reliability of a staging assessment system for recurrent respiratory papillomatosis. *Int J Pediatr Otorhinolaryngol*. 2003;67(5):505–509.

33. Kupfer RA, Cadalli Tatar E, Barry JO, Allen CT, Merati AL. Anatomic Derkay score is associated with voice handicap in laryngeal papillomatosis in adults. *Otolaryngol Head Neck Surg*. 2016;154(4):689–692.

34. Derkay CS, Hester RP, Burke B, Carron J, Lawson L. Analysis of a staging assessment system for prediction of surgical interval in recurrent respiratory papillomatosis. *Int J Pediatr Otorhinolaryngol*. 2004;68(12):1493–1498.

35. Kashima HK, Shah F, Lyles A, et al. A comparison of risk factors in juvenile-onset and adult-onset recurrent respiratory papillomatosis. *Laryngoscope*. 1992;102:9–13.

36. Hallden C, Majmudar B. The relationship between juvenile laryngeal papillomatosis and maternal condylomata acuminata. *J Reprod Med*. 1986;31:804–807.

37. Shah KV, Kashima H, Polk BF, et al. Rarity of cesarean delivery in cases of juvenile-onset respiratory papillomatosis. *Obstet Gynecol*. 1986;68:795–799.

38. Silverberg MJ, Thorsen P, Lindeberg H, et al. Condyloma in pregnancy is strongly predictive of juvenile-onset recurrent respiratory papillomatosis. *Obstet Gynecol*. 2003;101:645–652.

39. Zeitels SM. Phonomicrosurgical treatment of early glottic cancer and carcinoma in situ. *Am J Surg*. 1996;172(6):704–709.

40. Zeitels SM, Sataloff RT. Phonomicrosurgical resection of glotta papillomatosis. *J Voice*. 1999;13(1):123–127.

41. Uloza V. The course of laryngeal papillomatosis treated with endolaryngeal microsurgery. *Eur Arch Otorhinolaryngol*. 2000;257:498–501.

42. Kim HT, Baizhumanova AS. Is recurrent respiratory papillomatosis a manageable or curable disease. *Laryngoscope*. 2016;126(6):1359–1364.

43. Hermens JM, Bennett MJ, Hirshman CA. Anesthesia for laser surgery. *Anesth Analg*. 1983; 62(2):218–229.

44. Strong MS, Vaughan CW, Healy GB, et al, Clemente MACP. Recurrent respiratory papillomatosis management with the CO_2 laser. *Ann Otol*. 1976;85:508–516.

45. Wetmore SJ, Key JM, Suen JY. Complications of laser surgery for laryngeal papillomatosis. *Laryngoscope*. 1985;95:798–801.

46. Crockett DM, McCabe BF, Shive CJ. Complications of laser surgery for recurrent respiratory papillomatosis. *Ann Otol Rhinol Laryngol*. 1987;96:639–644.

47. Benjamin B, Parsons DS. Recurrent respiratory papillomatosis: a 10-year study. *J Laryngol Otol*. 1988;102:1022–1028.

48. Ossoff RH, Werkhaven JA, Dere H. Soft-tissue complications of laser surgery for recurrent respiratory papillomatosis. *Laryngoscope*. 1991;101:1162–1166.

49. Papaioannou VA, Lux A, Voigt-Zimmermann S, Arens C. Treatment outcomes of recurrent respiratory papillomatosis: retrospective analysis of juvenile and adult cases. *HNO*. 2017;65(11):923–932.

50. Preuss SF, Klussmann JP, Jungehulsing M, Eckel HE, Guntinas-Lichius O, Damm M. Long-term results of surgical treatment for recurrent respiratory papillomatosis. *Acta Otolaryngol*. 2007;127(11):1196–1201.

51. Hermann JS, Pontes P, Weckx LLM, Fujita R, Avelino M, Pignatari SSN. Laryngeal sequelae of recurrent respiratory papillomatosis surgery in children. *Rev Assoc Med Bras*. 2012;58(2):204–208.

52. Dedo HH, Yu KCY. CO_2-laser treatment in 244 patients with respiratory papillomas. *Laryngoscope*. 2001;111:1639–1644.

53. Myer III CM, Willging JP, McMurray S, et al. Use of laryngeal micro resector system. *Laryngoscope*. 1999;109:1165–116.

54. Mortensen M, Woo P. An underreported complication of laryngeal microdebrider: vocal fold web and granuloma: a case report. *Laryngoscope*. 2009;119(9):1848–1850.

55. Patel N, Rowe M, Tunkel D. Treatment of recurrent respiratory papillomatosis in children with the microdebrider. *Ann Otol Rhinol Laryngol*. 2003;112:7–10.

56. Pasquale K, Wiatrak B, Woolley A, et al. Microdebrider versus CO2 laser removal of recurrent respiratory papillomas: a prospective analysis. *Laryngoscope*. 2003;113:139–143.

57. El–Bitar MA, Zalzal GH. Powered instrumentation in the treatment of recurrent respiratory papillomatosis: an alternative to the carbon dioxide laser. *Arch Otolaryngol Head Neck Surg*. 2002;128(4):425–428.

58. McMillan K, Shapshay SM, Mcgilligan JA, et al. A 585-nanomater-pulse dye laser treatment of laryngeal papillomas: preliminary report. *Laryngoscope*. 1998;108:968–972.

59. Franco Jr RA, Zeitels SM, Farinelli WA, et al. 585-nm pulsed dye laser treatment of glottal papillomatosis. *Ann Otol Rhinol Laryngol*. 2002;111:486–492.

60. Hartnick CJ, Boseley ME, Franco Jr RA, Cunningham MJ, Pransky S. Efficacy of treating children with anterior commissure and true vocal fold respiratory papilloma with the 585-nm pulsed-dye laser. *Arch Otolaryngol Head Neck Surg*. 2007;133:127–130.

61. Kuo YR, Wu WS, Jeng SF, et al. Suppressed TGF-beta1 expression is correlated with up-regulation of matrix metalloproteinase-13 in keloid regression after flashlamp pulsed-dye laser treatment. *Lasers Surg Med*. 2005;36:38–42.

62. Ivey CM, Woo P, Altman KW, Shapshay SM. Office pulsed dye laser treatment for benign laryngeal vascular polyps: a preliminary study. *Ann Otol Rhinol Laryngol*. 2008;117(5):353–358.

63. Koufman JA, Rees CJ, Frazier WD, et al. Office based laryngeal laser surgery: a review of 443 cases using three wavelengths. *Otolaryngol Head Neck Surg*. 2007;137(1):146–151.

64. Centric A, Hu A, Heman-Ackah YD, et al. Office-based pulsed-dye laser surger for laryngeal lesions: a retrospective chart review. *J Voice*. 2014;28(2):262.

65. Zeitels SM, Akst LM, Burns JA, Hillman RE, Broadhurst MS, Anderson RR. Office-based 532-nm pulsed KTP laser treatment of glottal papillomatosis and dysplasia. *Ann Otol Rhinol Laryngol.* 2006;115(9):679–685.

66. Kuet ML, Pitman MJ. Photoangiolytic laser treatment of recurrent respiratory papillomatosis: a scaled assessment. *J Voice.* 2012;27:124–128.

67. Burns JA, Zeitels SM, Akst LM, et al. 532-nm pulsed potassium-titanyl-phosphate laser treatment of laryngeal papillomatosis under general anesthesia. *Laryngoscope.* 2007;117(8):1500–1504.

68. Broadhurst MS, Akst LM, Burns JA, et al. Effects of 532-nm pulsed-KTP laser parameters on vessel ablation in the avian chorioallantoic membrane: implications for vocal fold mucosa. *Laryngoscope.* 2007;117(2):220–225.

69. Zeitels SM, Lopez-Guerra G, Burns JA, et al. Microlaryngoscopic and office-based injection of bevacizumab (Avastin) to enhance 532-nm pulsed KTP laser treatment of glottal papillomatosis. *Ann Otol Rhinol Laryngol Supp.* 2009;201:1–13.

70. Zeitels SM, Barbu AM, Landau-Zemer T, et al. Local injection of bevacizumab (Avastin) and angiolytic KTP laser treatment of recurrent respiratory papillomatosis of the vocal folds: a prospective study. *Ann Otol Rhinol Laryngol.* 2011;120(10):627–634.

71. Piazza C, Del Bon F, Peretti G, et al. Narrow band imaging in endoscopic evaluation of the larynx. *Curr Opin Otolaryngol Head Neck Surg.* 2012;20(6):472–476.

72. Tjon Pian Gi RE, Halmos GB, van Hemel BM, et al. Narrow band imaging is a new technique in visualization of recurrent respiratory papillomatosis. *Laryngoscope.* 2012;122(8):1826–1830.

73. Ochsner MC, Klein AM. The utility of narrow band imaging in the treatment of laryngeal papillomatosis in awake patients. *J Voice.* 2015;29(3):349–351.

74. Adachi K, Umezaki T, Kiyohara H, et al. New Technique for laryngomicrosurgery: narrow band imaging-assisted video-laryngomicrosurgery for laryngeal papillomatosis. *J Laryngol Otol.* 2015;129(2):74–76.

75. Imaizumi M, Okano W, Tada Y, et al. Surgical treatment of laryngeal papillomatosis using narrow band imaging. *Otolaryngol Head Neck Surg.* 2012;147(3)522–524.

76. Bjork H, Weber C. Papilloma of the larynx. *Acta Otolaryngol.* 1956;46(6):499–516.

77. Majora M, Parkhill EMR, Devine KD. Papilloma of larynx in children. *Am J Surg.* 1964;108:470–475.

78. Singer DB, Greenberg SD, Harrison GM. Papillomatosis of the lung. *Am Rev Resp Dis.* 1966;94(5):777–783.

79. Strong MS, Vanghan CW, Cooper brand SR. Recurrent respiratory papillomatosis. *Ann Otol Rhinol Laryngol.* 1976;85:508–516.

80. Cohen SR, Seltzeer S, Geller KA, et al. Papilloma of larynx/trachea-bronchial tree in children. *Ann Otol Rhinol Laryngol.* 1980;89:497–503.

81. Weiss MD, Kashima HK. Tracheal involvement in laryngeal papillomatosis. *Laryngoscope.* 1983;93(1):45–48.

82. Wang J, Han DM, MA LJ, et al. Risk factors of juvenile onset recurrent respiratory papillomatosis in the lower respiratory tract. *Chin Med J.* 2012;125(19):3496–3499.

83. Harris K, Chalhoub M. Tracheal papillomatosis: what do we know so far. *Chron Respir Dis.* 2011;8(4):233–235.

84. Carney AS, Evans AS, Mirza S, et al. Radiofrequency coblation for treatment of advanced laryngotracheal recurrent respiratory papillomatosis. *J Laryngol Otol.* 2010; 124(5):510–514.

85. Shikowitz MJ, Abramson AL, Freeman K, et al. Efficacy of DHE photodynamic therapy for respiratory papillomatosis: immediate and long-term results. *Laryngoscope.* 1998;108(7):962–967.

86. Ulualp SO, Ryan MW, Wright ST. Microdebrider removal of tracheal papilloma via tracheostomy in the child with an obliterated larynx. *J Laryngol Otol.* 2007; 121(11):1070–1072.

87. Mohan KT, Greenheck J, Rubio ER. Recurring tracheal papillomatosis treated with cryosurgery. *South Med J.* 2008;101(9):967–968.

88. Zur KB, Fox E. Bevacizumab chemotherapy for management of pulmonary and laryngotracheal papillomatosis in a child. *Laryngoscope.* 2017;127(7):1538–1542.

89. Reitman E, Flood P. Anaesthetic considerations for non-obstetric surgery during pregnancy. *Br J Anaesth.* 2001;107 (suppl 1):i72–i78.

90. Hawkins JL, Chang J, Palmer SK, et al. Anesthesia-related maternal mortality in the United States:1979–2002. *Obstet Gynecol.* 2011;117(1):69–74.

91. Itskowitz J, LaGamma EF, Rudolph AM. The effect of reducing umbilical blood flow on fetal oxygenation. *Am J Obstet Gynecol.* 1983;145(7):813–818.

92. Dilts PV, Brinkman CR, Kirschbaum TH, et al. Uterine and systemic hemodynamic interrelationships and their response to hypoxia. *Am J Obstet Gynecol.* 1969;103 (1):138–157.

93. Pransky SM, Brester DF, Magit AE, et al. Clinical update on 10 children treated with intralesional cidofovir injections for severe recurrent respiratory papillomatosis. *Arch Otolaryngol Head Neck Surg.* 2000;126:1239–1243.

94. Pransky SM, Albright JT, Magit AE. Long-term follow-up of pediatric recurrent respiratory papillomatosis managed with intralesional cidofovir. *Laryngoscope.* 2003; 113:1583–1587.

95. Bielamowicz S, Villagomez V, Stager SV, et al. Intralesional cidofovir therapy for laryngeal papilloma in an adult cohort. *Laryngoscope.* 2002;112:696–699.

96. Akst LM, Lee W, Discolo C, et al. Stepped-dosed protocol of cidofovir therapy in recurrent respiratory papillomatosis in children. *Arch Otolaryngol Head Neck Surg.* 2003;129:841–846.

97. Chhetri DK, Shapiro NL. A schedule protocol for the treatment of juvenile recurrent respiratory papillomatosis

with intralesional cidofovir. *Arch Otolaryngol Head Neck Surg*. 2003;129:1081–1085.

98. Tanna N, Sidell D, Joshi AS, et al. Adult intralesional cidofovir therapy for laryngeal papilloma: a 10-year perspective. *Arch Otolaryngol Head Neck Surg*. 2008;134(5):497–500.

99. Wierzbicka M, Jackowska J, Bartochowska A, et al. Effectiveness of cidofovir intralesional treatment in recurrent respiratory papillomatosis. *Eur Arch Otorhinolaryngol*. 2011;268(9):1305–1311.

100. Durvasula VS, Richter GT. Intralesional cidofovir as adjuvant for the successful management of aggressive respiratory papillomatosis in an infant. *Int J Pediatr Otorhinolaryngol*. 2013;77(11):1912–1915.

101. Ksiazek J, Prager JD, Sun GH, et al. Inhaled cidofovir as an adjuvant therapy for recurrent respiratory papillomatosis. *Otolaryngol Head Neck Surg*. 2011;144(4):639–641.

102. Chhetri DK, Blumin JH, Shapiro NL, et al. Office-based treatment of laryngeal papillomatosis with percutaneous injection of cidofovir. *Otolaryngol Head Neck Surg*. 2002;126:642–648.

103. Co J, Woo P. Serial office-based intralesional injection of cidofovir in adult onset recurrent respiratory papillomatosis. *Ann Otol Rhinol Laryngol*. 2004;113:859–862.

104. El Hakim H, Waddell AN, Crysdale WS. Observations on the early results of treatment of recurrent respiratory papillomatosis using cidofovir. *J Otolaryngol*. 2002;31:333–335.

105. Milczuk HA. Intralesional cidofovir for the treatment of severe juvenile recurrent respiratory papillomatosis: long-term results in 4 children. *Otolaryngol Head Neck Surg*. 2003;128:788–794.

106. Peyton W, Wiatrak B. Is cidofovir a useful adjunctive therapy for recurrent respiratory papillomatosis in children. *Int J Pediatric Otorhinolaryngol*. 2004;68(4):413–418.

107. Shi ZP, Wang CH, Lee JC, et al. Cidofovir injection for recurrent respiratory papillomatosis. *J Chin Med Assoc*. 2008;71(3):143–146.

108. McMurray JS, Connor N, Ford CN. Cidofovir efficacy in recurrent respiratory papillomatosis: a randomized, double blind, placebo-controlled study. *Ann Otol Rhinol Laryngol*. 2008;117(7):477–483.

109. Tjon Pian Gi REA, Ilmarinen T, van den Heuvel ER, et al. Safety of intralesional cidofovir in patients with recurrent respiratory papillomatosis: an international retrospective study of 635 RRP patients. *Eur Arch Otorhinolaryngol*. 2013;270:1679–1687.

110. Derkay CS, Volsky PG, Rosen CA, et al. Current use of intralesional cidofovir for recurrent respiratory papillomatosis. *Laryngoscope*. 2013;123:705–712.

111. Man LX, Statham MM, Rosen CA. Mucosal bridge and pitting of the true vocal fold an unusual complication of cidofovir injection. *Ann Otol Rhinol Laryngol*. 2010;119(4): 236–238.

112. Dancey DR, Chamberlain DW, Krajden M, et al. Successful treatment of juvenile laryngeal papillomatosis-related multicystic lung disease with cidofovir: case report and review of the literature. *Chest*. 2000;118(4):1210–1214.

113. de Bilderling G, Bodart E, Lawson G, et al. Successful use of intralesional and intravenous cidofovir in association with indole-3-carbinol in an 8-year-old girl with pulmonary papillomatosis. *J Med Virol*. 2005;75(2):332–335.

114. Van Valckenborg I, Wellens W, De Boeck K, et al. Systemic cidofovir in papillomatosis. *Clin Infect Dis*. 2001;32 (3):E62–E64.

115. Inglis Jr AF. Editorial: cidofovir and the black box warning. *Ann Otol Rhinol Laryngol*. 2005;114(11):834–835.

116. Lott DG, Krakovitz, PR. Squamous cell carcinoma associated with intralesional injection of cidofovir for recurrent respiratory papillomatosis. *Laryngoscope*. 2009; 119:567–570.

117. Gupta HT, Robinson A, Murray RC, et al. Degress of dysplasia and the use of cidofovir in patients with recurrent respiratory papillomatosis. *Laryngoscope*. 2012; 120:698–702.

118. Lindsay F, Bloom D, Pransky S, et al. Histologic review of cidofovir-treated recurrent respiratory papillomatosis. *Ann Otol Rhinol Laryngol*. 2008;117(2):113–117.

119. Fusconi M, Grasso M, Greco A, et al. Recurrent respiratory papillomatosis by HPV: review of the literature and update on the use of cidofovir. *Acta Otorhinolaryngol Ital*. 2014;34(6):375–381.

120. Karatayli-Ozgursoy S, Bishop JA, Hillel A, et al. Risk factors for dysplasia in recurrent respiratory papillomatosis in adult and pediatric population. *Ann Otol Rhinol Laryngol*. 2016;125(3):235–241.

121. Broekema FI, Dikkers FG. Side-effects of cidofovir in the treatment of recurrent respiratory papillomatosis. *Eur Arch Otorhinolaryngol*. 2008;265(8):871–879.

122. Zeitels SM, Barbu AM, Landau-Zemer T, et al. Local injection of bevacizumab (Avastin) and angiolytic KTP laser treatment of recurrent respiratory papillomatosis of the vocal folds: a prospective study. *Ann Otol Rhinol Laryngol*. 2011;120(10):627–634.

123. Mohr M, Schliemann C, Biermann C, et al. Rapid response to systemic bevacizumab therapy in recurrent respiratory papillomatosis. *Oncol Lett*. 2014;8(5):1912–1918.

124. Best SR, Mohr M, Zur KB, et al. Systemic bevacizumab for recurrent respiratory papillomatosis: a national survey. *Laryngoscope*. 2017;127(10):2225–2229.

125. Best SR, Friedman AD, Landau-Zemer T, et al. Safety and dosing of bevacizumab (Avastin) of the treatment of recurrent respiratory papillomatosis. *Ann Otol Rhinol Laryngol*. 2012;121(9):587–593.

126. Rosen CA, Woodson GE, Thompson JW, et al. Preliminary results of the use of indole-3-carbinol for recurrent respiratory papillomatosis. *Otolaryngol Head Neck Surg*. 1998;118:810–815.

127. Rosen CA, Bryson PC. Indole-3-carbinol for recurrent respiratory papillomatosis: long term results. *J Voice.* 2003;18:248–253.

128. Haglund S, Lundquist PG, Cantell K, et al. Interferon therapy in juvenile laryngeal papillomatosis. *Arch Otolaryngol.* 1981;107(6):327–332.

129. Goepfert H, Sessions RB, Gutterman JU, et al. Leukocyte interferon in patients with juvenile laryngeal papillomatosis. *Ann Otol Rhinol Laryngol.* 1982;91(4pt1): 431–436.

130. McCabe BF, Clark KF. Interferon and laryngeal papillomatosis: the Iowa experience. *Ann Otol Rhinol Laryngol.* 1983;93:2–7.

131. Sessions RB, Goepfert H, Donovan DT, et al. Further observations on the treatment of recurrent respiratory papillomatosis with interferon: a comparison of sources. *Ann Otol Rhinol Laryngol.* 1983;92:456–461.

132. Lundquist PG, Haglund S, Carlsoo B, et al. Interferon therapy in juvenile laryngeal papillomatosis. *Otolaryngol Head Neck Surg.* 1984;92:386–391.

133. Deunas L, Alcantud V, Alvarez F, et al. Use of interferon-alpha in laryngeal papillomatosis: eight years of the Cuban national programme. *J Laryngol Otol.* 1997;111: 134–140.

134. Gerein V, Rastorguez E, Gerein J, et al. use of interferon-alpha in recurrent respiratory papillomatosis: 20-year follow-up. *Ann Otol Rhinol Laryngol.* 2005;114(6):463–471.

135. Kashima H, Leventhal B, Clark K, et al. Interferon alfa-N1 (Wellferon) in juvenile onset recurrent respiratory papillomatosis: results of a randomized study in twelve collaborative institutions. *Laryngoscope.* 1988;98:334–340.

136. Leventhal BG, Kashima HK, Mounts P, et al. Long-term response of recurrent respiratory papillomatosis to treatment with lymphoblastoid interferon alfa-n1. *N Engl J Med.* 1991;325:613–617.

137. Suter-Montano T, Montano E, Martinez C, et al. Adult recurrent respiratory papillomatosis: a new therapeutic approach with pegylated interferon alpha 2a (Peg-IFN-alpha-2a) and GM-CSF. *Otol Head Neck Surg.* 2013;148: 253–260.

138. Healy GB, Gelber RD, Trowbridge AL, et al. Treatment of recurrent respiratory papillomatosis with human leukocyte interferon: results of a multicenter randomized clinical trial. *N Engl J Med.* 1988;319:401–407.

139. Shibata M, Hoon D, Okun E, et al. Modulation of histamine type II receptors on CD8+ T cells b interleukin-2 and cimetidine. *Int Arch Allergy Immunol.* 1992;97:8–16.

140. Ershler WB, Hacker MP, Burroughs BJ, et al. Cimetidine and the immune response. *Clin Immunol Immunopathol.* 1983;26:10–17.

141. Ishikura H, Fukui H, Takeyama N, et al. Cimetidine activates interleukin-12 which enhances cellular immunity. *Blood.* 1999;93:1782–1783.

142 Harcourt JP, Worley G, Leighton SEJ. Cimetidine treatment for recurrent respiratory papillomatosis. *Int J Ped Otorhinolaryngol.* 1999;51:109–113.

143. Shikowitz MJ, Steinberg BM, Abramson AL. Hematoporphyrin derivative therapy of papillomas. Experimental study. *Arch Otolaryngol Head Neck Surg.* 1986;112: 42–46.

144. Abramson AL, Shikowitz MJ, Mullooly VM, et al. Clinical effects of photodynamic therapy on recurrent laryngeal papillomatosis. *Arch Otolaryngol Head Neck Surg.* 1992;188:25–29.

145. Abramson AL, Shikowitz MJ, Mulloly VM, et al. Variable light-dose effect on photodynamic therapy for laryngeal papillomas. *Arch Otolaryngol Head Neck Surg.* 1994;120:852–855.

146. Shikowitz MJ, Abramson AL, Freeman K, et al. Efficacy of DHE photodynamic therapy for respiratory papillomatosis: immediate and long-term results. *Laryngoscope.* 1998;108:962–967.

147. Lei J, Yu W, Yuexin L, et al. Topical measles-mumps-rubella vaccine in the treatment of recurrent respiratory papillomatosis: results of a preliminary randomized, controlled trial. *ENT J.* 2012:91:174–175.

148. Meacham RK, Thompson JW, et al. Comparison of cidofovir and the measles, mumps, and rubella vaccine in the treatment of recurrent respiratory papillomatosis. *Ear Nose Throat J.* 2017;96(2):69–74.

149. Derkay CS, Smith RJ, McClay J, et al. HspE7 treatment of pediatric recurrent respiratory papillomatosis: final results of an open-label trial. *Ann Otol Rhinol Laryngol.* 2005;114:730–737.

150. Vandepapeliere P, Barrasso R, Meijer CJLM, et al. Randomized controlled trial of an adjuvant human papillomavirus (HPV) type 6 L2E7 vaccine: infection of external anogenital warts with multiple HPV types and failure of the therapeutic vaccinations. *J Infect Dis.* 1995; 192(12):2099–2107.

151. Hocevar-Boltezar I, Maticic M, Sereg-Bahar M, et al. Human papilloma virus vaccination in patients with an aggressive course of recurrent respiratory papillomatosis. *Eur Arch Otorhinolaryngol.* 2014;271(12):3255–3262.

152. Tjon Pian Gi RE, San Giorgi MR, Pawlita M, et al. Immunological response to quadrivalent HPV vaccine in treatment of recurrent respiratory papillomatosis. *Eur Arch Otorhinolaryngol.* 2016;273(10):3231–3236.

153. Young DL, Moore MM, Halstead LA. The use of the quadrivalent human papillomavirus vaccine (Gardasil) as adjuvant therapy in the treatment of recurrent respiratory papilloma. *J Voice.* 2015;29(2):223–229.

154. Hermann JS, Weckx LY, Monteiro Nurmberger J, et al. Effectiveness of the human papillomavirus (types 6, 11, 16, and 18) vaccine in the treatment of children with recurrent respiratory papillomatosis. *Int J Pediatr Otorhinolaryngol.* 2016;83:94–98.

155. Baumannis MM, Elmaraghy CA. Intersurgical interval increased with use of quadrivalent human papillomavirus vaccine (Gardasil) in a pediatric patient with recurrent respiratory papillomatosis: a case report. *Int J Pediatr Otorhinolaryngol.* 2016;91:166–169.

156. Sullivan C, Curtis Curtis S, Mouzakes J. Therapeutic use of the HPV vaccine in recurrent respiratory papillomatosis: a case report. *Int J Pediatr Otorhinolaryngol.* 2017;93:103–106.

157. Meszner Z, Jankovics I, Nagy A, et al. Recurrent laryngeal papillomatosis with oesophageal involvement in a 2 year old boy: successful treatment with the quadrivalent human papillomatosis vaccine. *Int J Pediatr Otorhinolaryngol.* 2015;79(2):262–266.

158. Förster G, Boltze C, Seidel J, Pawlita M, Müller A. Juvenile laryngeal papillomatosis—immunisation with the polyvalent vaccine Gardasil. *Laryngorhinootologie.* 2008;87(11):796–799.

159. Cohen EG, Almahmeed T, Du B, et al. Microsomal prostaglandin E synthase-1 is overexpressed in head and neck squamous cell carcinoma. *Clin Cancer Res.* 2003; 9(9):3425–3430.

160. Yoshimatsu K, Golijanin D, Paty PB, et al. Inducible microsomal prostaglandin E synthase is overexpressed in colorectal adenomas and cancer. *Clin Cancer Res.* 2001;7(12):3971–3976.

161. Lucs AV, Wu R, Mullooly V, et al. Constitutive overexpression of the oncogene Rac1 in the airway of recurrent respiratory papillomatosis patients is a targetable host-susceptibility factor. *Mol Med.* 2012;18:244–249.

162. Limsukon A, Susanto I, Soo Hoo GW, et al. Regression of recurrent respiratory papillomatosis with celecoxib and erlotinib combination therapy. *Chest.* 2009; 136(3):924–926.

163. Vambutas A, Di Lorenzo TP, Steinberg BM. Laryngeal papilloma cells have high levels of epidermal growth factor receptor and respond to epidermal growth factor by a decrease in epithelial differentiation. *Cancer Res.* 1993;53(4):910–914.

164. Wu R, Abramson AL, Shikowitz MJ, et al. Epidermal growth factor-induced cyclooxygenase-2 expression is mediated through phosphatidylinositol-3 kinase, not mitogen-activated protein/extracellular signal-regulated kinase, in recurrent respiratory papillomas. *Clin Cancer Res.* 2005;11(17):6155–6161.

165. Cohen MH, Williams GA, Sridhara R, et al. FDA drug approval summary: gefitinib (ZD1839) (Iressa) tablets. *Oncologist.* 2003;8(4):303–306.

166. Kultan J, Kolek V, Fajkosova L, et al. Recurrent respiratory papillomatosis successfully treated with gefitinib: a case study. *AJMCR.* 2015;3(11):352–358.

167. Bostrom B, Sidman J, Marker S, et al. Gefitinib therapy for life-threatening laryngeal papillomatosis. *Arch Otolaryngol Head Neck Surg.* 2005;131(1):64–67.

168. Keir ME, Butte MJ, Freeman GJ, et al. PD-1 and its ligands in tolerance and immunity. *Annu Rev Immunol.* 2008;26:677–704.

169. Chen N, Fang W, Zhan J, et al. Upregulation of PD-L1 by EGFR activation mediates the immune escape in EGFR-driven NSCLC: implication for optional immune targeted therapy for NSCLC patients with EGFR mutation. *J Thorac Oncol.* 2015;10:910–923.

170. Liu T, Greenberg M, Wentland C, et al. PD-L1 expression and CD8+ infiltration shows heterogeneity in juvenile recurrent respiratory papillomatosis. *Int J Pediatr Otorhinolaryngol.* 2017;95:133–138.

171. Yang W, Song Y, Lu YL, et al. Increased expression of programmed death (PD)-1 and its ligand PD-L1 correlates with impaired cell-mediated immunity in high-risk human papillomavirus-related cervical intraepithelial neoplasia. *Immunology.* 2013;139(4):513–522.

172. Lyford-Pike S, Peng S, Young GD, et al. Evidence for a role of the PD-1:PD-L1 pathway in immune resistance of HPV-associated head and neck squamous cell carcinoma. *Cancer Res.* 2013;73(6):1733–1741.

173. Brahmer JR, Tykodi SS, Chow LQ, et al. Safety and activity of anti-PD-L1 antibody in patients with advanced cancer. *N Engl J Med.* 2012;366(26):2455–2465.

174. Le DT, Uram JN, Wang H, et al. PD-1 blockade in tumors with mismatch-repair deficiency. *N Engl J Med.* 2015;372(26):2509–2520.

CHAPTER 22

Vocal Granuloma

Declan Costello
With thanks to Dr. Marion Palmer for comments on the manuscript

BACKGROUND AND ONSET OF SYMPTOMS

A 50-year-old gentleman, who is usually fit and well, fell while on holiday and required emergency orthopedic surgery for a broken ankle. Under general anesthetic (ventilated with an oral endotracheal tube), he had an open reduction and internal fixation (ORIF) of his ankle.

In the subsequent months, he experienced a persistent irritation and pain on the left side of his throat. He did not experience any dysphagia, but his swallow was occasionally painful on the left side. His voice was mildly hoarse, and he experienced vocal fatigue in the course of a working day (his managerial job required significant voice usage).

PRESENTATION TO ENT

He consulted an ENT surgeon, and on fiberoptic laryngoscopy, a small swelling was noted over the vocal process of the left arytenoid. No pre-surgical treatments were attempted, he was admitted for microlaryngoscopy and excision biopsy under general anesthetic, and the lesion was excised with cold steel instruments. No postoperative voice rest was recommended, and no other treatments were instituted. The histopathology report showed features consistent with a vocal process granuloma.

For the first 2 weeks after his microlaryngoscopy, his throat symptoms improved, but they then returned over the subsequent 4 weeks. He was seen again by the same surgeon, who noted a recurrence of the granuloma (but this time the lesion was significantly larger

than previously) and he operated once more, using the same technique; a similar pattern followed, with a rapid recurrence of his symptoms.

The patient was referred for a second opinion. A large granuloma was now present, and the patient was admitted for a further microlaryngoscopy; on this occasion, a CO_2 laser was used to excise the lesion and ablate its base. Yet again, the symptoms recurred.

Comment

Chevalier Jackson was the first author to identify laryngeal contact ulcers,[1] but the first description of an intubation-related laryngeal granuloma was by Clausen in 1932.[2]

Laryngeal granulomas can occur when there is exposure of cartilage, usually around the vocal process of the arytenoid cartilage. The initial insult can be (as in this case) during intubation; in particular, in cases of emergency or hurried intubation, the endotracheal tube can cause shearing of the mucosa over the vocal process, leaving bare cartilage. As most anesthetists are right-handed, the endotracheal tube is usually directed toward the left side of the larynx, and hence granulomas are more common on the left than on the right.

Irritation and inflammation by reflux are known to be significant causative and propagatory factors in vocal process granulomas.[3]

It has also been suggested that untreated glottic insufficiency may be a contributory factor[4] in patients who prove refractory to conservative treatment.

Histopathologically, laryngeal granulomas are characterized by vessel proliferation, inflammation, and intra-cytoplasmic alterations in fibroblasts suggesting cellular dysfunction and damage.[5]

TERTIARY REFERRAL

At time of presentation to a tertiary center, the larynx was as shown below (Figure 22–1).

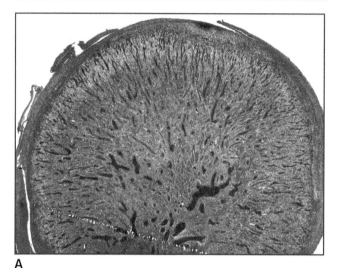

A

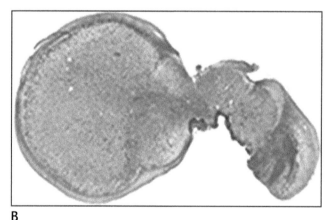

B

Figure 22–1. (A) Whole mount histological section of a large contact ulcer/granuloma demonstrating an exophytic, focally pedunculated, polypoidal architecture. There is global surface ulceration, surmounted by pyogenic coagulum. The core comprises exuberant, richly vascularized granulation tissue type response with radial symmetry (hematoxylin and eosin [H&E] stain; ultra-low magnification). (B) Close-up view, demonstrating the zoned symmetrical granuloma pyogenicum-like proliferation of small and medium caliber blood vessels characteristic of contact ulcer/granuloma. The native surface epithelium is comprehensively ulcerated and replaced by a superficial mantle of fibrino-purulent exudate (H&E stain; medium magnification).

A large vocal process granuloma is seen. By this stage, the lesion was of sufficient size to be causing airway symptoms: there was a reduction in exercise tolerance (the patient was a keen runner) and his vocal fatigue had started to cause difficulties with his work.

REFLUX SYMPTOMS

Close questioning demonstrated some heartburn and occasional acid brash; he had not yet been treated for this, so he was started on a twice daily proton pump inhibitor (PPI); he was also advised to use an alginate and was given written advice about reflux-inhibiting lifestyle measures.

Because of the airway limitation caused by the size of the granuloma, further surgery was planned; the patient was counseled that recurrence was likely, but he was very keen to pursue another operation.

Under general anesthetic, the patient was ventilated with supraglottic jet ventilation (to avoid further trauma from another endotracheal tube). On this occasion, the procedure focused on excision of the lesion, but taking care to avoid leaving any exposed cartilage. This necessitated leaving a small part of the stalk of the granuloma. Steroids (Depo-Medrone, 40 mg/mL) were injected into the base of the granuloma. Postoperatively, he was advised to rest his voice for 5 days. He was given strict instructions to avoid coughing, throat clearing, and vocal straining.

Initially, his symptoms remained at bay, and the larynx showed no significant sign of recurrence of the granuloma. At follow-up 4 weeks following surgery, it was noted that the surgical bed showed signs of ulceration, so there was clearly a concern that a recurrence may occur.

Indeed, 3 months later, his symptoms returned, along with a recurrence of the granuloma.

Comment

Vocal process granulomata are known to be recalcitrant to treatment, particularly if a cycle of trauma ensues, such as the repeated surgical removal and abrasion of the vocal process region. Ideally the granuloma should be treated as conservatively as possible to limit trauma to the region and minimize establishing chondritis with subsequent recurrent granulation tissue formation.

Treatment

A number of different treatment modalities have been employed over the years:

- simple observation
- antireflux treatment
- voice therapy
- steroid inhalers
- surgical excision
- laser
- cold steel
- can be combined with injection of steroid, and/or mitomycin C
- botulinum toxin injection

As noted above, antireflux treatment is usually initiated. Voice therapy, focusing on avoidance of further laryngeal trauma, should be offered.

It is important to eliminate any ongoing irritation of the posterior larynx. Hence, treatment of any extra-esophageal reflux is important, and the patient should be counseled to halt any vocally abusive behaviors.

Excision of vocal process granulomas exposes more cartilage, and hence recurrence is almost universal. Indeed, the recurrence is often more aggressive than the original lesion.

Cautious and painstaking monitoring is usually the best option in these cases, as surgery is usually doomed to failure and recurrence. However, in a few cases, where airway compromise is present, there may be no option but to operate.

A systematic review by Karkos et al[6] evaluated a range of different treatment options of treatment for vocal process granulomas including antireflux therapy, speech and language therapy, steroid, botulinum toxin and microlaryngeal surgery. They reported level 2A evidence for antireflux treatment as the main treatment strategy, with surgery reserved only for failures of medical treatment or airway obstruction, or when the diagnosis was in doubt. The authors noted that methodological issues prevented the undertaking of a formal meta-analysis and highlighted the need for randomized controlled trials in this area.[6]

In a large retrospective study ($n = 590$) of non-intubation granulomas in South Korea,[7] it was found that PPI antireflux treatment and voice therapy were more effective than simple observation (giving a "good response" rate of 44% versus 20%, respectively); the addition of botulinum toxin further enhances the response rate (good response rate of 74%). In this group, surgical excision led to a significantly higher recur-

rence rate than simple observation. Steroid inhalers resulted in a 32% good response rate.[7]

In a series of 168 patients,[8] it was found that 41.3% of cases were resolved with antireflux treatment, voice therapy, and observation. Patients who went on to have surgical excision and micro-flap mucosal transposition had a 70% response rate, and this increased to 95% when this was combined with injection of botulinum toxin.

If glottic insufficiency is found to coexist with the granuloma (Carroll et al found that 53% of patients with granuloma had an underlying diagnosis of glottic insufficiency), it may be important to treat the insufficiency to aid in resolution of the granuloma. This was also the finding in nine patients treated with fat augmentation.[9] It is suggested that glottic insufficiency results in laryngeal hyperfunction, hence increasing collision forces between the arytenoid cartilages.

It has even been suggested that radiotherapy can be used as a treatment, but this is certainly not in widespread usage in contemporary practice.[10]

Botulinum Toxin Injection

As shown, the primary site of origin of vocal process granulomas is the tip of the vocal process. For this reason, there is some logic in trying to limit the rotation of the arytenoid cartilage to avoid the tips of the vocal processes from making contact with each other. The lateral cricoarytenoid (LCA) muscle is the primary rotator of the arytenoid cartilage, so reducing the pulling force of the LCA should, in theory, reduce the contact between the arytenoid vocal processes. In practice, it is impossible to inject solely the LCA, but the effect can partially be achieved with a targeted injection of botulinum toxin into the lateral cricoarytenoid-thyroarytenoid (LCA-TA) complex of muscles.

At this point, an injection of botulinum toxin was offered: under local anesthetic and electromyographic (EMG) control, botulinum toxin A was injected into the LCA-TA muscles on the left side.

As is usual, there was no effect for 2 days, but subsequently this had the effect of inducing a very breathy voice for a period of 3 weeks. His larynx was not examined during this time, but it is clear that he was experiencing a pharmacologically induced vocal fold paralysis (or at least a paresis). When his voice returned, he continued his vocal hygiene and careful avoidance of vocally abusive behaviors.

His symptoms did not recur, and examination 6 months later showed no recurrence of his granuloma.

CONCLUSION

Vocal process granulomata remain difficult to treat and require a patient approach; the mainstay of management rests on elimination of laryngeal irritation, with a combination of voice therapy (targeted at removing abusive vocal behaviors) and antireflux treatment.

In cases of airway compromise, or where there is a doubt about the diagnosis, surgery may be required. However, recurrence rates are high after excision.

Further treatment with botulinum toxin can be effective but may be associated with side effects such as breathy voice or (occasionally) aspiration.

REFERENCES

1. Jackson C. Contact ulcer of the larynx. *Ann Otol Rhinol Laryngol.* 1928;37:227–230.
2. Clausen RJ. Unusual sequela of tracheal intubation. *Proc R Soc Med.* 1932;25:1507
3. Ogawa M, Hosokawa K, Iwahashi T, Inohara H. The results of Kaplan-Meier and multivariate analyses of etiological factors related to the outcome of combined pharmacological therapy against laryngeal granuloma. *Acta Oto-Laryngologica.* 2016;136(11): 1141–1146.
4. Carroll TL, Gartner-Schmidt J, Statham MM, Rosen CA. Vocal process granuloma and glottal insufficiency: an overlooked etiology? *Laryngoscope.* 2010;120:114–120.
5. Martins RH, Dias NH, Santos DC, Fabro AT, Braz JR. Clinical, histological and electron microscopic aspects of vocal fold granulomas. *Braz J Otorhinolaryngol.* 2009;75(1): 116–122.
6. Karkos PD, et al. Vocal process granulomas: a systematic review of treatment. *Ann Otol Rhinol Laryngol.* 2014; 123(5):314–320.
7. Lee SW, Hong HJ, Choi SH, et al. Comparison of treatment modalities for contact granuloma: a nationwide multicenter study. *Laryngoscope.* 2014;124 (5):1187–1191.
8. Ma L, et al. Analysis of therapeutic methods for treating vocal process granulomas. *Acta Oto-Laryngologica.* 2015;135(3): 277–282.
9. Hu HC, Hung YT, Lin SY, Chang SY. Office-based autologous fat injection laryngoplasty for vocal process granuloma. *J Voice.* 2016;30:758.e7–758.e11.
10. Harari PM, Blatchford SJ, Coulthard SW, Cassady JR. Intubation granuloma of the larynx: successful eradication with low-dose radiotherapy. *Head Neck.* 1991;13(3): 230–233.

CHAPTER 23

Anterior Glottic Webs

Matthew Broadhurst

INTRODUCTION

An anterior glottic web is a soft tissue connection between the left and right true vocal folds. It is most commonly acquired through endotracheal intubation, surgery to the glottis, or trauma. Congenital webs are rare and when large enough, present in early life as airway obstruction. Glottic webs can be classified as anterior, posterior, and complete. This chapter will address only *acquired* anterior glottic webs. Anterior glottic webs can be small and thin but range to thick, fibrous, or long, extending posterior toward the arytenoids. It is important to recognize that most anterior glottic webs contain fibrous tissue that has replaced the superficial lamina propria (SLP). As such, correction of a web would rarely improve the voice. It is important to treat the patient's symptoms rather than just treat the web. Prevention, of course, is better than cure, and certain key principals can be employed to minimize the formation of anterior glottic webs in glottic surgery. Treatments have evolved over decades dating back to Haslinger in 1924[1] with a silver keel and Jackson in 1930[2] with further innovations. McNaught introduced a keel through a laryngofissure using tantalum.[3] Other materials for a keel have included Teflon,[4] Silastic,[5–7] and silicone.[8] Various stents and mucosal flaps have also been utilized.[9,10] Over the past century the most common cause of an anterior glottic web is endotracheal tube trauma.[11]

DEFINITION

An anterior glottic web is the continuity of soft tissue across the anterior glottic angle (commissure) narrowing the airway with/without disturbance to the mucosal wave, usually resulting in hoarseness.

CASE PRESENTATION

History

A 64-year-old male presented with hoarseness and moderate airway restriction on walking up hills or stairs. He is a non-smoker and has no history of cardiovascular or respiratory disease. Speech therapy has not improved the voice quality.

Social history: non-drinker, never smoked.

Medications: nil regular

No known allergies.

Initial Assessment

History

Red flag symptoms (stridor with/without exertion, stridor while sleeping). Presence of these may warrant more urgent assessment with hospital admission to secure the airway. Fortunately, most cases are not considered airway emergencies and can be managed more methodically. It is important to obtain from the patient the true impact of the glottic web on daily activity, voice use, and quality of life.

Examination

Assessment of the voice and airway are critical in establishing the diagnosis and management plan. This patient had moderate roughness with reduced projection to conversational voice. There was no audible restriction in breathing or stridor and he had a normal cough. There was reduced maximal phonation time at 7 seconds and limited pitch range. Examination of the neck and oral cavity were unremarkable.

Endoscopy

A simple laryngoscopy is the minimum required. For true assessment of the vocal fold vibration and degree of glottal closure, videostroboscopy is required. Use of high definition video capture and adequate illumination enable a detailed laryngeal assessment. It is important to note the following on stroboscopy (Table 23–1):

Table 23–1. Important Findings on Videostroboscopy:

Vocal fold mobility:	normal, reduced, absent, unilateral, bilateral
Vocal fold edges:	straight, concave, convex
Vocal fold closure:	complete, incomplete
Surface pliability:	normal, reduced, increased
Presence of lesion(s):	cyst, polyp, nodules, neoplasia, web
Supraglottic constriction:	absent, mild, moderate, severe

If a lesion is present, and certain indications are met, then an office biopsy can be performed in this setting.

Scenario 1

A history was obtained of multiple treatments for laryngeal papillomatosis using CO_2 laser and microdebrider and involving the anterior commissure. There was incremental loss of vocal quality with repeated microlaryngeal surgeries and increasing difficulty walking up stairs and hills. His surgeries numbered nine and spanned 5 years. He has no residual papilloma, but a glottic web of moderate length and thickness is restricting his physical activity and voice use.

Videostroboscopy

Videostroboscopy found normal range of motion of the cricoarytenoid joints, reduced glottal aperture from an anterior glottic web extending partway toward the arytenoids, incomplete glottal closure, reduced mucosal wave of each vocal fold, and no evidence of papilloma (Figure 23–1; Video 23–1).

Diagnosis

Moderate length and thickness anterior glottic web, glottal insufficiency.

Management

Given there are symptoms from this anterior glottic web, intervention is a suitable option. After informed consent discussion with the patient, he can proceed to surgical reconstruction.

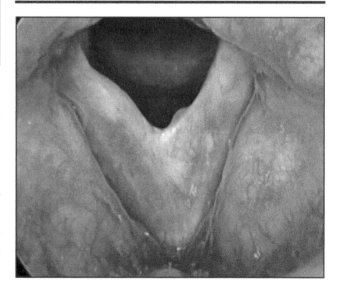

Figure 23–1. After extensive anterior commissure treatments for laryngeal papillomatosis using CO_2 laser, a moderate glottic web has formed. There is no papilloma but this has come at the expense of significant hoarseness and airway limitation.

He has a history of T1b glottic squamous cell carcinoma involving the anterior commissure. This was initially treated by partial excisional biopsy followed by curative intent radiotherapy. His voice never improved and over 2 years actually deteriorated. Although he remains cancer free, he has severe hoarseness, minimal volume and projection, and significantly reduced exercise tolerance. He is unable to work as a fruit market manager in a loud outdoor market environment.

Videostroboscopy

Videostroboscopy found normal range of motion of the cricoarytenoid joints, significantly reduced glottal aperture from an extensive anterior glottic web extending to the arytenoids, incomplete glottal closure, reduced mucosal wave of each vocal fold, multiple telangectasias, but no evidence of cancer. There is a large mucosal component to the web (Figure 23–2; Video 23–2a, 23–2b, Audio 23–2a, 23–2b).

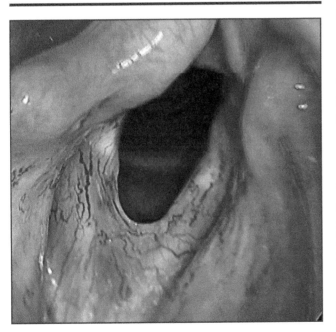

Figure 23–2. After curative intent radiation therapy for a glottic cancer, an extensive membranous glottic web has formed causing severe dysphonia and airway limitation. Although there is no cancer, it has come at severe cost to the airway and voice.

Diagnosis

Extensive membranous anterior glottic web, glottal insufficiency.

Management

Given there are symptoms from this anterior glottic web, intervention is a suitable option. After informed consent discussion with the patient, he can proceed to surgical reconstruction.

SCENARIO 3

He provided a history of an extensive T2 glottic squamous cell carcinoma involving the anterior commissure. This was treated by dual, staged potassium titanyl phosphate (KTP) laser ablation procedures, with complete resolution of the cancer. At 5 years, he remains disease free. Although he only has mild hoarseness, he has mildly reduced exercise tolerance. There is some erythroplasia on the right true vocal fold that will be ablated with KTP laser (Figure 23–3; Video 23–3).

Diagnosis

Moderate length and moderate thickness anterior glottic web, glottal insufficiency.

Management

Given he is minimally symptomatic from this anterior glottic web, intervention is not essential. This case highlights the fact that some glottic webs, even when moderately extensive, may need no treatment.

DIFFERENTIAL DIAGNOSIS

Most anterior glottic webs are iatrogenic but can also include neoplastic, infective, infiltrative, and congenital. Table 23–2 summarizes the causes but is not exhaustive.

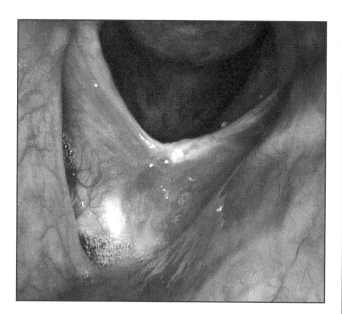

Figure 23–3. KTP laser was used to successfully treat an extensive anterior commissure T2 glottic SCC. Although there is only mild hoarseness he has reduced exercise tolerance and this moderate thickness glottic web will be repaired. Note the granulation on the cephalad surface which was reported as mild dysplasia and granulation at surgery.

Table 23–2. Summary of Causes for Most Anterior Glottic Webs

CONGENITAL:	Failure of complete canalization of laryngeal septum
ACQUIRED:	
Iatrogenic:	Traumatic placement of an endotracheal tube, instrumentation of the lower airway that inadvertently traumatizes the anterior glottic mucosa
Neoplastic:	Squamous cell carcinoma
Infective:	Laryngeal papilloma, diphtheria, mycobacterium tuberculosis
Inflammatory:	Wegener's, amyloidosis, sarcoidosis, pemphigoid
Intentional:	Transgender surgery, Wendler's glottoplasty

Management

The management of anterior glottic webs can be divided into: (1) approaches for prevention and (2) approaches for treatment once a web is established.

ANTERIOR WEB PREVENTION

In commonly performed microlaryngeal surgeries including cytoreduction of polypoid corditis, ablation of squamous cell carcinoma (SCC), or ablation of papillomatosis, simple measures can be utilized to minimize the chance of web formation. In polypoid corditis, careful preservation of at least 2 to 4 mm of epithelium on one side or 2 mm of epithelium on both sides will minimize web formation. Over the past 3 years, the author has been applying Bioglue (Cryolife, Kennesaw, Georgia, USA) to the treated anterior

commissure at the time of web resection. Although this bovine serum albumin product is an adhesive, it can minimize web formation. By applying a thin film over the treated surfaces, the Bioglue dries as a flexible dressing firmly adherent for 2 weeks in the author's experience. During this time, epithelialization occurs beneath the Bioglue while the opposing medial glottic surfaces are maintained apart (Figure 23–4A–C and Video 23–4a, b).

For treatment of anterior commissure SCC, ablation using KTP laser minimizes depth of tissue damage, allowing for minimal web formation if at all. Again, the addition of Bioglue can allow epithelial regeneration while the opposing raw surfaces heal, reducing the risk of web formation. Prevention of a web and preservation of the normal anterior commissure can be seen in the pre- and 12-month post-surgical images (Figure 23–5A–C; Video 23–5a, b, c).

In laryngeal papillomatosis, utilizing the properties of the KTP laser is highly effective at avoiding web formation when treating anterior commissure disease (Figure 23–6). In over 200 procedures performed by the author, involving the anterior commissure and treated with the KTP laser and more recently the addition of Bioglue, there have been only five web formations.

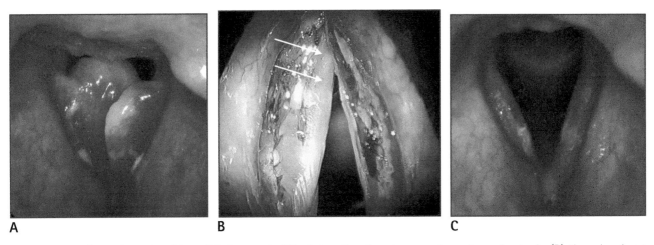

Figure 23–4. Extensive polypoid corditis is seen in (A) obstructing the airway and causing aphonia. In (B) there has been meticulous cytoreduction and preservation of 3 mm of vocal fold epithelium on the left anterior true cord. A thin film of Bioglue is then applied and provides a barrier to prevent adhesions between the raw surfaces as epithelialization occurs. At 6 months, the anterior commissure is entirely normal with no web in (C) although a right saccular cyst persists.

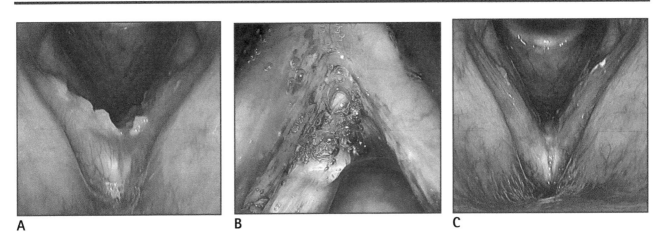

Figure 23–5. A T1b glottic SCC is seen in (A) before treatment centred on the anterior commissure. After KTP laser ablation there are de-epithelialized surfaces on the opposing anterior left and right medial vocal folds. A thin film of Bioglue is applied to prevent adhesions and subsequent web formation in (B). At 12 months, the office endoscopy shows an entirely normal anterior commissure and he has remained disease free with normal voice for over 5 years (C).

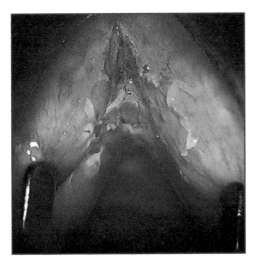

Figure 23–6. After treating laryngeal papilloma at the anterior commissure with KTP laser the de-epithelialized surfaces on the opposing anterior left and right medial vocal folds are covered with a thin film of Bioglue. This will prevent adhesions and subsequent web formation. The cord spreader in place lateralizes the medical vocal fold surfaces while the Bioglue dries.

ANTERIOR WEB TREATMENT

Once a web has been established, then attention turns from prevention to management. Management of anterior glottic webs depends on the underlying cause and the severity of the symptoms. Be sure to treat the patient as a whole, not just the anterior glottic web. Assuming there is airway limitation, which can be on exertion or even at rest, surgical intervention can be considered. The surgical procedure depends on the length, thickness, and composition of the web. Given that the glottal aperture is increasing with surgery, a temporary tracheotomy is rarely necessary but should always be consented for.

A minimally invasive approach is serial excision with dilation and steroids injection into the treated soft tissues.[12,13] This requires minimal specialized equipment so would be a suitable option for most ENT surgeons. This procedure is suitable for both longer and shorter symptomatic webs. The procedure does lack the precision of phonomicrosurgery and, multiple admissions with general anesthetic may be required, with results being less predictable than other more formal methods.

For a membranous web that has limited length, simple lysis may be adequate. Minimizing mucosal trauma by ensuring the incision is precise, and avoiding the heat of CO_2 laser can reduce the reformation rate. Application of Bioglue is useful here. It should be noted, however, that there are numerous reports with good outcomes utilizing CO_2 laser.[14,15]

If simple lysis and Bioglue are not sufficient or when there is generous mucosal tissue available that can be mobilized, then advancement flap(s) reconstruction is suitable. For short, long, thick, or thin webs, carefully planned incisions can preserve mucosa, allowing for resection of the subepithelial portion of the web. Using 6/0 polydioxanone suture, the flaps can be sutured to cover opposing glottic surfaces[9,10] (Figure 23–7). There are some situations where the free edge of each vocal fold is fibrosed and contracted into the midline, leaving inadequate mucosal tissue. As such, adequate mucosa cannot be raised as a flap and another option is chosen (Figure 23–8).

In such situations where mucosal surfaces are not salvageable to cover the lysed surfaces, a keel placed between the anterior opposing surfaces of the true cords is necessary.[16,17] This is particularly useful with a high vertical height web. The keel can be a formal implant made from silastic or polytetrafluoroethylene and placed endoscopically, or through a small laryngofissure. Alternatively, cardiac patch Gore-Tex (Gore, Flagstaff, Arizona, USA) can be cut to size and secured endoscopically avoiding a laryngofissure. Sutures are then passed anteriorly through the midline superior and inferior to the glottis and secured over a silastic button (Figures 23–9 and 23–10). External thyroid lamina perichondrium can also be used by dissecting and raising this flap from lateral to cross the midline.[18,19] A small vertical cartilage thyrotomy is made in the midline where the perichondrium has been dissected free (Figure 23–11). The perichondrium is then positioned through the thyrotomy to enter the anterior glottis forming the keel. A keel needs to enable adequate epithelialization to occur, so needs to remain in place for at least 4 weeks.

An anterior glottic web may be both high in vertical height and long in anterior-posterior dimension, composed of dense fibrous tissue. A formal resection of the anterior glottis is then required to normalize the anterior commissure contour. In this setting the pliable SLP is absent, there is no voice to salvage, and the surgical goal is solely improvement of the airway. Mitomycin C has been shown to be of benefit in this setting,[20] and simple keel can be inadequate. A stent instead can be used, although a temporary tracheotomy will be required. As such, a Montgomery Safe-T-Tube (Boston Medical, Shrewsbury, Massachusetts, USA) can accomplish the tracheotomy and the stenting. Alternatively, a separate tracheotomy with a soft silastic tube fashioned to size and secured at the glottic level can be used. The Eliashar laryngeal stent (Lucas Medical, Anaheim, California, USA) can be a large stent option for the glottis and is secured to a tracheotomy caudally to maintain it in position. As more tissue requires remodeling in the setting, the stent must remain for at least 2 months before removal.

Occasionally, there may be complete occlusion at the glottic level where there is no lumen through the glottis. The author received a tertiary referral of this nature. The entire glottis was occluded with a granulomatous web and the patient was tracheotomy dependent following multiple CO_2 laser attempts to resolve a laryngeal stenosis. His only communication was with an electrolarynx. A formal external approach with laryngofissure, resection, and silastic stenting was planned. This can be the only option at times, albeit rarely. In this case, however, a passage was created through the glottis endoscopically by careful instrumentation above and below the web, followed by dilations and endoscopic stent placement in the same sitting. The superior and partial medial vocal fold surfaces were uninvolved with the subcordal true folds being the level of the web. A formal laryngofissure was spared and the patient successfully decannulated 3 months later with more than satisfactory voice.

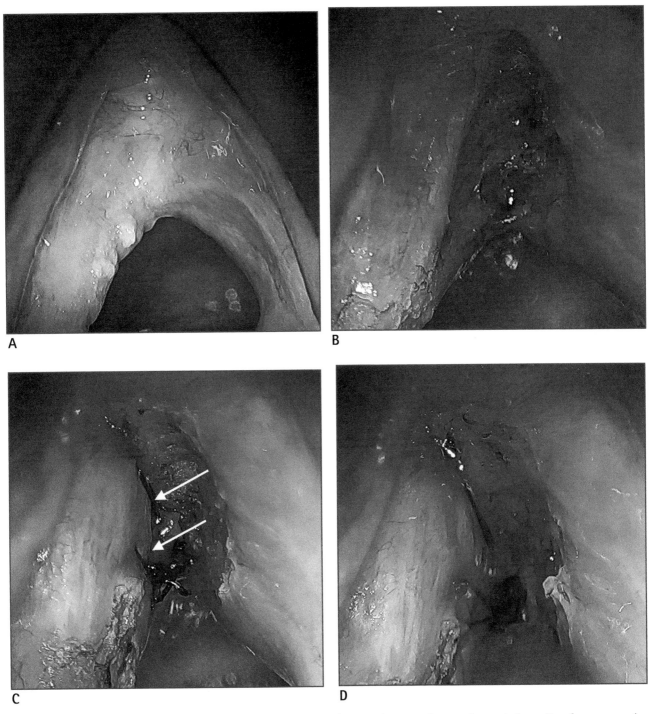

Figure 23–7. Mucosal flaps can be mobilized to reconstruct the anterior commissure after web formation from aggressive treatment. Careful preservation of mucosa is critical in planning the mucosal flaps and they are sutured in place with 6/0 polydioxanone suture. This will prevent adhesions and subsequent web formation. The large glottic web in (**A**) is divided in (**B**) preserving an inferior based left mucosal flap. Once sutured in place in (**C**), the left medial vocal fold is entirely lined by epithelium (*white arrows*). Bioglue is then applied in (**D**) to act as a flexible dressing to minimize web re-formation.

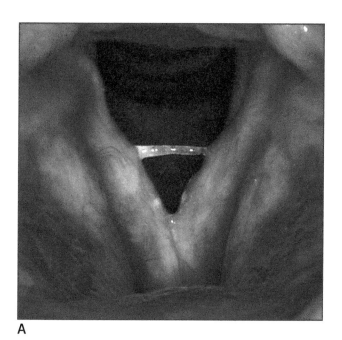

A

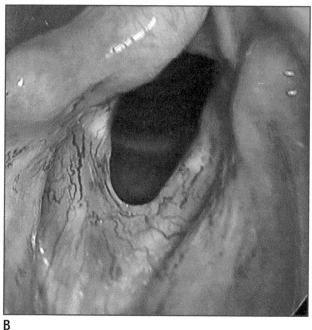

B

Figure 23–8. (A) shows an anterior glottic web with significant medialization of each true cord as the fibrotic process has contracted the left and right sides to the midline. As such, there is not adequate mucosa available to mobilize and utilize as flap coverage after web resection. Compare this to (B) where there is extensive mucosa and the underlying true cords remain much more lateralized beneath the fibrosis and web.

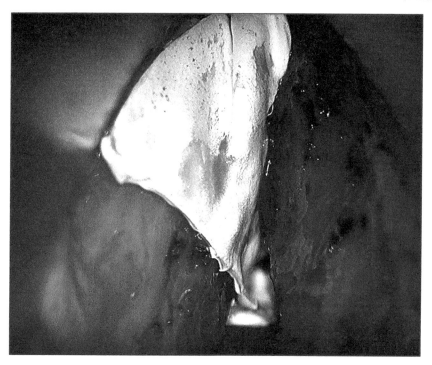

Figure 23–9. After resection of the anterior glottis with KTP laser for glottic cancer, a Gore-Tex implant has been sutured in place as a keel. It is tied anteriorly over a Silastic button placed under the skin on the anterior thyroid lamina.

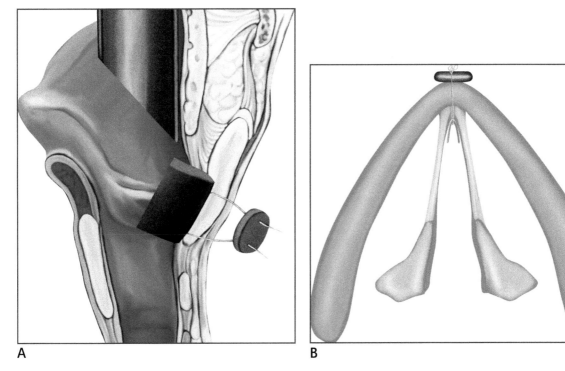

Figure 23–10. (A and B) show sagittal and axial sketches of the thyroid lamina with the Gore-Tex sutured over a silastic button. The Gore-Tex is firmly drawn into the anterior commissure to maintain separation of the left and right anterior vocal folds as healing occurs. See Figure 23–9 for endoscopic view of a 10 × 12 × 0.9-mm Gore-Tex keel in situ.

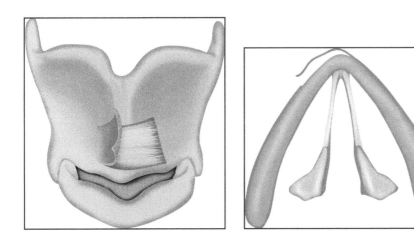
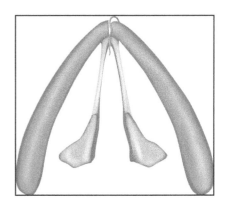

Figure 23–11. Axial and coronal views of the thyroid cartilage show the perichondrial flap raised and then passed through a midline laryngofissure to provide a biological keel. Note the flap is raised from at least 15 mm to one side of midline of the anterior thyroid lamina and dissected past the midline to be based at least 5 mm from the midline on the contralateral thyroid lamina.

PITFALLS

Assuming the presence of an anterior glottic web causes hoarseness and that reconstruction will improve the voice.

A glottic web is a marker of the presence of fibrosis in an area that is normally soft and pliable, the SLP. When the SLP becomes replaced with fibrosis, a simple division or even lysis with mucosal flap reconstruction will not restore pliability; it will only expose scar on each medial vocal fold edge. As such, efficiency of the mucosal wave is not enhanced, and may even establish areas of differential pliability with resultant diplophonia. As such, reconstruction of a web has the possibility of worsening the voice. Closure during phonation would not entrain vibration of healthy SLP but rather stiff scar with no resolution of the pre-surgery hoarseness. Therefore, patients must be fully educated under informed consent for such surgery that their voice may remain unchanged or worsen.

Allowing adhesions to form and progress to web re-formation.

Careful endoscopic evaluation in the office is critical to ensuring a successful outcome. The author sees patients weekly until the larynx has healed. This enables office removal of adhesions or debris in the anterior commissure to prevent granulation from progressing the fibrosis and resulting in re-formation of web, if not managed early (Figure 23–12).

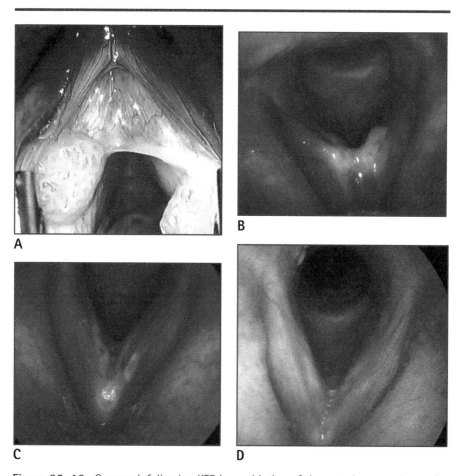

Figure 23–12. One week following KTP laser ablation of the anterior commissure for extensive dysplasia and simple lysis of an anterior glottic web (**A**), debris is noted on the office endoscopy in (**B**). If not removed, this forms adhesions which progress to mature fibrosis and web formation. It is essential to have regular post-surgery follow-up and remove the adhesions to prevent web formation or re-formation. At 2 weeks after office debridement, the anterior commissure has a more normal contour in (**C**). After 2 months, the anterior commissure has healed with normal appearance in (**D**).

DISCUSSION

Most anterior glottic webs result from bilateral anterior mucosal injury with subsequent inflammation, fibrosis, and web formation. The management approach can be endoscopic or open, with almost all surgery now being performed with the former. Rarely, a covering tracheotomy may be necessary. Realistic voice expectations are critical to convey to the patient, as often a web repair does not improve phonation.

As with many areas of medicine, prevention is better than cure. This applies strongly to the anterior commissure. With the left and right medial vocal fold surfaces in close apposition, minimal epithelial injury can cause web formation. The ideal prevention strategy is to limit mucosal disruption to one side during elective surgery—for example, in papilloma (see Figure 23–6), polypoid corditis (see Figure 23–4B), or dysplasia (see Figure 23–5). Use of the KTP laser can minimize the risk of web formation. In a setting of multiple treatments for anterior commissure papillomatosis using KTP laser ablation and Avastin, an anterior web can be avoided. Due to the unique interaction of the KTP laser and the glottic tissue and use of Bioglue in one typical patient, there has been no glottic web formation after 15 treatments over 5 years (Figure 23–13).

Bioglue can be an effective preventative flexible dressing. It is applied to the anterior commissure and remains adherent and effective for at least 2 weeks based on the author's experience in over 20 cases.

Many treatment modalities have been reported over the years using endoscopic or open approaches with or without stenting.[13,21–23] Treatment approaches therefore remain somewhat controversial, with all techniques having their own pros and cons.

Division of an anterior web was first described endoscopically in 1930 by Jackson et al.[2] Stasney then advanced these ideas coupled to new technology involving multiple dilations, but there were limitations to long-term success from recurrent scar tissue.[12] Although Haslinger placed the first keel in 1924,[1] Dedo in 1979 used a Teflon keel without tracheotomy with satisfactory outcomes.[4] Other materials have been used, including Silastic and then a stent after laser resection with good voice outcomes.[12] There does not seem to be any agreement around the duration of stenting but it would seem reasonable for the duration to be similar to that required for adequate epithelialization. This ranges from 2 to 6 weeks. If we consider more mature wound healing and fibrosis, then 2 to 3 months may be a better time frame.

The author's preference when using a keel is to place a small section of cardiac patch Gore-Tex ,which

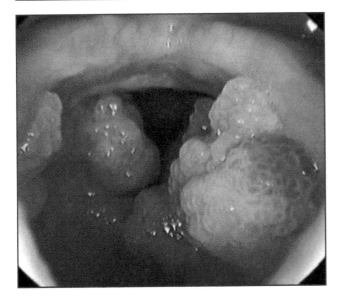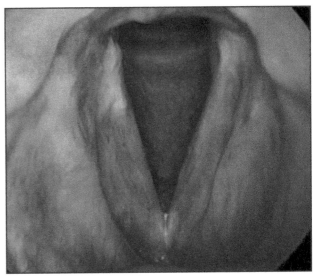

Figure 23–13. After extensive and repeated KTP laser treatments for recurrent papillomatosis of the anterior commissure, and use of Bioglue as a dressing, no significant web has formed and the voice remains entirely normal. Note the complete preservation of the anterior commissure.

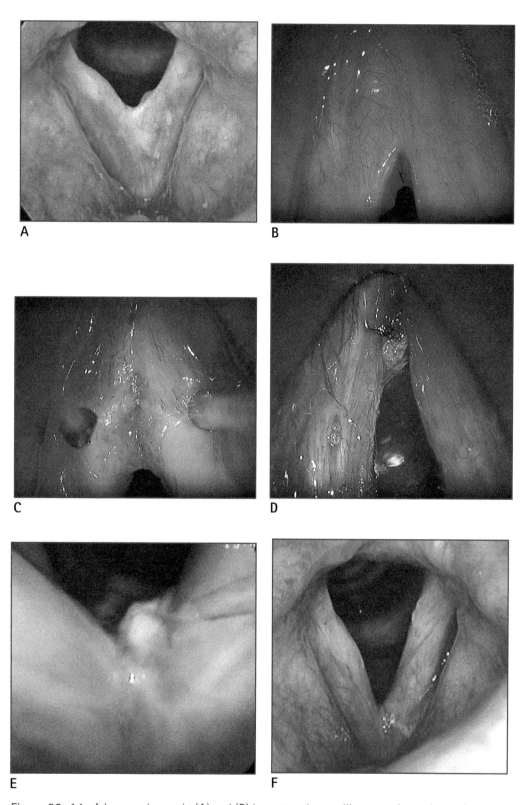

Figure 23–14. A large web seen in (A) and (B) has extensive papilloma on the under surface seen in (C). After the papilloma has been sutured into the anterior commissure in (D) as a biological keel, it is ablated 1 month later in the office under local anesthetic with KTP laser. The 300 micron laser fiber is seen on the right with the papilloma blanching from treatment in (E). The final result is shown 6 months later in (F).

is anchored caudal and cephalad to the true vocal folds anteriorly through the thyroid alar, with sutures. The patch is delivered to the anterior commissure through the laryngoscope with sutures passed endoscopically through the mucosa into the anterior neck. The sutures are then secured over a Silastic button for 2 months without a tracheotomy (see Figure 23–9). Gore-Tex is well tolerated as it is soft but still able to provide separation of the opposing mucosal surfaces, enabling them to heal with a normal contour.

There are options for host tissue to cover the resected tissue, which can also include using a mucosal advancement flap, pedicle flap, residual papilloma, or even a free mucosal graft. Results can be impressive with these approaches.[14,15,22,24] When choosing the mucosal flap technique, ensure there is adequate mucosa covering the web to form flaps large enough to cover the defects. Figure 23–8B shows a web with excessive mucosa to create flaps, in contrast to the web in Figure 23–8A, which has a fibrotic contracture between the left and right vocal folds with no adequate mucosa to create suitable flaps. This will require another technique utilizing a form of keel described below.

In some patients, a portion of papilloma at or near the anterior commissure can be preserved and dissected on a pedicle. This pedicle can then be sutured into the fully treated anterior commissure to act as a biological keel. At 1 month post-surgery, an office KTP laser procedure can be performed where the small residual papilloma is ablated with preservation of the anterior commissure contours (Figure 23–14A–F).

If a portion of papilloma is not available, then another option is a perichondrial flap. This was described by Izadi in 2010 and involved raising a perichondrial flap. The flap was then tunneled through a small laryngofissure to cover the resected web and sutured with 4/0 Vicryl.[19] The perichondrial flap is raised from one thyroid lamina, across the midline to the contralateral side (see Figure 23–11). The flap is then based 2 to 3 mm from the midline laryngofissure. This enables easy tunneling of the flap through the thyrotomy, where it can be sutured in place. Over 2 months the flap will become redundant after epithelialization has occurred and can then be trimmed endoscopically.

Topical agents to augment the reconstruction procedures have been used with varying degrees of success. These include mitomycin C[20] and steroids, but no adequate data are reported on the latter. The author has used Avastin in some patients based on its ability to block vascular endothelial growth factor but with unconvincing results.

SUMMARY

The best cure is prevention. Consider surgery at the anterior commissure carefully and minimize tissue trauma. This can be achieved by preserving mucosa across the anterior commissure to avoid opposing demucosalized areas or by using a KTP laser in place of the CO_2 laser or microdebrider to treat disease such as SCC or papilloma. Addition of Bioglue as a thin film across the anterior commissure is effective in allowing epithelialization without web formation, but for larger webs and resection, some form of keel may be required. Materials including Silastic and Gore-Tex have a good track record, but biological keels, including perichondrium, a pedicle of papilloma, or mucosal flaps can provide excellent outcomes.

Ensure the patient understands that web surgery does not routinely improve the voice, so the indication for surgery must be more aligned to airway improvement over voice restoration.

REFERENCES

1. Haslinger F. A case of membrane formation in larynx, a new method of safer recovery. *Monatsschr Ohrenheilkd Laryngorhinol* 1924;22:174–176.
2. Jackson C, Coates G. *The Nose, Throat and Ear and Their Diseases*. Philadelphia, PA: WB Saunders; 1930.
3. McNaught RC. Surgical correction of anterior web of the larynx. *Trans Am Laryngol Rhinol Otol Soc*. 1950;54th Meeting:232–242.
4. Dedo HH. Endoscopic Teflon keel for anterior glottic web. *Ann Otol Rhinol Laryngol*. 1979;88(4 Pt 1):467–473.
5. Parker DA, Das Gupta AR. An endoscopic silastic keel for anterior glottic webs. *J Laryngol Otol*. 1987;101(10):1055–1061.
6. Liyanage SH, Khemani S, Lloyd S, Farrell R. Simple keel fixation technique for endoscopic repair of anterior glottic stenosis. *J Laryngol Otol*. 2006;120:322–324.
7. Paniello RC, Desai SC, Allen CT, Khosla SM. Endoscopic keel placement to treat and prevent anterior glottic webs. *Ann Otol Rhinol Laryngol*. 2013;122(11):672–678.
8. Edwards J, Tanna N, Bielamowicz SA. Endoscopic lysis of anterior glottic webs and silicone keel placement. *Ann Otol Rhinol Laryngol*. 2007;116(3):211–216.
9. Xiao Y, Wang J, Han D, Ma L, Ye J, Xu W. Vocal cord mucosal flap for the treatment of acquired anterior laryngeal web. *Chin Med J (Engl)*. 2014;127(7):1294–1297.
10. Deganello A, Gallo O, Gitti G, de'Campora E, Mahieu H. New surgical technique for endoscopic management of anterior glottic web. *B–ENT*. 2010;6(4):261–264.

11. Lahav Y, Shoffel-Havakuk H, Halperin D. Acquired glottic stenosis—the ongoing challenge: a review of etiology, pathogenesis, and surgical management. *J Voice*. 2015; 29(5):646.e1–646.e10.

12. Stasney CR. Laryngeal webs: a new treatment for an old problem. *J Voice*. 1995;9(1):106–109.

13. Yoo MJ, Roy S, Smith LP. Endoscopic management of congenital anterior glottic stenosis. *Int J Pediatr Otorhinolaryngol*. 2015;79(12):2056–2058.

14. Casiano RR, Lundy DS. Outpatient transoral laser vaporization of anterior glottic webs and keel placement: risks of airway compromise. *J Voice*. 1998;12(4):536–539.

15. Benmansour N, Remacle M, Matar N, Lawson G, Bachy V, Van Der Vorst S. Endoscopic treatment of anterior glottic webs according to Lichtenberger technique and results on 18 patients. *Eur Arch Otorhinolaryngol*. 2012;269(9): 2075–2080.

16. Lichtenberger G, Toohill RJ. New keel fixing technique for endoscopic repair of anterior commissure webs. *Laryngoscope*. 1994;104(6 Pt 1):771–774.

17. Liyanage SH, Khemani S, Lloyd S, Farrell R. Simple keel fixation technique for endoscopic repair of anterior glottic stenosis. *J Laryngol Otol*. 2006;120(4):322–324.

18. Cheng AT, Beckenham EJ. Congenital anterior glottic webs with subglottic stenosis: surgery using perichondrial keels. *Int J Pediatr Otorhinolaryngol*. 2009;73(7):945–949.

19. Izadi F[1], Delarestaghi MM, Memari F, Mohseni R, Pousti B, Mir P. The butterfly procedure: a new technique and review of the literature for treating anterior laryngeal webs. *J Voice*. 2010;24(6):742–749.

20. Hartnick CJ[1], Hartley BE. Topical mitomycin application after laryngotracheal reconstruction: a randomized, double-blind, placebo-controlled trial. *Arch Otolaryngol Head Neck Surg*. 2001;127(10):1260–1264.

21. Dedo HH, Sooy CD. Endoscopic laser repair of posterior glottic, subglottic and tracheal stenosis by division or micro-trapdoor flap. *Laryngoscope*. 1984;94(4):445–450.

22. Isshiki N, Taira T, Nose K, Kojima H. Surgical treatment of laryngeal web with mucosa graft. *Ann Otol Rhinol Laryngol*. 1991;100(2):95–100.

23. Schweinfurth J. Single-stage, stentless endoscopic repair of anterior glottic webs. *Laryngoscope*. 2002;112(5):933–935.

24. Akst LM, Broadhurst MS, Burns JA, Zeitels SM. Microflap laryngosplasty for treating an anterior-commissure web with papillomatosis. *Laryngoscope*. 2007;117(8):1496–1499.

CHAPTER 24

Assessment and Management of Vocal Fold Paresis in a Singer

Lisa D'Oyley, Emily Wilson, and Albert Merati

Mrs. M is a 52-year-old female singer with history of enlarging thyroid mass 6 months status post hemi-thyroidectomy. She was referred to the multidisciplinary laryngology clinic for initial evaluation due to persistent voice changes status post thyroid surgery.

Background History

Mrs. M first noticed fullness in her right neck 1.5 years ago. She subsequently saw an otolaryngologist for evaluation. Thyroid ultrasound and fine needle aspirate biopsy indicated benign mass with no evidence of neoplasm. Initially, she and her surgeon elected for close surveillance. Over the course of 8 months, the mass had increased in size and she decided to proceed with hemi-thyroidectomy. She had no voice or swallowing concerns at that time. Preoperative flexible laryngoscopy was completed and judged to be largely within normal limits.

Mrs. M endorsed weak breathy voice and choking on thin liquids immediately following surgery. She was subsequently seen 2 weeks postoperatively by her surgeon. Initial postoperative laryngoscopy revealed right true vocal fold immobility in the paramedian position and modest laryngeal edema. Her surgeon discussed options for management, including surveillance versus right true vocal fold injection augmentation. She elected to continue with surveillance. Speech therapy was recommended to further evaluate her dys-

phagia but she did not pursue it at that time. When her symptoms did not return to premorbid baseline, Mrs. M was referred to our multidisciplinary laryngology clinic.

History of Present Illness

At the time of initial evaluation 6 months postoperatively, Mrs. M reported that her dysphagia symptoms had largely resolved, other than having to "think" about swallowing, particularly with pills and water. She otherwise tolerated a general diet. Voice had slowly improved in quality over the past 6 months; however, she reported that she continued to experience loss of upper range, decreased volume, and vocal fatigue. She was not particularly bothered by her speaking voice quality but she did notice vocal fatigue with extensive speaking voice use.

Mrs. M endorsed high vocal demands as an elementary school music teacher and an active member of her church choir with weekly performances. She reported that she is a mezzo-soprano. She has not been classically trained nor has she had any singing technique lessons in the last 15 years. Prior to becoming a voice and piano teacher, she received her degree in musical education and has done extensive singing with various companies. She has three teenage children.

Following thyroid surgery, she took several months off of work to recover but returned at the beginning of the school year. Since returning to work postoperatively, she realized she was unable to maintain her previous vocal demands. She decreased her number of private voice lessons and stopped leading worship at her church. She still continued to experience vocal fatigue at the end of each workday despite decreasing vocal demands.

Otherwise, Mrs. M denied dyspnea. She never smoked cigarettes. She enjoyed one cup of coffee daily and one glass of wine per night. She denied heartburn or regurgitation and did not take reflux medication.

Patient Questionnaires

Prior to initial evaluation, patient-reported questionnaires were provided to the patient, including Voice Handicap Index 10 (VHI-10),[1,2] Eating Assessment

Table 24–1. Self-Assessment Questionnaire Scores at Initial Evaluation

Questionnaire	Score	Range	Abnormal
VHI-10	18/40	0–40	Scores >11
EAT-10	6/40	0–40	Scores >2
RSI	14/45	0–45	Scores >13
SVHI-10	31/40	0–40	–

Tool 10 (EAT-10),[3] Reflux Severity Index (RSI),[4] and Singing Voice Handicap Index 10 (SVHI-10).[5] See Table 24–1.

Evaluation

Perceptual voice evaluation was completed by an experienced speech language pathologist. Consensus Auditory-Perceptual Evaluation of Voice (CAPE-V) was used for perceptual voice evaluation. Perceptual judgment was based on sustained phonation, speech tasks, and conversational speech.[6] Voice quality was judged to be mildly strained with intermittent posterior focus and glottal fry at the ends of phrases in conversation. Mild breathiness was noted with sustained phonation. Maximum phonation time (MPT) was 13 seconds. This was decreased compared with patient's age and gender norms (21 ± 5 SD).[7] Pitch measurements were also collected using Computerized Speech Lab Sona Speech. Habitual pitch was 192 Hz, which is the lower end of normal limits for patient's age and gender.[8] She presented with a pitch range of 135 737 Hz, which was decreased compared with age and gender normative data as well as her own premorbid pitch range.[9,10] See Figure 24–1.

Oral mechanism exam was normal for structure and function. Thyroid incision was healed. Laryngeal

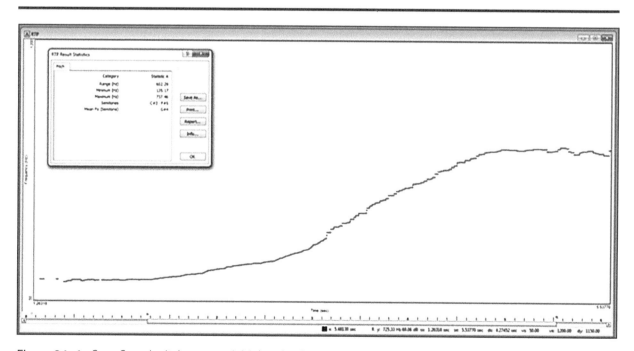

Figure 24–1. Sona Speech pitch range at initial evaluation.

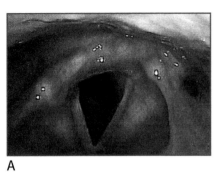 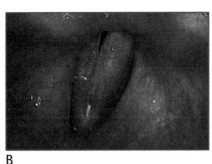 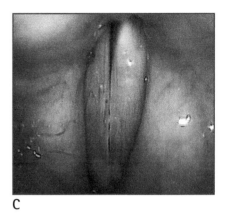

A   B   C

Figure 24–2. (A) Right true vocal fold hypomobility with abduction. (B) Posterior gap noted at habitual pitch. (C) Slight full-length gap noted with high pitch.

palpation revealed moderately reduced thyrohyoid space with bilateral tenderness reported upon palpation.

Laryngeal videostroboscopy revealed subtle right true vocal fold hypomobility with normal left true vocal fold mobility. See Figure 24–2A. Subtle posterior glottic gap noted at habitual pitch and slight full length glottic gap noted with high pitch. See Figures 24–2B and 24–2C. Right vocal fold did not appear to fully lengthen with increased pitch. No true vocal fold masses or lesions appreciated but slight bilateral irregular true vocal fold medial edge noted. Mucosal wave was present but asymmetrical with subtle chasing wave more pronounced with high pitch. Amplitude of mucosal wave was mildly increased on the right and judged to be within normal limits on the left. Maladaptive strain was noted in the form of mild false vocal fold compression with connected speech and high pitched sustained phonation. With singing tasks, increased base of tongue tension and posterior pharyngeal wall constriction was noted particularly within the upper register.

Diagnosis

Mrs. M was diagnosed with subtle right true vocal fold hypomobility in the setting of recent thyroid surgery suggestive of injury to the recurrent laryngeal nerve (RLN). Options for ongoing plan of care were then discussed with the patient at length, including (1) surveillance only, (2) imaging, (3) laryngeal electromyography (EMG), (4) behavioral intervention, and/or (5) surgical intervention.

DIAGNOSTIC AND MANAGEMENT OPTIONS

Surveillance Only

After discussing the findings with Mrs. M, she was pleasantly surprised to find that her right true vocal fold had regained some movement. This was consistent with her timeline of overall improvement in symptoms since initial onset. The majority of expected vocal fold recovery is anticipated to occur within 6 months of initial injury; however, the evidence for anticipated timeline of recovery varies in the literature.[11,12] As such, the team discussed with Mrs. M that it is difficult to predict the degree and timing of recovery from RLN injury. Due to possibility of ongoing spontaneous recovery, the first option presented to Mrs. M was to continue with surveillance only. However, she was interested in pursuing additional intervention given her high vocal demands and current voice limitations.

Imaging

Another potential etiology of vocal fold motion impairment could be tumor or mass effect on the vagus nerve and its branches. In cases without any obvious antecedent events that might explain new changes, imaging may be considered for further diagnostic information. CT scans are most commonly used; however, chest x-rays can also be informative but are not typically sufficient alone.[13,14] In this case, the patient's clinical history suggested that the etiology of her vocal fold motion impairment was likely iatrogenic in nature, which does not usually warrant a CT scan.[15] Subsequently, imaging was discussed but not recommended in Mrs. M's case.

Laryngeal EMG

Laryngeal EMG (LEMG) can be a useful diagnostic tool for determining possible neurologic etiology of vocal fold motion impairment compared with structural etiologies such as arytenoid dislocation or fixation.[16] Specifically, LEMG is used to assess electrical activity of laryngeal muscles by evaluating motor unit morphology and recruitment of motor unit potentials to determine electrophysiological evidence of denervation, reinnervation, or, in this case, a peripheral nerve injury.[16] The muscles most commonly evaluated in LEMG are the thyroarytenoid, posterior cricoarytenoid, lateral cricoarytenoid, interartyenoid, and cricothyroid.[17]

The utility of LEMG remains highly debated in clinical practice, particularly for predicting recovery of vocal fold motion.[16] Indicators of poor prognosis of vocal fold motion recovery include the presence of fibrillations or positive sharp waves and absent/reduced recruitment of motor unit potentials in the muscles. Conversely, the presence of voluntary recruitment and polyphasic potentials are used as indicators of possible good prognosis of recovery.[18,19] According to the literature, LEMG is more useful in predicting prognosis for poor functional outcomes but is not as useful in predicting prognosis of good functional outcomes.[14,18] For patients with unilateral vocal fold immobility, LEMG findings that suggest poor prognosis could influence patients to pursue permanent laryngeal framework surgery earlier during course of treatment, especially for patients with high vocal demands.[19] However, the advent of injection augmentation providing immediate relief while waiting for potential spontaneous recovery is now a popular management option which oftentimes is more appealing to patients and healthcare providers than an early LEMG.

Another consideration for completing LEMG is timing of the procedure after onset of injury. The literature generally suggests that the later LEMG is completed after onset, the more reliable the results can be. However, this is not always a feasible option for patients who are suffering from functional voice limitations. If prognosis is poor based on LEMG, these patients may be more likely to opt for surgical intervention rather than waiting for possible recovery even if LEMG was not completed during the ideal timeframe.[18]

Although LEMG may not always influence decision making, findings can be intellectually stimulating, specifically for determining degree of superior laryngeal nerve (SLN) versus RLN injury. In this case, we can likely infer that Mrs. M initially had both RLN and SLN injury, as evident by her complete right true vocal fold immobility, severe dysphonia with difficulty modulating pitch, and liquid dysphagia. Although some of her symptoms have improved with time, Mrs. M's remaining symptoms were suggestive of persistent SLN injury (ie, vocal fatigue, difficulty projecting, reduced pitch range).[20] If reduced recruitment of motor unit potentials was demonstrated primarily within the cricothyroid muscle on LEMG, this would suggest that Mrs. M's symptoms are related to SLN injury more so than RLN injury.[21] Although less common, there are procedures that can be pursued for exclusive SLN injury management. These include modified type IV thyroplasty, combined type I and IV thyroplasty, cricothyroid adduction, and selective cricothyroid muscle reinnervation.[20,22–24] Even if one of these procedures is not pursued, LEMG findings could be used in counseling and patient education to explain the functional impact SLN injury can have on the voice, particularly in regard to pitch range. If LEMG findings suggested RLN injury (with or without SLN injury), then more common interventions such as injection medialization, medialization thyroplasty, and laryngeal reinnervation might be pursued. These will be discussed in more detail in the next section.

After describing LEMG and the diagnostic information that this procedure could yield, Mrs. M reported that this was a consideration, although she wanted to learn more about behavioral and surgical interventions first.

Behavioral Intervention

Voice Therapy

Voice therapy with an experienced speech language pathologist can be an invaluable management option for patients with dysphonia of varying etiologies. For patients with partial or complete vocal fold motion impairment, voice therapy can be used as a primary treatment modality or completed in conjunction with medical and/or surgical intervention. Although there is a need for further research exploring the effect of voice therapy on voice outcomes in patients with vocal fold motion impairment, several studies have been published to support the efficacy of voice therapy with this patient population.[25] Studies have shown that voice therapy alone can result in satisfactory voice outcomes for patients with unilateral vocal fold paralysis to the extent that some patients are able to meet their vocal demands from behavioral intervention alone.[26] For example, voice therapy can improve glottic closure, MPT, acoustic measurements, and VHI scores.[25] For those who do elect to pursue surgical management, voice therapy can be helpful in providing preoperative, postoperative and sometimes intraoperative care. Preoperative voice therapy typically focuses on patient education, management of expectations, and instruction in postoperative voice use guidelines, including voice rest and exercises to facilitate healing and optimize voice use. The patient is also instructed in voice techniques to reduce maladaptive voice or breathing patterns that may interfere with surgical intervention and healing. Postoperative therapy typically focuses on maximizing postoperative phonatory efficiency in order to help patients meet their communicative needs and vocal demands. In some cases, intraoperative therapy may be pursued to assist the surgeon in facilitating best voice during awake procedures (ie, medialization thyroplasty).

Speech pathology intervention can also address swallowing concerns for patients with vocal fold motion impairment by providing swallowing strategies and techniques for improved airway protection. These often include postural adjustments, including chin tuck and head turn, dietary modifications, supraglottic swallow technique, and super-supraglottic technique.[14]

Singing Voice Rehabilitation

Often, singers also benefit from formal singing rehabilitation in conjunction with speaking voice therapy. Historically, the singing voice rehabilitation specialist is not well defined and can have varying backgrounds and training. Typically, professionals with this title include speech pathologists with advanced degrees in vocal pedagogy, voice teachers who work in a clinical setting, and voice teachers who have undergone supplementary training in vocal anatomy and physiology.[27] The laryngologist, speech pathologist, and/or singing voice rehabilitation specialist should work together as part of a multidisciplinary team in order to provide best treatment outcomes. Singing voice therapy should include specialized rehabilitative exercises tailored to each patient considering specific diagnoses, symptoms, singing styles, voice types, careers, training backgrounds, and performance schedules.[27] The reha-

bilitation plan is aimed to improve coordination and conditioning of singing voice, reduce inefficient or maladaptive singing behaviors, and develop strategies to promote healing and prevent further injury.

Surgical Intervention

After discussing less invasive approaches with Mrs. M, surgical interventions were then outlined in detail. Specifically, the team focused on temporary versus permanent vocal fold medialization; however, laryngeal innervation was also briefly discussed.

Temporary Vocal Fold Injection Medialization

Temporary vocal fold injection medialization has been used by otolaryngologists since the early 1900s and has continued to increase in popularity over time due to its ability to offer immediate improvement in voice and swallowing concerns for many patients. The primary objective of injection medialization is to alter the geometry of the impaired vocal fold by bringing the medial edge closer to midline for improved glottic closure. This is achieved by injecting material into the thyroarytenoid muscle in order to provide bulk to the affected vocal fold for improved contact with the contralateral side. Some studies have shown that injection medialization can also result in medial rotation and translation of the arytenoid cartilage.[28] Vocal fold injection medialization can be completed awake as an in-office procedure or under general anesthesia in the operating room. Surgical technique options include transoral, transnasal, transcricothyroid, and transthyrohyoid approaches. This varies by surgeon and patient needs. There are also a variety of injectable materials that can be used depending on surgeon preference, duration, cost, accessibility, and rheologic properties.[14] Commonly used materials include autologous fascia or fat, cadaveric micronized dermis, calcium hydroxylapatite, carboxymethylcellulose, hyaluronic acid gels, and porcine gelatin.[29] Polytetrafluoroethylene, more commonly known as Teflon, was a popular material used in the past due to its long-lasting effect; however, this material has been associated with increased risk of granulomatous inflammatory response and is now less commonly used.[29] Additionally, some studies have demonstrated that the use of hyaluronan leads to improved vibratory function and less resorption compared with other materials such as collagen.[30,31]

Vocal fold injection medialization is often used as an early intervention technique for vocal fold immobility while waiting for possible spontaneous recovery. Some studies also suggest that early injection medialization procedures can lead to shortened hospital stays, decreased risk of pneumonia, and potentially reduced need for permanent intervention in the future.[14,28,32] This could have been a beneficial early option for Mrs. M, who was significantly limited by her dysphonia and dysphagia for several months postoperatively. However, Mrs. M and her original surgeon had decided to forgo this option for observation only, as she was reluctant to pursue additional procedures at that time.

Six months postoperatively, Mrs. M's symptoms had improved but had not returned to premorbid baseline. She subsequently was interested in learning more about surgical intervention as observation alone was not sufficient to meet her extensive voice demands. Reliable expectations for vocal fold injection medialization were then thoroughly discussed with Mrs. M. Although this procedure commonly results in less vocal effort, decreased compensatory strain, and reduced vocal fatigue, it is less reliable in restoring full vocal range and improved singing voice quality. It was also explained to Mrs. M that although this procedure improves glottic closure, it does not necessarily return normal function, as she would continue to compensate for a partial vocal fold motion impairment. Often, self-assessment measures such as the VHI-10 may improve post-treatment, but the scores do not necessarily improve to within normal limits. Patients with subtle deficits do not always experience the same degree of benefit as those with more severe vocal deficits. As such, management of expectations was important when presenting this option to Mrs. M. Complications of injection medialization were also discussed, including overinjection or subepithelial injection. Although rare, this can result in temporarily worsened voice quality and/or stridor while waiting for the injectable material to reabsorb.[14]

Medialization Thyroplasty

Another option presented to Mrs. M was laryngeal framework surgery, specifically medialization thyroplasty. Similar to injection medialization, this procedure aims to improve glottic closure by bringing the impaired vocal fold closer to midline. This is achieved through surgical placement of an implant through a window in the thyroid cartilage in order to displace the vocal fold medially.[33,34] Unlike injection medialization, this procedure is meant to be permanent and is completed in the operating room under local anesthesia. The patient remains awake during this procedure, so the surgeon is able to make perceptual voice judgments in order to custom carve the implant for optimal results. See Figure 24–3. The materials most commonly used for medialization thyroplasty include carved Silastic, Montgomery prosthesis, and Gore-Tex implant.[14] This procedure can also be done in conjunction with arytenoid adduction for improved closure of the posterior glottis for those with vocal fold immobility.[35] Potential complications include edema, poor wound healing, extrusion of the implant, and need for tracheotomy.[14] Additionally, a number of patients may need to pursue revision thyroplasty at some point postoperatively due to suboptimal placement of the implant or changes to laryngeal anatomy over time (i.e., presbylaryngis).[36] The patient will oftentimes participate in preoperative, postoperative, and sometimes intraoperative voice therapy for optimal surgical results. Postoperative voice use guidelines can include a short period of voice rest followed by gradual return to voice use as determined appropriate by the surgeon and speech language pathologist. Although it is not always indicated, many patients choose to pursue

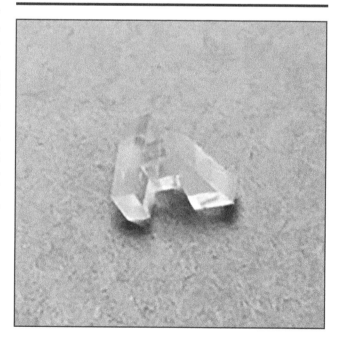

Figure 24–3. Carved Silastic implant used for type I medialization thyroplasty.

a trial injection medialization prior to committing to permanent medialization thyroplasty. In Mrs. M's case, medialization thyroplasty may help improve vocal stamina and reduce vocal fatigue, but, similar to injection medialization, this procedure may not necessarily improve vocal range or singing voice quality.

Laryngeal Reinnervation

Laryngeal reinnervation is another management technique for patients with vocal fold motion impairment, specifically complete vocal fold paralysis. This procedure allows the surgeon to use surrounding nerves to reinnervate the vocal fold to minimize laryngeal atrophy and improve tone of the paralyzed vocal fold.[37,38] The most commonly used nerve for reinnervation is the ansa-RLN, but other options may include phrenic, hypoglossal, and nerve-muscle pedicles.[29] Although this procedure can benefit some patients with known vocal fold paralysis, this would not be recommended for those with partial vocal fold motion impairment, as this would result in complete denervation of the vagus nerve. As such, the team did not recommend this procedure as a viable option for Mrs. M, who already demonstrated signs of innervation such as vocal fold movement with intact vocal fold tone.

INITIAL PLAN, TREATMENT, AND OUTCOMES

Plan

After discussing the aforementioned management options, Mrs. M decided to forgo additional diagnostic testing. Had her right vocal fold still been immobile, LEMG could have been used to assess prognosis and candidacy for early permanent intervention. However, partial recovery of vocal fold mobility was noted on laryngeal videostroboscopy. As such, it was felt that LEMG was less clinically meaningful, since it would not necessarily offer new diagnostic information that would change the plan of care. Instead, she preferred to start with treatment. Behavioral intervention was the most appealing option for her, as she had not yet pursued speech or singing rehabilitation postoperatively and she was interested in the least invasive options to begin with. She subsequently participated in voice therapy and singing voice rehabilitation with plans to follow up in the laryngology clinic after completion. However, Mrs. M reported that she was open

to surgical intervention in the future depending on outcomes from behavioral intervention.

Treatment

Mrs. M completed a course of voice therapy with an experienced speech language pathologist. The goal of voice therapy was to reduce Mrs. M's vocal fatigue and to increase vocal stamina. She was instructed in strategies to optimize vocal hygiene, particularly in relation to her daily schedule and prioritization of voice use.[39,40] She was encouraged to utilize voice amplification in the classroom to decrease vocal effort and fatigue. Voice exercises were aimed at improving coordination of respiration and phonation, optimizing resonance in speech, and reducing maladaptive compensation used during speech tasks.[39,40] Specific exercises included laryngeal massage, elements of flow phonation, straw phonation, and resonant voice therapy. First, laryngeal massage was indicated based on initial evaluation, which revealed reduced thyrohyoid space with bilateral tenderness reported upon palpation. Given Mrs. M's complaint of daily vocal fatigue, this technique was taught to Mrs. M to bring immediate relief of throat discomfort and to promote relaxation of laryngeal musculature.[41,42] After laryngeal massage, flow phonation was introduced to reduce breath holding patterns and to promote optimal airflow needed for efficient phonation during conversational speech.[43] Mrs. M was able to demonstrate diaphragmatic breathing accurately due to her singing background; however, she tended to conserve breath during speech, resulting in increased strain and inefficient voice use. Flow phonation was a tool used to promote awareness of consistent airflow and breath release during speech. Semi-occluded vocal tract techniques and resonant voice therapy were then introduced to increase forward focus of the voice without increased vocal strain.[44,45] She was provided with a structured hierarchy beginning with basic gestures such as humming, which were then advanced to conversational speech. Additionally, Mrs. M was instructed in vocal function exercises to promote strength, balance, and flexibility of the laryngeal musculature.[46,47] Literature suggests that vocal function exercises can lead to decreased airflow and increased maximum phonation times consistent with improved phonatory efficiency in singers.[48] Mrs. M was compliant with speech therapy recommendations and closely adhered to the prescribed home exercise program.

Of note, intermittent dysphagia symptoms were briefly discussed during therapy sessions. Although Mrs. M reported that she had to be careful when drinking thin liquids too quickly, this had largely improved and was not a primary concern of hers. She was provided with safe swallowing strategies, but otherwise speech language pathology did not focus on dysphagia intervention.

In addition to speech language pathology intervention, Mrs. M also pursued treatment with a singing voice rehabilitation specialist. This was focused on vocal pacing, body alignment, coordination of respiration and phonation (*appoggio*), and appropriate vocal tract configuration and resonance while singing.[27,49] She was not necessarily at risk for accruing damage by singing and so speaking voice and singing voice rehabilitation were recommended at the same time.

Outcomes

Mrs. M was then seen for reevaluation 9 months postoperatively with her laryngologist and speech language pathologist. She reported that although behavioral intervention resulted in reduced vocal fatigue and improved singing technique, she continued to feel limited compared with her premorbid baseline. Although she was able to get through her workday, she noticed that her voice sounded weaker and intermittently "airy." Although her voice was functional at work, Mrs. M continued to endorse slightly decreased pitch range and reduced singing stamina limiting her ability to perform solos at church and other engagements.

Self-assessment scores were re-administered. Mrs. M's VHI-10 decreased from 18 to 13 and her SVHI-10 score decreased from 31 to 21. Although these scores improved, they were still within the abnormal range. See Table 24–2. Her MPT was largely comparable to pre-

Table 24–2. Pre- and Post-Behavioral Intervention Self-Assessment Questionnaire Scores

Questionnaire	Initial Evaluation	Post-Behavioral Intervention
VHI-10	18/40	13/40
EAT-10	6/40	4/40
RSI	14/45	8/45
SVHI-10	31/40	21/40

Table 24–3. Pre- and Post-Behavioral Intervention Acoustic Measures

Acoustic Measure	Initial Evaluation	Post-Behavioral Intervention
Maximum phonation time (MPT)	13 seconds	14 seconds
Habitual pitch	192 Hz	196 Hz
Pitch range	135–737 Hz	130–780 Hz

therapy baseline at 14 seconds. Perceptual voice evaluation using the CAPE-V revealed mildly breathy voice quality with decreased strain and forward resonance. Pitch measurements were collected post-therapy using Computerized Speech Lab Sona Speech. Habitual pitch remained within normal limits at 196 Hz. Pitch range improved compared with pre-therapy measures but was still reduced compared with Mrs. M's premorbid baseline at 130 Hz to 780 Hz. See Table 24–3.

Repeat laryngeal videostroboscopy revealed persistent subtle right true vocal fold hypomobility and decreased lengthening with pitch increase that was largely unchanged compared with previous exam. Although her phonatory hyperfunction and laryngeal edema were significantly improved, her posterior glottic gap was more prominent with all speech tasks.

FOLLOW-UP PLAN, TREATMENT, AND OUTCOMES

Plan

After reviewing findings from Mrs. M's videostroboscopy, the team discussed potential management options regarding her ongoing plan of care. Mrs. M was interested in pursuing intervention that could offer immediate benefit given her long-standing voice limitations. Mrs. M appeared to be a good candidate for surgical intervention to improve glottic closure especially now that her compensatory muscle tension had been eliminated through behavioral management. Temporary vocal fold augmentation and medialization thyroplasty were then reviewed. Although medialization thyroplasty can reliably improve vocal fatigue and speaking voice quality, it is less predictable in restoring pitch range and singing voice quality. Due to her high vocal demands as a singer, Mrs. M was hesitant to proceed with permanent intervention without being sure of its benefit. She preferred to trial vocal fold injection augmentation first to assess the effect of medialization prior to committing to a permanent alteration in vocal fold anatomy.

Treatment

Mrs. M decided to pursue temporary vocal fold injection augmentation as an in-office procedure. She underwent trans-cricothyroid injection of 0.2 cc hyaluronic acid to the right true vocal fold. Immediately after this procedure, the right vocal fold appeared to be well medialized. See Figures 24–4A and 24–4B. She was

then instructed to limit voice use for the remainder of the day and return to voice therapy postoperatively.

Outcome

Mrs. M reported that her voice was tight and strained for several days following injection; however, she endorsed an overall stronger voice quality and improved vocal stamina with both teaching and singing. Although her vocal range was still reduced, she felt that it was easier to reach her upper register with less effort. This was consistent with her self-reported measures. Mrs. M's VHI-10, EAT-10, and RSI scores decreased to within normal limits. Her MPT also increased from 14 seconds to 18 seconds. Perceptual voice evaluation using the CAPE-V was largely normal. See Table 24–4.

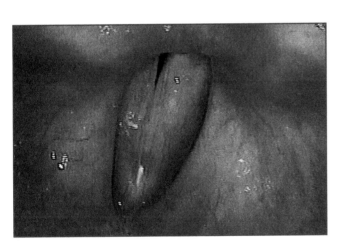
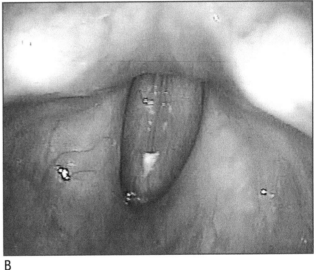

A   B

Figure 24–4. (A) Pre-injection glottic closure at habitual pitch. (B) Post-injection glottic closure at habitual pitch.

Table 24–4. Self-Assessment Questionnaire Scores for Initial Evaluation, Post-Behavioral Intervention, and Post-Injection Augmentation

Questionnaire	Initial Evaluation Score	Post-Behavioral Intervention	Post-Injection Augmentation	Abnormal
VHI-10	18/40	13/40	8/40	Scores >11
EAT-10	6/40	4/40	2/40	Scores >3
RSI	14/45	8/45	7/45	Scores >13
SVHI-10	31/40	21/40	17/40	–

ONGOING PLAN

Although her voice did not return to premorbid baseline, she noticed substantial benefit and ultimately made the decision to pursue medialization thyroplasty. The team decided to schedule this procedure in the future once the hyaluronic acid fully resorbed. It was also recommended that Mrs. M participate in 1 to 2 more sessions of voice therapy in order to provide preoperative counseling and postoperative voice use guidelines, and to ensure optimal phonation to be used intraoperatively.

CONCLUSIONS

Management of vocal fold motion impairment is a complex process with many different options for evaluation and treatment. As such, intervention should be customized to the patient depending on etiology, timing of injury, severity of symptoms, and functional needs. In Mrs. M's case, a conservative approach was initially pursued due to these individual factors as well as her demands as a professional voice user. Voice therapy and singing voice rehabilitation were the first methods of treatment selected. Although Mrs. M's voice improved, behavioral intervention alone was not sufficient and ultimately served as adjuvant treatment to surgical intervention. Additionally, the information gained from the results of therapy helped in the decision-making process to pursue surgical intervention. Based on the positive results of injection augmentation, Mrs. M elected to pursue medialization thyroplasty as the next course of intervention. The combination of behavioral and surgical intervention in this case highlights the importance of a multidisciplinary approach in the management of singers with vocal fold motion impairment.

REFERENCES

1. Rosen C, Lee A, Osborne J, Zullo T, Murry T. Development and validation of the Voice Handicap Index-10. *Laryngoscope*. 2004;114(9):1549–1556.
2. Arffa R, Krishna P, Gartner-Schmidt J, Rosen C. Normative values for the Voice Handicap Index-10. *J Voice*. 2012;26(4):462–465.
3. Belafsky P, Mouadeb D, Rees C, et al. Validity and reliability of the Eating Assessment Tool (EAT-10). *Ann Otol Rhinol Laryngol*. 2008;117(12):919–924.
4. Belafsky P, Postma G, Koufman J. Validity and Reliability of the Reflux Symptom Index (RSI). *J Voice*. 2002; 16(2):274–277.
5. Cohen S, Statham M, Rosen C, Zullo T. Development and validation of the Singing Voice Handicap-10. *Laryngoscope*. 2009;119(9):1864–1869.
6. Zraick R, Kempster G, Connor N, et al. Establishing validity of the Consensus Auditory-Perceptual Evaluation of Voice (CAPE-V). *Am J Speech Lang Pathol*. 2011;20 (1):14–22.
7. Kent R, Kent J, Rosenbek J. Maximum performance tests of speech production. *J Speech Hear Dis*. 1987;52(4): 367–387.
8. Brown W, Morris R, Hollien H, Howell E. Speaking fundamental frequency characteristics as a function of age and professional singing. *J Voice*. 1991;5(4):310–315.
9. Hollien H, Dew D, Philips P. Phonational frequency ranges of adults. *J Speech Lang Hear Res*. 1971;14(4):755–760.
10. Colton R, Hollien H. Phonational range in the modal and falsetto registers. *J Speech Lang Hear Res*. 1972;15(4): 708–713.
11. Chiang F, Wang L, Huang Y, Lee K, Kuo W. Recurrent laryngeal nerve palsy after thyroidectomy with routine identification of the recurrent laryngeal nerve. *Surgery*. 2005;137(3):342–347.
12. Jeannon J, Orabi A, Bruch G, Abdalsalam H, Simo R. Diagnosis of recurrent laryngeal nerve palsy after thyroidectomy: a systematic review. *Int J Clin Pract*. 2009;63(4): 624–629.
13. Merati A, Halum S, Smith T. Diagnostic testing for vocal fold paralysis: survey of practice and evidence-based medicine review. *Laryngoscope*. 2006;116(9):1539–1552.
14. Misono S, Merati A. Evaluation and management of unilateral vocal fold paralysis. *Otolaryngol Clin North Am*. 2012;45(5):1083–1108.
15. Glazer H, Aronberg D, Lee J, Sagel S. Extralaryngeal causes of vocal cord paralysis: CT evaluation. *Am J Roentgenol*. 1983;141(3):527–531.
16. Blitzer A, Crumley R, Dailey S et al. Recommendations of the Neurolaryngology Study Group on laryngeal electromyography. *Otolaryngol Head Neck Surg*. 2009; 140(6): 782–793.
17. Halum S, Patel N, Smith T, Jaradeh S, Toohill R, Merati A. Laryngeal electromyography for adult unilateral vocal fold immobility: a survey of the American Broncho-Esophagological Association. *Ann Otol Rhinol Laryngol*. 2005;114(6):425–428.
18. Rickert S, Childs L, Carey B, Murry T, Sulica L. Laryngeal electromyography for prognosis of vocal fold palsy: a meta-analysis. *Laryngoscope*. 2012;122(1):158–161.
19. Wang C, Chang M, De Virgilio A et al. Laryngeal electromyography and prognosis of unilateral vocal fold paralysis—a long-term prospective study. *Laryngoscope*. 2014;125(4):898–903.
20. Orestes M, Chhetri D. Superior laryngeal nerve injury. *Otolaryngol Head Neck Surg*. 2014;22(6):439–443.

21. Woo P. Laryngeal electromyography is a cost-effective clinically useful tool in the evaluation of vocal fold function. *Arch Otolaryngol Head Neck Surg.* 1998;124(4):472–475.

22. Shaw G, Searl J, Hoover L. Diagnosis and treatment of unilateral cricothyroid muscle paralysis with a modified Isshiki type 4 thyroplasty. *Otolaryngol Head Neck Surg.* 1995;113(6):679–688.

23. Nasseri S, Maragos N. Combination thyroplasty and the "twisted larynx": combined type IV and type I thyroplasty for superior laryngeal nerve weakness. *J Voice.* 2000;14(1):104–111.

24. El-Kashlan H, Carroll W, Hogikyan N, Chepeha D, Kileny P, Esclamado R. Selective cricothyroid muscle reinnervation by muscle-nerve-muscle neurotization. *Arch Otolaryngol Head Neck Surg.* 2001;127(10):1211–1215.

25. Schindler A, Bottero A, Capaccio P, Ginocchio D, Adorni F, Ottaviani F. Vocal improvement after voice therapy in unilateral vocal fold paralysis. *J Voice.* 2008;22(1):113–118.

26. Heuer R, Thayer Sataloff R, Emerich K, et al. Unilateral recurrent laryngeal nerve paralysis: the importance of "preoperative" voice therapy. *J Voice.* 1997;11(1):88–94.

27. Scearce L. *Manual of Singing Voice Rehabilitation.* San Diego, CA: Plural Publishing; 2016.

28. Mau T, Weinheimer K. Three-dimensional arytenoid movement induced by vocal fold injections. *Laryngoscope.* 2010;120(8):1563–1568.

29. Rubin A, Sataloff R. Vocal fold paresis and paralysis. *Otolaryngol Clin North Am.* 2007;40(5):1109–1131.

30. Hertegård S, Hallén L, Laurent C, et al. Cross-linked hyaluronan used as augmentation substance for treatment of glottal insufficiency: safety aspects and vocal fold function. *Laryngoscope.* 2002;112(12):2211–2219.

31. Hertegård S, Hallén L, Laurent C, et al. Cross-linked hyaluronan versus collagen for injection treatment of glottal insufficiency: 2-year follow-up. *Acta Oto-Laryngologica.* 2004;124(10):1208–1214.

32. Arviso L, Johns M, Mathison C, Klein A. Long-term outcomes of injection laryngoplasty in patients with potentially recoverable vocal fold paralysis. *Laryngoscope.* 2010;120(11):2237–2240.

33. Isshiki N, Okamura H, Ishikawa T. Thyroplasty type I (lateral compression) for dysphonia due to vocal cord paralysis or atrophy. *Acta Oto-Laryngologica.* 1975;80(1–6):465–473.

34. Isshiki N, Kojima H, Taira T, Shoji K. Recent modifications in thyroplasty type I. *Ann Otol Rhinol Laryngol.* 1989;98(10):777–779.

35. Isshiki N, Tanabe M, Sawada M. Arytenoid adduction for unilateral vocal cord paralysis. *Arch Otolaryngol Head Neck Surg.* 1978;104(10):555–558.

36. Woo P. Failed medialization laryngoplasty: management by revision surgery. *Otolaryngol Head Neck Surg.* 2001;124(6):615–621.

37. Tucker H. Long-term results of nerve-muscle pedicle reinnervation for laryngeal paralysis. *Ann Otol Rhinol Laryngol.* 1989;98(9):674–676.

38. Tucker H. Long-term preservation of voice improvement following surgical medialization and reinnervation for unilateral vocal fold paralysis. *J Voice.* 1999;13(2):251–256.

39. Colton RH, Casper JK. *Understanding Voice Problems: A Physiological Perspective for Diagnosis and Treatment.* Philadelphia, PA: Lippincott Williams & Wilkins; 1996.

40. Stemple J. *Voice Therapy: Clinical Studies.* San Diego, CA: Singular; 2000.

41. Roy N, Ford C, Bless D. Muscle tension dysphonia and spasmodic dysphonia: the role of manual laryngeal tension reduction in diagnosis and management. *Ann Otol Rhinol Laryngol.* 1996;105(11):851–856.

42. Roy N, Bless D, Heisey D, Ford C. Manual circumlaryngeal therapy for functionaldysphonia: an evaluation of short- and long-term treatment outcomes. *J Voice.* 1997;11(3):321–331.

43. Stone RE, Casteel R. Restoration of voice in nonorganically based dysphonia. In: Filter M, ed. *Phonatory Voice Disorders in Children.* Springfield, IL: CC Thomas; 1982:132–165.

44. Titze I. Voice training and therapy with a semi-occluded vocal tract: rationale and scientific underpinnings. *J Speech Lang Hear Res.* 2006;49(2):448–459.

45. Verdolini Abbott K. *Lessac-Madsen Resonant Voice Therapy.* San Diego, CA: Plural Publishing; 2008.

46. Stemple J. *Clinical Voice Pathology: Theory And Management.* Columbus, OH: Charles E. Merrill; 1984.

47. Stemple J, Lee L, D'Amico B, Pickup B. Efficacy of vocal function exercises as a method of improving voice production. *J Voice.* 1994;8(3):271–278.

48. Sabol JW, Lee L, Stemple J. The value of vocal function exercises in the practice regimen of singers. *J Voice.* 1995;9(1):27–36.

49. Wicklund K. *Singing Voice Rehabilitation: A Guide for the Voice Teacher and Speech-Language Pathologist: A Guide for the Voice Teacher and Speech-Language Pathologist.* Clifton Park, NY: Cengage Learning; 2010.

CHAPTER 25

Early Laryngeal Carcinoma Involving the Anterior Commissure

Mark G. Watson and Omar Mulla

CASE PRESENTATION

A 56-year-old male was referred urgently by his general practitioner with a 3-week history of persistent hoarseness. He was otherwise fit and well. Although he had smoked in the past, he had not done so for 10 years. He works as a senior corporate lawyer and frequently appears in court, so has a significant vocal demand. He has been unable to work for the last week due to his voice problem.

On examination his voice was very hoarse ($G_2R_2B_0A_0S_0$) but there was no stridor. Flexible digital laryngoscopy showed a lesion involving both vocal cords and crossing the anterior commissure. The vocal cords were fully mobile. No neck nodes were palpable. Microlaryngoscopy confirmed the extent of the lesion (as shown in Figure 25–1), and a biopsy was taken. This confirmed a moderately differentiated squamous carcinoma. An MRI scan of the neck demonstrated the lesion affecting the vocal cords, but there was no evidence of invasion of the laryngeal cartilages or extralaryngeal spread. A chest x-ray showed no abnormality.

His case was discussed at the multidisciplinary team meeting. Staging was confirmed as T1bN0M0. It was felt that both transoral laser resection of the lesion and radical radiotherapy would be possible treatments for this tumor, and both options should be discussed with the patient.

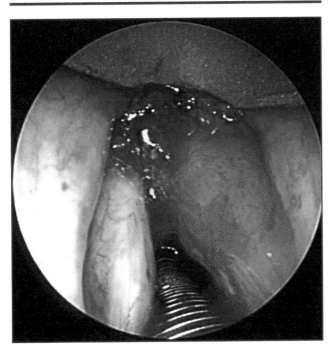

Figure 25–1. T1b tumor crossing anterior commissure of larynx.

DISCUSSION

Early laryngeal carcinoma is frequently encountered by most laryngologists and is typically seen in males over 50 years old with a history of past or present tobacco smoking. It is generally curable using single modality treatment in the form of either surgery (most commonly transoral CO_2 laser resection) or radical radiotherapy. Outcomes of either treatment, in terms of cure rate and vocal function, are good for T1a tumors, but anterior commissure (AC) involvement upstages the lesion to

T1b, with a worse prognosis in terms of both oncological and functional outcomes. Prognosis in terms of the Tumor, Node, Metastasis (TNM) stage is non-uniform and seems better for T2 lesions with no involvement of the AC than T1 lesions with AC involvement.

ANATOMICAL CONSIDERATIONS

The anterior commissure is a well-recognized but poorly defined area of the larynx. Rucci et al reviewed the anatomy and embryology of the AC region.[1] They found that AC structures develop from a single mesenchymal band in the midline of the embryo, present from about 7 weeks gestation. These structures include the intermediate lamina of the thyroid cartilage (IL) and the median process (MP), which lie above glottis level, and an area of loose connective tissue caudal to this level which contains many blood vessels. The MP later differentiates into Broyles' ligament, with fibers that penetrate deeply into the IL. The anterior insertion fibers of the vocal muscles fuse with the ligament fibers. The thyroepiglottic ligament was not considered to be a true AC structure as it has a different embryological origin.

It was suggested that superior spread of a tumor at the AC was restricted by the dense connective tissue cranial to the MP, with caudal spread into the loose vascular connective tissue described above being more likely.

The same group then went on to apply their classification of the AC to a group of 534 patients previously treated for primary laryngeal cancer involving the anterior two thirds of the vocal cords.[2] Three hundred and nine had AC involvement and 225 did not. Most patients were staged T1 or T2 but some higher-stage patients were included. Treatment involved a variety of surgical procedures, or radiotherapy. Only 24/534 (4.5%) had nodal involvement. Outcome was measured as local control at 36 months, with rates according to T stage as follows:

- T1a: 94.2%
- T1b: 70.8%
- T2: 83%
- T3: 100%
- T4: 89%

It can therefore be seen that the worst prognosis group was T1b, which are early tumors with AC involvement. Most treatment failures were salvaged by radical procedures (mainly total laryngectomy). The apparently favorable outcomes for T3 and T4 lesions is explained by the fact that these groups underwent primary radical rather than conservative surgery. The authors went on to describe a four-point system for classifying the extent of AC involvement, in order to address the apparent unreliability of the TNM system in this setting. They found that lesions with no AC involvement, or involvement of only one side but not actually crossing the midline, had a local control rate of >90% compared with those where the tumor crossed the midline (regardless of vertical extent), which had a local control rate of 75%.[2]

An international group confirmed the importance of AC involvement in terms of oncological outcome.[3] It was suggested that AC tumors may not impair vocal cord mobility due to lack of invasion into the vocalis/thyroarytenoid muscles. The importance of cross-sectional imaging in the management of AC tumors in order to rule out deep cartilage or soft tissue invasion was stressed.[3]

A German group looked at 119 T1-T2 laryngeal tumors, all treated surgically (either transoral laser microsurgery or open resection).[4] Total recurrence rate at 5 years was 24.5% if the AC was involved, compared with 5.7% if it was not.[4]

TREATMENT OPTIONS

Possible treatments for early laryngeal carcinoma involving the anterior commissure include surgery (endoscopic or open) or radical radiotherapy. A Cochrane review has been carried out on this subject but as is often the case with such studies, it was unable to reach any conclusions as to which treatment gave the best oncological or voice outcome.[5] An international review suggests that treatment should preferably be single modality but stressed that all patients would benefit from multidisciplinary assessment and discussion.[6] The review stressed that endoscopic surgical access can be difficult at the anterior commissure. Although open surgery will provide better anterior access, it does entail a much more invasive procedure, a neck scar, covering tracheostomy, nasogastric feeding, and a postoperative stay of 1 to 2 weeks, part of which may be in an intensive care setting.

OPEN SURGERY

Sachse et al[4] compared open surgery (OS) (external cordectomy or frontolateral partial laryngectomy) with transoral laser microsurgery (TLM) in a retrospective group of 119 patients with T1-T2 carcinoma of the larynx. They found no difference in outcome between the two modalities in terms of local control rate at 3 and 5 years.

Wolber et al reviewed 77 patients with T1-T2 glottic cancer involving the anterior commissure treated over a 10-year period using either OS (cordectomy or a range of partial laryngectomy techniques) or TLM.[7] In the presence of anterior commissure involvement, OS appeared to give a lower local recurrence rate than TLM (12.5% vs. 38.1%) with a median follow-up of 62 months.[7]

A Polish group reported a large group of 249 patients with anterior commissure involvement treated by a range of partial laryngectomy techniques.[8] A recurrence rate of 14.8% was quoted, but no other treatment modalities were included for comparison. All recurrences occurred within the first 36 months. In a later publication they concentrated on a group of 108 patients with T1b tumors involving the anterior commissure treated by OS and compared their outcomes with those of TLM and radiotherapy (RT) obtained from the available literature.[9] Their recurrence rate for OS was 16.7%, compared with 9 to 20% for TLM in the literature review. Their results were better than the 26% recurrence rate quoted for RT, but this figure was derived from a relatively old source, published in 1991.[9]

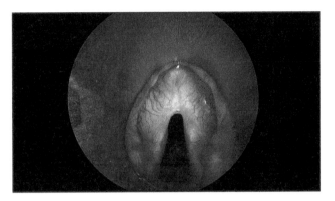

Figure 25–2. Anterior glottic web following transoral laser of a T1b cancer of the glottis.

TRANSORAL LASER MICROSURGERY

TLM is a widely used treatment for early glottic tumors, but may be more difficult with anterior commissure involvement due to access difficulties, and the resulting postoperative morbidity may be greater if it is necessary to resect the anterior portion of both vocal cords in a European Laryngological Society (ELS) type V cordectomy.[10] This can lead to a poor voice outcome or airway impairment due to web (Figure 25–2) or scar formation. This technique has the advantage of a short hospital stay, no external scarring, no covering tracheostomy, and no need for nasogastric feeding.

Steiner's group treated 153 patients with T1-T2 glottic tumors with anterior commissure involvement by TLM.[11] Local recurrence rate was 32% for T1b tumors with commissure involvement. Many patients required regular postoperative debridement in an attempt to prevent web formation.

A more recent report reported 51 cases of T1b glottis cancer treated by TLM. Five-year results showed a recurrence-free survival rate of 72.4%.[12] Twelve patients

suffered one local recurrence (23.5%), 5 patients had two recurrences (10%), and 2 patients suffered three recurrences (4%).

A Canadian multicenter study included 21 cases with T1b glottis tumors treated by TLM. Local control rate at 2 years was 95%, but no long-term data were available.[13]

A British group looked at cost-effectiveness of TLM compared with RT in a UK setting.[14] TLM was costed at £634 per case as opposed to £2654 for RT, although this does assume no second-look procedure for TLM, and does not include the use of intensity-modulated radiotherapy for RT patients. In terms of quality adjusted life years, TLM was felt to be superior to RT. The authors did comment that the optimal strategy for T1b tumors was uncertain.[14]

RADIOTHERAPY

Primary radiotherapy is frequently used to treat early laryngeal cancer. A Japanese group reported a group of 163 patients with T1 tumors of the glottis (115 T1a and 48 T1b) who underwent RT between 1976 and 2002.[15] Five-year local control rate was 92.3% for T1a and 85% for T1b. Further analysis of the T1b group showed that total dose of radiotherapy was important: a dose of <66 Gy gave a 5-year local control rate of 76.2% compared with 100% when the total dose was >66 Gy.[15] As a result, the authors recommended a dose of 67–70 Gy for T1b tumors.

Results from the Cleveland Clinic for 141 patients with T1-T2 treated with RT alone showed a 5-year local control rate of 83% for T1b tumors.[16] Most patients had a hoarse voice at diagnosis, and 73% of subjects reported voice improvement after treatment. A degree of laryngeal edema persisted in 18.4% of individuals but was severe in only one, who required tracheostomy. Some swallowing difficulty was reported by 6.4%, but only one needed tube feeding.[16]

Concurrent chemoradiotherapy (CRT) is not widely used to treat early laryngeal tumors. Hirasawa et al reported 279 patients with T1-T2 tumors, of whom 93 underwent CRT and 186 had RT alone.[16] For the 64 patients with T1b tumors, 5-year local control rates were 78.6% for CRT and 83.8% for RT alone, so there was clearly no advantage in offering combined modality treatment for this patient group.[16] Only T2 tumors showed a benefit from CRT, with a 5-year local control rate of 80.7% compared with 64.4% for RT alone. Taylor et al compared 42 patients with T1b tumors treated by RT with 21 who had TLM.[17] Outcome was measured at 2 years: local control rate was 85.9% for RT and 95% for TLM, but the numbers are small and there was no statistical analysis. No long-term outcomes were measured. Remmelts et al reported a 5-year local control rate of 75% for TLM and 86% for RT, which was on the cusp of statistical significance ($p = 0.07$).[18,19] This trend toward higher local control rates for RT compared with TLM was supported in a systematic review.[20] This suggested a 3-year local control rate (for T1b tumors) of 76.8% for TLM and 86.2% for RT.

VOICE OUTCOMES

As well as oncological outcome, the functional result in terms of voice is critical for patients treated for early laryngeal tumors, as most will be cured of their disease. This is especially so for the professional voice user. Poor vocal outcomes may be related to inadequate glottic closure during phonation or excessive scarring, fibrosis, or edema interfering with the mucosal wave.

For T1a tumors, an excellent voice outcome can be expected from either TLM or RT. For T1b tumors, especially those involving the anterior commissure, resection via TLM would normally require an ELS type V cordectomy, which is likely to lead to either limited glottic closure during phonation or excessive scarring with web formation.

Bahannan et al looked at 62 patients who had resection of early glottic tumors.[20] For cordectomy types I–III the voice outcome was good, but for types IV–V the post-treatment Voice Handicap Index (VHI) score was four times greater than for types I to III.[20] Bajaj et al described 19 patients treated for T1-T2 glottic cancer by

TLM.[21] Anterior commissure resection was required in 10 patients. Eight of these (80%) developed significant scarring in the form of an anterior glottic web. Voice outcomes, as measured by the Voice Symptom Scale (VoiSS), were significantly worse in those who developed a web (VoiSS outcome, $p = 0.05$).[21]

For T1b patients, Taylor et al showed little difference in average VHI score between their RT and TLM groups, but the overall result based on average values may have been skewed by one patient in the RT group who needed a tracheostomy.[17]

Remmelts et al found that patients with T1b tumors treated by TLM had a significantly worse vocal outcome than those treated by RT.[19] Average VHI score was 16.7 for TLM versus 4.9 for RT ($p < 0.05$). Cohen et al found that anterior commissure resection was the key factor in predicting a worse voice outcome.[22] VHI was 6.2 if the commissure was preserved, compared with 15.7 if it was resected.

Voice outcomes following OS may be expected to be worse than for TLM. Szyfter et al, in their series of open horizontal glottectomy for T1b tumors, reported an average VHI score of 28.[9] In addition, maximum phonation time was reduced to 10 seconds (20–30 seconds would be regarded as normal).

PATIENT CHOICE AND CASE RESOLUTION

After the case had been discussed at the multidisciplinary team meeting, the option of either transoral laser microlaryngoscopy or primary RT was discussed with the patient. The implications for oncological outcome for T1b tumors (70–75% local control rate for TLM versus 80–85% for RT) and worse voice outcomes were clearly described. The patient asked for time to study the evidence himself, and so was seen again 7 days later. At that stage, he stated that if his tumor were T1a with no commissure involvement, he would have opted for TLM, but because of the AC disease he had decided to have radical radiotherapy.

REFERENCES

1. Rucci L, Gammarota L, Cirri MBB. Carcinoma of the anterior commissure of the larynx: I. embryological and anatomic considerations. *Ann Otol Rhinol Laryngol.* 1996; 105:303–309.

2. Rucci L, Gammarota L, Gallo O. Carcinoma of the anterior commissure of the larynx: II. proposal of a new staging system. *Ann Otol Rhinol Laryngol.* 1996;105:391–396.

3. Bradley PJ, Rinaldo A, Suarez C, et al. Primary treatment of the anterior vocal commissure squamous carcinoma. *Eur Arch Otorhinolaryngol.* 2006;263:879–888.

4. Sachse F, Stoll W, Rudack C. Evaluation of treatment results with regard to initial anterior commissure involvement in early glottic carcinoma treated by external partial surgery or transoral laser microresection. *Head Neck.* 2009;31:531–537.

5. Warner L, Chudasama J, Kelly CG, Loughran S, McKenzie K, Wight R, Dey P. Radiotherapy versus open surgery versus microlaryngeal surgery (with or without laser) for early laryngeal squamous cell carcinoma. *Cochrane Database.* 2014; doi:10.1002/14651858.CD002027.pub2

6. Hartl DM, Ferlito A, Brasnu DF, Langendijk JA, Rinaldo A, Silver CE, Wolf GT. Evidence-based review of treatment options for patients with glottis cancer. *Head Neck.* 2011; doi:10.1002/hed

7. Wolber P, Schwarz D, Strange T, Ortmann M, Balk M, Anagiotos A, Gostian AO. Surgical treatment of early stage glottic carcinoma with involvement of the anterior commissure. *Otolaryngol Head Neck Surg.* 2018;158: 295–302.

8. Syzfter W, Wierzbicka M, Leszcznska M, Mlodkowska A. Treatment of glottic cancer with involvement anterior commissure by supracricoid laryngectomy: our experiences with group 249 patients. *Eur Arch Otorhinolaryngol.* 2012;269:1394.

9. Syzfter W, Leszcznska M, Wierzbicka M, Kopec T, Bartochowska A. Value of open horizontal glottectomy in the treatment for T1b glottic cancer with anterior commissure involvement. *Head Neck.* 2013;35:1738–1744.

10. Remacle M, Eckel HE, Antonelli A, et al. Endoscopic cordectomy. A proposal for a classification by the working committee. European Laryngological Society. *Eur Arch Otorhinolaryngol.* 2000;257:227–231.

11. Rodel RMW, Steiner W, Muller RM, Kron M, Matthias C. Endoscopic laser surgery of early glottic cancer: involvement of the anterior commissure. *Head Neck.* 2009; 31:583–592.

12. Weiss BG, Ihler F, Pilavakis Y, Wolff HA, Canis M, Welz C, Steiner W. Transoral laser microsurgery for T1b cancer:

13. Prettyjohns M, Winter S, Kerawala C, Paleri V. Transoral laser microsurgery versus radiation therapy in the management of T1 and T2 laryngeal glottic carcinoma: which modality is cost-effective within the UK? *Clin Otol.* 2017; 42:404–415.

14. Nomiya T, Nemoto K, Wada H, Takai Y, Yamada S. Long-term results of radiotherapy for T1a and T1bN0M0 glottic carcinoma. *Laryngoscope.* 2008;118:1417–1421.

15. Khan MK, Koyfman SA, Hunter GK, Reddy CA, Saxton JP. Definitive radiotherapy for early glottis squamous cell carcinoma: a 20-year Cleveland clinic experience. *Radiat Oncol.* 2012;7:193. doi: 10.1186/1748-717X-7-193

16. Hirasawa N, Itoh Y, Naganawa S, Ishihara S, Suzuki K, Koyama K, et al. Multi-institutional analysis of early glottic cancer from 2000-2005. *Radiat Oncol.* 2012;7:122. doi:10.1186/1748-717X7-122

17. Taylor SM, Kerr P, Fung K, Aneeshkumar MK, Wilke D, Jiang Y, Scott J, Phillips J, Hart RD, Trites JRB, Rigby MH. Treatment of T1b glottic SCC: laser vs radiation—a Canadian multicentre study. *J Otolaryngol Head Neck Surg.* 2013;42:22. doi:10.1186/1916-0216-42-22

18. Remmelts AJ, Hoebers FJP, Klop WMC, Balm AJM, Hamming-Vrieze O, van den Breckel MWM. Evaluation of laser surgery and radiotherapy as treatment modalities in early stage laryngeal carcinoma: tumour outcome and quality of voice. *Eur Arch Otorhinolaryngol.* 2013;270: 2079–2087.

19. O'Hara J, Markey A, Homer JJ. Transoral laser surgery versus radiotherapy for tumour stage 1a or 1b glottis squamous cell carcinoma: systematic review of local control outcomes. *J Laryngol Otol.* 2013;127:732–738.

20. Bahannan AA, Slavicek A, Cerny L, et al. Effectiveness of transoral laser microsurgery for precancerous lesions and early glottic cancer guided by analysis of voice quality. *Head Neck.* 2014;36:763–767.

21. Bajaj Y, Uppal S, Sharma RK, et al. Evaluation of voice and quality of life after transoral endoscopic laser resection of early glottis carcinoma. *J Laryngol Otol.* 2011;125:706–713.

22. Cohen SM, Garrett CG Dupont WD, et al. Voice-related quality of life in T1 glottic cancer: irradiation versus endoscopic excision. *Ann Otol Rhinol Laryngol.* 2006;115: 581–586.

review of 51 cases. *Eur Arch Otorhinolaryngol.* 2017; 274: 1997–2004.

CHAPTER 26

Laryngeal Dysplasia and Early Glottic Cancer

Valeria Silva Merea, Rebecca C. Nelson, and Michael S. Benninger

INTRODUCTION

The larynx is a critical structure for basic physiologic functions such as breathing, speech, and swallowing. Although premalignant and malignant laryngeal lesions may have an impact on any of those functions, involvement of the vocal folds with loss of voice may lead to symptoms at earlier stages than other cancers of the head and neck. However, benign conditions may lead to similar symptoms and have a similar appearance on exam, making it essential to obtain a detailed history and perform a complete physical examination with an endoscopic examination of the larynx.

Laryngeal cancer is the second most common head and neck cancer worldwide.[1] In the United States, there is an estimated 13,360 new cases diagnosed yearly.[2] Squamous cell carcinoma (SCC) is the most common cancer in the larynx.[3] It is more common in men than women, although the gap has become smaller over time.[2,3] Among patients with laryngeal dysplasia, a trend toward younger age at diagnosis and less severe grade at diagnosis has been reported.[4]

DEFINITION

Dysplasia is the term used to describe cells that look abnormal under the microscope. The World Health Organization (WHO) defines dysplasia in the upper aerodigestive tract as "a spectrum of architectural and cytological epithelial changes caused by an accumulation of genetic changes that can be associated with an increased likelihood of progression to squamous cell carcinoma."[5] Previously classified as mild, moderate, and severe dysplasia, and carcinoma in situ, the WHO now recognizes two types: low-grade and high-grade dysplasia.[5] Once dysplastic cells invade through the basement membrane, the diagnosis changes to SCC.

CASE PRESENTATION #1

A 60-year-old man presents with a 2-month history of progressive hoarseness in the absence of any inciting events. He has no history of vocal abuse. He has mild dysphagia with food sticking in his throat and has lost a few pounds because of this. He has no odynophagia or otalgia and no difficulty breathing.

Past medical history: Hypertension, peripheral vascular disease status post bypass graft to his left leg

Medications: Metoprolol, aspirin, and clopidogrel

No known drug allergies

Social: Current smoker, 30 to 40 pack year history; social alcohol use

Initial Assessment

History—Hoarseness or voice change, dysphagia or aspiration, odynophagia, stridor, sore throat, chronic cough, hemoptysis, otalgia, weight loss, and globus sensation are signs and symptoms that may be associated with premalignant and malignant lesions. In addition, risk factors for these lesions include smoking, alcohol use, radiation exposure, gastroesophageal reflux, history of human papilloma virus (HPV) infection or recurrent respiratory papillomatosis.

In this patient, concerning features are his progressive hoarseness, which did not have an inciting event, and dysphagia leading to weight loss. His significant smoking history, as well as alcohol use, also place him at increased risk of malignancy. It is also important to pay attention to this patient's past medical history of a revascularization procedure to his leg and need for dual antiplatelet therapy. If surgery is required, the patient would likely need to discontinue clopidogrel to decrease the risk of bleeding complications.

Examination—Assessment of the patient's voice, followed by a complete head and neck examination including cranial nerves is performed. Visualization of the larynx may be accomplished by mirror exam; however, more commonly now, a flexible fiberoptic laryngoscopy is preferred.

Endoscopy—Given that the primary complaint is hoarseness, at minimum a flexible fiberoptic laryngoscopy should be performed; however, if available, either flexible or rigid videostroboscopic evaluation would allow for more complete assessment of vocal fold pliability and provide information regarding depth of invasion in any present vocal fold lesion. Given his significant history of smoking, alcohol use, and dysphagia with associated weight loss, an esophagoscopy is recommended to rule out an esophageal mass, lesion, or stricture. This can be performed in the office as a flexible transnasal esophagoscopy (TNE) or in the operating room with a rigid or a flexible esophagoscope.

SCENARIO 1

The patient's voice is rough and mildly breathy. Head and neck examination is normal; there is no cervical lymphadenopathy and no cranial nerve deficits. Flexible fiberoptic examination demonstrates a right true vocal fold mass and normal bilateral vocal fold mobility with glottic insufficiency secondary to the mass preventing full glottic closure. On videostroboscopic evaluation, the mucosal wave is reduced on the right and there is vibratory asymmetry. Transnasal esophagoscopy in the office was within normal limits.

Preliminary diagnosis: Right true vocal fold mass

Management 1

The patient should be immediately counseled to stop smoking, and resources to aid with smoking cessation should be provided to the patient. Given the patient's risk factors and the characteristics of the mass, surgical excision is recommended. Options include direct microlaryngoscopy with biopsy and possible excision of the vocal fold mass via either microdissection or with carbon dioxide (CO_2) or potassium titanyl phosphate (KTP) laser. The specific techniques and tools would depend in part on the depth of the lesion and the confirmation of the pathology. Microdissection or KTP laser is a better option for superficial lesions requiring a type I or type II cordectomy, while a CO_2 laser might be preferred for deeper resections. There is some evidence that functional voice outcomes may be better following a type II cordectomy with resection of the vocalis ligament than with a type I with removal of the entire epithelium.[6]

Extended T1a lesions or T2 lesions might be candidates for definitive radiation therapy. The choice between primary resection or primary radiation as definitive treatment depends on a number of factors: (1) the depth of resection and how it will impact long-term voice and swallowing; (2) the specific histology, with verrucous or spindle carcinomas having better outcomes with surgery; (3) the patient's desire to balance time and expense of treatment with functional outcomes.

In this case, complete excision of the mass via microdissection was performed. See Figure 26–1.

Pathology: T1a squamous cell carcinoma, HPV negative

Management 2

- Computed tomography (CT) of the neck with contrast depending in part on the stage of the lesion to evaluate surgical site and cervical lymph nodes. For a T1a lesion, CT is not necessary. In this case, CT was obtained and it was negative.
- Chest x-ray to evaluate for lung metastasis or a secondary lung primary; negative.
- Reflux management to prevent further inflammation secondary to refluxate. In a patient taking clopidogrel, proton pump inhibitors should be avoided, a histamine H2 receptor antagonist such as ranitidine can be used.

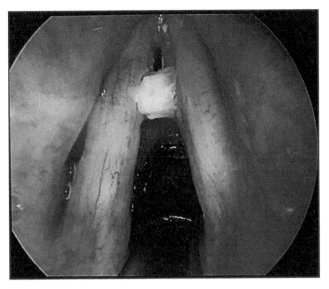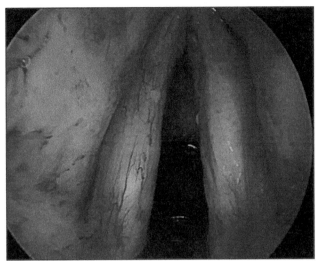

Figure 26–1. Intraoperative view of the glottis before and after excision. Right vocal fold mass seen in left image.

- Close follow-up: Every 2 months during the first year, 3 months during the second year, 4 months in the third year, 6 months during the fourth and fifth years, then yearly; or sooner as needed. No recurrence of disease on long-term follow-up.

Final diagnosis: T1aN0M0 (Stage I) right glottic squamous cell carcinoma

SCENARIO 2

Hoarse voice. Head and neck examination is within normal limits. Flexible fiberoptic laryngoscopy demonstrated full bilateral vocal fold mobility with complete glottic closure and bilateral vocal fold leukoplakia.

Preliminary diagnosis: Bilateral true vocal fold leukoplakia

Management 1

- Smoking cessation
- Reflux control with a histamine H2 receptor antagonist given clopidogrel use

- Antifungal therapy typically with daily oral fluconazole, but given interaction between fluconazole and clopidogrel, another antifungal such as itraconazole should be considered.
- Follow-up

At follow-up: Persistent bilateral true vocal fold leukoplakia

Management 2

Direct microlaryngoscopy with excision of bilateral vocal fold leukoplakia via microdissection given superficial nature of lesions. See Figure 26–2.

Pathology: High-grade dysplasia, HPV negative

Final diagnosis: High-grade laryngeal dysplasia

Management 3

- Chest x-ray: Negative
- Close monitoring in the office: Patient found to have recurrent leukoplakia multiple times over 15 years

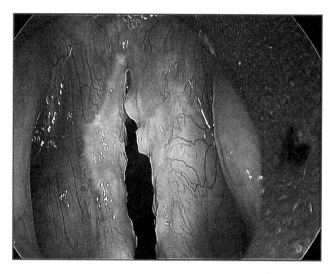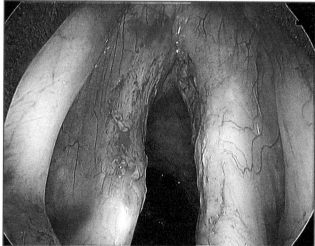

Figure 26–2. Intraoperative images before and after excision. Leukoplakia involves both true vocal folds.

- In-office KTP laser ablation of recurrent leukoplakia performed when mild recurrent disease. Under local anesthesia, bilateral lesions treated with a 0.4 mm KTP laser fiber, at the following settings: 30 watts, 15 milliseconds, 2 pulses per second.
- Repeat microlaryngoscopy with microexcision performed when more extensive recurrence. Pathology always consistent with high-grade dysplasia/carcinoma in situ.

CASE PRESENTATION #2

A 36-year-old man presents with a 3-month history of progressive hoarseness. Voice initially changed in the setting of an upper respiratory infection with coughing. As his cough resolved, his voice remained intermittently hoarse. Initially, throat clearing momentarily improved the quality of his voice, over time the dysphonia has become constant. No dysphagia, odynophagia, dyspnea, or otalgia. No history of vocal abuse.

Past medical history: No chronic medical problems; history of septoplasty many years prior.

Medications: None

No known drug allergies

Social history: Works in information technology; never smoker, three alcoholic beverages per week

Initial Assessment

History—Similar to case #1, hoarseness has been progressive but this time it started in the setting of an upper respiratory infection. In the setting of severe coughing, benign processes such as a granuloma are in the differential. Moreover, this is a much younger patient and there is no smoking history. Other than the constant change in voice, there are no other red flag features.

Examination—Voice assessment and a complete head and neck examination should be performed.

Endoscopy—A flexible fiberoptic laryngoscopy with videostroboscopy would provide enough detail to narrow the differential diagnosis. Rigid stroboscopy could also be performed, which may provide some additional light for anatomic assessment, but would limit the full evaluation of the voice throughout the entire vocal range and with running speech or singing that might be required in this patient. In addition, the high resolution or high definition (HD) distal tip cameras on the flexible scopes provide nearly equivalent anatomic evaluation.

SCENARIO 3

Dysphonia present (class III, moderate). The head and neck exam is unremarkable. Flexible fiberoptic examination shows normal bilateral vocal fold mobility. There is an irregular mass with some papillomatous

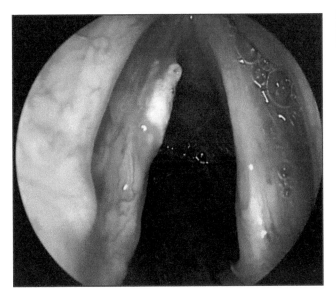 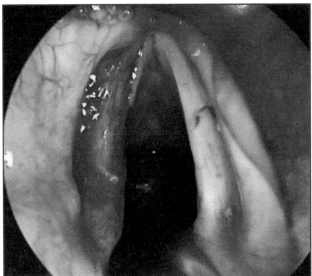

Figure 26–3. Intraoperative images before and after excision. Note the mass on the medial aspect of the left true vocal fold, with papillomatous changes extending laterally.

change emanating from the upper surface of the left vocal fold and it interferes with closure and vibration on videostroboscopy.

Preliminary diagnosis: Left true vocal fold mass

Management 1

Direct microlaryngoscopy with excision of left vocal fold mass. See Figure 26–3.

Pathology: HPV+, p16+, at least carcinoma in situ

At follow-up: Persistent focal area of leukoplakia on left true vocal fold. Re-excision recommended.

Management 2

Direct microlaryngoscopy with excision of left vocal fold mass via microdissection

Pathology: Moderately differentiated squamous cell carcinoma

Management 3

- Computed tomography of the neck with contrast: negative
- Chest x-ray: negative
- Close follow-up for recurrence

Final diagnosis: T1aN0M0 left glottic squamous cell carcinoma, HPV positive

CASE PRESENTATION #3

An 83-year-old man with a history of a stage I T1b squamous cell carcinoma of the glottis surgically excised 8 months prior, presented to the office for routine surveillance. Voice has continued to improve since the surgery and he has no complaints. No dysphagia, odynophagia, otalgia, or weight loss. See Figure 26–4.

Past medical history: Glottic SCC, bladder cancer treated with surgery, HTN, hyperlipidemia

Medications: Atenolol, Olmesartan, Rosuvastatin, omeprazole, ranitidine

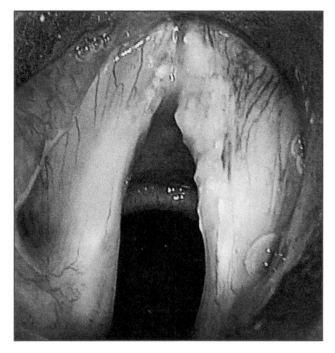
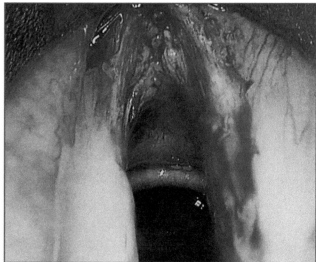

Figure 26–4. Intraoperative photos from original resection of T1b glottic squamous cell carcinoma with involvement of the anterior commissure.

No known drug allergies

Social history: Remote 15-pack year smoking history, no alcohol use

Initial Assessment

History

Given the history of a prior early stage laryngeal carcinoma, the patient is being followed closely. Sensitivity to mucus is a common complaint among patients with prior vocal fold surgery. There are no worrisome symptoms or complaints at follow-up.

Examination

Voice assessment and a complete head and neck examination should be performed.

Endoscopy

Laryngoscopy with videostroboscopy is essential in this situation of early glottic cancer surveillance as changes in vocal fold pliability may indicate a recurrent lesion. As previously discussed, either flexible or rigid examination could be performed.

SCENARIO

Voice is abnormally high-pitched. Head and neck evaluation is within normal limits. No palpable cervical masses or lymphadenopathy. On flexible fiberoptic laryngoscopy with videostroboscopy, true vocal fold movement is intact bilaterally with complete glottic closure. Small slightly irregular subepithelial mass on the superior surface of the vocal fold over an anterior commissure web. Mucosal wave was noted to be present and equal bilaterally. Amplitude decreased, likely because of the shortened vocal folds secondary to the glottic web but preserved phase symmetry.

Preliminary diagnosis: Anterior commissure mass on surface of anterior glottic web, concern for recurrent glottic squamous cell carcinoma

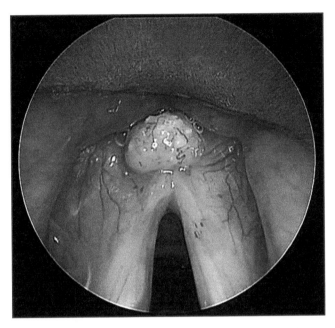 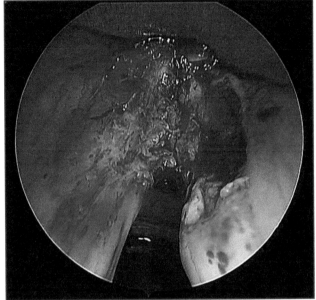

Figure 26–5. Intraoperative images showing the anterior commissure mass and the surgical bed post excision.

Management 1

Given that there was a significant change from one surveillance visit to the next less than 2 months apart, direct microlaryngoscopy with excision was recommended as recurrence could not be ruled out. Because of the location of the lesion as well as possibility of cancer recurrence necessitating aggressive resection, risk of permanently worsening his voice was discussed with the patient. See Figure 26–5.

Pathology 1: Invasive moderately differentiated squamous cell carcinoma, negative margins. HPV negative.

At follow-up: Voice is near normal but there is slight breathiness. Head and neck evaluation is within normal limits. No palpable cervical masses or lymphadenopathy. On flexible fiberoptic laryngoscopy with videostroboscopy, anterior commissure healing well, with recurrent anterior glottic web.

Management 2

Continued close surveillance.

DIFFERENTIAL DIAGNOSIS

Once a laryngeal lesion is identified, the laryngologist must consider all potential disease entities in his or her differential diagnosis, rather than just premalignant or malignant lesions. This may include infectious, rheumatological, or inflammatory lesions of the laryngeal epithelium. Laryngeal papillomatosis can present with an irregular mass, but is often readily distinguished by its characteristic papillary appearance on laryngoscopy. Though malignant transformation can occur, it is rare.[7] Benign lesions such as nodules, cysts, and polyps are often sited along the free edge of the vocal fold. Granulomata typically occur in the posterior larynx. Less common lesions may include pyogenic granuloma of the larynx or laryngeal hemangioma.[8] Teflon granuloma, from previous vocal fold augmentation, may also present with an irregular appearance. Often lesions can be distinguished with history and laryngoscopy; however, at times, tissue diagnosis may be required.

LARYNGEAL DYSPLASIA

Dysplasia is a histologic diagnosis which requires tissue for definitive categorization. The distinction between benign, premalignant, and malignant diagnoses is crucial for guiding management and is reported by the histopathologist. Clinical presentation is diverse, as is the endoscopic appearance. Descriptive terms such as leukoplakia, erythroplakia, and mixed erythroleukoplakia describe the color of the plaque seen macroscopically. Plaques may be localized or diffuse, flat or exophytic and continuous or discontinuous. Approximately 50% of patients with laryngeal leukoplakia demonstrate dysplasia on histopathologic evaluation.[9] Laryngeal leukoplakia is often recurrent and multifocal.

The overall rate of progression of laryngeal dysplasia to malignancy has been estimated as 13.6% according to a meta-analysis.[10] However, a more recent large, 20-year single institution study found this rate to be 8.4%.[4] Low-grade dysplasia shows malignant transformation in about 2% of cases, while high-grade dysplasia has been associated with up to 40% rate of malignant progression.[4,11,12]

Latency period between initial diagnosis and development of cancer has been found to be approximately 4 years for those patients with mild dysplasia, 3 years for those with moderate dysplasia, and 2 years for patients with severe dysplasia.[9]

Tobacco smoke is the most important risk factor and when alcohol is also present there is a synergistic effect.[13,14] Gastroesophageal reflux disease is also considered a risk factor.[15]

Diagnosis and Histopathology

Symptoms vary widely according to the location and size of the lesions. Patients may be asymptomatic or may complain of voice changes, sore throat or irritation, chronic cough,[5] otalgia or dysphagia, with dysphonia often being the first sign of glottic pathology.[16] Diagnosis is usually made by evaluation of the larynx in the office setting detecting a lesion followed by tissue sampling for confirmation of histological diagnosis, which may be performed in the office or the operating room.

Histopathologic diagnosis and grading of premalignant laryngeal lesions have been shown to be subjective and lack reproducibility.[17–19] With the recent changes by the WHO, what used to be considered mild dysplasia is now "low grade," and moderate and severe dysplasia, together with carcinoma in situ, are all "high grade" dysplasia.[5]

Immunohistochemistry markers have been used to differentiate low-grade from high-grade dysplasia and dysplasia from malignancy, but findings have been inconsistent, at least partly because immunohistochemistry overexpression does not necessarily correlate to molecular alterations in the progression of disease.[20] For instance, increased p53 expression is higher in carcinoma than dysplasia, while p27 follows the opposite pattern[20,21]; CD163+ tumor-associated macrophages (TAMs) infiltrating epithelium are significantly higher in high-grade dysplasia than in low-grade dysplasia, while Ki67 is overexpressed in the basal layer of lesions with high-grade dysplasia.[22]

Genetics

Multiple genetic alterations in laryngeal dysplastic lesions involving chromosomal changes and loss of heterozygosity have been described, with cyclin-dependent kinase inhibitor 2A (CDKN2A) gene alterations being the most frequently identified and associated with tumor protein 53 (TP53).[23] Cyclin-D1 overexpression and activated telomerase activity are also involved in early phases of neoplastic transformation.[24] At this time, tests to detect these genetic abnormalities are not routinely used.

Management

The management of laryngeal dysplasia is not standardized and varies with disease burden and grade of dysplasia. In addition, one must balance treatment aggressiveness versus voice outcomes.[4] Approaches to management of dysplasia include expectant observation, vocal fold stripping, phonomicrosurgical excision with cold instruments, laser excision, and radiation therapy.[25] Suspicious laryngeal lesions are usually managed with phonomicrosurgical technique or with the use of lasers such as the carbon dioxide CO_2 or KTP lasers.[26–29] Availability of intraoperative frozen section analysis allows for a single-stage intervention for diagnosis and management.

The CO_2 laser is frequently used for excision of premalignant or malignant lesions of the larynx. Although CO_2 lasers reduce bleeding when deeper muscular resections are performed, utilizing a laser to excise more superficial lesions has some limitations. The laser artifact can obscure the margins of the resection and thereby require additional specimens to ensure negative margins, thereby increasing the overall amount of tissue resected. There is also a loss of tactile sensation of the surgeon that is present with microdissection, which may focus the surgeon's suspicion as to deeper areas of invasion. The pulse dye laser (PDL) and KTP laser are photoangiolytic and do not provide a specimen. Thus, tissue sampling for diagnosis of dysplasia and mapping of the lesion should be done prior to initiating treatment with PDL or KTP.[16] Patients with recurrent leukoplakia can be transitioned from the operating to the office setting for outpatient management with photoangiolytic lasers as needed.[4,30] This is an appealing option for patients who present with chronic and indolent disease and would like to avoid recurrent trips to the operating room.

Radiation therapy (RT) has been used in cases of field cancerization resulting from chronic exposure to carcinogens over a wide area or in recurrent high-grade dysplasia.[15,31] However, more recent studies suggest that these lesions can be well managed by in-office KTP laser with decreased morbidity.[30,32] RT may be reserved for refractory cases.

Elimination of risk factors such as tobacco smoking, alcohol use, and gastroesophageal reflux is also an important aspect of management of laryngeal dysplasia. Recently, metformin and folic acid supplementation have been suggested to have a role in chemoprevention for patients with laryngeal dysplasia.[33,34]

EARLY GLOTTIC CANCER

The term "early glottic cancer" refers to T1 and T2 malignancy without evidence of local lymph node or metastatic spread. These tumors can be treated differently than their more advanced counterparts due to the unique anatomical structure of the larynx, which has implications for the behavior of tumors, and in turn their management. Even embryological development is important when considering locoregional spread: The glottis develops from the sixth branchial arch, from paired structures that fuse midline. Drainage, and therefore malignant lymphatic spread, is unilateral, unlike in the supraglottis, which embryologically forms without midline union, explaining its bilateral lymphatic drainage pattern.[35,36]

There are few lymphatic channels in the vocal folds, and therefore glottic tumors typically do not spread through this route until there is deep local invasion. Consequently T1-2 glottic carcinomas are known to have a low incidence of lymph node metastasis, reported as 0 to 10%.[37] Additionally, a study by Pressman in 1956 was performed where dyes and radio-isotopes were injected into specific locations within the larynx and subsequently demonstrated relatively limited avenues for spread and have implications for glottic tumor development.[38] Anatomic barriers, such as the vocal ligament, conus elasticus, and thyroid perichondrium may also play a role in halting locoregional tumor spread. Broyle's ligament at the anterior commissure, however, attaches to the thyroid cartilage where there is no inner perichondrium, and therefore can serve as a pathway for extralaryngeal spread.[36]

However, due to overall lower rates of metastatic and locoregional spread, surgeons have a unique opportunity for procedural staging and structure preservation when managing early glottic cancer. Probability of cure for carcinoma in situ/high-grade dysplasia (Tis), T1, and T2 lesions is 80 to 90% in contrast to more advanced laryngeal disease, which is closer to 60%.[39]

Risk Factors

Similar to dysplasia, smoking and alcohol use are known to be risk factors for laryngeal cancer,[39] and gastroesophageal reflux has also been implicated as a risk factor.[40] HPV is also known to be associated with laryngeal SCC. Prevalence has been reported to be 20 to 30% of laryngeal squamous cell cancers, though it may vary with geographic location and HPV detection method. The most common subsite of HPV-related laryngeal cancer is in fact the glottis, likely due to the squamo-columnar epithelial junction. However, it remains unclear what HPV status means for management and prognosis.[41]

Diagnosis and Histopathology

As with dysplasia, evaluation begins in the office with flexible or rigid laryngoscopy and videostroboscopy. This step is critical in that it provides information about vocal fold mobility, which is important when determining clinical staging. Narrow-band light filters may be used to aid in evaluation of lesions to highlight microvascular abnormalities, which should raise suspicion for a neoplastic process. Patients who present with suspicious lesions should be taken to the operating room for direct laryngoscopy for further examination under anesthesia as well as biopsy. Diagnosis is confirmed with tissue sampling, and careful mapping of the tumor is useful for staging. If there is concern for the possibility of lymph node metastasis for more distant spread, imaging is warranted and typically includes CT of the neck with IV contrast as well as chest x-ray.

The American Joint Committee on Cancer tumor (T) staging criteria for glottic malignancy can be found in Table 26–1.

A variety of malignancies can exist in the larynx, including adenocarcinoma, spindle cell carcinoma, adenoid cystic carcinoma, among others; however, SCC is by far the most common, accounting for over 95% of all primary cancers.[42] Pathologic diagnosis can typically be made with hematoxylin and eosin (H&E) stain and conventional light microscopy.[39] Histologic analysis can also differentiate laryngeal verrucous carcinoma, a well-differentiated subtype of SCC that most frequently presents in early stages in the glottis. Though this often can be identified by a "warty" appearance, definitive diagnosis can only be made with biopsy with pathological features showing well-differentiated carcinoma, with local invasion via intrastromal invaginations with thin, vascular cords. It accounts for 1–4% of all laryngeal carcinomas and has a predilection for males, with a 13.8:1 male to female ratio. Additionally, association with HPV has been found in 65 to 85% of tested specimens. Surgical resection is the preferred treatment method for this subtype.[43]

Genetics

Laryngeal cancer is thought to be a progression from precancerous lesions. Molecular studies have shown that cell aneuploidy, overexpression of p53, microsatellite instability, and loss of heterozygosity are involved in the transformation from benign to dysplastic to malignant cells.[44] Cyclin-D1 is a critical protein involved in the cell cycle, and deregulation of this protein in the CCND1 gene was found to be potentially implicated in the risk of laryngeal cancer development and prognosis.[45]

Management

For reasons stated above, the prognosis for early stage glottic cancer is favorable and may generally be treated with single modality therapy. Typically, this is either radiation therapy or surgical therapy, and functional preservation is often kept in high consideration.

Radiation Therapy

Definitive RT is an effective treatment option for early stage lesions, with 5-year local control rates ranging 82 to 94% for T1a, 80 to 93% for T1b, 62 to 94% for T2a (mobile vocal folds), and 23 to 73% for T2b (impaired vocal fold mobility),[46] with 5-year survival rates as high as 94 to 98% for T1 lesions and 90 to 95% for T2. The use of concurrent chemotherapy has been studied and is reported to improve outcomes in T2 cancer.[47] Although there is some debate about RT voice outcomes

Table 26–1. American Joint Committee on Cancer (AJCC) 8th ed. Staging Criteria for SCC Glottis

Clinical Stage	
Tis	Carcinoma in situ
T1	Tumor limited to the vocal cord(s) (may involve anterior or posterior commissure) with normal mobility
T1a	Tumor limited to one vocal cord
T1b	Tumor involves both vocal cords
T2	Tumor extends to supraglottis and/or subglottis, and/or with impaired vocal cord mobility
T3	Tumor limited to the larynx with vocal cord fixation and/or invasion of the paraglottic space, and/or the inner cortex of the thyroid cartilage
T4	Moderately advanced or very advanced
T4a	Moderately advanced local disease: Tumor invades through the outer cortex of the thyroid cartilage and/or invades tissues beyond the larynx (e.g. trachea, soft tissues of the neck including deep extrinsic muscle of the tongue, strap muscles, thyroid, or esophagus)
T4b	Very advanced local disease: Tumor invades prevertebral space, encases carotid artery, or invades mediastinal structures

Table 26–2. Endoscopic Cordectomy Classification

Type	Extent
I	Subepithelial cordectomy, resection of epithelium only
II	Subligamental cordectomy, includes epithelium, Reinke's space, and vocal ligament
III	Transmuscular cordectomy, proceeds through vocalis muscle
IV	Total cordectomy
Va	Extended cordectomy encompassing anterior commissure and contralateral vocal fold
Vb	Extended cordectomy including arytenoid
Vc	Extended cordectomy encompassing the subglottis
Vd	Extended cordectomy including ventricle

compared with a surgical approach, the literature suggests that patient reported voice outcomes may be comparable for T1 carcinomas.[48]

Although counseling for radiation is an option that should be discussed with all patients, it is a particularly good option for elderly patients or those with significant medical comorbidities that increase surgical risk. Similarly, radiation may be preferred if a surgeon feels he or she cannot resect the tumor without causing significant voice compromise. Radiation is often avoided in younger patients, due to radiation-related changes such as chronic laryngeal edema, dysphagia, skin changes, and radiation-induced malignancy. Additionally, recurrence after radiation may necessitate a salvage total laryngectomy, so often younger patients will opt for initial surgical management to save the potential need for radiation for the future.

Surgical Management

Surgical management includes a range of techniques from endoscopic cold-steel resection to endoscopic laser resection/ablation to open partial laryngectomy procedures. In recent years, endoscopic approaches have been increasingly supplanting open partial laryngectomy approaches. In addition to lower postsurgical morbidity, endoscopic approaches are effective, with local control rates of 80 to 94% and laryngeal preservation rates of 94% with transoral laser microsurgery for Tis, T1, and T2 tumors.[49] Initially CO_2 lasers were introduced in the 1960s and more recently KTP lasers have gained popularity, in part due to their angiolytic nature and ability to target abnormal vasculature associated with tumors.[50] The extent of endoscopic resection depends on tumor depth and involvement and it can be classified into eight types of cordectomies.[51] Table 26–2 lists all cordectomy types.

Perhaps the most distinct advantage of endoscopic surgical management is that it does not preclude the use of future RT, future endoscopic surgery, or even future open laryngeal preservation procedures. It is relatively non-invasive with low morbidity and is tolerated by most patients. Additionally, office-based procedures are appealing in select patients who require additional treatment. Ultimately, all options should be discussed with the patient prior to initiation of treatment, and consultation with a radiation oncology specialist may be beneficial as well.

REFERENCES

1. Ferlay J, Shin HR, Bray F, Forman D, Mathers C, Parkin DM. Estimates of worldwide burden of cancer in 2008: Globocan 2008. *Int J Cancer*. 2010;127:2893–2917.
2. SEER Cancer stat facts: laryngeal cancer. National Cancer Institute. Bethesda, MD, http://seer.cancer.gov/statfacts/html/laryn.html
3. Schultz P. Vocal fold cancer. *Eur Ann Otorhinolaryngol Head Neck Dis*. 2011;128:301–308.
4. Karatayli-Ozgursoy S, Pacheco-Lopez P, Hillel AT, Best SR, Bishop JA, Akst LM. Laryngeal dysplasia, demographics, and treatment: a single-institution, 20-year review. *JAMA Otolaryngol Head Neck Surg*. 2015;141:313–318.
5. Gale N, Hille J, Jordan RC, Nadal A, Williams MD. Precursor lesions. In: El-Naggar AK, Chan JKC, Grandis JR, Takata T, Slootweg PJ, eds. *WHO Classification of Head*

and Neck Tumors (4th ed). Lyon, France: International Agency for Research on Cancer; 2017.

6. Hillel AT, Johns MM 3rd, Hapner ER, Shah M, Wise JC, Klein AM. Voice outcomes from subligamentous cordectomy for early glottic cancer. *Ann Otol Rhinol Laryngol.* 2013;122:190–196.

7. Aaltonen L-M, Rihkanen H, Vaheri A. Human papillomavirus in larynx. *Laryngoscope.* 2002;112:700–707.

8. Bastian R. Benign vocal fold mucosal disorders. In: Flint PW, Haughey BH, Lund VJ, et al, eds, *Cummings Otolaryngology* (6th ed). Philadelphia, PA: Elsevier Saunders.

9. Ricci G, Molini E, Faralli M, Simoncelli C. Retrospective study on precancerous laryngeal lesions: long-term follow-up. *Acta Otorhinolaryngol Ital.* 2003;23:362–367.

10. Weller MD, Nankivell PC, McConkey C, Paleri V, Mehanna HM. The risk and interval to malignancy of patients with laryngeal dysplasia; a systematic review of case series and meta-analysis. *Clin Otolaryngol.* 2010;35(5): 364–372.

11. Gale N, Blagus R, El-Mofty SK, et al. Evaluation of a new grading system for laryngeal squamous intraepithelial lesions—a proposed unified classification. *Histopathology.* 2014;65:456–464.

12. Zhang HK, Liu HG. Is severe dysplasia the same lesion as carcinoma in situ? 10-year follow-up of laryngeal precancerous lesions. *Acta Otolaryngol.* 2012;132:325–328.

13. Sereg-Bahar M, Jerin A, Hocevar-Boltezar I. Higher levels of total pepsin and bile acids in the saliva as possible risk factor for early laryngeal cancer. *Radiol Oncol.* 2015;49: 59–64.

14. Altieri A, Garavello W, Bosetti C, Gallus S, La Vecchia C. Alcohol consumption and risk of laryngeal cancer. *Oral Oncol.* 2005;41:956–965.

15. Sadri M, McMahon J, Parker A. Laryngeal dysplasia: aetiology and molecular biology. *J Laryngol Otol.* 2006; 120:170–177.

16. Russell JO, Scharpf J. Premalignant and early malignant lesions of the larynx. In: Sataloff RT, Benninger MS, eds, *Sataloff's Comprehensive Textbook of Otolaryngology: Head & Neck Surgery: Laryngology* (Vol 4). New Delhi, India: Jaypee Brothers Medical Publishers; 2016.

17. Blackwell KE, Fu YS, Calcaterra TC. Laryngeal dysplasia. A clinicopathologic study. *Cancer.* 1995;75:457–463.

18. Bosman FT. Dysplasia classification: pathology in disgrace? *J Pathol.* 2001;194:143–144.

19. Johnson FL. Management of advanced premalignant laryngeal lesions. *Curr Opin Otolaryngol Head Neck Surg.* 2003;11:462–466.

20. Thompson LDR. Laryngeal dysplasia, squamous cell carcinoma, and variants. *Surg Pathol.* 2017;10:15–33.

21. Mondal D, Saha K, Datta C, Chatterjee U, Sengupta A. Ki67, p27 and p53 expression in squamous epithelial lesions of larynx. *Indian J Otolaryngol Head Neck Surg.* 2013;65:126–133.

22. Su C, Jia S, Liu H. Immunolocalization of CD163+ tumor-associated macrophages and symmetric proliferation of Ki-67 as biomarkers to differentiate new different grades of laryngeal dysplasia. *Am J Clin Pathol.* 2017;149:8–16.

23. Yoo WJ, Cho SH, Lee YS, et al. Loss of heterozygosity on chromosomes 3p,8p,9p and 17p in the progression of squamous cell carcinoma of the larynx. *J Korean Med Sci.* 2004;19:345–351.

24. Nadal A, Campo E, Pinto J, et al. p53 expression in normal, dysplastic, and neoplastic laryngeal epithelium. Absence of a correlation with prognostic factors. *J Pathol.* 1995;175:181–188.

25. Paleri V, Mackenzie K, Wight RG, Mehanna H, Pracy P, Bradley PJ; ENT-UK Head and Neck Group. Management of laryngeal dysplasia in the United Kingdom: a web-based questionnaire survey of current practice. *Clin Otolaryngol.* 2009;34:385–389.

26. Zeitels SM. Premalignant epithelium and microinvasive cancer of the vocal fold: the evolution of phonomicrosurgical management. *Laryngoscope.* 1995;105(3):1–51.

27. Johnson FL. Management of advanced premalignant laryngeal lesions. *Curr Opin Otolaryngol Head Neck Surg.* 2003;11:462–466.

28. Mehanna H, Paleri V, Robson A, Wight R, Helliwell T. Consensus statement by otorhinolaryngologists and pathologists on the diagnosis and management of laryngeal dysplasia. *Clin Otolaryngol.* 2010;35:170–176.

29. Kishimoto Y, Suzuki R, Kawai Y, Hiwatashi N, Kitamura M, Tateya I, Hirano S. Photocoagulation therapy for laryngeal dysplasia using angiolytic lasers. *Eur Arch Otorhinolaryngol.* 2016;273:1221–1225.

30. Zeitels SM, Akst LM, Burns JA, Hillman RE, Broadhurst MS, Anderson RR. Office-based 532-nm pulsed KTP laser treatment of glottal papillomatosis and dysplasia. *Ann Otol Rhinol Laryngol.* 2006;115(9):679–685.

31. Sengupta N, Morris CG, Kirwan J, Amdur RJ, Mendenhall WM. Definitive radiotherapy for carcinoma in situ of the true vocal cords. *Am J Clin Oncol.* 2010;33:94095.

32. Sheu M, Sridharan S, Kun M, et al. Multi-institutional experience with the in-office potassium titanyl phosphate laser for laryngeal lesions. *J Voice.* 2012;26:806–810.

33. Lerner MZ, Mor N, Paek H, Blitzer A, Strome M. Metformin prevents the progression of dysplasticmucosa of the head and neck to carcinoma in nondiabetic patients. *Ann Otol Rhinol Laryngol.* 2017;126:340–343.

34. Mesolella M, Iengo M, Testa D, Ricciardiello F, Iorio B. Chemoprevention using folic acid for dysplastic lesions of the larynx. *Mol Clin Oncol.* 2017;7:843–846.

35. Armstrong W, Vokes D, Verma S. Malignant tumors of the larynx. In: Flint PW, Haughey BH, Lund VJ, et al, eds, *Cummings Otolaryngology* (6th ed). Philadelphia, PA: Elsevier Saunders.

36. Mor N, Blitzer A. Functional anatomy and oncologic barriers of the larynx. *Otolaryngol Clin North Am.* 2015; 48(4):533–545.

37. Yang C, Andersen P, Everts E, Cohen J. Nodal disease in purely glottic carcinoma: is elective neck treatment worthwhile? *Laryngoscope.* 1998;108(7):1006–1008.

38. Pressman J, Dowdy A, Libby R, Fields M. Further studies upon the submucosal compartments and lymphatics of the larynx by the injection of dyes and radioisotopes. *Ann Otol Rhinol Laryngol.* 1956;65(4):963–980.

39. Marioni G, Marchese-Ragona R, Cartei G, Marchese F, Staffieri A. Current opinion in diagnosis and treatment of laryngeal carcinoma. *Cancer Treat Rev.* 2006;32(7):504–515.

40. Coca-Pelaz A, Rodrigo J, Takes R, et al. Relationship between reflux and laryngeal cancer. *Head Neck.* 2013;35(12): 1814–1818.

41. Erkul E, Yilmaz I, Narli G, Alparslan Babyigit M, Gungor A, Demirel D. The presence and prognostic significant of human papilloamvirus in squamous cell carcinoma of the larynx. *Eur Arch Otorhinolaryngol.* 2017;274: 2921–2926.

42. Shah J, Karnell L, Hoffman H, et al. Patterns of care for cancer of the larynx. *Arch Otolaryngol Head Neck Surg.* 1997;123:475–483.

43. Echanique K, Desai S, Marchino E, et al. Laryngeal verrucous carcinoma: a systemic review. *Otolaryngol Head Neck Surg.* 2017;156(1):38–45.

44. Veltman J, Van Weert I, Aubele M, et al. Specific steps in aneuploidization correlate with loss of heterozygostiy of 9p21, 17p13 and 18q21 in the progression of pre-malignant laryngeal lesions. *Int J Cancer.* 2001;91:193–199.

45. Rydzanicz M, Golusinski P, Mielcarek-Kuchta D, Golusinski W, Szyfter K. Cyclin D1 gene (CCND1) polymorphism and the risk of squamous cell carcinoma of the larynx. *Eur Arch Otorhinolaryngol.* 2006;263:43–48.

46. Khan M, Koyfman S, Reddy C, Saxton J. Definitive radiotherapy for early (T1-T2) glottic squamous cell carcinoma: a 20-year Cleveland Clinic experience. *Radiat Oncol.* 2012;7:193.

47. Nishimura G, Tsukuda M, Mikami Y, et al. Efficacy of concurrent chemoradiotherapy for T1 and T2 laryngeal squamous cell carcinoma regarding organ preservation. *Anticancer Res.* 2009;29(2):661–666.

48. Misono S, Merati A. Are patient-reported voice outcomes better after surgery or after radiation for treatment of T1 glottic carcinoma? *Laryngoscope.* 2011;121(3):461–462.

49. Ambrosch P. The role of laser microsurgery in the treatment of laryngeal cancer. *Curr Opin Otolaryngol Head Neck Surg.* 2007;15:82–88.

50. Zeitels S. Transoral and transcervical surgical innovations in the treatment of glottic cancer. *Otolaryngol Clin North Am.* 2015;48(4):677–685.

51. Remacle M, Eckel HE, Antonelli A, et al. Endoscopic cordectomy. A proposal for a classification by the Working Committee, European Laryngological Society. *Eur Arch Otorhinolaryngol.* 2000;257:227–231.

CHAPTER 27

Laryngeal Leukoplakia

Natasha Quraishi and Michael Petrou

LEUKOPLAKIA

Laryngeal leukoplakia may be defined as white lesions on the laryngeal mucosa. Traditionally this was considered to be due to abnormal keratosis in the squamous epithelial cells of the larynx.[1] However, more recently it has been found that leukoplakia is not always associated with keratosis.[2] It may vary in appearance from being clearly demarcated and exophytic (Figure 27–1) to being flat and diffuse (see Figure 27–4), which is partially related to the amount of keratin produced. Leukoplakia may seem speckled due to varying thickness of the surface keratin layer.[3]

Leukoplakia of the larynx was first described by Durant in 1880 as "white cicatrices" where it was seen next to laryngeal malignancy.[4] It was then Chevalier Jackson who in 1923 hypothesized on the "undoubted clinical fact that there is a class of morbid conditions in the larynx the cure of which will diminish the incidence of cancer," citing keratosis of the larynx as one such condition.[5]

Leukoplakia is a clinical manifestation of a number of different cellular processes such as dysplasia, metaplasia, carcinoma-in-situ (CIS), and squamous cell carcinoma (SCC) and benign conditions such as fungal infection. A meta-analysis by Isenberg et al showed that approximately 53.6% of biopsies of laryngeal leukoplakia were associated with no dysplasia, 33.5% were associated with mild or moderate dysplasia, and 15.2% were associated with severe dysplasia or SCC in situ.[6] Therefore while hyperkeratosis in the form of leukoplakia is often considered to be cause for concern as a premalignant lesion, it is not always associated with dysplasia at the time of biopsy.

Malignant conversion has been noted to occur in cases of leukoplakia with an overall conversion rate of

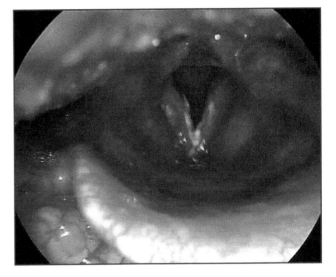

Figure 27–1. Laryngeal leukoplakia.

8.2%. Higher rates of progression to malignancy were noted in cases with more severe dysplasia. Although it would appear that almost half of cases involving laryngeal leukoplakia are not associated with dysplasia, this does not mean that these lesions do not have the potential to progress toward malignancy, with a conversion rate of 3.7% being seen in cases with no dysplasia.[6]

ERYTHROPLAKIA

Laryngeal erythroplakia denotes red lesions of the larynx (Figures 27–2 and 27–3), which are characterized by apparent increased vascularity in the form of dilated subepithelial vessels as well as thinner epithelium.[7] Like leukoplakia, erythroplakia is a clinical finding associated with the possibility of dysplasia or malignancy. It is believed to be more commonly associated with severe dysplasia, CIS, or invasive carcinoma[8] and therefore a higher risk of progression to malignancy, particularly in the anterior and posterior commissures of the larynx.[3] However, it should be noted that there is no rate of conversion in the literature of laryngeal erythroplakia, which appears to cite evidence relating to oral erythroplakia.[9,10] It has been suggested that laryngeal erythroplakia has been neglected due to possible confounding laryngeal erythema seen in patients who smoke.[1]

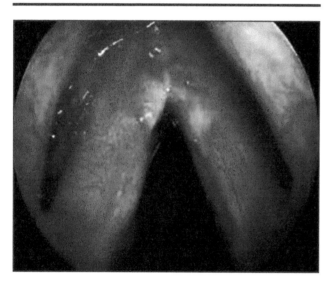

Figure 27–2. Laryngeal erythroplakia and leukoplakia.

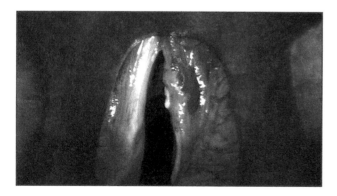

Figure 27–3. Laryngeal erythroplakia associated with an exophytic lesion.

RISK FACTORS FOR LARYNGEAL DYSPLASIA

As laryngeal dysplasia is considered part of the process of development of laryngeal carcinoma, the risk factors are the same:

- Tobacco smoking[11]
- Alcohol, particularly in combination with tobacco smoking[12–14]
- Geographic
- Lower socio-economic class
- Air pollution
- Asbestos
- Malnutrition
- Previous radiotherapy
- Laryngopharyngeal reflux (LPR)/ gastroesophageal reflux disease (GERD)

  - It has been proposed that LPR may cause laryngeal SCC,[15] but any direct etiological role requires further clarification[7]

- Human papilloma virus

  - Considered to be more of a risk factor for oropharyngeal rather than laryngeal malignancy[16,17]

EVOLVING CLASSIFICATION OF LARYNGEAL DYSPLASIA

Despite the apparent associations between leukoplakia and erythroplakia and the possibility of malignancy, as previously discussed, these are merely clinical manifestations of a variety of different degrees of dysplasia. Therefore, histopathology is essential in procuring a more definitive diagnosis.[3]

It is known that epithelial dysplasia incurs an increased risk of development of malignancy, in comparison with epithelium with no dysplasia. A meta-analysis by Weller and coworkers found the rate of transformation to malignancy to be 14% occurring over an average of 5.8 years.[18] Similarly it is also known that early recognition of preneoplastic changes confers better outcomes,[19] as greater severity of dysplasia is associated with a higher rate of conversion to malignancy.[18] There have been numerous attempts to grade dysplasia in a manner that may be used to indicate prognosis and risk of conversion to malignancy.

Box 1: Kleinsasser (1963)

The first such attempt at grading dysplasia was by Kleinsasser,[20] who proposed the following grades:

- Class 1: Squamous hyperplasia
- Class 2: Hyperplasia with atypia
- Class 3: Carcinoma-in-situ (CIS)

Box 2: Ljubljana (1971)

This was then followed by the Ljubljana classification, with the following grading:

- Simple hyperplasia (benign)
- Abnormal hyperplasia (benign)
- Atypical hyperplasia ("risky" epithelium)
- Carcinoma-in-situ (malignant)

Box 3: WHO (2005)

The World Health Organization attempted further definition in 2005:

- Squamous cell hyperplasia (increased cell numbers in basal layer of epithelium but no cell atypia)
- Mild dysplasia (cell atypia limited to lower third of epithelium)
- Moderate dysplasia (cell disturbance to middle third, prominent nucleoli but no abnormal mitoses)
- Severe dysplasia (atypia and cell disturbance high up in epithelium)
- Carcinoma-in-situ (full thickness architectural abnormalities, pronounced atypia, atypical mitotic figures, and abnormal mitoses)

Box 4: Amended Ljubljana (2014)

A new grading system for squamous intraepithelial lesions (SIL) was proposed by the European Working Group together with the American Working Group of pathologists to provide a unified classification that would be reproducible in terms of research and therapy.[21] It was termed the amended Ljubljana classification and is graded as follows:

- Low-grade SIL

  - Defined as "most often benign, with low malignant potential, and characterized by a spectrum of morphological changes ranging from a simple hyperplastic process with retention of the basal layer and an increased prickle cell layer, up to augmentation of basal and parabasal cells occupying up to the lower half of the epithelium, with the upper part remaining unchanged, containing regular prickle cells"

- High-grade SIL

  - Defined as "a potentially premalignant lesion, with ≥12% patients subsequently developing malignancy. Morphologically, it is characterized by a spectrum of changes, including augmentation of immature epithelial cells, which occupy the lower half or more of the epithelial thickness"

- Carcinoma-in-situ (CIS)

  - Defined as "lesions showing features of conventional carcinoma, e.g., structural and cellular abnormalities but without invasion (intraepithelial carcinoma)"

It was found to have improved interobserver agreement when used in the assessment of a set of SILs and was also shown to have prognostic value by demonstrating a significant difference in the risk of progression to malignancy between low-grade and high-grade SILs.[21] However, it should be noted that this does not appear to be consistently utilized across the UK.[22]

Box 5: WHO (2017)
In 2017, WHO proposed a new classification system based on the amended Ljubljana classification. This new system consisted of two tiers for diagnostic purposes (low-grade dysplasia/SIL and high-grade dysplasia/SIL) but may be changed to three tiers when considering treatment, with the third tier being derived when a distinction is made between high-grade dysplasia/SIL and carcinoma–in-situ (see below).[23]

- Low-grade dysplasia/SIL

  - (previous categories squamous hyperplasia, mild dysplasia)—low malignant potential—spectrum of morphological changes ranging from squamous hyperplasia to an augmentation of basal/parabasal cells, occupying up to the middle of the epithelial thickness, upper part unchanged

- High-grade dysplasia/SIL

  - (previous categories moderate and severe dysplasia, carcinoma-in-situ)— high malignant potential—spectrum of atypical epithelial cells, occupying at least lower epithelial half up to the whole epithelial thickness

- Carcinoma-in-situ

  - distinguished from high-grade dysplasia if three-tier system is used—showing features of conventional carcinoma, e.g., structural and cellular abnormalities but without invasion

This classification system may appear to show better interrater agreement than previous systems such as the 2005 WHO classification system; however, its reliability has been debated.[24]

MANAGEMENT OF LARYNGEAL DYSPLASIA

The management of laryngeal dysplasia is a balance between reduction of malignancy risk and preservation of vocal function. There is a broad range of choice regarding management of preneoplastic lesions of the larynx.[25] A survey in 2009 found considerable variation in practice in the UK.[26] This led to a UK consensus meeting of otolaryngologists and pathologists in 2010 where standards of practice were discussed. They advocated a multidisciplinary approach to management of premalignant laryngeal lesions, with further advice depending on the number of leukoplakic lesions and the degree of spread and methods of surgical management (described below).[27] This was supplanted by the most recent national guidance on head and neck cancer,[28] which advises:

- Management of leukoplakia is not informed by high-level evidence, but consensus supports targeted use of biopsy and histopathological assessment.
- The management of biopsy proven dysplastic lesions favors:

  - advice to reduce known environmental carcinogens such as tobacco and alcohol
  - surgical excision when the size of the lesions and the patient's function allows
  - long-term surveillance

They also advise that "management decisions should take account of the microscopic severity of the lesion and its clinically assessed extent."

Conservative

Management of risk factors for laryngeal malignancy, particularly management of smoking and LPR, is recommended.[27]

Surgical

Surgical management has traditionally been deemed the "treatment of choice."[29] It is generally recommended that excision be performed endoscopically via either sharp or "cold steel" excision or CO_2 laser resection, although it should be noted that the latter is discouraged due to inability to obtain biopsy specimens.[27] CO_2 lasers may be used in conjunction with micromanipulating scanning devices, which give greater precision and thus reduce the risk of local damage. Hydrodissection is an adjunctive technique that may assist in preservation of the vocal cords during cold steel resection. Vocal testing pre- and post-intervention is recommended.[7]

Other

Surgical management may not be appropriate in all cases for a number of reasons. Therefore, alternative modalities of treatment may be required.

Radiotherapy has been considered for treatment of widespread high grade lesions and shows greater local control rate (93.52%) in comparison with CO_2 laser excision (80.88%) and vocal cord stripping (77.37%).[30] It should be noted that vocal cord stripping is no longer recommended practice.[27] Radiotherapy may also be used for primary lesions that have not previously been treated. However, this is only in select cases—for example, where surgical management may be difficult and must be a multidisciplinary team decision given its implications, such as radiotherapy no longer being an option should the patient then develop carcinoma.[3,7]

Another developing treatment modality is photodynamic therapy, which has been used in the treatment of early laryngeal cancer.[29,31] Fiber-based pulsed dye lasers have also been suggested, particularly in the context of recurrent laryngeal procedures, although 532-nm pulsed potassium titanyl phosphate (KTP) laser may be a better alternative.[32,33] However, the CO_2 laser remains the laser type of choice in the UK.[27]

CASE

A 57-year-old gentleman presented to an ear, nose, and throat clinic having been referred by his general practitioner for a 7-month history of worsening hoarseness and sore throat. His past medical history included chronic obstructive pulmonary disorder (COPD) and GERD. He had newly been initiated on treatment for GERD and had recently self-medicated with levofloxacin for a presumed upper respiratory tract infection. His other regular medication included inhaled corticosteroids. He smoked an average of 40 cigarettes a day and drank approximately 12 units of alcohol a week.

On external examination of the head and neck, there were no findings of note. Oral cavity and oropharyngeal examinations were unremarkable. On examination with flexible nasendoscope (FNE), there were

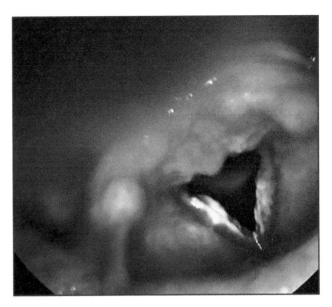

Figure 27–4. Bilateral laryngeal leukoplakia.

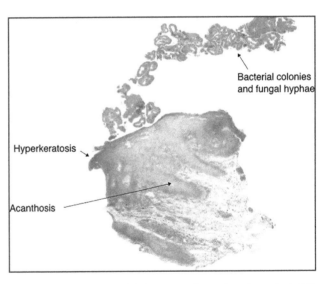

Figure 27–5. Biopsy with hemotoxylin and eosin stain (x40). Image courtesy of Consultant Pathologist Dr. Justin Weir.

white irregular plaques on both vocal cords with underlying erythema. The patient underwent microlaryngoscopy and biopsy due to the concern of possible malignancy. Appearances on microlaryngoscopy were consistent with the previous examination, once again showing bilateral leukoplakia (Figure 27–4).

A biopsy was taken and sent for histopathology. It showed hyperkeratosis and epithelial hyperplasia (Figure 27–5). The specimen was also tested for fungal infection and use of periodic acid–Schiff (PAS) stain

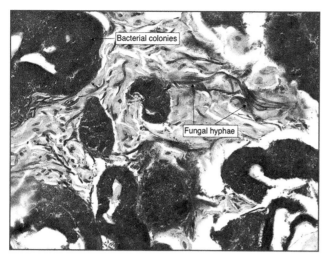

Figure 27–6. PAS stained sample (x400). Image courtesy of Consultant Pathologist Dr. Justin Weir.

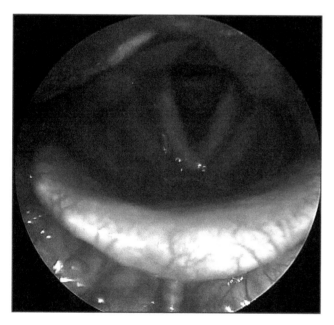

Figure 27–7. Laryngeal appearance after treatment with fluconazole.

revealed the presence of candidiasis and Gram-staining revealed the presence of bacteria (Figure 27–6).

The patient was advised on good hygiene while using his inhaler and to consult his general practitioner regarding changing his corticosteroid inhaler and smoking cessation. He was commenced on oral nystatin gel (10,000 units, four times daily) for 2 weeks.

At follow-up 2 weeks later, the patient reported no improvement in his symptoms. He was therefore commenced on oral fluconazole (200 mg daily for 2 weeks). One month later, the patient reported an improvement in his voice and that his pain had resolved. Repeat examination with FNE showed normal appearances of the larynx (Figure 27–7).

FUNGAL INFECTIONS OF THE LARYNX

Introduction

Fungal infections of the larynx may be focal affecting the vocal cords or larynx in isolation, or may be part of a systemic fungal disease. Fungal laryngitis is often noted within the context of a wider fungal infection of the upper respiratory tract. Isolated fungal laryngitis appears to be rare, although this may in part be attributed to poor recognition.[34–37]

The most common fungal pathogens are Candida, Aspergillus, Cryptococcus and Histoplasma. Usual presentation is with non-specific laryngeal and pharyngeal symptoms. A high index of suspicion is necessary to differentiate it from other pathologies such as laryngeal carcinoma. Management is dependent upon a number of factors, such as the presence of surface mucosal disease or invasive fungal disease, the knowledge as to whether the fungus is a yeast or a mold, and the immunodeficiency status of the patient.

Risk Factors

Fungal infection of the larynx has often been considered to be a disease of immunocompromised patients. However, there has been increasing recognition of fungal laryngitis in the immunocompetent as well. Therefore, it has been suggested that risk factors for fungal laryngitis may be categorized into two broad groups: immunocompetent patients and immunocompromised patients.

Risk factors for fungal laryngitis in immunocompetent patients include factors that affect the mucosal barrier. These may include GERD,[38] previous radiotherapy, inhaled corticosteroids, and prolonged antibiotic use. The latter is felt to cause fungal infection through alteration and suppression of mucosal flora.[34,39–41] Another group of risk factors for fungal laryngitis in immunocompetent patients are those which confer local trauma, such as intubation, smoking, and thermal injury.[42,43]

In contrast to this, risk factors of fungal infection of the larynx in patients with immunocompromise involve anything that may alter immune response such as diabetes mellitus, nutritional deficiency, immunodeficiency status, and immunosuppressive medication i.e., chemotherapy or corticosteroids.

Etiology

A variety of organisms have been found to cause fungal laryngitis, the most common being Candida, Aspergillus, Cryptococcus, Histoplasma, and Blastomyces. Other notable pathogens causing fungal infections of the larynx include *Coccidioides immitis*, *Paracoccidioides brasiliensis*, and Mucormycetes. More specifically, it has been suggested that yeasts such as Candida, Cryptococcus, Histoplasma, and Blastomyces are more likely to be implicated in primary laryngeal disease.[35]

Candidiasis

Candidiasis is an endogenous infection caused by the Candida species, which is a commensal organism of the oropharynx and the gastrointestinal and genital tracts.[44] Candida is typically opportunistic, causing infection in patients who are immunocompromised, those on long-term antibiotics, or surgical patients (Figure 27–8).[34,35] Between 1968 and 2005, there were 14 cases

of isolated laryngeal candidiasis reported in the literature.[44] Candida may affect the glottis, the supraglottis, or the hypopharynx.[45]

Aspergillosis

Aspergillosis is an infection caused by the Aspergillus species, typically *Aspergillus fumigatus* (Figures 27–9 and 27–10) or *Aspergillus flavus* (Figure 27–11).[46] Aspergillus is ubiquitous, found in soil, vegetable matter, and decaying matter across the world.[47] Transmission is via airborne spores, particularly during demolition of old buildings.[46] However, the larynx is usually resistant to aspergillosis, despite the abundance of spores.[47,48] Laryngeal aspergillosis commonly occurs due to pulmonary aspergillosis.[47] Aspergillosis of the larynx in the context of wider infection such as invasive Aspergillus tracheobronchitis, appears to be extremely rare, with only 3 cases reported in literature.[49] Isolated laryngeal aspergillosis also appears to be rare, with less than 50 cases being reported in the literature.[39]

Like candidiasis, aspergillosis is often considered to be an opportunistic infection occurring in immunocompromised patients.[34,35,46] There have been 14 to 22 such cases in patients who were immunocompetent.[39,47]

Cryptococcus

Cryptococcus neoformans is an encapsulated yeast found in the fecal matter of pigeons, fruit, and vegetables and soil all over the world that can cause pulmonary infection through inhalation (Figure 27–12).[50–52] Like

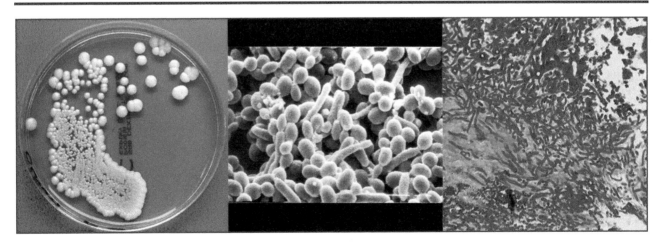

Figure 27–8. *Candida albicans*, culture, left, culture scanning electron microscopy also showing Germ tubes, middle, and from tissue biopsy, right.

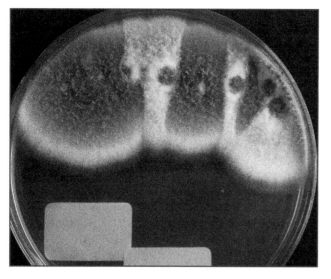

Figure 27–9. *Aspergillus fumigatus* from a respiratory specimen. Note the different types of colonial morphology.

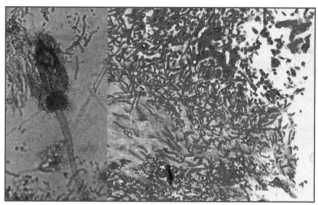

Figure 27–10. *Aspergillus fumigatus* from culture, left and from tissue biopsy, right.

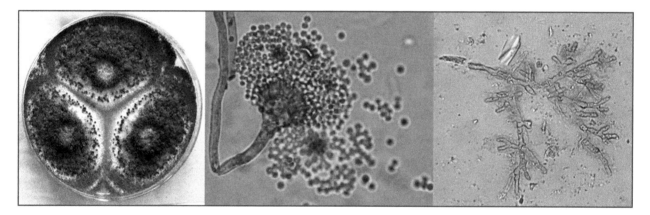

Figure 27–11. *Aspergillus flavus*, culture, left, culture microscopy, middle, and from tissue biopsy, right.

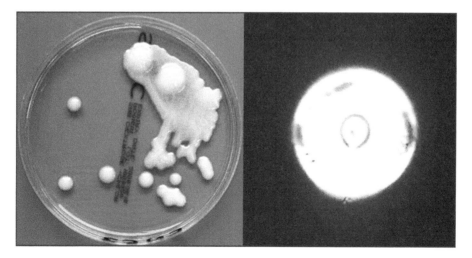

Figure 27–12. *Cryptococcus neoformans* in culture and as seen with india ink microscopy from a CSF.

other organisms causing mycotic laryngitis, Cryptococcus can affect both the immunocompromised and the immunocompetent.[51] The latter are mostly infected by *Cryptococcus gattii*, found mainly in trees and thought to account for 70 to 80% of cryptococcal infections.[50,53] The distribution of *Cryptococcus gattii* is across tropical and subtropical regions including South America and Australia; however, it has been isolated in many other parts of the world.[12,51] In contrast to this, *Cryptococcus neoformans* is believed to be an opportunistic infection affecting the immunocompromised.[54] It is estimated that approximately 17–23 cases of cryptococcal laryngitis have been reported in the literature.[51,52,54]

Histoplasmosis

Histoplasmosis, also known as Cave disease, Darling's disease, Ohio Valley disease, reticuloendotheliosis, Spelunker's lung, and Caver's disease, is an infection by *Histoplasma capsulatum*, an endemic dimorphic fungus (ie, a fungus that can be found in specific areas around the globe and exists in two forms: mould in nature <30 °C and yeast during infection; Figures 27–13 and 27–14).[55,56] *Histoplasma capsulatum* is typically found in acidic soil with high nitrogen content. Bird and bat droppings improve sporulation of *Histoplasma capsulatum*, and thus raise its growth rate.[55] Transmission, like most molds, is usually through fungal spore inha-

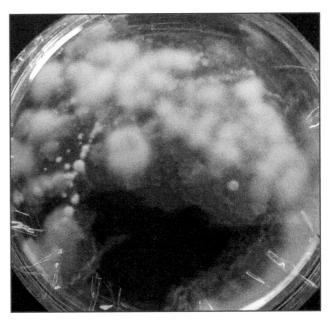

Figure 27–14. *Histoplasma capsulatum* 30°C culture.

lation.[56] It has been estimated that less than 100 cases of laryngeal histoplasmosis have been reported in the literature.[57]

Blastomycosis

Blastomycosis is infection caused by *Blastomyces dermatitidis*, which is an endemic dimorphic fungus that is commonly found in decaying matter such as wood. It is transmitted through the inhalation of fungal spores. Blastomycosis of the larynx may occur although it may be through primary infection rather than through hematogenous spread from pulmonary infection.[58]

PRESENTATION

Symptoms

Fungal laryngitis commonly manifests with nonspecific laryngeal and pharyngeal symptoms. These typically range from hoarseness, dysphagia, dysphonia, odynophagia, and cough to signs of airway compromise such as stridor and respiratory distress.[59] Of all these symptoms regardless of causative pathogen, hoarseness appears to be the most frequent, with a variable duration (typically over months).[44,49,52,59] It is

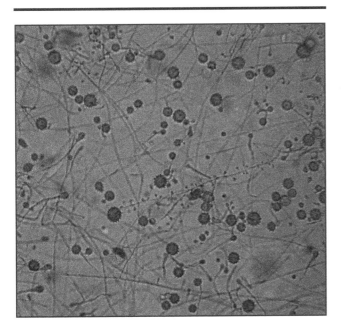

Figure 27–13. *Histoplasma capsulatum* microconidia, chlamydospores from a 30°C culture.

interesting to note that while inhaled corticosteroids are considered to be a risk factor for fungal laryngitis which causes hoarseness, they may also cause hoarseness themselves by inducing laryngeal inflammation.[60]

Patients may have systemic symptoms such as fever, malaise, and weight loss.[55-57,61] Laryngotracheal mucormycosis was also noted to be associated with headache, facial pain, dyspnea, and hemoptysis.[61,62]

Signs

The pattern of oral with laryngopharyngeal fungal infection is easy to recognize. Typically signs of isolated fungal laryngitis are best appreciated via flexible or stroboscopic laryngoscopy.[44] The most commonly reported findings on examination regardless of causative pathogen are leukoplakia and exophytic growth on one or both vocal cords.[39,44,52,54,55-57,61] Ulcerated lesions of the vocal cords have also been reported, particularly in cases of laryngeal aspergillosis and histoplasmosis.[39,55,56] There may also be more diffuse features such as laryngeal edema and erythema.[44,52,54,55,61] Pseudomembranes across the vocal cords have also been noted in cases of laryngeal candidiasis and histoplasmosis.[44,59]

LEUKOPLAKIA IN FUNGAL INFECTION

It is important to understand the way a microorganism can achieve colonization, particularly of a sterile site, and formation of a thick film seen as leukoplakia.

When bacteria, yeasts, and fungal spores enter the body of a host, they must adhere to cells of a tissue surface, usually epithelial cells. In the respiratory tract, a film of mucus covers the surface and is constantly being driven upward by ciliated cells toward the natural orifices. Therefore, if the microorganisms did not adhere, they would be swept away by mucus and other fluids that bathe the tissue surface and dispose of them. Adherence, which is only one step in the infectious process, is followed by the development of microcolonies, also called biofilms, and subsequent steps in the pathogenesis of infection.

The interactions between bacteria and tissue cell surfaces in the adhesion process are complex. For some microorganisms, the first step in infection is their attachment to surface epithelial cells by means of adhesive surface proteins. Several factors play important roles, including surface hydrophobicity and net surface charge, binding molecules on the microorganism and host cell receptor interactions. Microorganisms, such as bacteria, yeast, and fungal spores, and host cells commonly have net negative surface charges and therefore repulsive electrostatic forces. These forces are overcome by hydrophobic and other more specific interactions between microorganisms and host cells—in general, the more hydrophobic the microorganisms' cell surface, the greater the adherence to the host cell. Different strains of bacteria within a species and the spores of fungi (Aspergillus spores are highly hydrophobic) may vary widely in their hydrophobic surface properties and ability to adhere to host cells and this might explain why so few fungi manage to attach to the respiratory tract surfaces.

After adherence occurs, conformational changes in the host cell ensue that can lead to cytoskeletal changes allowing organism uptake by the cell. Bacterial and yeast biofilms may or may not invade deep into the tissue, whereas the molds after spore germination will penetrate with destructive force that varies according to the fungus; the greater damage is caused by Mucormycetes.

Sometimes changes in the adhesin molecule after attachment may trigger activation of virulence genes that promote invasion or result in other pathogenic changes (seen primarily with bacteria); however, if the cells have immunoglobulin A antibody on their surfaces—a host resistance mechanism—attachment may be prevented; some microorganisms can overcome this resistance mechanism by breaking down the antibody with a protease.

The mucociliary apparatus for removal of bacteria, yeasts, and fungal spores in the respiratory tract is also aided by the pulmonary macrophages. Special protective mechanisms in the respiratory tract include the hairs at the nares and the cough reflex, which prevents aspiration. Saliva contains numerous hydrolytic enzymes, thus a microorganism that manages to adhere to the oral mucosa and forms a biofilm for protection will be killed when it is detached from the biofilm.

It must be remembered that most mucous membranes, such as those of the oral cavity, carry a constant normal microbiota that itself opposes establishment of pathogenic microorganisms ("bacterial interference") and has important protective and physiologic functions.

Fungal infections can be divided into endogenous and exogenous. Endogenous are those fungi, like Candida spp., that are part of the normal microflora of humans, whereas exogenous are fungi acquired from the environment, primarily by inhalation, such as Aspergillus, Mucormycetes, and many others.

Fungi must also be viewed as yeasts and molds, as these are the morphologies in which they are encountered in nature and during infection. There are, however, fungi that can exist both as yeast and as mold depending on the growth conditions and are known as dimorphic fungi. The majority of the dimorphic fungi are classified as Biological Safety Level 3, as they are primary or true pathogens. Dimorphic fungi are also called endemic fungi, as their distribution is restricted to specific geographical areas.

DIAGNOSIS

Diagnosis of fungal laryngitis is often influenced by history and examination. As previously discussed, a common risk factor is being immunocompromised, the presence of which may make diagnosis easier. However, given that fungal laryngitis may arise in immunocompetent patients, a higher level of suspicion is required in this population of patients. This is further confounded by the common examination findings described above, which cause consideration of important differentials such as laryngeal malignancy, tuberculosis, and other granulomatous conditions, particularly in cases of isolated laryngeal disease in comparison to cases where laryngeal involvement forms part of more disseminated disease with oropharyngeal involvement. Therefore, definitive diagnosis of fungal laryngitis relies on further investigations, such as culture, tissue biopsy, or fungal staining, to provide proof of fungal spores, hyphae, or pseudohyphae. In some cases, fungal laryngitis has only been diagnosed following tissue biopsy and fungal staining.[34]

Regardless of causative pathogen, histopathology characteristically demonstrates hyperkeratosis, epithelial hyperplasia, neutrophils present in upper epithelial layers, plasma cells, lymphocytes, and submucosal stromal scarring. This typical appearance of fungal laryngitis is known as "pseudoepitheliomatous hyperplasia."[43,59] These appearances may be difficult to distinguish from preneoplastic lesions and carcinoma.[44]

A number of fungal stains may be utilized to identify the causative pathogen. For example, aspergillosis may be identified through hematoxylin and eosin staining which reveals hyphae characterized by being basophilic, narrow (3 to 6 μm), and regularly septate. The hyphae show regular, progressive, and dichotomous branching that will develop at acute angles from the parental hypha. Other types of stains that may aid diagnosis include methenamine silver staining, in which fungi appear black and PAS staining, where they appear magenta.[47] Gomori methenamine silver stain and mucicarmine stain have also been used in the identification of Cryptococcus.[54]

It has been suggested that galactomannan assay for Aspergillus and respiratory secretion cultures for all fungi may also be used to aid diagnosis in situations where biopsy is not possible.[49]

MANAGEMENT

Conservative

Given the common differential of malignancy and the fact that fungal laryngitis may have serious consequences such as destruction of the vocal cords and further dissemination resulting in more severe invasive disease, conservative management of fungal laryngitis is not a treatment option. Alongside active management detailed below, optimization of risk factors is recommended, such as review of inhaled corticosteroids and consultation with the appropriate specialist for possible alternatives or possible reduction of immunosuppressive medication where appropriate.[54]

Medical

In addition to removal of risk factors as discussed above, antifungal agents are the mainstay of medical management of fungal laryngitis. The choice of agent and route is dependent on a number of factors. Topical nystatin is mentioned in the literature to be considered as possible topical treatment in superficial candidiasis infections or in patients who are immunocompetent.[43,44,59] Nystatin oral gel works by direct contact and has no systemic action. In patients with a normal swallow it will be swallowed past the glottis with no treatment effect on the vocal cords.[63] Furthermore, once the patients wash the mouth or eat and drink, nystatin concentration in the oral cavity will be negligible, as the drug does not adhere to the cells of the oral cavity. Review of the literature suggests that systemic antifungals such as oral azoles and triazoles appear to be the preferred choice of management for fungal laryngitis, being deemed the "first line of treatment."[42] Systemic antifungals are further indicated in more severe and disseminated infection and in immunocompromised patients. Choice of systemic antifungals varies depending upon the causative organism.

Fluconazole, itraconazole, or ketoconazole may be considered with an escalation to intravenous amphotericin B in cases of laryngeal candidiasis particularly in the immunocompromised.[40,44,46] It is worth mentioning that oral ketoconazole, which has been used by millions for over four decades, is no longer available in Europe and the USA as there are equivalent and safer alternatives. Voriconazole is recommended for cases of invasive aspergillosis by the Infectious Diseases Society of America and the American Thoracic Society, highlighting the need to know the nature of the fungal pathogen.[64] Once again, escalation from this may be to options including liposomal amphotericin B, an echinocandin, and combination therapy.[49]

Cryptococcal laryngitis appears to resolve frequently with medical management alone. The Infectious Diseases Society of America provides guidance for management of cryptococcal infection based on a number of variables, such as whether the patient is immunocompromised and whether there is meningeal infection as well. They advise fluconazole (400 mg once a day for 6 to 12 months) for immunocompetent and immunocompromised patients with nonmeningeal disease and without cryptococcemia.[51,52,65] Similarly to previous mycotic pathogens, histoplasmosis may also be treated with systemic antifungals such as fluconazole, itraconazole, and ketoconazole, although intravenous amphotericin B is also favored.[46,56,66] Blastomycosis may also be treated with oral itraconazole over a long period of time or liposomal amphotericin B.[46,47]

It should be noted that all the aforementioned antifungal agents are associated with a risk of adverse effects on the liver, and at-risk patients should have their liver function assessed both prior to and during treatment. Both fluconazole and ketoconazole have been associated with transaminitis and subsequent jaundice. Itraconazole may cause hepatocellular and cholestatic injury; however, the drug has excellent activity against yeasts, including Candida and Cryptococcus, as well as molds such as Aspergillus and the Mucormycetes. Amphotericin B may cause renal failure, whereas hepatocellular injury appears to be rare.[67]

Surgical

One aspect of surgical management in fungal laryngitis is the need for tracheostomy in situations of airway obstruction.[51] However, in general, surgery is utilized where there is concern (and possibly misdiagnosis) of malignancy or where there has been a lack of response to medical management in order to prevent further dissemination of fungal disease and possible necrosis.[34,44,46] This may be in the form of "cold-steel" endoscopic removal of any masses or endoscopic polypectomy.[34,54] There may be a need for debridement of necrotic tissue such as in cases of mucormycosis.[61]

There is also the possibility of laser resection in the surgical management of fungal laryngitis. Potassium titanyl phosphate (KTP) laser ablation has been utilized in the management of cryptococcal laryngitis refractory to medical management.[51]

DISCUSSION

Isolated fungal infection of the larynx appears to be rare, with relatively few cases reported in the literature. However, it is interesting to note that there is a possibility of underdiagnosis for a number of reasons. One reason may be that both on examination with laryngoscope and on histopathology, fungal laryngitis appears to mimic laryngeal dysplasia or carcinoma. There have been cases where patients have been treated for malignancy before the definitive diagnosis of fungal etiology has been found.[34]

Another possible cause for lack of recognition of fungal infection of the larynx is that traditionally fungal laryngitis, alongside many other mycotic infections, has been associated with immunocompromised patients, with causative pathogens being viewed as "opportunistic." Therefore, diagnosis of fungal laryngitis in immunocompetent patients may have been missed. There is increasingly a greater understanding of the possible risk factors contributing to fungal infection of the larynx in such patients. Clinicians should therefore maintain a high degree of suspicion for fungal laryngeal infection regardless of the patient's immunodeficiency status.

Improved recognition and understanding of fungal laryngitis is ultimately beneficial to the patient given the potentially devastating consequences of untreated fungal infection which may have local destructive effects as well as causing disseminated fungal infection. Early diagnosis may also mean that the patient requires only medical management. While surgical management is possible and has been associated with relatively favorable outcomes, evidence for some methods is based on a small number of cases.[51]

Better understanding and recognition of fungal laryngitis may also be of benefit as possible risk factors for fungal infection of the larynx in both immunocompetent and immunocompromised individuals increase in prevalence.[64]

CONCLUSION

In cases of isolated laryngeal leukoplakia, where the patient is immunocompetent but has a number of risk factors for laryngeal dysplasia or malignancy, one must explore and investigate this etiology in the first instance. The fact remains that fungi are a rare but important class of pathogens that may cause laryngitis and leukoplakia. Isolated fungal infections of the larynx are very rare. The apparently low incidence of fungal laryngitis may be related to underdiagnosis, particularly in immunocompetent individuals. Similarly, diagnosis may be delayed in cases where there has been a misdiagnosis of malignancy on the basis of a laryngeal lesion associated with premalignancy. While methods for definitive diagnosis may be relatively simple, a high degree of suspicion is required for consideration of fungal laryngitis. In patients with an increased risk of fungal infections, one can consider a 1- to 2-week trial of a drug such as fluconazole or itraconazole if a mold is suspected, especially if there is no evidence of an invasive laryngeal neoplasm. This short delay is unlikely to alter the treatment outcome for patients with an eventual diagnosis of high-grade dysplasia. Timely treatment of a fungal infection will reduce the risk of serious adverse consequences for the patients.

REFERENCES

1. Bouquot, JE, Gnepp DR. Laryngeal precancer: a review of the literature, commentary, and comparison with oral leukoplakia. *Head Neck*. 1991;13(6):488–497.
2. Frangez I, Gale N, Luzar B. The interpretation of leukoplakia in laryngeal pathology. *Acta Otolaryngol Suppl*. 1997;527:142–144.
3. Gale N, Zidar N, Paljak M, Cardesa A. Current views and perspectives on classification of squamous intraepithelial lesions of the head and neck. *Head Neck Pathol*. 2014;8(1):16–23.
4. Durant G. Case of cancer of the larynx. *Arch Otolaryngol*. 1880;1:61–62.
5. Jackson C. Cancer of the larynx: is it preceded by a recognizable precancerous condition? *Ann Surg*. 1923;77(1):1–14.
6. Isenberg J, Crozier D, Dailey S. Institutional and comprehensive review of laryngeal leukoplakia. *Ann Otol Rhinol Laryngol*. 2008;117(1):74–79.
7. Ahmed J, Ghufoor K. Premalignant lesions of the larynx. In: Battacharyya A, ed, *Otorhinolaryngology–Head and Neck Surgery Series*. Noida, Uttar Pradesh: Thieme Medical and Scientific Publishers; 2014.
8. Wenig BM. Squamous cell carcinoma of the upper aerodigestive tract: precursors and problematic variants. *Mod Pathol*. 2002;15(3):229–254.
9. Mashberg A, Feldman L. Clinical criteria for identifying early oral and oropharyngeal carcinoma: erythroplasia revisited. *Am J Surg*. 1988;156(4):273–275.
10. Amagasa T, Yamashiro M, Uzawa N. Oral premalignant lesions: from a clinical perspective. *Int J Clin Oncol*. 2011;16(1):5–14.
11. Polesel J, et al. Tobacco smoking and the risk of upper aero-digestive tract cancers: A reanalysis of case-control studies using spline models. *Int J Cancer*. 2008;122(10):2398–2402.
12. Maier H, Tisch M. Epidemiology of laryngeal cancer: results of the Heidelberg case-control study. *Acta Otolaryngol Suppl*. 1997;527:160–164.
13. Talamini R, et al. Combined effect of tobacco and alcohol on laryngeal cancer risk: a case–control study. *Cancer Causes Control*. 2002;13(10):957–964.
14. Hashibe M, et al. Interaction between tobacco and alcohol use and the risk of head and neck cancer: pooled analysis in the International Head and Neck Cancer Epidemiology Consortium. *Cancer Epidemiol Biomarkers Prev*. 2009;18(2):541–550.
15. Olson N. The effects of stomach acid on the larynx. *Proc Am Laryngol Assoc*. 1983(104):108–112.
16. Hobbs CG, et al. Human papillomavirus and head and neck cancer: a systematic review and meta-analysis. *Clin Otolaryngol*. 2006;31(4):259–266.
17. Lewis JS, et al. Transcriptionally-active high-risk human papillomavirus is rare in oral cavity and laryngeal/hypopharyngeal squamous cell carcinomas—a tissue microarray study utilizing E6/E7 mRNA in situ hybridization. *Histopathology*. 2012;60(6):982–991.
18. Weller MD, et al. The risk and interval to malignancy of patients with laryngeal dysplasia; a systematic review of case series and meta-analysis. *Clin Otolaryngol*. 2010;35(5):364–372.
19. Ferlito A, et al. What is the earliest non-invasive malignant lesion of the larynx? *ORL J Otorhinolaryngol Relat Spec*. 2000;62(2):57–59.
20. Kleinsasser O, The classification and differential diagnosis of epithelial hyperplasia of the laryngeal mucosa on the basis of histomorphological features. II. *Z Laryngol Rhinol Otol*. 1963;42:339–362.
21. Gale N, Blagus R, El-Mofty SK, et al. Evaluation of a new grading system for laryngeal squamous intraepithelial lesions—a proposed unified classification. *Histopathology*. 2014;65(4):456–464.

22. Helliwell TR, Giles T. Pathological aspects of the assessment of head and neck cancers: United Kingdom National Multidisciplinary Guidelines. *J Laryngol Otol.* 2016;130(S2):S59–S65.

23. Gale N, Poljak M, Zidar N. Update from the 4th edition of the World Health Organization classification of head and neck tumours: what is new in the 2017 WHO blue book for tumours of the hypopharynx, larynx, trachea and parapharyngeal space. *Head Neck Pathol.* 2017;11(1):23–32.

24. Mehlum CS, Larsen SR, Kiss K, et al. Laryngeal precursor lesions: interrater and intrarater reliability of histopathological assessment. *Laryngoscope.* 2018; 128:2375-2379.

25. Ferlito A, et al. Squamous epithelial changes of the larynx: diagnosis and therapy. *Head Neck.* 2012;34(12):1810–6.

26. Paleri V, et al. Management of laryngeal dysplasia in the United Kingdom: a Web–based questionnaire survey of current practice. *Clin Otolaryngol.* 2009;34(4):385–389.

27. Mehanna H, et al. Consensus statement by otorhinolaryngologists and pathologists on the diagnosis and management of laryngeal dysplasia. *Clin Otolaryngol.* 2010; 35(3):170–176.

28. Shaw R, Beasley N. Etiology and risk factors for head and neck cancer: United Kingdom National Multidisciplinary Guidelines. *J Laryngol Otol.* 2016;130(S2):S9–S12.

29. Panwar A, Lindau R, Wieland A. Management of premalignant lesions of the larynx. *Expert Rev Anticancer Ther.* 2013; 13(9):1045–1051.

30. Sadri M, McMahon J, Parker A. Management of laryngeal dysplasia: a review. *Eur Arch Otorhinolaryngol,* 2006; 263:843-852.

31. Biel MA. Photodynamic therapy of head and neck cancers. *Methods Mol Biol.* 2010;635:281–293.

32. Koufman JA, et al. Office-based laryngeal laser surgery: a review of 443 cases using three wavelengths. *Otolaryngol Head Neck Surg.* 2007;137(1):146–151.

33. Zeitels SM, et al. Office-based 532-nm pulsed KTP laser treatment of glottal papillomatosis and dysplasia. *Ann Otol Rhinol Laryngol.* 2006;115(9):679–685.

34. Mäkitie AA, et al. Fungal infection of the epiglottis simulating a clinical malignancy. *Arch Otolaryngol Head Neck Surg.* 2003. 129(1):124–126.

35. Vrabec DP. Fungal infections of the larynx. *Otolaryngol Clin North Am.* 1993;26(6):1091–1114.

36. Bolivar R, et al. Aspergillus epiglottitis. *Cancer.* 1983;51(2):367–370.

37. Richardson BE, Morrison VA, Gapany M, Invasive aspergillosis of the larynx: case report and review of the literature. *Otolaryngol Head Neck Surg.* 1996;114(3):471–473.

38. Forrest LA, Weed H. Candida laryngitis appearing as leukoplakia and GERD. *J Voice.* 1998;12(1):91–95.

39. Saha A, Saha K, Chatterjee U. Primary aspergillosis of vocal cord: long-term inhalational steroid use can be the miscreant. *Biomed J.* 2015;38(6):550–553.

40. Neuenschwander MC, et al. Laryngeal candidiasis. *Ear Nose Throat J.* 2001;80(3):138–139.

41. Gleeson M, Scott-Brown W. *Scott-Brown's Otorhinolaryngology, Head and Neck Surgery.* CRC Press, Boca Raton, FL, 2008.

42. Mehanna HM, et al. Fungal laryngitis in immunocompetent patients. *J Laryngol Otol.* 2004;118(5):379–381.

43. Ravikumar A, et al. Fungal laryngitis in immunocompetent patients. *Indian J Otolaryngol Head Neck Surg.* 2014; 66(suppl 1):375–378.

44. Sulica, L., Laryngeal thrush. *Ann Otol Rhinol Laryngol.* 2005;114(5):369–375.

45. Wong KK, et al. Laryngeal candidiasis in the outpatient setting. *J Otolaryngol Head Neck Surg.* 2009;38(6):624–627.

46. Turner AL. Logan Turner's diseases of the nose, throat and ear: head and neck surgery.11th edition. 2016: CRC Press. Boca Raton, FL.

47. Gangopadhyay M, et al. Invasive primary aspergillosis of the larynx presenting as hoarseness and a chronic nonhealing laryngeal ulcer in an immunocompetent host: a rare entity. *Ear Nose Throat J.* 2014;93(7):265–268.

48. Fairfax A, David V, Douce G. Laryngeal aspergillosis following high dose inhaled fluticasone therapy for asthma. *Thorax.* 1999;54(9):860–861.

49. Barry ME, et al. Invasive aspergillus laryngotracheobronchitis in an adult with primary cns lymphoma. *Mycopathologia.* 2017;182(7–8):733–737.

50. Levitz S. The ecology of Cryptococcus neoformans and the epidemiology of cryptococcosis. *Rev Infect Dis.* 1991; 13(6):1163–1169.

51. Jeng JY, et al. Laryngeal cryptococcosis: Literature review and guidelines for laser ablation of fungal lesions. *Laryngoscope.* 2016;126(7):1625–1629.

52. Ihenachor E, Dewan K, Chhetri D. Pulsed dye laser treatment of primary cryptococcal laryngitis: a novel approach to an uncommon disease. *Am J Otolaryngol.* 2016; 37(6):572–574.

53. Mittal N, et al. Cryptococcal infection of the larynx: case report. *J Laryngol Otol.* 2013;127(suppl 2):S54–S56.

54. Lu X, Wang Q, Xiao S. Laryngeal cryptococcus infection: Literature review and a case study. *Int J Clin Exp Med.* 2016;9(9):18632–18636.

55. Ansari HA, Saeed N, Khan N, Hasan N. Laryngeal histoplasmosis. *BMJ Case Rep.* 2016. doi: 10.1136/bcr-2016-216423

56. Teoh J, Hassan F, Mohamad Yunus M. Laryngeal histoplasmosis: an occupational hazard. *Singapore Med J.* 2013;54(10):e208–e210.

57. Elias A, et al. Case report: histoplasmosis: first autochthonous case from Israel. *Am J Trop Med Hyg.* 2018;98(1):278–280.

58. Witorsch P, Utz J. North American blastomycosis: a study of 40 patients. *Medicine (Baltimore).* 1968;47(3):169–200.

59. Swain S, Nahak B, Sahu M. Fungal laryngitis in asthmatic boy treated with inhalatory corticosteroids: a case report. *Polish Annals of Medicine.* 2017;23(2):161–164.

60. Chmielewska M, Akst L. Dysphonia associated with the use of inhaled corticosteroids. *Curr Opin Otolaryngol Head Neck Surg.* 2015;23(3):255–259.

61. Mattioni J, et al. Laryngotracheal mucormycosis: report of a case. *Ear Nose Throat J*. 2016;95(1):29–39.

62. Alkan S, et al. Coexistence of laryngeal mucormycosis with retropharyngeal abscess causing acute upper airway obstruction. *J Otolaryngol Head Neck Surg*. 2008;37(3): E73–E75.

63. Kornblut A. An evolution of therapy for mucocutaneous candidiasis. *Laryngoscope*. 1980;90(7 Pt 2 Suppl 22):1–30.

64. Walsh TJ, et al. Treatment of aspergillosis: clinical practice guidelines of the Infectious Diseases Society of America. *Clin Infect Dis*. 2008;46(3):327–360.

65. Perfect JR, et al. Clinical practice guidelines for the management of cryptococcal disease: 2010 update by the Infectious Diseases Society of America. *Clin Infect Dis*. 2010;50(3):291–322.

66. Wheat LJ, et al. Clinical practice guidelines for the management of patients with histoplasmosis: 2007 update by the Infectious Diseases Society of America. *Clin Infect Dis*. 2007;45(7):807–825.

67. Zimmerman HJ, Hepatotoxicity: *The Adverse Effects of Drugs and Other Chemicals on the Liver. 2nd ed.* 1999: Lippincott Williams & Wilkins.

CHAPTER 28

Irradiated Larynx and Voice Issues

Timothy M. McCulloch and Matthew R. Hoffman

Radiation is a common primary or adjuvant treatment for head and neck cancer, including laryngeal and non-laryngeal primary tumors. For T1 glottic cancers, radiation alone is an effective treatment, with curative rates exceeding 90%.[1-3] Some providers prefer a primary radiation approach for T1 and T2 lesions, citing a potentially superior voice outcome.[4-6] However, it is important to realize that radiation has deleterious effects on the larynx and voice. Potential laryngeal side effects from radiation include thyroarytenoid muscle atrophy, mucosal dryness, and fibrosis.[7] These changes can result in short- and long-term dysphonia characterized by breathiness, increased vocal effort, strain, and impaired quality of life.[7-10] Treatment of non-laryngeal primary tumors can also result in levels of radiation exposure capable of impairing laryngeal function.[11-13] In this chapter, we review the effects of radiation on the larynx and voice production and discuss a management approach which can be applied to this patient population.

CASE PRESENTATION #1

A 68-year-old female with history of left T1aN0 squamous cell carcinoma of the left true vocal fold underwent primary radiotherapy (68 Gy) and completed treatment about 2 months ago (Figure 28–1A). She presents for scheduled oncologic surveillance and would also like to discuss her voice. She describes increased effort with voice production, difficulty with projection and communicating via telephone, and fear that her voice could drop out at any moment. She participated in voice therapy for a few sessions during her radiation course, but was limited by discomfort and dryness. She is worried about potential for persistent cancer.

Social history: 40 pack/year smoking history, quit a few years ago; four caffeinated beverages daily

Medications: Alendronate, calcium, vitamin D

On exam, there was significant glottic and subglottic edema, blunting of the vallecular spaces, and evidence of an anterior glottic web (Figure 28–1B). She was treated with a short course of oral steroids and antibiotics. At additional follow-up visits, she exhibited recovery of the acute radiation changes and did not show any recurrence. At 1-year follow-up visit she exhibited persistent mild dysphonia with slight strain and roughness, but good endurance. Her laryngeal exam showed persistence of the anterior glottic web and stable mild supraglottic edema.

Management: Vocal hygiene, including hydration and limitation of caffeine intake, is discussed. Voice therapy is provided including resonance voice therapy, straw therapy, and stretch and flow therapy. The anterior glottic web is relatively small and should be observed. The Reflux Symptom Index (RSI)[14] is administered to evaluate for any laryngopharyngeal reflux. If laryngopharyngeal reflux is present, lifestyle modifications are recommended, including avoiding eating or alcohol for 3 hours before bedtime and elevation of the head of bed by 4 to 6 inches using wood blocks, and a 2-month course of proton pump inhibitors (eg, omeprazole, 20 mg twice daily) is prescribed.

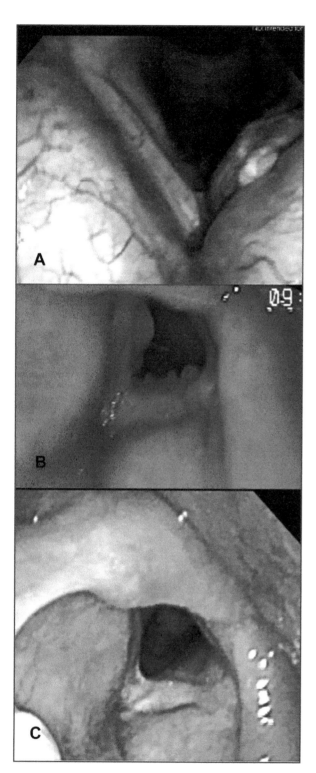

Figure 28–1. T1 glottic cancer prior to and after radiation therapy. (A) Lesion as seen in clinic before biopsy, (B) laryngeal exam 8 weeks after completing radiation treatment, (C) laryngeal exam 1 year later.

This case reveals that acute radiation changes involve all aspects of the larynx within the radiation field. Also, presence of radiation mucositis at points of contact like the anterior commissure can lead to tissue adherence and long-term scar formation. Yet, as with this patient, enough normal tissue in the posterior two thirds of the larynx allow for a functional voice.

CASE PRESENTATION #2

A 55-year-old male with a 25-year history of smoking three to five cigarettes per day developed slowly progressive hoarseness leading to a clinic exam with laryngoscopy.

The initial laryngeal exam identified an infiltrative lesion with involvement of the entire right vocal fold with limited arytenoid mobility (Figure 28–2A).

The workup revealed a T3N2c right glottic squamous cell carcinoma. Treatment included radiation to 70 Gy in 33 fractions with concurrent weekly cisplatin.

Three months after radiation, he was described as having a moderately hoarse voice without airway concerns or dysphagia. Laryngeal exam revealed right-sided complete tumor regression and improved arytenoid mobility but significant stiffness of the right true vocal fold, primarily in the anterior two thirds (Figure 28–2B). After 1 year and several sessions of voice therapy, the patient's voice was described as mildly hoarse with hyperemia and thickening of the vocal fold, right greater than left, mild stiffness on the right but good gross mobility and widely a patent airway and no lesions or masses present. The vocal fold mobility improved but did not normalize. The anterior right vocal fold remains without apparent mucosal wave, consistent with loss of the lamina propria after tumor development and treatment (Figures 28–2C-D).

Management: A trial of vocal hygiene and voice therapy is recommended. A key component of vocal hygiene in this population is emphasis on hydration, which can be challenging in the setting of radiation-related mucosal dryness. Modifiable behaviors include reducing caffeine intake and carrying a water bottle at all times. Supplementary options include xylitol chewing gum[15] and topical sialogogue spray containing 1% malic acid.[16]

Voice therapy has been shown to be helpful for patients following radiation.[17–18] In this scenario, dryness and stiffness is a driving factor for the dysphonia. It can also lead to dysphagia, particularly with thin liquids. If voice therapy is inadequate additional interventions can be considered. If the stiffness and

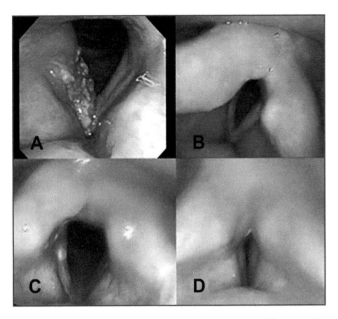

Figure 28–2. (A) T3 glottic lesion prior to biopsy, (B) 3 months post treatment, (C, D) 15 months post treatment breathing and phonating.

bowing results in glottic insufficiency, an office-based injection can be performed. Injections with calcium hydroxyapatite and micronized dermis are safe in the irradiated larynx.[19] Even if injection laryngoplasty is performed, voice therapy serves an important role in addressing the supraglottic hyperfunction and associated muscle tension dysphonia that often accompanies glottic insufficiency.

This case highlights the limitations of tissue recovery after radiation therapy. Stiffness and mucosal dryness will interfere with vocal quality. These changes in tissue elasticity and the loss of laryngeal mucus glands are irreversible side effects of radiation once dose exceeds 25 Gy.

CASE PRESENTATION #3

A 58-year-old male with history of a T2N2c p16+ squamous cell carcinoma of left tonsil underwent primary chemoradiation 8 years ago (70 Gy in 33 fractions, weekly cisplatin at 30 mg/m²). Seven years after treatment, he is referred by his radiation oncologist for evaluation of slowly progressive dysphonia present for 2 months. The patient reports mild ongoing xerostomia and describes his voice as rough and requiring

additional effort to produce. He works in manufacturing and has limited occupational voice demands, but is having difficulty communicating with his spouse, friends, and family. He has never had any voice therapy. He reports mild dysphagia and sensation of residue and sometimes requires a double swallow to clear the bolus. Prior swallow study reported radiation effect with reduced laryngeal closure during swallows, though use of a chin tuck strategy appeared to eliminate aspiration risk. There is occasional coughing, but he has not had any pneumonia or weight loss. He further denies any persistent throat pain, hemoptysis, otalgia, or neck masses. He also has slight trismus and low-grade hypothyroidism treated with levothyroxine.

Social history: former smoker, having quit 10 years prior to his cancer diagnosis, social drinker; one caffeinated beverage daily.

Laryngeal exam revealed persistent low-grade laryngeal edema which included the arytenoids, false vocal folds, and epiglottis, widespread post-radiation vascular changes (telangiectasia) within areas of edema, and mucosal dryness. His right true vocal fold presented a mid-fold lesion with leukoplakia.

Management: A biopsy identified parakeratosis and low-grade dysplasia. Figure 28–3A shows the larynx prior to radiation at the time of the tonsil biopsy and Figure 28–3B shows the chronic laryngeal changes 8 years after treatment as well as the new true vocal fold lesion. Vocal hygiene, voice therapy, and ongoing laryngoscopic surveillance is performed to monitor the epithelial changes.

This case highlights the long-term changes that occur when the larynx is a part of the radiation field required to deliver appropriate curative doses to adjacent structures. It also highlights the need to monitor the patient after cancer treatment and to remain aware that new onset vocal changes need to be investigated, with heightened attention to patients with baseline hoarseness.

APPROACH TO ASSESSMENT

History

When evaluating a patient with history of radiation for head and neck cancer who is presenting with dysphonia, it is essential to consider a recurrent or second primary malignancy. Comorbid symptoms which may suggest this include otalgia, neck mass, hemoptysis,

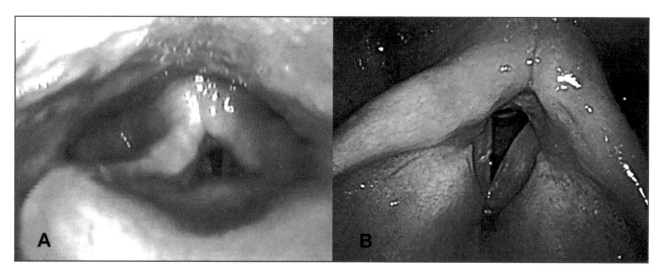

Figure 28–3. (A) shows the larynx prior to radiation at the time of the tonsil biopsy and (B) shows the chronic laryngeal changes 8 years post treatment as well as a new true vocal fold lesion.

pain, weight loss, and dysphagia (red flag or alarm symptoms).

If the patient's primary symptom is dysphonia and there are no concerning comorbid symptoms, one can focus on a description of the dysphonia as primarily rough (implying impaired vibration) or breathy (implying impaired glottic closure), onset timing, whether it is constant/progressive or fluctuating, associated xerostomia which may suggest laryngeal dryness, history of tobacco and alcohol use, caffeine use, and prior surgical interventions, including vocal fold biopsy which could result in scar, current voice demands, and effects on communication.

Examination

If history raises concern for recurrent or second primary malignancy, next steps in assessment can include a comprehensive head and neck exam, flexible laryngoscopy, potential flexible esophagoscopy, videofluoroscopy, and CT neck with contrast. In-office versus operative biopsy may be performed if indicated based on physical exam. Maintaining a record of patient laryngeal examinations over the course of treatment and follow-up simplifies the identification of new lesions.

If history is not concerning for malignancy, exam can focus on vocal function. A comprehensive head and neck examination is performed including mirror exam of the larynx. The clinician should assess the patient's conversational voice during the visit using targeted tasks, such as a loud "hello" to assess projection, maximum phonation time to assess glottic efficiency, and upward and downward glissandos to address frequency range.

Formal subjective and objective voice assessment should be performed. This includes patient-reported questionnaires (eg, Voice Handicap Index, Voice-Related Quality of Life),[20,21] perceptual assessment (grade, roughness, breathiness, asthenia, strain [GRBAS]; Consensus Auditory-Perceptual Evaluation of Voice [CAPE-V]), aerodynamic assessment, and acoustic assessment.

Endoscopy

Flexible laryngoscopy is performed to evaluate the pharynx and larynx for evidence of recurrent or new malignant lesions. Any suspicious lesions can be biopsied in the clinic using topical anesthetic or in the operating room during direct laryngoscopy.

Videolaryngostroboscopy is then performed to evaluate for epithelial lesions, vocal fold mobility, endolaryngeal mucous stranding, vocal fold pliability, and vibratory amplitude and symmetry.

An effort should be made to store the images of the larynx with each visit providing the clinician and patient the opportunity to identify the structural changes that occur with treatment and therapy and over time. These images can help guide therapy and educate the patient and family members.

DISCUSSION

Management of Dysphonia in the Irradiated Larynx

The rate of dysphonia after radiation is high, with 88% of patients reporting slight-to-moderate vocal dysfunction.[22–23] Changes include reduced loudness, decreased fundamental frequency, decreased breath support, roughness, breathiness, variability, unpredictability, and fatigue.[6,24–26] Improvements after treatment are expected to occur, particularly within the first few months, but patients do not usually return to a normal voice.[27] Thus, evaluation and management of dysphonia can remain an issue throughout the patient's period of oncologic surveillance and beyond.

All patients can be counseled on vocal hygiene. Relevant aspects for this patient population include an emphasis on smoking cessation and addressing mucosal dryness. Steam inhalation, drinking water throughout the day, and medications or supplements that improve salivation should be employed. Contributing factors that worsen dryness should be identified and modified. This can include caffeine and medications, particularly anticholinergics and diuretics. Review of medications is particularly important in elderly patients, in whom polypharmacy is common and susceptibility to medication side effects is increased.[28]

In addition to vocal hygiene, voice therapy can be recommended. Though results on efficacy are somewhat mixed,[29–32] it is generally safe and can help as either a primary treatment or adjunct if surgery is considered.

Lastly, surgical intervention may be considered. This has been evaluated primarily for post-radiation glottic insufficiency, including vocal fold paralysis.[33–36] Traditional concern regarding potential for increased rate of complications and implant extrusion has largely been alleviated by recent studies demonstrating both safety and effectiveness of injection laryngoplasty and type I thyroplasty.[19,34–37]

Physiologic and Anatomic Changes to the Larynx After Radiation

The range of changes which occur to the larynx following radiation was described by Chandler.[38] Most patients will exhibit mild dysphonia and mucosal dryness with edema and telangiectasias. A more severe reaction may include slight mobility impairment and endolaryngeal erythema. Even more severe reactions may result in comorbid dysphagia with overlying skin changes. Finally, the most dramatic reactions, including chondroradionecrosis (Figure 28–4), can result in severe pain, fistula, and respiratory distress with airway obstruction.

Laryngeal Chondroradionecrosis

Radiation exposure, particularly for a laryngeal primary tumor, can lead to laryngeal chondroradionecrosis.[39–40] Most cases will occur within the first year after radiation[41] but can occur years after treatment.[42] Radiation-induced inflammatory changes can result in arteritis and small vessel thrombosis around the laryngeal cartilages, followed by ischemia, fibrosis, scarring, and tissue death.[43–44] Presentation may be subtle or dramatic, and ranges from dysphonia and mucosal dryness with edema and hyperemia on exam (Figure 28–5)—all common findings in patients with history of radiation. Extension of necrosis leads to severe dysphonia, dyspnea, and laryngeal obstruction.[38,45] Risk factors for chondroradionecrosis include cartilage invasion by tumor and ongoing alcohol and tobacco use after treatment.[45] Appearance on CT is non-specific, and it can be difficult to distinguish chondroradionecrosis from recurrence.[39] Key findings suggesting the diagnosis include sloughing of the arytenoid cartilage, collapse of the thyroid cartilage, and gas around the laryngeal cartilages.[39]

Treatment depends on disease severity. The primary concern should be confirming or establishing the presence of a safe airway. Following this, antibiotics, steroids, and hyperbaric oxygen can be helpful in controlling the disease process and maintaining a functional larynx.[46–48] If the disease is advanced, total laryngectomy can be considered.

Figure 28–4 demonstrates the CT and PET findings in a 65-year-old male with chondroradionecrosis. Prior treatment included high-dose intensity-modulated radiation treatment (IMRT) to 70 Gy for stage III (T2N1M0) p16 negative squamous cell carcinoma of the left hypopharynx extending into the left pyriform sinus. Radiation was delivered to the hypopharynx and bilateral neck along with concurrent weekly cisplatin. Post-radiation course was complicated by hypopharyngeal obstruction requiring restoration of the hypopharyngeal lumen with a rendezvous procedure followed by repeated dilations. He presented 18 months after completion of radiation with severe pain, tenderness, and worsened swallow dysfunction.

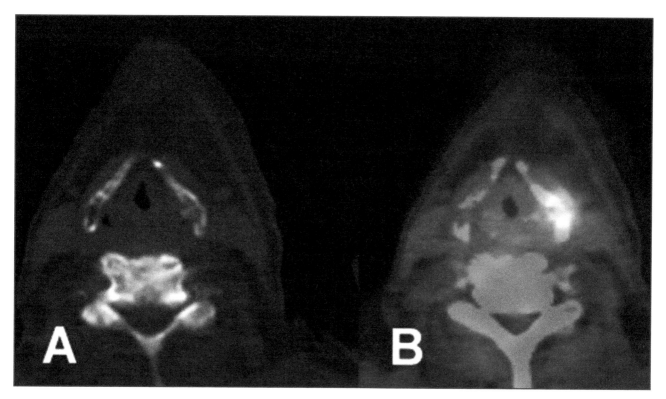

Figure 28–4. Chondroradionecrosis of the larynx 1 year after comprehensive chemoradiation treating a T3 hypopharyngeal cancer, (A) is bone-windowed CT scan, (B) fused PET.

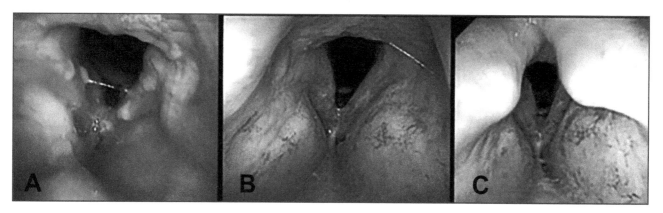

Figure 28–5. (A) Pretreatment T1 left anterior glottis tumor, (B) 7 years post treatment, (C) 9 years post treatment.

Effect on Voice Parameters

Commonly observed post-radiation changes on acoustic voice assessment include increased jitter and shimmer as well as reduced signal- or harmonic-to-noise ratio.[7,49] These values can improve over the first year after treatment,[5] but will still often remain below the normative range.[27] Degree of impairment is related to primary tumor site, with tumors below the hyoid bone often having a greater impact than those above the hyoid bone.[7]

On perceptual voice assessment, increased grade, particularly early after treatment, is common.[11] Maximum phonation time is decreased.[5] Videostroboscopy may demonstrate reduced mucosal wave amplitude, phase asymmetry, and a posterior glottic gap. Dysphonia plicae ventricularis, or supraglottic hyperfunction, may be evident, which can occur more commonly in patients receiving radiation for non-laryngeal tumors.[12]

Patients will perceive voice impairment, reporting abnormal values on the Voice Handicap Index[7] and voice symptoms scale.[11] Such changes can persist even 10 years after treatment.[50]

PITFALLS

The main pitfall to avoid is failure to recognize dysphonia as the presentation for malignancy. This can be avoided with careful laryngoscopy at each clinic visit, and short-term follow-up or biopsy for any abnormal finding. If the patient is presenting to a clinician not able to visualize the larynx, prompt referral to otolaryngology should be made. Causes of dysphonia other than those related to radiation should also be considered. This includes laryngopharyngeal reflux, chronic rhinorrhea, muscle tension dysphonia, presbylaryngis, tremor, and medication side effect.

SUMMARY

Changes to the larynx following radiation, including dryness, muscular atrophy, fibrosis, and edema, cause predictable changes in voice, including breathiness, strain, and a propensity for compensatory supraglottic hyperfunction. Careful exam to rule out recurrent or primary malignancy is of the utmost importance. After ruling out malignancy and dysplasia, full voice evaluation and consideration of other causes contributing to dysphonia is appropriate. Management includes vocal hygiene, voice therapy, and in some cases surgery, and can have a positive impact on the quality of life in this patient population.

REFERENCES

1. Rosier JF, Gregoire V, Counoy H, et al. Comparison of external radiotherapy, laser microsurgery and partial laryngectomy for the treatment of T1N0M0 glottic carcinomas: a retrospective evaluation. *Radiother Oncol.* 1998;48(2):175–183.
2. Yoo J, Lacchetti C, Hammond JA, Gilbert RW. Role of endolaryngeal surgery (with or without laser) compared with radiotherapy in the management of early (T1) glottic cancer: a clinical practice guideline. *Curr Oncol.* 2013;20(2):e132–e135.
3. Mendenhall WM, Amdur RJ, Morris CG, Hinerman RW. T1-T2N0 squamous cell carcinoma of the glottic larynx treated with radiation therapy. *J Clin Oncol.* 2001;19(20):4029–4036.
4. Fung K, Lyden TH, Lee J, et al. Voice and swallowing outcomes of an organpreservation trial for advanced laryngeal cancer. *Int J Radiat Oncol Biol Phys.* 2005;63:1395–1399.
5. Kazi R, Venkitaraman R, Johnson C, et al. Electroglottographic comparison of voice outcomes in patients with advanced laryngopharyngeal cancer treated by chemoradiotherapy or total laryngectomy. *Int J Radiat Oncol Biol Phys.* 2008;70:344–352.
6. Lazarus CL. Effects of chemoradiotherapy on voice and swallowing. *Curr Opin Otolaryngol Head Neck Surg.* 2009;17:172–178.
7. Kraaijenga SA, van der Molen L, Jacobi I, Hamming-Vrieze O, Hilgers FJ, van den Brekel MW. Prospective clinical study on long-term swallowing function and voice quality in advanced head and neck cancer patients treated with concurrent chemoradiotherapy and preventive swallowing exercises. *Eur Arch Otorhinolaryngol.* 2015;272(11):3521–3531.
8. Schuster M, Stelze F. Outcome measurements after oral cancer treatment: speech and speech-related aspects—an overview. *Oral Maxillofac Surg.* 2012;16:291–298.
9. Lazarus CL, Husiani H, Hu K, et al. Functional outcomes and quality of life after chemoradiotherapy: baseline and 3 and 6 months post-treatment. *Dysphagia.* 2014;229:365–375.
10. Harrison LB, Solomon B, Miller S, et al. Prospective computer-assisted voice analysis for patients with early stage glottic cancer: a preliminary report of the functional result of laryngeal irradiation. *Int J Radiat Oncol Biol Phys.* 1990;19:123–127.
11. Paleri V, Carding P, Chatterjee S, et al. Voice outcomes after concurrent chemoradiotherapy for advanced nonlaryngeal head and neck cancer: a prospective study. *Head Neck.* 2012;34:1747–1752.
12. Fung K, Yoo J, Leeper HA, et al. Vocal function following radiation for non-laryngeal versus laryngeal tumors of the head and neck. *Laryngoscope.* 2001;111(11 pt 1):1920–1924.
13. Hamdan AL, Geara F, Rameh C, et al. Vocal changes following radiotherapy to the head and neck for non-laryngeal tumors. *Eur Arch Otorhinolaryngol.* 2009;266:1435–1439.
14. Belafsky PC, Postma GN, Koufman JA. Validity and reliability of the reflux symptom index (RSI). *J Voice.* 2002;16(2):274–247.
15. Martin M, Marin A, Lopez M, Linan O, Alvarenga F, Buchser D, Cerezo L. Products based on olive oil, betaine, and xylitol in the post-radiotherapy xerostomia. *Reports Practical Oncol Radiother.* 2017;22:71–76.
16. Gomez-Moreno G, Cabrera-Ayala M, Aguilar-Salvatierra A, et al. Evaluation of the efficacy of a topical sialogue spray containing malic acid 1% in elderly people with xerostomia: a double-blind, randomized clinical trial. *Gerodontology.* 2014;31(4):274–280.

17. Tuomi L, Bjorkner E, Finizia C. Voice outcome in patients treated for laryngeal cancer: efficacy of voice rehabilitation. *J Voice*. 2014;28(1):62–68.

18. Ouyong LM, Swanson MS, Villegas BC, Damodar D, Kokot N, Sinha UK. ABCLOVE: voice therapy outcomes for patients with head and neck cancer. *Head Neck*. 2016; 38:E1810–E1813.

19. Tirado Y, Lewin JS, Hutcheson KA, Kupferman ME. Office-based injection laryngoplasty in the irradiated larynx. *Laryngoscope*. 2010;120:703–706.

20. Jacobson BH, Johnson A, Grywalski C, et al. The voice handicap index (VHI): development and validation. *Am J Speech Lang Pathol*. 1997;6(3):66–70.

21. Hogikyan ND, Sethuraman G. Validation of an instrument to measure voice-related quality of life (V-RQOL). *J Voice*. 1999;13(4):557–569.

22. Sjogren EV, va Rossum MA, Langeveld TPM. Voice outcome in T1a midcord glottic carcinoma:laser surgery versus radiotherapy. *Arch Otolaryngol Head Neck Surg*. 2008; 134:965–972.

23. Siupsinskiene N, Vaitkus S, Grebliauskaite M, et al. Quality of life and voice in patients treated for early laryngeal cancer. *Medicina (Kaunas)*. 2008;44:288–295.

24. Stoicheff ML. Voice following radiotherapy. *Laryngoscope*. 1975;85:608–618.

25. Morris MR, Canonico D, Blank C. A critical review of radiotherapy in the management of T1 glottic carcinoma. *Am J Otolaryngol*. 1994;15:276–280.

26. Orlikoff RF, Kraus RH. Dysphonia following nonsurgical management of advanced laryngeal carcinoma. *Am J Speech Lang Pathol*. 1996;5:47–52.

27. Bibby JRL, Cotton SM, Perry A, Corry JF. Voice outcomes after radiotherapy treatment for early glottic cancer: assessment using multidimensional tools. *Head Neck*. 2008; 30:600–610.

28. Bostock C, McDonald C. Antimuscarinics in older people: dry mouth and beyond. *Dent Update.*. 2016;43(2):186–188.

29. Van Gogh CDL, Verdonck-de Leeuw IM, Langendijk JA, Kuik DJ, Mahieu HF. Long-term efficacy of voice therapy in patients with voice problems after treatment of early glottic cancer. *J Voice*. 2012;226(3):398–401.

30. Fex S, Henriksson B. Phoniatric treatment combined with radiotherapy of laryngeal cancer for the avoidance of radiation damage. *Acta Otolaryngol Suppl*. 1969;263:128–129.

31. Zwirmer P, Michaelis D, Kruse E. On documentation of voice rehabilitation after laser surgery laryngeal carcinoma resection. *HNO*. 1996;44:514–520.

32. Sittel C, Eckel HE, Eschenburg C. Phonatory results after laser surgery for glottic carcinoma. *Otolaryngol Head Neck Surg*. 1998;119:418–424.

33. Crawley BK, Sulica L. Vocal fold paralysis as a delayed consequence of neck and chest radiotherapy. *Otolaryngol Head Neck Surg*. 2015;153(2):239–243.

34. Rosow DE, Al-Bar MH. Type I thyroplasty in previously irradiated patients: assessing safety and efficacy. *Otolaryngol Head Neck Surg*. 2015;153(4):582–585.

35. Kubik M, Rosen C. Laryngeal framework surgery in the irradiated neck: a retrospective matched cohort study. *Ann Otol Rhinol Laryngol*. 2016; 125(10):823–828.

36. White JR, Orbelo DM, Noel DB, Pittelko RL, Maragos NE, Ekbom DC. Thyroplasty in the previously irradiated neck: a case series and short-term outcomes. *Laryngoscope*. 2016;126:1849–1853.

37. Chang J, Courey MS, Al-Jurg SA, Schneider SL, Yung KC. Injection laryngoplasty outcomes in irradiated and non-irradiated unilateral vocal fold paralysis. *Laryngoscope*. 2014;124:1895–1899.

38. Chandler JR. Radiation fibrosis and necrosis of the larynx. *Ann Otol Rhinol Laryngol*. 1979;88(4 Pt 1):509–514.

39. Keene M, Harwood AR, Bryce DP, van Nostrand AWP. Histopathological study of radionecrosis in laryngeal carcinoma. *Laryngoscope*. 1982;92:173–180.

40. O'Brien P. Tumour recurrence or treatment sequelae following radiotherapy for larynx cancer. *J Surg Oncol*. 1996; 63:130–135.

41. Hermans R, Pameijer FA, Mancuso AA, Parsons JT, Mendenhall WM. CT findings in chondroradionecrosis of the larynx. *AJNR Am J Neuroradiol*. 1998;19:711–718.

42. Lederman M. Radiation therapy in cancer of the larynx. *JAMA*. 1972;221:1253–1254.

43. Calcaterra TC, Stern F, Ward PH. Dilemma of delayed radiation injury of the larynx. *Ann Otol Rhinol Laryngol*. 1972;81:501–507.

44. Filntisis GA, Moon RE, Kraft KL, Farmer JC, Scher RL, Piantadosi CA. Laryngeal radionecrosis and hyperbaric oxygen therapy: report of 18 cases and review of the literature. *Ann Otol Rhinol Laryngol*. 2000;109:554–562.

45. Gessert TG, Britt CJ, Maas AMW, Wieland AM, Harari PM, Hartig GK. Chondroradionecrosis of the larynx: 24-year University of Wisconsin experience. *Head Neck*. 2017;39:1189–1194.

46. Ferguson BJ, Hudson WR, Farmer JC. Hyperbaric oxygen therapy for laryngeal necrosis. *Ann Otol Rhinol Laryngol*. 1987;96:1–6.

47. Feldmeier JJ, Heimbach RD, Davolt DA, Brakora MJ. Hyperbaric oxygen as an adjunctive treatment for severe laryngeal necrosis: a report of nine consecutive cases. *Undersea Hyperbaric Med*. 1993;20:329–335.

48. Rowley H, Walsch M, McShane D, Fraser I, O'Dwyer TP. Chondroradionecrosis of the larynx: still a diagnostic dilemma. *J Laryngol Otol*. 1995;109:218–220.

49. Lehman JL, Bless DM, Brandenburg JH. An objective assessment of voice production after radiation therapy for stage I squamous cell carcinoma of the glottis. *Otolaryngol Head Neck Surg*. 1988;98:121–129.

50. Kraaijenga SAC, Oskam IM, van Son RJJH, Hamming-Vrieze O, Hilgers FJM, van den Brekel MWM, van der Molen L. Assessment of voice, speech, and related quality of life in advanced head and neck cancer patients 10-years+ after chemoradiotherapy. *Oral Oncology*. 2016; 55:24–30.

CHAPTER 29

Laryngeal Chondrosarcoma

Jahangir Ahmed and Chadwin Al Yaghchi

INTRODUCTION

Chondrosarcomas are rare malignant mesenchymal tumors mostly arising from hyaline cartilage. They commonly occur in cartilage avid areas of the thoracic cage, pelvis, and appendicular skeleton (90% collectively). It is the second most prevalent primary malignant bone neoplasm following osteosarcoma, accounting for 11% of such tumors. Although difficult to ascertain accurately, 1 to 12% of cases occur in the head and neck, representing 0.2% of all neoplasms of the head and neck.[1] Primary chondrosarcoma of the larynx per se comprises 1% of all laryngeal malignancies, but remains the third most prevalent in this subsite, behind squamous cell carcinoma (SCC) and adenocarcinoma.

DEFINITION

Chondrosarcomas are malignant neoplasms of mesenchymal origin characterized by a cartilaginous tumor matrix.

CASE PRESENTATION

A 53-year-old man presented to the ENT clinic with progressive dysphonia over the last 4 months. In addition, he noticed exertional dyspnea in association with a reduced exercise tolerance. He denied dysphagia, odynophagia, otalgia, hemoptysis, or weight loss. He was on a statin and was a never-smoker and con-sumed 20 units of alcohol per week. He had no known allergies.

INITIAL ASSESSMENT

History

Dysphonia lasting over 4 weeks in a patient over 40 years of age warrants an urgent referral to ENT for endoscopic laryngeal examination primarily to exclude malignant laryngeal pathology. Associated "red flag" symptoms including stridor, dysphagia, odynophagia, otalgia, hemoptysis, and weight loss should raise the suspicion of malignancy prompting further investigations. Patients with progressive dyspnea may also require a respiratory consult. It is important to directly inquire about swallowing difficulties and potential aspiration as these may significantly influence treatment options. A referral to speech and language therapy (SLT) for clinical, endoscopic, and radiological swallowing assessment should be instigated in such circumstances. A smoking and alcohol history is mandatory.

Examination

A full head and neck examination, including endoscopic evaluation of all the mucosal surfaces of the upper aero-digestive tract, should be performed in the clinic, and ideally photo/video documented. Vocal fold appearance, mobility, and phonatory gaps should be looked for and recorded. The neck should be systematically palpated to exclude mass lesions and lymphadenopathy.

Investigations

These will be directed by history and examinations. A plain chest radiograph (CXR) should be requested in all patients with dyspnea. Cross-sectional imaging in the form of computed tomography (CT) and/or magnetic resonance imaging (MRI) are required to investigate head and neck mass lesions. These often offer complementary diagnostic information. CT has the added benefit of clearer anatomical detail of the laryngotracheal cartilaginous framework and, due to rapid sequence acquisition, is the preferred modality for imaging the chest when investigating concurrent dyspnea, hemoptysis, or vocal cord paralysis.

SCENARIO 1

Flexible nasolaryngoscopy demonstrated left vocal cord immobility with asymmetric arytenoid cartilages with normal overlying mucosa. There was a mass apparent in the lower glottis and subglottis. There were no other suspicious upper aerodigestive tract mucosal lesions or palpable neck masses.

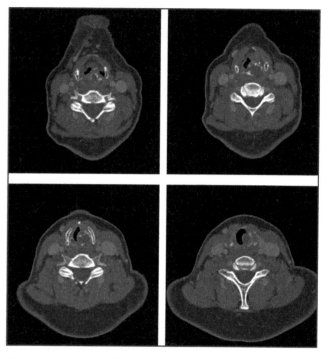

Figure 29–1. Axial CT scan images demonstrate a mass arising from the left cricoid plate extending to the left arytenoid.

Investigations

A CT scan of the neck and chest showed an expansile calcified lesion arising from the posterior cricoid plate and displacing the left arytenoid laterally. There was a narrowing of the airway at this level. There were no pathological lymph nodes and chest imaging was normal (Figure 29–1).

Management

An urgent microlaryngoscopy (ML) and carbon dioxide (CO_2) laser-assisted biopsy was performed. The authors advocate suspension ML using a Dedo-Pilling laryngoscope with high frequency jet-ventilation delivered via a supraglottic jetting needle. As part of the assessment the entire laryngotracheal complex should be visualized and the cricoarytenoid joints should be palpated to check for mobility. The CO_2 laser was used in a super-pulsed continuous mode, on high wattage (10–12 watts) with a finely focused point to cut through the cartilaginous mass.

Histopathology demonstrated a lobular chondroid matrix, surrounded by a rim of fibrofatty connective tissue. There were cytologic atypia and binucleation of chondrocytes. Focal chondrocytes clusters were apparent on a background of thinly dispersed chondrocytes within the stroma. No active mitotic cells were seen. The appearance was consistent with the diagnosis of a grade 1 (G1) chondrosarcoma.

The case was discussed in the head and neck cancer multidisciplinary team meeting (MDT). In view of the histopathological classification of low grade chondrosarcoma, laryngeal preservation surgery was advocated. This initially consisted of CO_2 laser debulking and subsequent close monitoring in the clinic (Figure 29–2).

Follow-Up

Surveillance consisted of monthly flexible nasal endoscopy, with suspension laryngoscopy at 3 months. Subsequently clinic review intervals were increased to 6-monthly, as the tumor demonstrated slow clini-

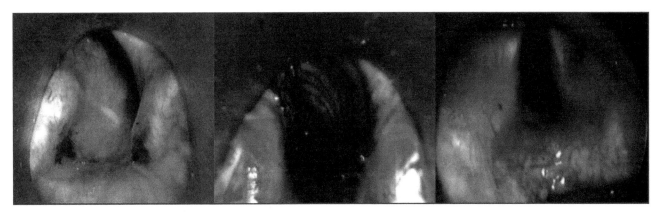

Figure 29–2. Endoscopic view of chondrosarcoma arising from cricoid plate in subglottis. Left, prior to resection. Center, immediately following laser resection. Right, at time routine review 3 months later.

cal progression. Over the subsequent 5 years, the patient underwent three further ML procedures to debulk the disease and maintain an adequate airway. This also improved his voice, although he remained mildly dysphonic. The left vocal cord remained immobile but there was good glottic approximation following speech therapy guidance. His swallow was normal throughout. The patient currently remains healthy, leading an active lifestyle, despite small volume residual disease. The adoption of this treatment approach allowed him to continue to work as a managing director, for which he requires good verbal communication.

SCENARIO 2

A 61-year-old man presented to his local ENT unit with acute onset stridor and dyspnea. He underwent an emergency tracheostomy under local anesthesia followed by ML and biopsy of a left subglottic mass.

Histopathology demonstrated loss of normal cartilaginous architecture with high cellularity. There were multiple cells within each lacuna; they exhibited nuclear atypia, hyperchromasia, and prominent nucleoli. There was invasion within ossified bone. These features were consistent with a grade 2 (G2) chondrosarcoma.

The patient was referred to our center for further management. Endoscopic evaluation demonstrated a left subglottic mass which occupied most of the subglottic airway. The vocal folds looked healthy and were bilaterally mobile. There were no other mucosal lesions in the upper aerodigestive tract or clinically palpable neck lymphadenopathy.

Investigations

A CT scan of the neck and chest demonstrated a calcified mass that replaced the left cricoid cartilage. It measured 25 × 30 × 32 mm. Posteriorly, the mass extended and just crossed the midline. At the level of the glottis, the airway had narrowed to a slit, measuring 3 mm in diameter. The ipsilateral arytenoid cartilage was superiorly displaced. There was no pathological lymph node enlargement. The lungs and pleural spaces were clear. In summary, radiology was consistent with a differentiated chondrosarcoma arising from the cricoid (Figure 29–3).

Management

Following discussion at the head and neck MDT, the patient underwent a two-stage laryngofissure approach to effect a submucosal resection of the tumor. Under general anesthesia, a horizontal skin incision was made at the level of the cricothyroid membrane; skin flaps were elevated in the subplatysmal plane and strap muscles were separated in the midline exposing the thyroid lamina. An extended laryngofissure from the thyroid notch and encompassing the upper two tracheal rings in the midline was performed. Inside the airway, the cricoid mucosa was divided horizontally below the tumor mass, and elevated superiorly off the tumor. The exposed tumor was debulked with a surgical drill, using both cutting and diamond burrs. The intention was to leave normal airway contours inside the larynx. Inevitably there was some mucosal

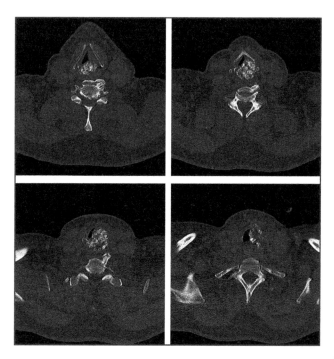

Figure 29–3. Axial CT scan demonstrates large chondrosarcoma arising from the cricoid plate.

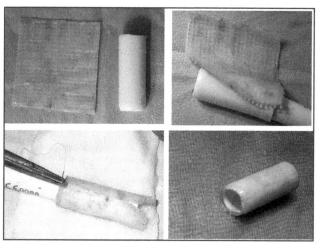

Figure 29–4. A superficial skin graft, backed by a paraffin gauze sheet, stitched to a silicone stent derived from a T-tube.

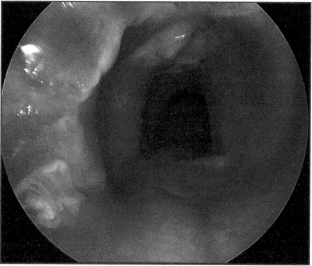

Figure 29–5. Mucus collecting in a small cavity in the subglottis where the tumor was overresected. The airway remains excellent.

loss when this was laid back over the tumor bed. A soft Silastic stent was fashioned from the cut vertical limb of a Montgomery T-tube. The stent was sized to extend from just inferior to the vocal folds to the pre-existing tracheotomy. A split-thickness skin graft (0.25 mm thickness) was harvested from a prepared outer thigh using an electric dermatome; it was backed by a paraffin-gauze sheet and both were sutured around the Silastic stent (with the epidermis side facing the stent) using 4/0 polydioxanone sutures (PDS) (Figure 29–4). This composite stent was inserted into the airway and sutured in place through the adjacent trachea and straps using a 2/0 PDS. The laryngofissure was then closed in a normal fashion.

The skin and stent were removed endoscopically at 2 weeks. Keratinocytes colonized the parts of the airway where the epithelium was missing at the time of surgery and prevented healing by contracture. The patient was successfully decannulated.

Follow-Up

The patient had a repeat microlaryngoscopy assessment at 2 months, where there was no evidence of active disease growth. The patient's airway and voice have thus far been excellent postoperatively. However, there remains a small cavity in the subglottis at the location of the previous tumor which collects mucus (Figure 29–5) and is managed with the regular saline nebulization. The patient remains under long-term clinic surveillance.

DEFINITION

Etiology and Histology

Chondrosarcoma encompasses a broad range of heterogeneous lesions that differ in terms of morphology, biology, and clinical aggressiveness. Histologically, the term "chondrosarcoma" should be reserved for a malignant neoplasm in which the tumor matrix is predominantly cartilaginous.[2] Tumors with bone forming elements and primitive mesenchymal elements behave biologically like aggressive osteosarcomatous neoplasms and should be managed as such. Primary chondrosarcomas occur de novo in normal cartilage; secondary chondrosarcomas arise in previously benign but neoplastic lesions, although the two entities are similar in all other respects. Given their indolent nature and delayed presentation, it is not clear whether laryngeal chondrosarcomas pass through a benign chondroma phase and it has been suggested that ischemic changes within these lesions might trigger transformation.[3]

The World Health Organization (WHO) classifies chondrosarcomas[2] into:

1. Conventional chondrosarcomas

   1.1. Central chondrosarcoma—approximately 75% of all chondrosarcomas; primary or secondary, usually occurs over the age of 50. There is a slight male predominance.
   1.2. Peripheral chondrosarcoma—approximately 10%, arise within the cartilage cap of a pre-existing osteochondroma; occur in younger patients.
   1.3. Periosteal chondrosarcoma—less than 1%; arise on the surface of a bone, usually have a good prognosis after adequate local surgery despite histologic features of a high-grade lesion.

2. Rare chondrosarcoma subtypes

   2.1. Dedifferentiated chondrosarcoma—approximately 10% percent, contain two juxtaposed components: a well-differentiated cartilage tumor and a high-grade non-cartilaginous sarcoma; they are biologically aggressive and have a poor prognosis.
   2.2. Mesenchymal chondrosarcoma—highly malignant tumors; occur in a younger age group than that of other types of chondrosarcoma, approximately 20% have metastasized at diagnosis.
   2.3. Clear cell chondrosarcoma—a rare low-grade variant of chondrosarcoma; they feature late recurrence and thus require long-term follow-up.

Histological grading criteria were initially described by Liechtenstein and Jaffe[4] and later modified by Evans[5] based on non–head and neck skeletal chondrosarcomas. Grading is dependent on the assessment of cellularity, cytological and nuclear atypia (bi and multinucleation), and local invasiveness. They are classified into three grades:

1. Grade 1 (G1, low grade)—can be difficult to distinguish from enchondroma. Chondrosarcomas have higher cellularity with occasional prominent nuclei.
2. Grade 2 (G2, intermediate grade)—characterized by increased cellularity. Most cells show distinct nucleoli and foci of myxoid change may be seen.
3. Grade 3 (G3, high grade)—characterized by high cellularity. Tumors show prominent nuclear atypia and mitosis.

Infiltration and metastatic potential increase with the grade of tumor. The most abundant type of chondrosarcoma in the head and neck is conventional G1, comprising over 90% at this site. These rarely metastasize, in contrast to G3 lesions from which over 50% have metastasized at presentation, most commonly to the lungs. Although rare in the head and neck, de-differentiation is lethal, with less than <10% 1-year survival.[6] Up to 13% of recurrent cases in the head and neck show a worse histological grade than at their original diagnosis,[7] raising the question of a spectrum of progression, with de-differentiation representing the end manifestation of a progressive accumulation of genetic mutations. Histologically, de-differentiated tumors demonstrate sharp biphasic morphology with high grade sarcomatous spindle-cell abundant lesions on a background of lower grade conventional chondrosarcoma matrix. In keeping with the progression model, higher grade and de-differentiated subtypes share similar genetic mutations, implying a common origin.[2] Other histologically distinct chondrosarcoma such as the mesenchymal type have distinct genetic signatures and are likely different entities.[1]

Symptoms and Presentation

Presenting symptoms will reflect the location of the lesion, and as most are slowly growing, their clinical manifestation may take considerable time. As they are locally aggressive, most symptoms in the head and neck are consequent to compression or destruction of bony, vascular, or nervous structures.[8]

The mean age of presentation of laryngeal chondrosarcoma is 62.5 years (range, 15–93), with a 3:1 male predilection.[9] In a recent systematic review, the primary sites in decreasing order were cricoid 56.3%, thyroid cartilage 11.5%, arytenoid 2.7%, and glottis 1.5%. Tumors arose simultaneously from multiple cartilaginous sites in a further 5.2%.[9]

Laryngeal chondrosarcoma commonly present with chronic dysphonia (47.2%) and mild stridor and dyspnea (25.8%)[9]; particularly with involvement of the subglottis. It is not uncommon for these symptoms to have been attributed to and thus treated as asthma and/or other chronic lower respiratory tract conditions. The mean duration from onset of symptoms to diagnosis was just over 24 months.[9] A prominent neck mass may be seen or felt, especially if the lesion originated in the thyroid laminae or anterior cricoid cartilage (9.5%). As the hyoid is bone, primary chondrosarcoma of the hyoid is rare.

Cervical lymphadenopathy occurs in less than 5% of laryngeal chondrosarcoma and will reflect a more aggressive histological subtype and or de-differentiation. Metastatic lesions, when they do occur, usually disseminate to the lungs.[10,11]

Diagnosis

As previously discussed, the histological appearance of low grade lesions may cause some diagnostic uncertainly. However, it is important to establish a correct diagnosis for management and prognostication. Macroscopic appearances are non-specific, with a differential that includes a wide spectrum of bony and soft tissue benign and malignant lesions, although suspicion in the larynx should be raised with a smooth submucosal soft mass located in the posterior subglottis.

Unlike for skeletal chondrosarcoma, plain x-ray images in the head and neck are not very helpful, with the exception of those arising in the mandible. In laryngeal chondrosarcomas, cross-sectional imaging is the initial investigative modality of choice. Both CT and MRI play important diagnostic roles.

CT will demonstrate local bony and cartilaginous destruction and outline the extent of the lesion. Calcifications in the tumor matrix add to the diagnostic certainty. A CT neck, chest, and possibly abdomen (if clinical or biochemical suspicion of liver involvement) is also recommended to exclude metastatic dissemination.

MRI is useful at delineating the extent of surrounding soft tissue involvement; the T2 weighted images in particular show high signal intensity, reflecting the high water content of the hyaline cartilaginous tumor matrix.[12] Diffusion weighted (DW) MRI is based on the Brownian motion of water molecules, which is impaired in hypercellular tissues, resulting in low apparent diffusion coefficient (ADC) values. DW MRI has been shown to be a useful modality in diagnosing de-differentiation in laryngeal chondrosarcoma.[13]

Fluorodeoxyglucose (FDG)-based PET scanning may be of additional help but due to low metabolic activity in lower grade lesions, they cannot reliably distinguish between low grade chondrosarcoma and benign chondromatous or other lesions. They may be useful in characterizing higher grade and de-differentiated lesions with high metabolic activity as well as associated metastatic dissemination. De-differentiated lesions demonstrate high FDG tracer uptake.[14] Hybrid PET-CT and most recently PET-MRI systems may demarcate areas of de-differentiation within low grade morphology tumors.[13] MRI and PET based imaging protocols are also useful in determining recurrence post-surgery.

Other imaging modalities such as ultrasonography with or without fine needle aspiration cytology and modified barium swallow are utilized as appropriate. A formal swallow assessment by SLT with either or both video fluoroscopy (VF) and functional endoscopic evaluation of swallow (FEES) is vital in the preoperative planning of a major endoscopic or open laryngeal resection. If swallow is doubtful preoperatively, then organ preservation should be reconsidered.

Ultimately, definitive diagnosis can only be achieved by performing a truly representative incisional biopsy and histological examination. In the larynx this usually entails suspension microlaryngoscopy under general anesthesia. The biopsy should be directed to areas that on high-resolution cross-sectional imaging are likely to yield the most aggressive foci of tumor. Thus, aim for areas adjacent to soft tissue or bony destruction with little calcification on corresponding imaging. A core needle biopsy may yield results similar to an open procedure, but there is a risk of seeding within the resulting tract. Indeed, when a direct incision biopsy is taken, it should be planned such that the resulting defect will be entirely included in the definitive excision. In some situations, if the lesion is very well localized, complete excision biopsy with margins should be contemplated if there is minimal risk of leaving a functional disability. As for all tumor biopsies, they should be correctly labeled, orientated, and marked if necessary.

Where reported, the mean laryngeal tumor size in a systematic review of laryngeal chondrosarcoma was 3.78 cm in greatest dimension (0.5 to 13 cm). Histologically, 67.8% were G1, 23.5% G2, and only 3.8% poorly differentiated.[9] Other variants were rarer and included clear cell, mesenchymal, and de-differentiated. De-differentiated laryngeal chondrosarcoma is extremely rare, with only 15 cases reported in the literature at the time of writing.[15]

As no universal guidelines currently exist, all cases should be discussed at a tumor MDT prior to establishing a consensus regarding management.

Management

The first-line treatment modality for chondrosarcoma is surgical. Although total laryngectomy has been used to treat 29.4% of cases in the reported literature, this analysis incorporated historic reports where tumor eradication with clear margins was the primary goal. Jones in 1973 outlined indications for total laryngectomy for laryngeal chondrosarcoma[16]:

1. Extensive tumor with the inability to preserve airway patency
2. Recurrence
3. Anaplastic histology

Furthermore, as most laryngeal chondrosarcoma occur in the posterior cricoid lamina, any tumor involvement greater than 50% of this cartilage has traditionally been approached with a total laryngectomy for fear of leaving significant disability and risk of recurrence. However, as these lesions are often of low grade and indolent biological behavior, endoscopic techniques and limited open excision with functional reconstructive techniques have been the mainstay in managing this rare tumor in the last two decades. The aim has shifted to enhancing quality of life with organ and function preservation. A balance therefore needs to be struck between the latter versus incomplete clearance with close clinical and radiological monitoring. This

shift in treatment paradigm may have contributed to the relatively high rate of local recurrence of 40% reported in the literature.[9]

Tiwari et al demonstrated that low grade chondrosarcoma of the cricoid can be successfully treated with a laryngofissure approach. In their series, one out of the five patients eventually needed a total laryngectomy to obtain control.[17] Zeitels et al similarly reported that low grade chondrosarcoma can be treated endoscopically or via a transcervical laryngofissure approach to excise the lesion and reconstruction by either tracheal advancement, free dermis, fat, or aortic homograft.[18] Seven out of eight patients were tracheostomy free at last follow-up. All patients retained good swallow function. The voice outcome was inversely correlated with extent of surgical resection. Importantly the authors demonstrated that total laryngectomy can be avoided even though all their patients had some disease-related impairment of at least one of the cricoarytenoid joints (CAJs).

The largest reported single multicenter case series was the AFIP study reported in 2002 by Thompson and Gannon[3] that analyzed 111 cases. The authors demonstrated that functional organ preserving laryngeal surgery for patients with low grade chondrosarcoma allowed for prolonged preservation of quality of life with no adverse impact on long term survival. The paper clearly highlighted the fact that chondrosarcoma in the larynx is a different biological entity to its epithelial counterpart, and that the treatment paradigms should therefore be similarly dichotomized.

Open/partial laryngeal extirpation procedures do, however, post a significant risk to vocal performance and potential airway obstruction from scarring, particularly in revision scenarios, as attested by the hitherto mentioned studies. Technological advances in anesthesia and visualization have popularized the recent trend for endoscopic extirpation and ablation with or without the aid of a laser. Many laryngeal lesions arise from the luminal surface of the posterior plate of the cricoid cartilage and if localized to this subsite would be readily accessible to initial endoscopic treatment. Ideally this would be performed under suspension laryngoscopy with supra or subglottic jet ventilation to enable optimal access and visualization without the need for temporary tracheostomy; jetting will also clear the laser plume intraoperatively. External manipulation of the larynx in our experience enables a clear view of nearly all subsites to the direct line of a CO_2 laser mounted on an operating microscope. However, a flexible fiber mediated laser system may also be utilized if necessary. The aim is to excise and/or ablate the lesion from the involved cricoid plate, ideally until the external perichondrium is reached. Preservation of at least one functional CAJ is imperative to achieve the goal of function preservation and one would have confirmed its preoperative functionality before embarking on surgery. Endoscopic procedures can also be safely repeated for residual or recurrent disease. Open procedures should be held in reserve for disease that is difficult to access or control endoscopically.

More extensive tumors will require an open surgical approach at the onset. Extensive involvement of the cricoid ring makes radical removal of these tumors very difficult without affecting laryngeal function. Resection of a significant section of the posterior cricoid interrupts laryngeal support, causing collapse of the glottis and ensuing laryngeal stenosis. De Vincentiis et al described three patients with laryngeal chondrosarcoma that were treated with total cricoidectomy with end to end thyro-tracheopexy.[19] Although long term oncological clearance and oral diet were achieved, two of three patients were tracheostomy dependent in the long term. Functional organ preservation generally requires the preservation of at least one uninvolved cricoarytenoid joint and muscle complex (posterior cricoarytenoid) along with an intact recurrent laryngeal nerve. Chondrosarcomas limited to the ipsilateral half of the cricoid would therefore be good candidates. Damiani et al described six patients in whom supratracheal partial laryngectomy procedures were performed with preservation of at least half of the cricoid and its associated cricoarytenoid functional unit.[20] Four of six patients regained normal swallow after 1 year and in all, their covering tracheostomies were successfully decannulated. All patients were reported to have dysphonic but comprehensible speech.

Rovo et al described a rotational tracheal reconstruction technique in four patients who had total or subtotal cricoidectomies for low grade chondrosarcoma emanating from the central posterior lamina of the cricoid cartilage.[21] The posterior and lateral cricoarytenoid muscles of both joints were sacrificed but the arytenoids were spared. The distal trachea was rotated 90° clockwise, pivoting at the level of the 3/4th tracheal ring to enable the creation of a cartilaginous platform that substituted the posterior cricoid plate upon which the arytenoids were stably fixed. As the only functional intrinsic muscles were inter and thyroarytenoids, endoscopic abduction lateropexy procedures were required to counter the tendency for adduction prior to tracheostomy decannulation. Swallow was reported to be safe and patients were rehabilitated to achieve a socially acceptable voice.

Numerous other methods of reconstructing the laryngeal framework following partial reconstruction have been described with variable success. Techniques have included autologous rib graft augmentation, local advancement and rotation of the residual cricotracheal framework, and tracheal autotransplantation. Regarding the latter, Delaere et al described the use of a two-stage tracheal autotransplant procedure to reconstruct laryngeal defects following chondrosarcoma ablation.[22] During the first stage, a radial forearm fascial flap is wrapped around the upper cervical trachea. In the second stage, a patch of this neo-vascularized cervical trachea on its new vascular pedicle was used to reconstruct the laryngeal defect. They treated seven patients in this way with good function preservation and long term disease control.

The important principle common to all these techniques is to augment or replace a stable posterior cricoid support upon which the arytenoids sit. Lesions located inferiorly on the cricoid and/or trachea may be amenable to partial cricotracheal or tracheal resection with end to end anastomosis, and such surgery in expert centers has led to good long term disease control and excellent functional outcomes.

Unless extremely localized with no evidence of dissemination, G3 and de-differentiated laryngeal chondrosarcomas should be treated with a curative total laryngectomy, as the risks of leaving behind microscopic disease outweigh functional organ preservation. Previous low grade (G1 and G2) tumors, which start to grow more rapidly after a period of slow growth, must be suspected of de-differentiation and treated with radical surgery and curative intent.

Concurrent therapeutic cervical lymph node clearance will be dictated by staging investigations, but prophylactic neck dissection in an N0 neck is not advocated in low to moderate grade lesions and should be the subject of an MDT discussion for higher grade and de-differentiated lesions. There are no conclusive data regarding the rate of occult metastasis for the different grades of laryngeal chondrosarcoma.

As most laryngeal chondrosarcomas are slow growing lesions, they are theoretically radiotherapy resistant. A lack of p16, a cell cycle regular protein, has been associated with resistance to radiotherapy (RT).[23] Conventional fractionated external beam radiotherapy is usually reserved for residual lesions post surgically and in a palliative context for irresectable disease or where patient infirmity precludes a surgical option.[24] Adjuvant radiotherapy is advocated following surgery for high grade or de-differentiated lesions and in rare cases has shown benefit as primary treatment for these highly mitotic lesions.[25] As RT fields narrow and become more conformal, e.g., with intensity modulated radiotherapy (IMRT) and indeed with the availability of newer types of RT (proton and stereotactic) which deliver highly focused dosages of radiation, sparing collateral structures, RT may play a bigger role in these conditions in the future.

There is no benefit of current chemotherapy protocols in the management of low to moderate grades of laryngeal or head and neck chondrosarcoma. Chemotherapy may play a role in the adjuvant treatment of higher grade and disseminated lesions.[26]

Outcomes and Prognosis

There has been a recent paradigm shift in the management of low grade laryngeal chondrosarcoma with evidence suggesting that curative resection at the expense of functional organ preservation does not necessarily alter prognosis. Furthermore, more and more endoscopic extirpative and debulking procedures are also being performed in suitable patients. In our unit the majority of patients are managed in this way. They are disease free, or with relatively stable disease, on longterm follow-up and importantly with excellent preservation of speech, swallow, and a laryngeal airway.

It must, however, be stressed that close follow-up and having a low threshold for reintervention is key to management. More aggressive resections are advocated if endoscopic techniques are not possible as local recurrence is still the major cause of death. Pathology will also dictate the course of management as higher grade tumors and certain histological subtypes, as previously discussed, are more locally destructive, have a higher propensity to metastasize, and thus carry a poorer prognosis.

In the systematic review conducted by Chin et al, the average follow-up duration was 61.9 months (0–360).[9] Overall survival for laryngeal chondrosarcoma ranged from 79.4% to 88.6% at 5 years. Diseasespecific survival at 1, 5, 10, and 20 years was 97.7, 91.4, 81.8, and 68%, respectively, confirming the good overall prognosis with laryngeal chondrosarcoma.[9] Although there was no significant differences in 5-year survival when comparing subsite, histological grade, and therapeutic intervention, the heterogeneity in diagnostic and therapeutic reporting from predominantly small case series and reports makes for difficult meaningfully interpretation. Other studies have suggested 5-year survival figures of 90, 81, and 43% for G1, 2, and 3 laryngeal chondrosarcomas, respectively.[20]

Patients presenting with laryngeal chondrosarcoma should be followed up indefinitely with interval cross sectional radiology, as recurrence and distant metastasis may occur many years following the initial diagnosis, even in those that have been treated with total laryngectomy.

SUMMARY

Laryngeal chondrosarcomas are a rare clinical entity. They are mostly low grade with indolent biology. Due to disease rarity and limited research, there is no unified consensus on management. Historical management objectives of margin-free complete disease clearance, often via a total laryngectomy, was based on treatment principles of SCC of the larynx. In recent decades the treatment paradigm has shifted. Many authors would argue that the main treatment objective is organ and function preservation for as long as oncologically possible. Although this paradigm shift is related to the high risk of local recurrence, it has no effect on long term survival. In low grade tumors, endoscopic debulking/ablation should be considered as a first line of treatment. In more advanced cases, an open surgical approach such as laryngofissure, cricotracheal resection, or partial laryngectomy should be adopted. The fundamental factor for the success of this pathway in preserving laryngeal function is to keep at least one intact cricoarytenoid joint. Total laryngectomy should therefore be reserved for salvaging aggressive recurrence, high grade undifferentiated tumors, or nonfunctional larynges.

REFERENCES

1. Coca-Pelaz, A, Rodrigo JP, Triantanfyllou A et al. Chondrosarcomas of the head and neck. *Eur Arch Otorhinolaryngol*. 2014;271(10):2601–2609.
2. Hogendoorn P, Bovee J, Nielsen G. Chondrosarcoma (grades I-III), including primary and secondary variants and periosteal chondrosarcoma. In: Fletcher C et al (eds), *World Health Organization Classification of Tumours of Soft Tissue and Bone*. Lyon, France: IARC; 2013:264.
3. Thompson L, Gannon F. Chondrosarcoma of the larynx: a clinicopathologic study of 111 cases with a review of the literature. *Am J Surg Pathol*. 2002;26(7):836–851.

4. Lichtenstein L, Jaffe H. Chondrosarcoma of bone. *Am J Pathol*. 1943;19(4):553–589.

5. Bathala, S., et al., Chondrosarcoma of larynx: review of literature and clinical experience. *J Laryngol Otol*. 2008; 122(10):1127–1129.

6. Dorfman H, Czerniak B. Bone cancers. *Cancer*. 1995;75 (1 Suppl):203–210.

7. Grimer RJ, Gosheger G, Taminiau A, et al. Dedifferentiated chondrosarcoma: prognostic factors and outcome from a European group. *Eur J Cancer*. 2007;43(14): 2060–2065.

8. Weber AL, Brown EW, Hug EB, Liebsch NJ. Cartilaginous tumors and chordomas of the cranial base. *Otolaryngol Clin North Am*. 1995;28(3):453–471.

9. Chin OY, Dubal PM, Sheikh AB et al. Laryngeal chondrosarcoma: A systematic review of 592 cases. *Laryngoscope*. 2017;127(2):430–439.

10. Hong P, Taylor SM, Trites JR, et al. Chondrosarcoma of the head and neck: report of 11 cases and literature review. *J Otolaryngol Head Neck Surg*. 2009;38(2):279–285.

11. Lee SY, Chen KC, Chen HY, Chen CY. Chondrosarcoma of the head and neck. *Yonsei Med J*. 2005;46(2):228–232.

12. Murphey MD, Vidal JA, Fanburg-Smith JC, Gajweski DA. From the archives of the AFIP: imaging of primary chondrosarcoma: radiologic-pathologic correlation. *Radiographics*. 2003;23(5):1245–1278.

13. Purohit BS, Dulguerov P, Burdhardt K, Becker M. Dedifferentiated laryngeal chondrosarcoma: combined morphologic and functional imaging with positron-emission tomography/magnetic resonance imaging. *Laryngoscope*. 2014;124(7):E274–E277.

14. Feldman F, Van Heertum R, Saxena C, Parisien M. 18FDG-PET applications for cartilage neoplasms. *Skeletal Radiol*. 2005;34(7):367–374.

15. Fidai SS, Ginat DT, Langerman AJ, Cipriani NA. Dedifferentiated chondrosarcoma of the larynx. *Head Neck Pathol*. 2016;10(3):345–348.

16. Jones HM. Cartilaginous tumours of the head and neck. *J Laryngol Otol*. 1973;87(2):135–151.

17. Tiwari R, Mahieu H, Snow G. Long-term results of organ preservation in chondrosarcoma of the cricoid. *Eur Arch Otorhinolaryngol*. 1999;256(6):271–276.

18. Zeitels SM, Burns JA, Wain JC, Wright CD, Rosenberg AE. Function preservation surgery in patients with chondrosarcoma of the cricoid cartilage. *Ann Otol Rhinol Laryngol*. 2011;120(9):603–607.

19. de Vincentiis M, Greco A, Fusconi M, Pagliuca G, Martellucci S, Gallo A. Total cricoidectomy in the treatment of laryngeal chondrosarcomas. *Laryngoscope*. 2011;121(11): 2375–2380.

20. Damiani V, Crosetti E, Rizzotto G, Camaioni A, Succo G. Well and intermediate differentiated laryngeal chondrosarcoma: toward conservative surgery? *Eur Arch Otorhinolaryngol*. 2014;271(2):337–344.

21. Rovó L, Back Á, Sztanó B, Matievics V, Szegesdi I, Castellanos PF. Rotational thyrotracheopexy after cricoidectomy for low-grade laryngeal chrondrosarcoma. *Laryngoscope*. 2017;127(5):1109–1115.

22. Delaere P, Vertriest R, Hermans R. Functional treatment of a large laryngeal chondrosarcoma by tracheal autotransplantation. *Ann Otol Rhinol Laryngol*. 2003;112(8):678–682.

23. Moussavi-Harami F, Mollano A, Martin JA et al. Intrinsic radiation resistance in human chondrosarcoma cells. *Biochem Biophys Res Commun*. 2006;346(2):379–385.

24. McNaney, D, Lindberg RD, Ayala AG, Barkely HT Jr, Hussey DH. Fifteen year radiotherapy experience with chondrosarcoma of bone. *Int J Radiat Oncol Biol Phys*. 1982;8(2):187–190.

25. Dailiana T, Nomikos P, Kapranos N et al. Chondrosarcoma of the larynx: treatment with radiotherapy. *Skeletal Radiol*. 2002;31(9):547–549.

26. Ruark D, Schlehaider U, Shah J. Chondrosarcomas of the head and neck. *World J Surg*. 1992;16(5):1010–1015; discussion 1015–1016.

CHAPTER 30

Bilateral Vocal Fold Mobility Impairment

Colin R. Butler

INTRODUCTION

The vocal cords have quite diverse physiological functions not only important in generating voice but also vital in protecting the airway against aspiration. At the same time the vocal cords regulate airflow by changing the aperture of the airway on a breath-by-breath basis. A number of conditions can lead to vocal cord immobility, and since the larynx is at the gateway to the aerodigestive tract, poor mobility of both cords can lead to dysfunction in swallowing and voice, as well as shortness of breath. Impaired movement can be considered as secondary to either neurological insults or those related to restricted movement of the cricoarytenoid joints. This chapter focuses on the latter, with restricted movement unrelated to neurology. Restricted movement can be due to cricoarytenoid joint ankylosis secondary to rheumatoid arthritis, trauma, or radiotherapy. More commonly, interarytenoid scarring, as result of endotracheal intubation, can lead to impaired abduction of the vocal cords. Treatment options include both endoscopic and open approaches and these are tailored according to the etiology and extent of disease.

DEFINITION

Bilateral vocal fold mobility impairment (BVFMI) is a reduction or fixation of the movement of both vocal folds. It is a finding typically identified by direct observation of the vocal cords during respiration and/or attempted phonation. The patient is asked to repeat the sound "eeee" followed by a sniff in through the nose. The degree of restriction of abduction should be noted for each cord. Sometimes there is a mixed pattern, or restricted abduction and adduction with the cords lying in the paramedian position.

CASE PRESENTATION

A 54-year-old gentleman presents with 4-month history of persistent dysphonia and increasing shortness of breath particularly on climbing stairs or when attempting gentle exercise. A recent upper respiratory tract infection led to more noisy and labored breathing, which improved with resolution of the infection. The patient had not declared any odynophagia, dysphagia, neck lumps, or weight loss. He had no other neurological symptoms. Of relevance was the fact that he had an admission, 6 months previously, for acute pancreatitis. This resulted in a prolonged intensive care unit (ICU) stay, where he was intubated for 3 weeks. Below, three potential scenarios of glottic injury and their management are presented.

The past medical history included rheumatoid arthritis, hypertension, and hypercholesterolemia. His general practitioner had recently started him on a bronchodilator inhaler for his shortness of breath.

Social history: He is an ex-smoker who drinks moderate amounts of alcohol. He is a company director.

Medications: Methotrexate, bisoprolol, Simvastatin, Salbutamol inhaler.

INITIAL ASSESSMENT

History

A standard history is taken focusing on the nature of complaint, duration, and exacerbating factors. The clinician should inquire about previous airway intubation and determine its duration and traumatic episodes. A history of previous neck surgery including thyroidectomy or neck trauma is also relevant. Arthropathies such as rheumatoid arthritis and previous radiotherapy to the head and neck region should be determined. Red flag symptoms include persistent odynophagia, marked dysphagia, repeat chest infections, weight loss, and noisy breathing at rest.

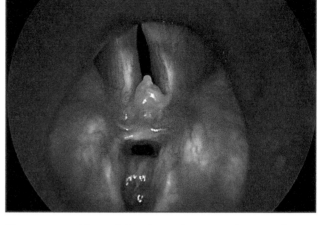

Figure 30–1. View of the glottis demonstrating an adhesion between the vocal processes of the arytenoids.

Examination

Head and neck examination should include identifying previous neck or airway surgery and exclude palpable neck lesions.

Flexible nasal endoscopy (FNE) is recommended in the clinic setting to evaluate the airway and identify the vocal folds (cords) and to confirm the presence of impaired vocal fold movement. Assessment should include the position of the folds in relation to the midline, and attempted movement (if any) during respiration or phonation. Evidence of an impaired swallow, such as excessive residue or pooling of secretions, should lead to formal assessment of the swallow. This can be through fiberoptic endoscopic evaluation of swallow (FEES) or videofluoroscopy (a modified barium swallow).

A computerized tomography (CT) scan of the neck and chest should always be considered, both to rule out changes in the lungs and to screen for other areas of airway stenosis.

SCENARIO 1

The patient had quiet stridor at rest and he was mildly dysphonic. With a reduced phonation time, he could not complete full sentences. Head and neck examination was normal. Flexible nasal endoscopy revealed bilateral impaired vocal cord movements, held in an adducted position. An interarytenoid adhesion was seen fixing vocal cord abduction. The vocal cords adducted on phonation. The remaining supraglottis and glottis were otherwise normal (Figure 30–1).

Diagnosis

Bilateral vocal fold (cord) immobility secondary to interarytenoid scarring or posterior glottic web formation.

Investigations

Nil.

Management

Surgery was performed under general anesthesia using suspension laryngoscopy and supraglottic jet ventilation. Definitive assessment of the glottis was made under the microscope using microlaryngeal instruments. A 0-degree endoscope was passed via the laryngoscope to visualize the subglottis and trachea and rule out other areas of airway damage. Division of the interarytenoid adhesion was performed with the carbon dioxide (CO_2) laser delivered through a micromanipulator attached to the microscope (Figure 30–2). As the cricoarytenoid joints can become ankylosed after prolonged fixation, a dilatation was performed using

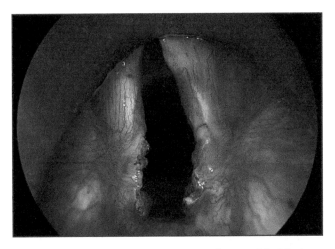

Figure 30–2. Division of interarytenoid scar with CO_2 laser and balloon dilation.

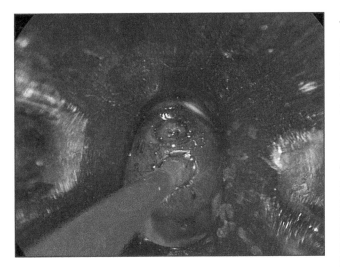

Figure 30–3. Balloon dilatation of the interarytenoid space.

a pulmonary balloon dilatator (Figure 30–3). In this clinical case, the arytenoids were seen to be mobile on the operating table at the end of the procedure.

SCENARIO 2

The clinical history is as described above with prolonged intubation on the ICU. During his hospital admission for pancreatitis a tracheostomy was inserted. It is now a year later and the tracheostomy remains. There have been multiple attempts to decannulate the patient despite downsizing to a size 6.0 fenestrated, non-cuffed, tracheostomy tube. The patient is able to voice with the use of a speech valve but only for limited periods. He cannot tolerate capping of the tracheostomy tube. Flexible nasal endoscopy revealed dense interarytenoid scar with the vocal folds fixed in an adducted position. There was a subtle "rocking" movement of the arytenoids on attempted phonation. The remainder of the supraglottis and glottis had a normal appearance (Figure 30–4).

Diagnosis

Bilateral vocal fold immobility secondary to interarytenoid scarring or a posterior glottic web.

Investigations

Baseline swallow assessment, in anticipation that a large laser resection or posterior glottic augmentation might be required for decannulation. This was normal. Electromyography (EMG) studies demonstrated normal nerve conductivity.

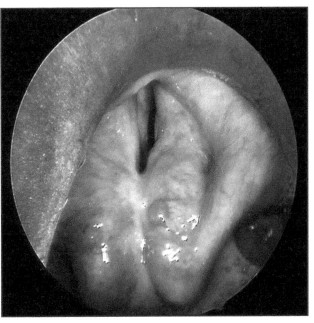

Figure 30–4. Dense interarytenoid scarring fixing the vocal cords.

Management

Microlaryngoscopy and division of interarytenoid scar with the CO_2 laser and balloon dilatation as for scenario 1. A biopsy was taken and sent for histology. There were no further lesions found. The scar was nearly a centimeter thick but did not extend into the subglottis. There remained limited mobility at the cricoarytenoid joints.

At Review

The patient had initial improvement of voice and tolerated periodic "capping" of the tracheostomy tube. Over a 3-month period this deteriorated and his symptoms returned to their preoperative state. Flexible nasal endoscopy confirmed recurrent interarytenoid scar and persistent vocal fold immobility.

Management 2

Where an interarytenoid scar fails to respond to simple division and there is ankylosis of the cricoarytenoid joints, a different surgical approach needs to be considered. Approaches toward this include combining division of the scar with a posterior cricoid split and placing a piece of costal cartilage within this split, to act as a biological "spacer." This can be performed as an open procedure (via a laryngofissure) or as an endoscopic procedure. The tracheostomy would be left in situ for several weeks post-surgery until the airway is stable.

SCENARIO 3

The history is as described above. The patient has had a tracheostomy inserted during a long term ICU admission for pancreatitis. It has been 1 year since the tracheostomy was inserted and there have been failed attempts to decannulate. Of note is treatment for his rheumatoid arthritis, which has required further optimization of his medications. Flexible nasal endoscopy reveals a normal appearance to the vocal cords, but they are held in an adducted position (Figure 30–5). No movement was seen on phonation or respiration.

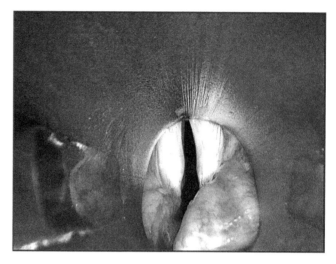

Figure 30–5. Bilateral vocal fold immobility with cricoarytenoid joint ankylosis.

EMGs demonstrated normal nerve conduction. Swallow assessment was also normal.

Diagnosis

Bilateral vocal cord (fold) immobility with cricoarytenoid joint ankylosis secondary to rheumatoid arthritis.

Investigations

Swallow study and laryngeal EMG studies.

Management

Suspension microlaryngoscopy and laser partial arytenoidectomy (Figure 30–6).

PITFALLS

Identifying the underlying cause is key to the surgical approach. Cricoarytenoid joint fixation can occur in isolation or in combination with scar formation and it is necessary to fully assess joint mobility in all such

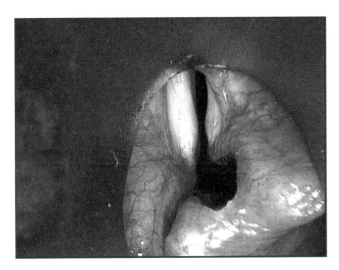

Figure 30–6. Microlaryngoscopy and partial arytenoidectomy.

cases. EMG studies are necessary if it is unclear if there is a neurogenic cause to the immobility.

DISCUSSION

Bilateral vocal fold immobility (BVFI) can be due to bilateral laryngeal denervation; bilateral cricoarytenoid joint fixation; or interarytenoid scarring. The impact of BVFI is often quite considerable, since the posterior glottis is the site of maximal airflow due to its large cross-sectional area. As such, any amount of limited mobility can have quite detrimental effects on the airway. Classification of BVFI can be considered according to etiology types 1 to 5 (Table 30–1); however, in some settings the etiology can be mixed. Treatment strat-

Table 30–1. Classification of Fixation in Bilateral Vocal Cord Immobility

Type 1	Neurogenic
Type 2	Cricoarytenoid joint ankylosis
Type 3	Early posterior glottic web (early granulation tissue formation)
Type 4	Late posterior glottic web (dense scar tissue formation). Type 4a is a band of fibrosis between the arytenoids, 4b is dense scar.
Type 5	Glottic and subglottic scar formation

egies are dependent on the etiology, the potential reversibility, and the extent of the pathological process. A complete and complex assessment is necessary to determine an optimal treatment strategy.[1] Interventions can be considered broadly as either resection of anatomical structures, refashioning of existing structures with tissue removal, displacement of existing structures without tissue removal, and restoration of innervation. Treatment options are considered briefly below according to etiology.

The most common etiology for type 1 BVFIs are conditions that lead to bilateral recurrent laryngeal nerve injury. Typically, these are iatrogenic injuries (secondary to thyroid surgery) but include others such as thoracic and cervical spinal surgery. Surgical approaches include cordotomies and partial arytenoidectomies[2-5] (Figure 30–7).

Type 2 BVFIs are conditions that cause cricoarytenoid joint ankylosis. These are often secondary to interarytenoid scar, but also due to rheumatoid arthritis. They can occur as a result of trauma, prolonged intubation, or irradiation injury. Initial treatment can include ballooning of the glottis; however, a partial laser arytenoidectomy may be necessary. Other strategies include suture lateralization, which increases the glottic aperture by repositioning the vocal cords in a abducted position.

Types 3 and 4 BVFI lead to posterior glottic webs or scars. They can both be an early or late phase development, secondary to a post-intubation inflammatory

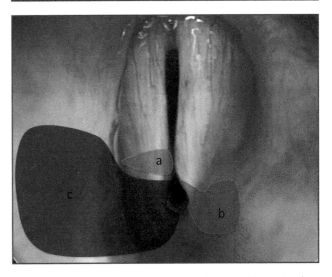

Figure 30–7. Cordotomies and partial arytenoidecomies (a = Kashima 1989, b = Crumley 1993, c = Ossoff 1983).

process. Type 3 impairment occurs early after endotracheal extubation on the ICU with the presence of significant granulation at the posterior commissure and between the arytenoids. Ongoing inflammation and ulceration, with attempted fibrosis, lead to dense interarytenoid scarring. Early intervention with steroid injection and granulation debulking can minimize the risk of mature scar.

Type 4 lesions can be further divided, based on whether there is a band of scar (type 4a) between the arytenoids (see Figure 30–1) or scar filling the posterior commissure (type 4b), as shown in Figure 30–4. Type 4a if identified early enough can be readily divided and ballooned with restoration of normal function. Type 4b lesions, due to the distribution and location of the scar, do not respond as well to this approach. Often the cricoarytenoid joint will be fixed after a prolonged period of immobility. Often Type 4b lesions will require a posterior costal cartilage "spacer" placed in a posterior cricoid split. This can be placed endoscopically or through an open approach via a laryngofissure. Other approaches can be considered, which include endoscopic division of the scar with the use of post-cricoid mucosal advancement flaps.

Type 5 BVFI is immobility due to dense glottic scar extending into the subglottis. These cases are rare but challenging to treat. Surgical strategies are often limited and scar formation often recurs despite attempts to address this with both endoscopic and open approaches.

It is worth noting that posterior glottic stenosis can also be classified according to Bodasarian et al,[6] who describe the type and extent of scar formation. These are as follows:

Type I: interaytenoid synechia

Type II: posterior commissure stenosis

Type III: posterior commissure stenosis with one cricoarytenoid joint ankylosis

Type IV: posterior commissure stenosis with bilateral cricoarytenoid joint ankylosis.

The advantage of this classification is that it reflects the complexity and anticipates the difficulty with surgical repair.

POSTERIOR GLOTTIC CARTILAGE SPACER

Posterior glottic spacer with autologous costal cartilage (Figure 30–8) can be used in cases of posterior glottic stenosis where dense scar formation or considerable joint ankylosis is present. In such cases there are high recurrence rates, and the use of a spacer reduces the potential scar reformation by the splitting of the posterior cricoid and increasing the posterior glottic

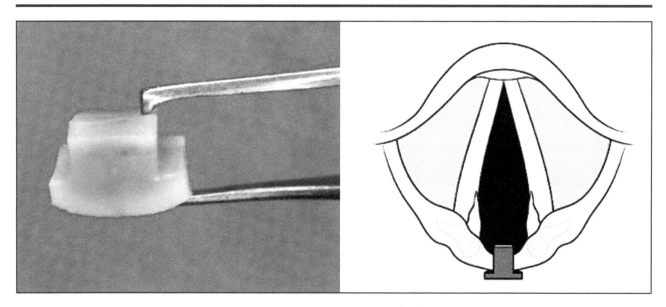

Figure 30–8. Posterior glottic cartilage spacer to maintain scar separation (*left*). Proposed placement site (*right*).

diameter. This has traditionally been performed as an open procedure through a laryngofissure[7,8] and in some cases requires a stent to hold such grafts in place.

With improved instrumentation, there has been a move toward endoscopic placement of such grafts. This experience has been seen mostly in the pediatric population, where an isolated posterior cricoid split (without an anterior division) is arguably easier to perform. It is also easier to distract the cricoid laterally in a child where the cartilage is more pliable. The advantage of endoscopic placement is that it avoids a laryngofissure, thus avoiding possible vocal fold malalignment and anterior webbing. Increasingly there have been reports of surgery where a covering tracheostomy has not been required. Outcomes from pediatric cases of isolated posterior glottic webbing suggest that it can be used successfully, leading to decannulation of tracheostomized patients.[9,10]

VOCAL CORD LATERALIZATION

Vocal cord lateralization has been used as an alternative method in both the acute and chronic setting and for very different etiologies. As with other interventions on the larynx, open approaches were traditionally used but have evolved toward endoscopic methods. One of the first reports of vocal cord lateralization was with a laryngofissure.[11] The procedure would involve removal of some interarytenoid and lateral cricoarytenoid muscle. The arytenoids with overlying mucosa would be sutured and pulled laterally, with placement of the suture on the neck skin surface.[11] Other open approaches have included lateral approaches to the larynx. These have included muscle transposition with omohyoid to the arytenoid cartilage.[12] Others have lateralized the vocal process by creating a thyroid window through which a suture can be placed.[13] Open procedures that have been popular include the Shobel technique,[14] which involves turning and tilting of the arytenoid cartilage laterally so that it approximates the thyroid cartilage. Suture fixation would be to the posterior aspect of the thyroid cartilage.

Endoscopic suture placement has more recently grown in popularity. One of the first reports of endoscopic suture lateralization included removal of the thyroarytenoid muscle combined with wires passed above and below the cord to create a loop around the cord.[15] This technique was later refined to creating loops around the vocal process.[16–20] Tissue resection can be combined with these approaches, and includes submucosal cordectomy and/or arytenoidectomy, depending on joint mobility.[21] Suture loops would be tightened over an external silicon tube. The results of suture fixation at mid-thyroid level have been mixed, and it is clear that attempting to fix to the lower parts of the thyroid cartilage, along a maximal abduction position, can lead to an increased glottis aperture.[22] Suture fixation is challenging; however, endoscopic instruments have evolved such that it is possible to pass sutures through these regions of thickened cartilage in the desired curvilinear direction.[23]

In acute neurogenic cases where it may be possible for recovery, suture lateralization has been used with good effect instead of a tracheostomy, with demonstrable reversibility after release of the sutures when there is evidence of nerve recovery.[18,24] The disadvantages of sutures are that in many cases they do not yield adequate improvement in glottis aperture. Re-medialization can occur, either due to the suture "slipping" or cutting through the vocal cord mucosa or cartilage. This occurs more readily if there is selective reinnervation of the adductor muscles. With the potential for re-medialization, revision or secondary tracheostomy is necessary in up to 38% of cases in some series.[17,25] Nonetheless, this procedure is minimally invasive and can be considered an additional strategy for BVFI, with the advantage of reversibility.

ENDOSCOPIC DIVISION OR RESECTION WITH MUCOSAL ADVANCEMENT FLAP

Severe posterior glottic webs can be extremely challenging to treat and other methods can be considered. A variety of methods have been attempted, but generally the procedure aims to fully remove the scar and cover the defect with a mucosal advancement flap, thus reducing the chance of scar reformation.[26] Typically, the interarytenoid scar is divided and extended to mobilize the joint. The interarytenoid muscle is often taken off one of the arytenoid bodies and the perichondrium shaved down. Dilatation with a balloon or bougie is often performed to fully mobilize the cricoarytenoid joints. Full resection of the posterior web scar is performed but there is often an attempt to leave a flap attached to the vocal process. The post-cricoid region is used to create the advancement flap that is used to fill the interarytenoid region. The advancement flap is sutured in place, endoscopically, covering all exposed cartilage.

SUMMARY

BVFI can be extremely challenging to treat with numerous strategies. A thorough assessment is necessary, with the etiology an important consideration in determining treatment. The extent and site of the disease, and the maturity of the injury, will determine the successful approach. Endoscopic techniques are gaining popularity.

Most surgical approaches lead to a compromise between voice, airway, and swallowing safety. For this reason consideration should be given to earlier tracheostomies on the ICU to reduce the incidence of this condition.

REFERENCES

1. Sittel C, et al. Prognostic value of laryngeal electromyography in vocal fold paralysis. *Arch Otolaryngol Head Neck Surg*. 2001;127(2):155–160.
2. Bosley B, et al. Medial arytenoidectomy versus transverse cordotomy as a treatment for bilateral vocal fold paralysis. *Ann Otol Rhinol Laryngol*. 2005;114(12):922–926.
3. Kashima HK. Bilateral vocal fold motion impairment: pathophysiology and management by transverse cordotomy. *Ann Otol Rhinol Laryngol*. 1991;100(9 pt 1):717–721.
4. Lawson G, et al. Posterior cordectomy and subtotal arytenoidectomy for the treatment of bilateral vocal fold immobility: functional results. *J Voice*. 1996;10(3):314–319.
5. Remacle M, et al. Subtotal carbon dioxide laser arytenoidectomy by endoscopic approach for treatment of bilateral cord immobility in adduction. *Ann Otol Rhinol Laryngol*. 1996;105(6):438–445.
6. Bogdasarian R, Olson N. Posterior glottic laryngeal stenosis. *Otolaryngol Head Neck Surg* (1979). 1980;88(6):765–772.
7. Zalzal GH. Rib cartilage grafts for the treatment of posterior glottic and subglottic stenosis in children. *Ann Otol Rhinol Laryngol*. 1988;97(5 pt 1):506–511.
8. McIlwain JC. Clinical aspects of the posterior glottis: a review. *J Otolaryngol*. 1991;20(2):74–87.
9. Provenzano MJ, et al. Pediatric endoscopic airway management with posterior cricoid rib grafting. *Laryngoscope*. 2011;121(5):1062–1066.
10. Dahl JP, et al. Endoscopic posterior cricoid split with costal cartilage graft: a fifteen-year experience. *Laryngoscope*. 2017;127(1):252–257.
11. Rethi A. Losung der bei der beiderseitigen Postikuslahmung bestehenden medianlage. *Mschr Ohr Laryngorhinol*. 1922;56:200–204.
12. King B. A new and function-restoring operation for bilateral abductor paralysis. *JAMA*. 1939;112:814–823.
13. Newman M, Work W. Arytenoidectomy revisited. *Laryngoscope*. 1976;86:840–849.
14. Schobel H. Glottiserweiterung bei beidseitiger Stimmlippenlaehmung. *HNO*. 1986;34:485–495.
15. Cancura W. [A new method for laterofixation. (Report on preliminary animal experiments)]. *Monatsschr Ohrenheilkd Laryngorhinol*. 1969;103(6):264–271.
16. Lichtenberger G. Endo-extralaryngeal needle carrier instrument. *Laryngoscope*. 1983;93:1348–1350.
17. Hyodo M, Nishikubo K, Motoyoshi K. Laterofixation of the vocal fold using an endo-extralaryngeal needle carrier for bilateral vocal fold paralysis. *Auris Nasus Larynx*. 2009;36(2):181–186.
18. Jóri J, Rovó L, Czigner J. Endolaryngeal laterofixation versus tracheostomy for treatment of acute bilateral vocal cord paralyses. *Magyar Sebészet*. 1997;50:227–229.
19. Jóri J, Rovó L, Czigner J. Vocal cord laterofixation as early treatment for acute bilateral abductor paralysis after thyroid surgery. *Eur Arch Otorhinolaryngol*. 1998;255:375–378.
20. Rovó L, et al. Minimally invasive surgery for posterior glottic stenosis. *Otolaryngol Head & Neck Surgery*. 1999;121:153–156.
21. Lichtenberger G, Toohill R. Endo-extralaryngeal suture technique for endoscopic lateralization of paralyzed vocal cord. *Head and Neck Surgery*. 1998;9(3):156–161.
22. Rovo L, et al. Airway complication after thyroid surgery: minimally invasive management of bilateral recurrent nerve injury. *Laryngoscope*. 2000;110(1):140–144.
23. Rovo L, et al. A new thread guide instrument for endoscopic arytenoid lateropexy. *Laryngoscope*. 2010;120(10):2002–2007.
24. Ejnell H, Tisell L. Acute temporary laterofixation for treatment of bilateral vocal cord paralyses after surgery for advanced thyroid carcinoma. *World J Surg*. 1993;17(2):277–281.
25. Lichtenberger G. Reversible immediate and defintive lateralization of paralyzed vocal cords. *Eur Arch Otorhinolaryngol*. 1999;256:407–411.
26. Goldberg AN. Endoscopic postcricoid advancement flap for posterior glottic stenosis. *Laryngoscope*. 2000;110(3 pt 1):482–485.

CHAPTER 31

Bilateral Recurrent Laryngeal Nerve Injury and Selective Laryngeal Reinnervation

Kate J. Heathcote

A 38-year-old caucasian man with a history of bilateral vocal fold paralysis was referred to us for consideration of laryngeal bilateral selective reinnervation (BSR). The paralysis dated back to a total thyroidectomy for papillary carcinoma when he was 22 years old. At age 23 he had had a left cordotomy to improve his airway and facilitate his work as a laborer. However, he continued to struggle with his voice and airway and had been unable to work since the thyroidectomy. He reported occasionally choking when drinking and had a history of recurrent chest infections. His general doctor reported that he was being treated for depression and had suicidal thoughts.

Discussion Points

- Bilateral vocal fold paralysis is most commonly a complication of thyroid surgery but may also occur following other bilateral neck procedures and in neurofibromatosis type 2. In children it may be idiopathic or due to surgical procedures such as tracheo-esophageal fistula repair.
- Immediately after thyroidectomy there will be some edema of the vocal cords related to the presence of an endotracheal tube during the procedure. This will resolve in the following hours/days and may be improved with steroids. During this time, if there has been bilateral nerve damage, the patient will be stridulous and sometimes a tracheostomy is required. However, there is general relaxation of the larynx following bilateral nerve injury and so once this initial phase of edema has passed, there is likely to be a period of adequate airway but severe breathy dysphonia and aspiration. As spontaneous, synkinetic reinnervation occurs in the following months, the vocal cords will medialize, the voice will improve and the aspiration risk diminish. Patients are often reassured at this time that the nerves are recovering, when in fact the improvement in voice and swallow is at the cost of the airway and increasing dyspnea occurs.
- A differentiation should be made between bilateral recurrent laryngeal nerve (RLN) palsy and bilateral vagal palsy. In the later condition the clinical picture is more complex due to additional sensory and motor deficits with loss of superior laryngeal nerve (SLN) function. In thyroidectomy the SLNs may also be damaged on one or

both sides. There is a view that loss of the external branch of the SLN may provide enough relaxation in the vocal fold to improve the airway and so the technique of injecting the cricothyroid muscle with botulinum toxin in cases where the SLN is intact has been proposed as a way to improve the airway in patients with bilateral RLN paralysis.[1] The major disadvantage with the loss of the SLN is that there will be a sensory loss and increased risk of aspiration. This will be more problematic if both sides are affected.

- Bilateral vocal fold paralysis is most commonly a complication of thyroid surgery but may also occur following other bilateral neck procedures and in neurofibromatosis type 2 and as a result of skull base surgery. In children it may be due to surgical procedures such as tracheo-esophageal fistula repair. In congenital/idiopathic paralysis, recovery may occur spontaneously in the next few years.

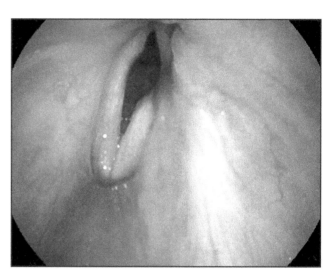

Figure 31–1. Bilaterally medialized vocal folds with left cordotomy.

procedure and stroboscopy enabled us to analyze the extent and impact of the scarring. See Figure 31–1.

The cordotomy was performed anterior to the vocal process with limited scarring, suggesting that it would be amenable to augmentation to improve voice if inspiratory abduction were to be achieved with BSR. There was also a reasonable chance that the cricoarytenoid joint on the side of the arytenoid was still mobile.

INITIAL EVALUATIONS

As in this case, patients requiring BSR have usually had an unexpected and devastating complication of thyroid surgery. Sixteen years later, this gentleman had not come to terms with his disabilities and, despite a healthy fear of undergoing any surgical procedure, was desperate to be considered for BSR. It is absolutely vital that his preoperative status is evaluated in detail to inform discussions regarding the potential gains and losses involved with the surgery. It is also important to have a record for purposes of surgical audit, research, and medicolegal protection.

SWALLOW ASSESSMENT

A flexible endoscopic evaluation of swallowing was performed and demonstrated aspiration on rapid liquid swallow. He performed a 100 mL water swallow test which showed a reduced speed of 18 seconds (normal ≤10 sec) and three coughs within 1 minute of finishing the test.

VOICE ANALYSIS

A GRBAS score was recorded as Grade 3, Roughness 2, Breathiness 3, Asthenia 2, and Strain 3. His Voice Handicap 10 score was 35 out of 40. Voice analysis was carried out using the Operavox app. His maximum phonation time was 3 seconds.

VIDEOLARYNGOSTROBOSCOPY

It is essential to have videolaryngostroboscopy to assess and record the state of the larynx. In this case there was scarring from a previous glottic enlargement

The intention here is to quantify the degree of upper airway restriction as well as to assess the underlying lung function. Maximal inspiratory peak flow is significantly diminished with glottic narrowing.

In the procedure of bilateral selective laryngeal reinnervation, the upper root of one of the phrenic nerves is transected and diverted to supply inspiratory innervation to the posterior cricoarytenoid (PCA) muscles. Although full recovery of diaphragmatic function is anticipated,[2–4] it is important to establish preoperatively that the patient's lung function is adequate to support the temporary effects of transecting one phrenic root. Of particular interest in this regard is the maximal inspiratory pressure, which reflects the strength of the diaphragm.

LARYNGEAL ELECTROMYOGRAPHY (LEMG)

We performed LEMG under local anesthetic at the time of his initial clinic assessment. It is the author's practice to do this by instilling 2% lignocaine through the cricothyroid membrane. A concentric needle electrode can then be inserted through the membrane and introduced in turn into the thyroarytenoid (TA) and PCA muscles on both sides. The PCAs are accessed by passing the electrode through the membrane, across the lumen of the subglottis, and then piercing the posterior cricoid cartilage to enter the muscle. A flexible nasendoscope can be useful for verifying the position of the electrode in this maneuver. The patient was asked to "sniff" and say "ahh" and the LEMG readings were recorded and interpreted by a consultant neurophysiologist on site. The cricothyroid (CT) muscles were also assessed by asking the patient to perform a glissando.

The purpose of the LEMG is to confirm that the movement disorder is of neurological origin. There is the possibility that the disability has been caused by bilateral cricoarytenoid joint fixation or interarytenoid scarring secondary to intubation trauma at the time of the thyroid surgery. In this situation the LEMG will be normal with full interference patterns in the PCAs on inspiration only and the TAs on phonation only. It must be remembered that there may be both paralysis and secondary ankylosis which has occurred over time as a result of prolonged immobility of the joints or glottic enlargement procedures.

The other important fact to establish is that the laryngeal muscles are not completely atrophied. With sustained denervation, muscles undergo fibrotic change and atrophy. This is unusual in the larynx, which is supplied by a plexus of nerves, and the denervated muscles will usually attract nerves from the vicinity to provide innervation and prevent fibrosis and atrophy. In addition, the RLN injuries are often crush injuries and nerve regeneration occurs through the conduit of the RLN, albeit synkinetic. Once fibrotic, the muscle will not regenerate and surgical reinnervation will fail.

In this case there were typical features of a partial reinnervation in both PCAs and both TAs. There were big motor units with reduced activity, firing spontaneously and synkinetically, and some polyphasia.

Both CT muscles showed normal, full interference patterns on glissando, confirming that the SLNs were not damaged at the time of thyroidectomy.

It is Professor Marie's practice to perform the LEMG at the same time as the suspension laryngoscopy (see below). He inserts the needle electrode transorally via a suspended laryngoscope. The patient must be cooperative enough to perform breathing and phonatory tasks and this is achieved using remifentanil and hypnosis. In children LEMG is performed with the child breathing spontaneously under general anesthesia with suspension laryngoscopy. Some voluntary activity may be captured as the anesthetic is lightened with the electrode still in place as the child will make deep inspiratory and phonatory efforts. Hook-wire needle electrodes are an option that can be left in both TAs and removed once the patient is fully awake and some voluntary activity has been recorded

ASSESSMENT OF THE LARYNX UNDER GENERAL ANESTHETIC

This is required to assess cricoarytenoid joint mobility and exclude interarytenoid scarring. Even if the LEMG confirms that the immobility is due to nerve injury, there is the concern that secondary joint fixation may occur as a result of prolonged immobility. In practice this seems to occur very rarely. In this case, the bilateral paralysis had been present for 16 years and he had had a cordotomy with resultant scarring. Whereby the LEMG had reassured us that this was a true case of denervation, it was essential to examine the larynx and establish that the joints were still mobile. Ultimately, inspiratory abduction is only essential on one side to dramatically improve the airway, but of course the chances of a successful outcome are doubled if both sides are still capable of movement.

In this gentleman, the previous glottic enlargement procedure was found to be a simple cordotomy with no arytenoidectomy and with scarring limited to the vocal fold. There was minimal reduction in joint mobility on the side of the cordotomy and no interarytenoid scarring. If interarytenoid scarring is identified, bilateral reinnervation is not an option unless the joints can be successfully re-mobilized.

BASIS OF DECISION TO PROCEED WITH BILATERAL SELECTIVE LARYNGEAL REINNERVATION

Traditional treatment options for bilateral laryngeal paralysis are either a permanent tracheostomy or a glottic enlargement procedure. The impact of tracheostomy tubes on quality of life is very significant and even more so in younger patients. Many patients refuse tracheostomy in favor of dramatically reducing their levels of activity and accepting occasional hospital admissions to manage episodes of stridor brought on by upper respiratory tract infections.

Glottic enlargement procedures can provide an adequate airway for reasonable daily activities but this still falls a long way short of creating an airway that would allow a young person a full sporting life. If the procedure is pushed in pursuit of this goal, the outcome will inevitably result in a very breathy voice and aspiration.

This patient had what must be judged a "good" outcome from his cordotomy in that he managed without a tracheostomy and had an audible voice and a minimally restricted diet. However, he judged his life to be intolerable as a result of his diminished voice and persistent reduction in exercise tolerance. His upper airway restriction prevented him returning to his laboring job and other physical employment and his grade 3 dysphonia precluded him from many other more sedentary occupations. For a person in early adulthood, this is particularly devastating and the negative impact on mental health is to be expected.

In addition, repeated aspiration pneumonia has an acute and chronic morbidity and mortality associated with it,[4] and the resultant lung damage further reduces the tolerance of the restricted upper airway.

This patient had heard about selective reinnervation and was desperate that he should be given the opportunity to have the surgery.

In some ways he was not an ideal candidate for the procedure. The paralysis had been present for 16 years and the glottic scarring from his previous cordotomy reduced the chances of creating adequate inspiratory abduction on that side. Moreover the quality of his voice will remain poor because of the previous cordotomy. However, he was adamant that his current quality of life was insufferable and that he needed to feel that everything had been tried to improve his situation.

The patient was counseled very carefully with regard to the likelihood of success in his case. It was explained to him that he would undergo a 6 to 8 hour operation under general anesthetic. He would need to have a covering tracheostomy tube for 5 to 7 days and a nasogastric feeding tube for 7 to 10 days. He would remain on the hospital ward for up to 2 weeks and may have to be careful with swallowing liquids for some months afterward.

Beyond the acute postoperative period, the chances of long-term negative effects are limited to a long skin crease scar at the level of the cricothyroid membrane, a tracheostomy scar (if not already present, as in this case), and numbness of one earlobe associated with harvesting the great auricular nerve.

What is reassuring, to both the patient and the surgeon, is that it is unlikely that the patient will be left in a worse condition than the preoperative state. This, of course, comes with the proviso that adequate training in the technique has been undertaken by the operating surgeon.

Consent
Indications:

    To improve the airway

    To improve/maintain voice

    To prevent aspiration

Risks:

    A long skin crease scar in the neck

    Temporary tracheostomy and scar

Wound infection
Intraoperative blood loss

Numbness of one earlobe
A period of nasogastric feeding
Postoperative aspiration risk for 14 days but possibly up to 3 months
Unilateral diaphragmatic paralysis
Approximate 25% risk of no significant improvement in airway*
Approximate 15% risk of some deterioration in voice*

*Reflects the results of Professor JP Marie's case series, although better results have been reported by Song et al in China.[5]

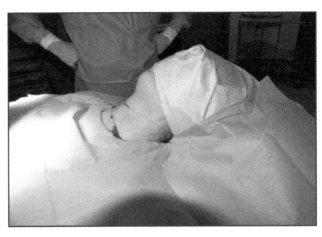

Figure 31–2. Ready to go. I apologize for the hand on hips pose. I am inevitably keen to get going and am sometimes impatient with photographs!

DESCRIPTION OF THE TECHNIQUE[6–9]

- The patient is supine on the operating table with neck extended using a shoulder bolster. The patient must be unparalyzed to facilitate the use of a nerve stimulator. See Figure 31–2.
- A tracheostomy is fashioned (unless already present). This is ideally through the third tracheal ring or lower so that it is separate from the main surgical wound and can be sealed off from the main operative site with a bio-occlusive dressing. It is necessary to avoid any communication between the tracheostomy and main operative wounds to minimize the risk of infection in the area of the nerve anastomoses.
- The neck is re-scrubbed and re-draped with the head in the midline and shoulder bolster still in place.
- A skin crease incision is made that extends from just lateral to the anterior border of the sternocleidomastoid muscle to the same point on the other side. This is done at the level of the cricothyroid membrane
- A further 3-cm skin crease incision is made two finger-breadths below the pinna on the right side. The great auricular nerve is harvested through this incision. An 8-cm "Y" graft is required and so the nerve is followed into the parotid for about 2 cm so that a short length of bifurcated nerve is harvested as part of the graft. This will be used as the extension

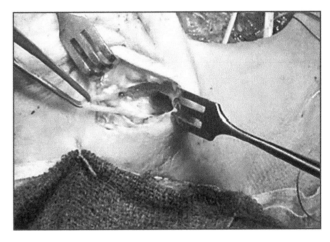

Figure 31–3. The right great auricular nerve is being retracted through the wound using nerve forceps. A length of 8 to 10 cm is required, including 2 cm where the graft is bifurcated.

graft from the root of the phrenic to the PCAs. The graft is stored in saline until required. See Figure 31–3.
- Surgery continues on the right side of the patient with lateral retraction of the sternocleidomastoid muscle and dissection lateral to the carotid sheath and down to the pre-vertebral fascia to identify the main trunk of the phrenic nerve where it rests on the

anterior scalene. The nerve stimulator is used to confirm its identity, placing a hand on the abdomen to feel contraction of the diaphragm.

- The main trunk of the right phrenic is followed superiorly. Here the roots can be seen as they exit the spinal foramina. The precise anatomy is variable, and in this gentleman, only a C3 and C4 root could be seen with no obvious contribution from C5. The C3 (uppermost) root was selected as the donor nerve and a sling placed around the root for identification purposes, but the nerve is left intact at this stage. In some cases there is an accessory phrenic which may be utilized and occasionally there is only one root. In this situation it may be best to explore the other side, which may have more favorable anatomy before deciding whether or not to proceed with utilizing the main trunk. See Figure 31–4.

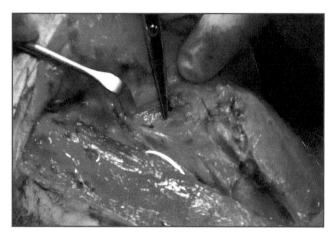

Figure 31–5. The tip of the scissors indicates the small nerve to thyrohyoid as it enters the muscle. The muscle runs from the hyoid bone (indicated by the finger) to the superior border of the thyroid cartilage. The muscle is noted to contract when the stimulator is applied to the nerve.

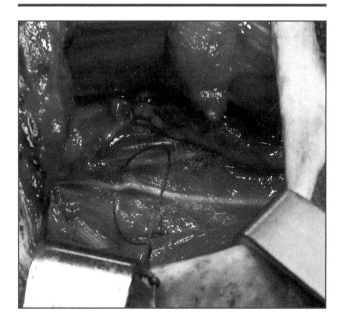

Figure 31–4. Superior is to the left of the picture. The sling is around the C3 root of the phrenic as it joins the C4 root to form the main trunk which descends, lying on the anterior scalene muscle. The root is transected just above its union with the C4 root. This allows continued innervation of the main phrenic trunk through the C4 root. If the C3 root is not present, the most superior root evident should be utilized.

- The next step is to identify the nerve to the right thyrohyoid (TH) muscle. This is a small branch of the ventral ramus of C1 from the cervical plexus which runs with the hypoglossal nerve. It can be identified as it leaves the hypoglossal nerve and descends inferomedially to reach the thyrohyoid muscle. The nerve stimulator is used to confirm its identity. This small nerve will provide innervation to the main trunk of the RLN and has been selected specifically for this function as it is not active on inspiration and so will not produce contraction of the adductor muscles on inspiration, which would compete with the newly established contraction of the PCA muscles required to achieve inspiratory glottic opening. A sling is placed around the nerve. See Figure 31–5.
- The larynx is then rotated using a skin hook placed behind the posterior border of the thyroid cartilage. The inferior constrictor muscle is removed from the posterior border of the thyroid cartilage with diathermy to expose the RLN as it enters the larynx. A sling is placed around it. We stimulated the nerve and noted contraction of the PCA muscle, confirming our LEMG findings of

spontaneous reinnervation. This natural reinnervation of the muscle has served the purpose of maintaining muscle bulk and preventing atrophy, although function has been lost through misdirection of abductor and adductor fibers resulting in synkinetic movements only. See Figure 31–6.

- A retrolaryngeal pocket is created between the larynx and esophagus on the right side and a length of dyed 1/0 thread is placed into it.
- The surgeon then moves to the left side of the patient and the left RLN and TH nerves are similarly identified.
- With the larynx rotated from the left side, a retrolaryngeal dissection is performed until the dyed thread is found and a complete tunnel is formed with the thread lying in the tunnel with an end visible on either side.
- The single end of the "Y" graft is attached to the thread on the left side of the larynx. The graft can then be pulled through so that the bifurcated ends lie adjacent to the PCA muscles.
- A pocket is then created in the vertical (more lateral) belly of the left PCA and one of the bifurcated ends of the graft is inserted into

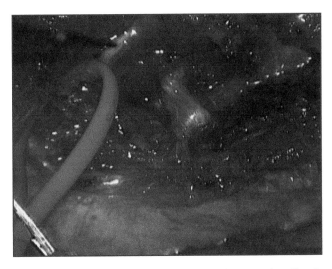

Figure 31–7. Right of picture superior. The vascular sling is around the left RLN, which remains in its original location. One of the bifurcated ends of the "Y" shaped free graft can be seen in the center of the picture, having been sutured into a pocket in the left PCA muscle.

the pocket, sutured in place, and secured with tissue glue. See Figure 31–7.

- The left RLN is then ligated and swung upward toward the TH nerve. There is usually a gap of several centimeters between the RLN and TH nerves and this is bridged using a free interposition graft that may be harvested from the ansa. A small quantity of fat can be wrapped around the anastomosis before applying the glue with a view to enhancing the healing of the neurorrhaphy.
- The surgeon moves to the right side of the patient for the final steps.
- The second bifurcated end of the "Y" graft is inserted into a pocket in the right PCA and secured with a suture and tissue glue.
- The right RLN is ligated, rotated upward, and anastomosed to the TH nerve via another free interposition graft harvested from the ansa. As on the other side, it is secured with fat and tissue glue. See Figure 31–8.
- The single end of the Y-shaped graft is tunneled behind the right carotid sheath to reach the previously identified root of the right phrenic. The root of the phrenic is transected and the final neurorrhaphy

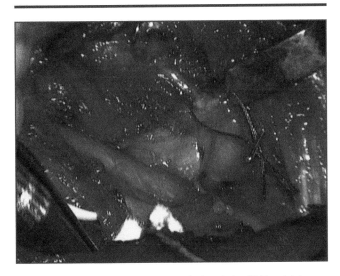

Figure 31–6. The sling is around the right RLN, which can be seen to pass inferiorly into scar tissue from the previous thyroidectomy. The skin hook is in the posterior border of the thyroid cartilage in order to rotate the larynx.

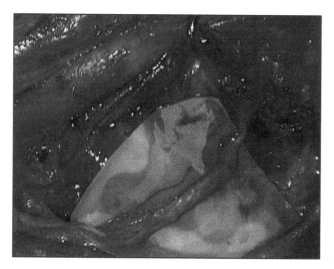

Figure 31–8. The neurorrhaphy between the right RLN and a free interposition graft can be seen on the right-hand side of the small piece of surgical glove that is being used as a stage for the suturing. The RLN is inferior, on the right-hand side of the picture, and the skin hook is in the posterior border of the thyroid cartilage in order to rotate the larynx. To the left of the picture, superior in the patient, this end of the free graft will be anastomosed to the TH nerve.

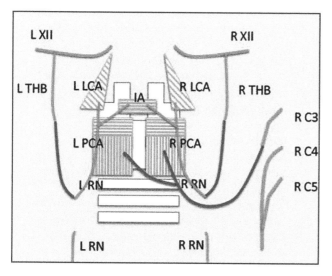

Figure 31–9. A schematic representation of selective laryngeal reinnervation for treating bilateral vocal palsy. C3–5 cervical nerve roots; IA, interarytenoid muscle; LCA, lateral cricoarytenoid; PCA, posterior cricoarytenoid; RN, recurrent nerve; THB, thyrohyoid branch; XII, hypoglossal nerve.

performed between the single end of the Y graft and the root of the phrenic. See Figure 31–9.

COMMENT

Transection of the RLNs during BSR should achieve total denervation of the abductor and adductor muscles of the larynx. It is essential that this is achieved, as a muscle fiber can only receive innervation from one nerve, and if already innervated it will not accept innervation from another nerve. By denervating the laryngeal muscles, they are prepared for targeted reinnervation by the selected donor nerves.

POSTOPERATIVE RECOVERY

A postoperative chest x-ray, performed post to confirm the position of the feeding tube, demonstrated elevation of the right hemi-diaphragm as would be predicted following transection of the upper nerve root of the phrenic.

In this case the tracheostomy was required for 7 days. In fact his airway was adequate throughout and the tracheostomy was required more for the management of his secretions and aspiration. It is really only needed to cover the immediate postoperative vocal fold edema that will have settled in a few days. After this period the glottic gap is likely to be better than the preoperative state as the RLNs have been transected again, removing any synkinetic reinnervation resulting in denervation of the larynx such that the vocal folds are flaccid and lie in a more lateralized position.

The aspiration risk following the surgery is an important symptom to manage. This issue is routinely overlooked at the time of the original nerve injury and there is good evidence to suggest that it is overlooked in many cases of unilateral nerve palsy, a significant percentage of which remain undiagnosed.[5] The advantage of the postoperative laryngeal relaxation is that the tracheostomy can be quickly removed, but this obviously comes at an increased risk of aspiration and with worsening of voice. However, these are also the risks of a glottic enlargement procedure.

This gentleman was discharged 12 days postoperatively. He had a good cough reflex and had stopped using fluid thickener, although he had to take liquids cautiously to avoid aspiration. His voice was very breathy on discharge, with a maximum phonation time (MPT) of 3 seconds.

FOLLOW-UP

1 Month Postop

- Videolaryngostroboscopy: mildly increased glottic gap.
- Swallow: managing a normal diet but remaining cautious with liquids. Cough occurred on rapid drinking.
- MPT, Voice Handicap Index 10 (VHI-10), and Voice Intensity scores: slightly worse than preop values. This is due to persistent laryngeal relaxation resulting in a slightly larger glottic gap.
- Maximal inspiratory peak flow: slightly increased from the preoperative value, reflecting laryngeal relaxation.
- Maximal inspiratory pressure: slightly reduced. This is due to residual weakness of the diaphragm following transection of the right upper root of the phrenic.
- 6 min walk test: slightly improved from the preop value.

6 Months Postop

- Videolaryngostroboscopy: glottic gap equivocal to preop. No inspiratory abduction observed.
- Swallow: managing a normal diet but remaining cautious with liquids. Cough occurred on rapid drinking.
- MPT, VHI-10, and Voice Intensity scores: equipoised with preop values.
- Maximal inspiratory peak flow: no change from the preoperative value.
- Maximal inspiratory pressure: improved from 1 month postop but still slightly below preop level. This is due to residual weakness of the diaphragm following transection of the right upper root of the phrenic.
- 6 min walk test: slightly improved from the preop value.

12 Months Postop

- Videolaryngostroboscopy: inspiratory abduction observed on the left side. Improved glottic closure.
- Swallow: managing a normal diet including rapid drinking, occasional cough with liquids but no penetration witnessed on FEES.
- MPT, VHI-10, Voice Intensity scores: minimal improvement from preop values.
- Maximal inspiratory peak flow: improved from the preoperative value.
- Maximal inspiratory pressure: recovered to preop values.
- 6 min walk test: significantly improved from the preop value.

2 Years Postop

- Videolaryngostroboscopy: wide inspiratory abduction observed on the left side. Good glottic closure other than at site of previous cordotomy. No significant arytenoid abduction observed on the left.
- Swallow: managing a normal diet, including rapid drinking and occasional cough with liquids, but no penetration witnessed on FEES.
- MPT, VHI-10, Voice Intensity scores: improved from preop values.
- Maximal inspiratory peak flow: improved from the preoperative value.
- Maximal inspiratory pressure: recovered to preop values.
- 6 min walk test: significantly improved from the preop value and the 12 month value.

At this stage the patient was extremely happy with the improvement in his exercise tolerance, but there remained the issue of his voice. It was felt that the abduction achieved on the left was adequate to consider injection augmentation at the site of the previous left cordotomy. This was performed under local anesthetic in the outpatient clinic. Hyaluronic acid was injected with a significant improvement. This will need repeating at intervals in the future.

Note: This is a fictional patient with elements of the case drawn from the pool of patients that we have treated. Please see the bibliography below for more information regarding clinical outcomes and further details related to the technique.

Acknowledgment: We would like to thank all members of our clinical team who support this work with great commitment and enthusiasm; in particular our speech therapy and neurophysiology colleagues. In addition, we acknowledge Professor Marie's dedicated research team, who spent years of trials and development required to devise this operative technique.

REFERENCES

1. Benninger MS, Hanick A, Hicks DM. Cricothyroid muscle botulinum toxin injection to improve airway for bilateral recurrent laryngeal nerve paralysis, a case series. *J Voice*. 2016;30(1):96–99.
2. Marie JP, Lacoume Y, Laquerrière A, Tardif C, Fallu J, Bonmarchand G, Vérin E. Diaphragmatic effects of selective resection of the upper phrenic nerve root in dogs. *Respir Physiol Neurobiol*. 2006;154(3):419–430.
3. Verin E, Marie JP, Similowski T. Cartography of human diaphragmatic innervation: preliminary data. *Respir Physiol Neurobiol*. 2011;176(1–2):68–71.
4. Nouraei SAR, Allen J, Kaddour H, Middleton SE, Aylin P, Darzi A, Tolley NS. Vocal palsy increases the risk of lower respiratory tract infection in low-risk, low-morbidity patients undergoing thyroidectomy for benign disease: a big data analysis. *Clin Oto*. 2017;42(6):1259–1266.
5. Song W, Li M, Zheng HL, et al. Treatment of bilateral vocal cord paralysis by hemi-phrenic nerve transfer. *Zhonghua Er Bi Yan Hou Tou JingWai Ke Za Zhi*. 2017;52:245–252.
6. Marina MB, Marie JP, Birchall MA. Laryngeal reinnervation for bilateral vocal fold paralysis. *Curr Opin Otolaryngol Head Neck Surg*. 2011;19(6):434–438.
7. Fancello V, Nouraei SAR, Heathcote KJ. Role of reinnervation in the management of recurrent laryngeal nerve injury: current state and advances. *Curr Opin Otolaryngol Head Neck Surg*. 2017;25(6):480–485.
8. Marie JP. Nerve reconstruction. In: Remacle M, Eckel HE, eds, *Surgery of Larynx and Trachea*. Heidelbergerman: Springer; 2010:279–294.
9. Marie JP. Reinnervation: new frontiers. In: Rubin JS, Sataloff RT, Korovin GS, eds, *Diagnostic and Treatment of Voice Disorders*. 4th ed. San Diego, CA: Plural Publishing; 2014.

CHAPTER 32

Atypical Spasmodic Dysphonia with Tremor

Daniel Novakovic

Ms K is a 47-year-old female who presents to a tertiary laryngology center with acute deterioration of her voice 3 months ago associated with an upper respiratory tract infection characterized by a hacking/non-productive cough. She lost her voice completely at that stage and it has not returned to normal despite resolution of her cough after a few months. She presents with symptoms of severely increased vocal effort and vocal fatigue which are exacerbated by minimal voice usage and relieved somewhat by rest. She experiences excessive neck muscle tightness/strain and pain on speaking (odynophonia). The voice quality remains poor throughout the day. She reports occasional mild dyspnea with noisy breathing which is not exacerbated by exercise.

She is employed as a primary school teacher and teaches groups of up to 60 children in a large area classroom without amplification. She has been unable to perform her duties at work due to an inability to meet the vocal demands associated with her job. She ceased work completely 6 weeks ago. A diagnosis of vocal nodules has been given by a general otolaryngologist and she has been undergoing voice therapy sessions with a voice specialized speech pathologist one or two times per week with minimal improvement in her voice over this period. Prior to the vocal deterioration she reports a 3- to 4-year history (since she began teaching in large classrooms) of intermittent hoarseness and rough voice with mild vocal fatigue worse toward the end of the school week which improved on weekends and school holidays.

She has past medical history of recurrent acute sinusitis, which is often associated with cough and dyspnea. She has had previous endoscopic sinus sur-

gery and remains on topical nasal therapy with saline and intranasal steroids for medical management of chronic rhinosinusitis with oral antibiotics reserved for flare-ups. A trial of acid suppression therapy with reflux dietary and lifestyle advice has been undertaken over the past 6 weeks with no appreciable effect upon her voice. No known drug allergies. There is a family history of rheumatoid arthritis and thyroid disorders. Her daughter underwent thyroidectomy at age 15.

There is no family history of voice disorder, tremor, dystonia, or other neurological condition. Her voice "relaxes" and becomes more fluid with alcohol but never reaches its baseline state. Her voice may be slightly better in the morning, although this varies. She does not sing. There are no other neurological symptoms, and respiratory review has excluded any lung pathology. She can, however, shout spontaneously with normal voice at most times and laughing is relatively preserved.

INTRODUCTION

Professional voice users are known to be at greater risk of developing voice problems.[1] Teachers have the highest incidence of voice disorders among all of the professional voice groups.[1,2] In an Australian cohort of 877 teachers, the prevalence of self-reported voice problems was as high as 20%, with females more likely to report voice problems than males.[3] Risk factors for teachers developing voice problems include loud voice use[4] as well as poor acoustic and noise conditions, including large classrooms and high background noise along with other factors, including longer working hours.[5] Teachers reporting voice problems have a higher rate of organic lesions, the most common pathology being vocal nodules.[6] Nodules can be a manifestation of functional dysphonia; however, this entity can also present with a normal videolaryngoscopy seen in 25% of teachers with voice complaints.[7]

Hoarseness associated with upper respiratory tract infection is most often due to acute viral laryngitis.[8] This condition is typically self-limiting and short lasting. Viral infections have also been implicated in hypofunctional neurological voice problems, including vocal fold palsy and post-viral vagal neuropathy, which can present with persistent symptoms similar to the above case, including dysphonia, vocal fatigue, and chronic cough or throat irritation, and typically presenting in the fifth decade of life in females.[9]

The above patient's symptoms are non-specific but are also consistent with a presentation of muscle tension dysphonia (MTD), which can manifest as a primary functional problem or secondary to organic pathology. Typical features exhibited in this case include vocal fatigue, hoarseness, and tightness in the laryngeal region exacerbated by speaking, thought to be related to hyperfunction/imbalance of perilaryngeal musculature.[10] In the author's experience, preceding upper repiratory tract infection is a common cause of exacerbation of symptoms in people with diagnoses of MTD. The presentation above is not typical, however, of MTD with or without vocal nodules, which will characteristically respond well to speech therapy treatment,[11] raising the possibility of an alternative diagnosis.

Alcohol responsiveness, better morning voice, and preservation of shouting suggest that spasmodic dyphonia (SD) should be considered in the list of differentials. Onset associated with upper respiratory tract infection is reported in 30% of SD patients,[12] with this patient exhibiting typical age and sex demographics for this condition. Eliciting family history is important, as 12% of patients with primary laryngeal dystonia have a family history of dystonia.[13]

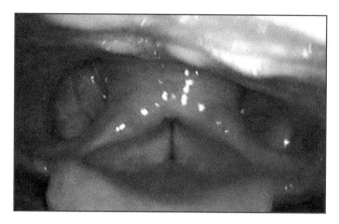

Figure 32–1. False vocal fold approximation at phonation onset.

CLINICAL EXAMINATION

The Voice Handicap Symptom Index 10 (VHI-10) score is elevated at 40/40. Her Reflux Symptom Index (RSI) score is elevated at 20/45. Perceptually her voice is severely abnormal and sounds breathy and tremulous and rated G2 R1 B2 A2 S3 on the GRBAS scale,[14] with frequent nonspecific voice breaks. Maximal phonation time is 15 seconds. General examinations of the ear, nose, and oral cavity/oropharynx are normal. She has significant laryngeal elevation on both phonation and connected speech with perilaryngeal muscle tenderness on palpation. Other neck examination was normal with no palpable masses or thyroid tenderness.

Laryngoscopy shows a structurally normal appearing larynx with equal and appropriate vocal fold movement that is full range and symmetrical. There is no sign of mucosal inflammation or edema. There is intermittent mild paradoxical vocal fold movement with inspiration and occasional short periods of inspiratory phonation. Laryngeal stroboscopy shows minimal mid-vocal fold thickenings with little to no effect upon mucosal wave, which is equal and symmetrical with a suggestion of mild glottal insufficiency (Video 32–1, see companion website). There is severe supraglottal constriction at the onset of connected speech (sentences and words) with complete false vocal fold approximation (Figure 32–1) which responds well to speech therapy de-constriction maneuvers. Connected speech is poorly coordinated with poor volume and breathiness even after speech therapy exercises. The voice sounds tremulous but only mild irregular vocal fold tremor can be demonstrated endoscopically on sustained phonation, which remains relatively preserved. Sentences designed to unmask spasmodic dysphonia were globally difficult and not specific for either the adductor or abductor variants using phonetically loaded sentences with nonspecific tight and breathy pitch breaks (Video 32–2, see companion website).

Her speech pathologist and referring otolaryngologist have suggested recalcitrant muscle tension dysphonia (possibly secondary to vocal nodules) as the primary diagnosis. Although significant neuromuscular incoordination is noted, the diagnosis of MTD (without nodules) is initially supported with a differential diagnosis of unspecified neurological voice condition. Further speech therapy is recommended with a trial of return to work on modified vocal duties at reduced hours with the assistance of amplification. Neurological consultation is suggested should she fail to make progress with voice therapy.

Patient self-reported outcome tools are useful in assessing the impact of a voice disorder upon quality of life and/or functional status and for tracking patient perceived response to treatment over time. There are numerous such measures available and we routinely utilize the VHI-10[15] as a validated measure of voice handicap in addition to the RSI[16] as a surrogate marker of throat irritation. This lady exhibits a maximal VHI-10 score indicating severe voice dysfunction as perceived by the patient.

Stroboscopy is a valuable voice assessment tool and frequently results in an altered diagnosis.[17] In this case the mid-vocal fold swellings previously described as nodules were found to be soft with normal mucosal vibration parameters and no significant effect upon glottal closure, thereby unlikely to be the main causative factor in her dysphonia.

MTD is one of the most common diagnoses for people presenting to specialized voice clinics. In its primary form it represents a functional voice disorder but can also occur secondary to underlying vocal pathology.

Spasmodic dysphonia (SD) is a rare (1–6 per 100,000) focal laryngeal dystonia affecting voice production during speech. It is more common in women and peak incidence is between the fourth and sixth decades.[18] Adductor spasmodic dysphonia (AdSD) is the most commonly reported form (80%) manifesting as tight and strained voice secondary to inappropriate adductor muscle complex activity. Abductor spasmodic dysphonia (AbSD) is less common (10–15%) and presents with breathy voice secondary to inappropriate posterior cricoarytenoid muscle abductor activity during phonation.[19] There also exists a poorly described mixed form of spasmodic dysphonia exhibiting features of both AdSD and AbSD. Concomitant vocal tremor is present in approximately 25% of SD cases[20,21] and is thought to be a marker for poorer response to treatment. SD is typically diagnosed based upon clinical history along with recognition of characteristic patterns of vocal spasms which can be unmasked using voice tasks specific to the adductor or abductor variants.

Distinguishing between SD and MTD can be challenging especially in atypical presentations. Both entities can present with similar symptoms of increased vocal effort and vocal fatigue. A careful directed history can help elicit the diagnosis. SD is task specific and predominantly affects the function of speech, although singing, breathing, and cough variants of laryngeal dystonia have also been described.[22–24] Speaking on the telephone or in high stress situations typically aggravate voice symptoms of SD. Non-speech voice functions such as laughing, crying, and singing are typically preserved in SD patients, and they may report better voice fluidity when speaking in a foreign accent or when shouting. Patients with SD frequently report that the voice is better for the first half an hour or so after they wake up. Symptom severity in MTD tends to be preserved across all vocal tasks and tends to be aggravated by usage. Up to 58% of people with SD report improvement of the voice with ingestion of alcohol,[25] which is not typical with MTD.

It can be difficult to distinguish between spasmodic dysphonia and muscle tension dysphonia based upon clinical examination. Lateral supraglottal compression (although not specific to MTD[26]) is recognized as a classic pattern of muscle tension constriction seen in MTD. A similar pattern of supraglottal hyperfunction may be seen in up to 25% of patients with AdSD.[27] An increase in dysphonia severity using phonetically loaded sentences (voiced for AdSD and voiceless for AbSD) is typical for SD compared with MTD,[28] in which dysphonia severity tends to remain constant across all phonatory tasks.

INVESTIGATIONS

Baseline routine blood tests and autoimmune screen have been normal. Thyroid function tests including thyroid antibodies are ordered and normal. Copper and ceruloplasmin levels are normal.

In the absence of a definitive diagnosis, alternative causes for dysphonia must be explored. Patients presenting with dysphonia have often already undergone ultrasound imaging of the thyroid gland via the primary care physician. Thyroid pathology may be seen more frequently in people with vocal fold paresis,[29] and in the author's experience, thyroiditis can be an underlying cause of both vocal fold paresis and laryngeal sensory dysfunction manifesting as dysphonia. Clinical examination of the neck and thyroid blood tests (including antibodies) may be useful in the diagnostic process.

When considering a potential diagnosis of spasmodic dysphonia, investigations to rule out rare underlying neurological problems causing secondary SD such as Huntington's or Wilson's disease may be appropriate. Early referral to a movement disorders neurologist can be useful to help elicit the presence of other neurological signs, which may assist with the diagnosis and to establish baseline neurological status, as 16% of people with primary laryngeal involvement can develop dystonia in other regions of the body.[13]

PROGRESS

Ms K returns 4 weeks later with further deterioration of her voice and limited further response to speech therapy. She is finding it increasingly difficult to work and becomes exhausted by effort when trying to speak for more than a few minutes at a time. Review by a general neurologist has suggested a possible diagnosis of spasmodic dysphonia (variant unspecified). Repeat laryngovideostroboscopy shows ongoing supraglottal squeeze at phonation onset with poor coordination of speech but no obvious glottal insufficiency. Management options were discussed including the potential diagnosis of spasmodic dysphonia vs muscle tension dysphonia with supraglottal squeeze as a primary feature.

The role of botulinum toxin (BTX) was discussed in each of these conditions and the patient elected to trial BTX therapy.

Patients with MTD typically respond to behavioral modification via voice therapy.[30,31] Minimal response to voice therapy in this case suggests an alternative diagnosis; however, MTD recalcitrant to voice therapy is well recognized. The second opinion from a neurologist in this case has further highlighted the possibility of SD as the primary diagnosis in this case, although the clinical features are not typical for either AdSD or AbSD. In a setting where the diagnosis is unclear and there has been limited response to voice therapy, it is reasonable to offer a trial of laryngeal BTX therapy to the patient.

BTX is established as the gold standard of treatment for SD, with efficacy demonstrated in double blind, placebo controlled trials.[32] Adductor SD is the most common variant, which is classically treated with BTX injections into the adductor muscle complex. Given the presence of extreme supraglottal constriction in this case, we elected to perform false vocal fold BTX injection as described by Young and Blitzer.[27] There is also some evidence that BTX may be useful in refractory MTD.[33]

OFFICE-BASED SUPRAGLOTTIC BOTULINUM TOXIN INJECTION

Under endoscopic and electromyography (EMG) guidance, 3.75 U of onabotulinum toxin type A (Botox®, Allergan, Irvine, CA, USA) was injected into the supraglottic larynx on each side via a trans-thyrohyoid approach under a regional laryngeal block.

The dose of Botox given was based upon personal experience and that of Young and Blitzer,[27] who used between 2.5 and 5.0 units per false vocal fold. Simpson et al described both a transoral and extramucosal trans-thyrohyoid approach to false vocal fold BTX treatment for AdSD injection, proposing that it would provide more gradual onset with less severe breathiness as a side effect. They utilized a higher dose averaging 7.6 units of Botox per false vocal fold in the subepithelial plane. Superior laryngeal nerve block via an external approach is a simple and effective method of providing regional anesthesia to the supraglottic region for such an approach,[34] although infiltration of the pre-epiglottic space with local anesthetic is a useful alternative/adjunct.

PROGRESS AFTER SUPRAGLOTTIC BOTULINUM TOXIN INJECTION

She is reviewed 6 weeks later, and the voice remains very inconsistent. She reports that some of the tightness is better and there is more intermittent fluidity and clarity in the voice, but she now suffers from increased breathiness and increased difficulty getting words out, which she describes as "stuttering," with difficulty speaking above background noise. Her percentage normal scale shows a characteristic dip in the first 2 weeks (type 2 curve as described by Novakovic et al[35]), suggesting effect of the BTX before returning to just above baseline. Laryngoscopy shows ongoing lateral supraglottal compression and mild glottal insufficiency on sustained phonation (Video 32–3, see companion website). Perceptually there appear to be intermittent breathy pitch breaks on voiceless weighted sentences. She continues voice therapy with an experienced speech pathologist with limited improvement. The options of further BTX (possibly into the abductor musculature) versus a trial augmentation laryngoplasty are discussed. The patient is keen for augmentation injection laryngoscopy to try to improve her symptoms of glottal insufficiency.

Breathy voice occurs frequently after BTX treatment for AdSD and can be a marker of technical success in treating the adductor complex as well as a predictor of successful treatment.[36] Treatment effect is best tracked by examining longitudinal functional outcomes, and the percentage normal function (PNF) scale (Figure 32–2) is a useful tool which we routinely used for this purpose.[35] Approximately 29% of AdSD patients will report an initial decrease in their PNF after BTX-A treatment (type II curve), which typically lasts for up to 2 weeks.[35] The characteristic decrease in PNF in this case suggests a technically successful BTX-A injection. Failure of the PNF to improve beyond baseline suggests that AdSD is not the primary/sole diagnosis. Breathiness is a common side effect of BTX-A treatment for AdSD experienced in 51% of cases,[35] which is thought to be related to glottal insufficiency secondary to adductor muscle weakness. In this case, however, it is unclear whether the ongoing breathiness is a result of BTX-A side effect or possibly abductor pitch breaks, suggesting the possibility of abductor or mixed spasmodic dysphonia.

OFFICE–BASED AUGMENTATION INJECTION LARYNGOPLASTY

Four months after the initial botulinum toxin injection, the patient undergoes augmentation injection laryngoplasty under local anesthetic: 0.4 cc of hyaluronic acid gel is injected into each paraglottic space via an endoscopically guided, transcutaneous, extramucosal cricothyroid approach.

On review 2 weeks later, she reports that her voice temporarily improved 5 days after the augmentation with decreased vocal effort and improved volume followed by deterioration in the past day or two and return of voice tightness. The VHI-10 score has improved to 28/40 and the voice sounds stronger with intermittent tight pitch breaks (and ongoing false vocal fold compression at phonation onset). Further voice therapy is recommended to target laryngeal constriction. She remains off work for medical reasons (6 months down the track). She is seen 8 weeks later and feels that there was some improvement after the augmentation procedure, with less breathlessness, vocal fatigue, and odynophonia.

Vocal fold augmentation injection laryngoplasty using a temporary biocompatible material is a useful tool for treatment of glottal insufficiency and can help guide diagnosis and management. The partial voice improvement seen in this patient after vocal fold augmentation raises the possibility of muscle tension dysphonia secondary to underlying glottal insufficiency. Belafsky et al[37] reported a higher incidence of abnormal muscle tension pattern in people with underlying glottal insufficiency. In this author's experience, augmentation injection laryngoplasty can be beneficial in both primary and secondary forms of recalcitrant MTD, facilitating improved response to ongoing voice therapy. The resolution of odynophonia after vocal fold injection augmentation suggests the possibility of underlying glottal insufficiency. Kuper et al[38] have reported on the utility of medialization laryngoplasty as a successful treatment in patients presenting with odynophonia.

PROGRESS

A further 8 weeks later Ms K feels that the voice has deteriorated with recurrent odynophonia and increased vocal effort and recurrent breathy pitch breaks. An opinion is obtained from a movement disorders neurologist with an interest in voice. Four-muscle laryngeal electromyography was performed as part of this assessment and is reported as normal. A diagnosis of adductor spasmodic dysphonia is made by the neurologist and she receives bilateral EMG guided Botox injections into the thyroarytenoid (TA) muscles (0.5 U each side). The voice deteriorates after this and 4 weeks later she remains aphonic with severe breathiness and ongoing mild dysphagia to fluids. There is mild glottal insufficiency on laryngovideostroboscopy with ongoing lateral supraglottal squeeze (Video 32–4, see companion website). She undergoes further vocal fold injection augmentation (while she has botulinum toxin on board) with hyaluronic acid crosslinked gel (0.3 cc each side). Exploratory microlaryngoscopy at the time reveals very mild subepithelial thickening on the left vocal fold but no sign of hidden pathology such as sulcus vocalis or vocal fold scar after subepithelial saline infusion of the superficial layer of lamina propria (SLLP). The symptoms of breathiness improve after vocal fold augmentation with a sensation that the voice is the best it had been since the problem began but still severely disordered (Video 32–5, see

Botulinum Toxin/Spasmodic Dysphonia Homework Sheet   Name: _____

CURRENT PERCENTAGE OF NORMAL FUNCTION

(No function)   0%-5%-10%-15%-20%-25%-30%-35%-40%-45%-50%-55%-60%-65%-70%-75%-80%-85%-90%-95%-100%   *(Normal function)*

DAY

__/__/__ 0   0%-5%-10%-15%-20%-25%-30%-35%-40%-45%-50%-55%-60%-65%-70%-75%-80%-85%-90%-95%-100%

__/__/__ 1   0%-5%-10%-15%-20%-25%-30%-35%-40%-45%-50%-55%-60%-65%-70%-75%-80%-85%-90%-95%-100%

__/__/__ 2   0%-5%-10%-15%-20%-25%-30%-35%-40%-45%-50%-55%-60%-65%-70%-75%-80%-85%-90%-95%-100%

__/__/__ 3   0%-5%-10%-15%-20%-25%-30%-35%-40%-45%-50%-55%-60%-65%-70%-75%-80%-85%-90%-95%-100%

__/__/__ 4   0%-5%-10%-15%-20%-25%-30%-35%-40%-45%-50%-55%-60%-65%-70%-75%-80%-85%-90%-95%-100%

__/__/__ 5   0%-5%-10%-15%-20%-25%-30%-35%-40%-45%-50%-55%-60%-65%-70%-75%-80%-85%-90%-95%-100%

__/__/__ 6   0%-5%-10%-15%-20%-25%-30%-35%-40%-45%-50%-55%-60%-65%-70%-75%-80%-85%-90%-95%-100%

__/__/__ 7   0%-5%-10%-15%-20%-25%-30%-35%-40%-45%-50%-55%-60%-65%-70%-75%-80%-85%-90%-95%-100%

__/__/__ 8   0%-5%-10%-15%-20%-25%-30%-35%-40%-45%-50%-55%-60%-65%-70%-75%-80%-85%-90%-95%-100%

__/__/__ 9   0%-5%-10%-15%-20%-25%-30%-35%-40%-45%-50%-55%-60%-65%-70%-75%-80%-85%-90%-95%-100%

__/__/__ 10   0%-5%-10%-15%-20%-25%-30%-35%-40%-45%-50%-55%-60%-65%-70%-75%-80%-85%-90%-95%-100%

__/__/__ 11   0%-5%-10%-15%-20%-25%-30%-35%-40%-45%-50%-55%-60%-65%-70%-75%-80%-85%-90%-95%-100%

__/__/__ 12   0%-5%-10%-15%-20%-25%-30%-35%-40%-45%-50%-55%-60%-65%-70%-75%-80%-85%-90%-95%-100%

__/__/__ 13   0%-5%-10%-15%-20%-25%-30%-35%-40%-45%-50%-55%-60%-65%-70%-75%-80%-85%-90%-95%-100%

__/__/__ 14   0%-5%-10%-15%-20%-25%-30%-35%-40%-45%-50%-55%-60%-65%-70%-75%-80%-85%-90%-95%-100%

WEEK

__/__/__ 3   0%-5%-10%-15%-20%-25%-30%-35%-40%-45%-50%-55%-60%-65%-70%-75%-80%-85%-90%-95%-100%

__/__/__ 4   0%-5%-10%-15%-20%-25%-30%-35%-40%-45%-50%-55%-60%-65%-70%-75%-80%-85%-90%-95%-100%

__/__/__ 5   0%-5%-10%-15%-20%-25%-30%-35%-40%-45%-50%-55%-60%-65%-70%-75%-80%-85%-90%-95%-100%

__/__/__ 6   0%-5%-10%-15%-20%-25%-30%-35%-40%-45%-50%-55%-60%-65%-70%-75%-80%-85%-90%-95%-100%

__/__/__ 7   0%-5%-10%-15%-20%-25%-30%-35%-40%-45%-50%-55%-60%-65%-70%-75%-80%-85%-90%-95%-100%

__/__/__ 8   0%-5%-10%-15%-20%-25%-30%-35%-40%-45%-50%-55%-60%-65%-70%-75%-80%-85%-90%-95%-100%

__/__/__ 9   0%-5%-10%-15%-20%-25%-30%-35%-40%-45%-50%-55%-60%-65%-70%-75%-80%-85%-90%-95%-100%

__/__/__ 10   0%-5%-10%-15%-20%-25%-30%-35%-40%-45%-50%-55%-60%-65%-70%-75%-80%-85%-90%-95%-100%

__/__/__ 11   0%-5%-10%-15%-20%-25%-30%-35%-40%-45%-50%-55%-60%-65%-70%-75%-80%-85%-90%-95%-100%

__/__/__ 12   0%-5%-10%-15%-20%-25%-30%-35%-40%-45%-50%-55%-60%-65%-70%-75%-80%-85%-90%-95%-100%

__/__/__ 13   0%-5%-10%-15%-20%-25%-30%-35%-40%-45%-50%-55%-60%-65%-70%-75%-80%-85%-90%-95%-100%

__/__/__ 14   0%-5%-10%-15%-20%-25%-30%-35%-40%-45%-50%-55%-60%-65%-70%-75%-80%-85%-90%-95%-100%

__/__/__ 15   0%-5%-10%-15%-20%-25%-30%-35%-40%-45%-50%-55%-60%-65%-70%-75%-80%-85%-90%-95%-100%

__/__/__ 16   0%-5%-10%-15%-20%-25%-30%-35%-40%-45%-50%-55%-60%-65%-70%-75%-80%-85%-90%-95%-100%

__/__/__ 17   0%-5%-10%-15%-20%-25%-30%-35%-40%-45%-50%-55%-60%-65%-70%-75%-80%-85%-90%-95%-100%

__/__/__ 18   0%-5%-10%-15%-20%-25%-30%-35%-40%-45%-50%-55%-60%-65%-70%-75%-80%-85%-90%-95%-100%

__/__/__ 19   0%-5%-10%-15%-20%-25%-30%-35%-40%-45%-50%-55%-60%-65%-70%-75%-80%-85%-90%-95%-100%

__/__/__ 20   0%-5%-10%-15%-20%-25%-30%-35%-40%-45%-50%-55%-60%-65%-70%-75%-80%-85%-90%-95%-100%

__/__/__ 21   0%-5%-10%-15%-20%-25%-30%-35%-40%-45%-50%-55%-60%-65%-70%-75%-80%-85%-90%-95%-100%

__/__/__ 22   0%-5%-10%-15%-20%-25%-30%-35%-40%-45%-50%-55%-60%-65%-70%-75%-80%-85%-90%-95%-100%

__/__/__ 23   0%-5%-10%-15%-20%-25%-30%-35%-40%-45%-50%-55%-60%-65%-70%-75%-80%-85%-90%-95%-100%

__/__/__ 24   0%-5%-10%-15%-20%-25%-30%-35%-40%-45%-50%-55%-60%-65%-70%-75%-80%-85%-90%-95%-100%

__/__/__ 25   0%-5%-10%-15%-20%-25%-30%-35%-40%-45%-50%-55%-60%-65%-70%-75%-80%-85%-90%-95%-100%

__/__/__ 26   0%-5%-10%-15%-20%-25%-30%-35%-40%-45%-50%-55%-60%-65%-70%-75%-80%-85%-90%-95%-100%

Figure 32–2. Percentage normal function scale.

companion website). The voice deteriorates once again after the effect of the botulinum toxin has worn off and further once the augmentation material has resorbed. Review of the case with another senior laryngologist suggests the presence of abductor posterior cricoarytenoid (PCA) muscle activity, greater on the right side during periods of supraglottal squeeze, suggesting the possibility of abductor or mixed spasmodic dysphonia with compensatory muscle tension constriction.

Exploratory microlaryngoscopy with palpation and subepithelial saline injection can be useful in cases of dysphonia recalcitrant to standard treatment to exclude underlying pathologies such as vocal fold scar or sulcus vocalis which may be missed on office examination. In this case the patient's voice deteriorated significantly after BTX-A treatment of the TA muscles (even at low dose) and vocal fold augmentation was offered at the same time as an exploratory procedure with an improvement in her voice. As the case evolves based upon response to treatment, pure adductor SD becomes an unlikely diagnosis as the clinical features of breathiness become more prominent following Botox injection. Abductor spasmodic dysphonia is a rarer form of SD responsible for 10 to 15% of focal laryngeal dystonia with a higher male predominance compared with AdSD and a less favorable response to BTX-A treatment.[19] Lateral supraglottal constriction and inhalational speech (both seen in this patient) have been described as compensatory maneuvers to abnormal abductor muscle activity.[39]

OFFICE-BASED TREATMENT OF THE ABDUCTOR MUSCLE COMPLEX

Right PCA muscle injection of Botox (3.75 U) is performed under EMG guidance. Two weeks later there is no improvement with full vocal fold mobility. A larger dose of 5.0 units was given into the left PCA muscle; 2 weeks later there is only mild hypomobility on this side. Chemodenervation of the abductor muscle complex is the preferred treatment for laryngeal dystonia presenting with abductor muscle spasms. Ludlow et al have also described chemodenervation of the cricothyroid muscles for AbSD[40]; however, we tend to reserve this for cases recalcitrant to standard treatment. Access to the PCA muscle is technically more difficult than the adductor complex due to the anatomical location at the posterior portion of the larynx. The lateral rotational approach described by Blitzer et al[19] provides

PCA muscle access without breach of the laryngeal mucosa but can be technically challenging. Alternatively, a transmucosal, transcricoid technique via the cricothyroid membrane can be utilized as described by Meleca et al.[41] Both techniques require the use of EMG muscle localization. Reported doses of Botox vary from 3.75 U to 15 U with unilateral and bilateral techniques described. Mild dysphagia is reported in 6% of cases[42] and thought to be related to diffusion of BTX into the inferior constrictor muscle. Technical success can be confirmed on laryngoscopy with a decrease in abductor activity. In the author's experience vocal fold injection augmentation can be a useful adjunct for symptomatic treatment of breathiness associated with AbSD, although it is not expected to stop the abductor pitch breaks.

We proceed with 10.0 units of BTX-A into the right PCA muscle under general anesthesia (Figure 32–3) along with repeat vocal fold augmentation. Two weeks later the breathy voice has improved but she has ongoing adductor type spasms of the voice (Video 32–6, see companion website). The voice is functional for work at low volume phonation and she returns to one on one and small group teaching part time. The diagnosis of mixed spasmodic dysphonia is discussed along with the role of further BTX into the adductor and abductor musculature. The patient is unwilling to undergo adductor complex BTX treatment given the previous side effects of aphonia and asks about surgical options.

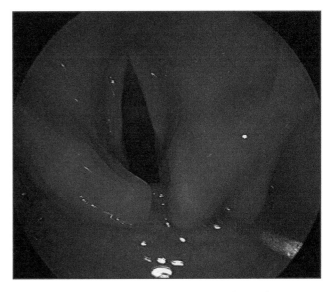

Figure 32–3. Right posterior cricoarytenoid muscle injection under general anesthetic.

For patients with poor response to in-office chemodenervation of the PCA muscle, a more direct approach under general anesthetic allows for injection into the PCA muscle under direct vision. The response to PCA BTX with ongoing adductor pitch breaks suggests mixed spasmodic dysphonia is a possible diagnosis.

Mixed spasmodic dysphonia is a rare form of laryngeal dystonia which is poorly characterized in the literature. The diagnosis relies on exclusion of other organic pathology and the presence of both abductor and adductor pitch breaks on perceptual phonatory analysis. These may become more noticeable after treatment of the opposing muscle group is undertaken as in the above case. Management of both adductor and abductor pitch breaks is required for symptomatic control.

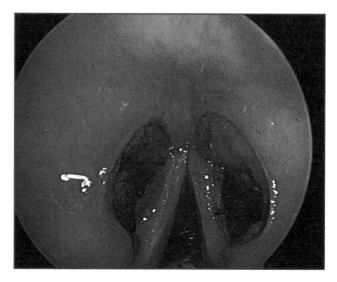

Figure 32–5. Endoscopic view of larynx after bilateral thyroarytenoid muscle myectomy.

SURGICAL TREATMENT OF ADDUCTOR SPASMODIC DYSPHONIA

Three months later the patient elects to undergo bilateral TA muscle myectomy for treatment of her symptoms of tightness and adductor type pitch breaks (Video 32–7, see companion website). The ventricular fold is removed for access using a carbon dioxide (CO_2) laser. Following this the entire TA muscle is removed endoscopically while preserving the mucosa, vocal ligament, and lateral cricoarytenoid muscle (Figures 32–4 and 32–5). She

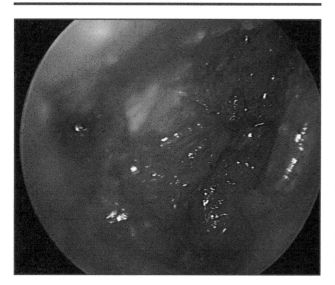

Figure 32–4. Endoscopic view of left paraglottic space after TA muscle myectomy.

initially experiences increased symptoms of glottal insufficiency which improve at the 2-month mark. The voice fluidity and symptoms of strangulated phonation are significantly improved and perceptually she shows improvement of adductor pitch breaks.

Various surgical approaches for the treatment of adductor spasmodic dysphonia have been reported in the literature. Laryngeal nerve section was first advocated by Dedo in 1976[43]; however, long-term outcomes were not favorable. Aronson and DeSanto[44] followed patients for 3 years after this procedure and found that almost 2/3 failed over time, with approximately half of these having a worse voice compared with before the surgery. Selective laryngeal adduction and denervation (SLAD/R) was described by Berke et al[45] as a method of preserving abductor activity. Type II thyroplasty using autologous cartilage[46] and later a titanium implant[47] has been proposed by Isshiki et al; however, this technique has not been reproducible, with Chan et al[48] reporting that only 5 of 17 patients (29%) undergoing Isshiki's originally procedure achieved moderate to good voice improvement with four early failures. Thyroarytenoid muscle myectomy has more recently gained favor[49] as a potential treatment for AdSD. After review of the options, the patient elected to undergo this procedure due to the significant side effects she experienced with previous adductor complex BTX treatments. The patient was counseled that long-term results of TA muscle myectomy are still not well established. Expected side effects of breathiness lasting up to 6 months or more after the surgical procedure were discussed prior to proceeding.

PROGRESS AFTER TA MUSCLE MYECTOMY: ONGOING TREATMENT OF ABDUCTOR SD SYMPTOMS

Two months following transoral TA muscle myectomy, the patient reports that symptoms of voice tightness and adductor pitch breaks are improved with better speech fluidity. She is still experiencing symptoms of glottal insufficiency with low volume and phonatory dyspnea which are improving over time. Laryngoscopy with stroboscopy shows a mild glottal gap. She has ongoing abductor pitch breaks on voiceless weighted sentences (Video 32–8, see companion website). A further EMG guided, office-based Botox injection (7.5 units) is performed into the left PCA muscle with good improvement in her overall voice quality at 2-week assessment (VHI-10 = 28). At this stage the left vocal fold has sluggish abduction compared with the right but full range of movement is preserved. She upgrades work to 3 days per week on modified duties. Two months later the breathy voice breaks return. Endoscopic assessment shows ongoing mild hypomobility of the left vocal fold. The right PCA muscle is treated with 10 units of Botox. The patient develops dyspnea and inspiratory stridor 4 days after the procedure and presents to the emergency department for review. Overnight monitoring shows the oxygen to be stable and repeat laryngoscopy shows a reasonable airway with only mild restriction. The symptoms of breathlessness improve over the next week.

TA muscle myectomy appears to have controlled the adductor pitch breaks in this person with mixed spasmodic dysphonia and improved overall fluidity of the voice. Longer term outcomes are yet unknown. Effectively this surgical procedure has managed to convert and simplify our treatment approach from a diagnosis of mixed spasmodic dysphonia to abductor spasmodic dysphonia, with chemodenervation of the PCA muscle the only required ongoing treatment.

In AbSD about 25% of patients will achieve satisfactory voice outcomes with unilateral treatment of the PCA muscles with BTX.[19] Dosing is adjusted individually and increased until symptoms are controlled, or complete immobilization of the vocal fold is endoscopically confirmed 2 to 4 weeks after treatment. If unilateral treatment is successful, then the same approach is adopted at each subsequent treatment cycle. The decision about whether to alternate sides or treat the same side each time is left up to the patient. Anecdotally, some patients feel that treatment of one particular side is more "successful" compared with the contralateral side. Approximately 3/4 of patients will require bilateral PCA chemodenervation for successful symptomatic control of abductor pitch breaks. We progress to this treatment if breathy voice breaks persist despite immobilization of the vocal fold or if the duration of treatment effect is too short using unilateral dosing. There are obvious theoretical concerns regarding airway compromise with bilateral PCA denervation. For this reason, we prefer staged treatment after successful immobilization of the more active PCA muscle. Smaller doses of Botox are given to the contralateral PCA (0.625 to 2.5 U) with the goal being to weaken but not completely immobilize its abduction. Bilateral synchronous denervation of the PCA muscle has been described, generally using lower doses in the range of 0.9 to 2.5 units of Botox. Significant dyspnea is a recognized side effect of this approach, reported in 5% of cases by Stong et al.[50] Furthermore, Meleca et al reported a case of airway distress requiring tracheostomy soon after treatment with such an approach.[41]

In this case the patient's abductor pitch break returned at 2 months while there was ongoing hypomobility of the treated vocal fold. The decision to treat the contralateral side was made based upon adequate abduction of the previously treated side to minimize the risk of airway compromise. Peak effect of Botox occurs 4 to 7 days after treatment, which is consistent with the patient's onset of dyspnea. She presented appropriately for airway assessment and management as counseled at the time of treatment. The finding of an adequate airway on laryngoscopy suggests an element of sensory dysfunction rather than true airway obstruction as the cause of her dyspnea. In the author's experience, mild dyspnea despite adequate airway is reported commonly after even unilateral PCA chemodenervation.

FINAL STATUS

Her voice improves once again and is stronger and more fluent. Her vocal fatigue has also improved. She has ongoing laryngoscopic signs of lateral supraglottal squeeze at phonation onset (Video 32–9, see companion website). She makes plans for ongoing future BTX treatment into alternating left and right PCA muscles 2 weeks prior to the beginning of each school term (three times per year). She remains employed teaching one on one and small group classes. The VHI remains elevated at 28/40 but the voice is functional and improved compared with the baseline state.

DISCUSSION

This case illustrates the systematic approach to a patient presenting with a complex, atypical voice disorder, with suspected neurological etiology which is non-responsive to standard management. MTD is one of the most common vocal pathologies and must remain in the list of differential diagnoses even when recalcitrant to standard voice therapy. In cases where the distinction between functional voice disorder and laryngeal dystonia is unclear, a directed history with awareness of the typical features of laryngeal dystonia is of paramount importance. Phonetically loaded vocal tasks are an important assessment tool for unmasking the adductor or abductor variants of spasmodic dysphonia. Stroboscopy ± exploratory microlaryngoscopy are useful in excluding underlying vocal pathology which may cause secondary muscle tension dysphonia. A multidisciplinary approach to treatment is advised, with early consultation with a movement disorders neurologist to help exclude rarer forms of neurological voice disorder. Functional overlay can coexist in conjunction with spasmodic dysphonia, further complicating the picture, and there is great value in the ongoing involvement of an experienced voice specific speech pathologist during treatment despite initial non-response to voice therapy. In challenging cases a stepwise trial of logical therapeutic approaches may help establish diagnosis based upon response to treatment. Repeated clinical assessment along with longitudinal self-reported functional outcome scales will help judge response over time and direct further management. Mixed spasmodic dysphonia can be challenging to diagnose; however, persistent antagonist muscle pitch breaks may become more evident after chemodenervation of the adductor or abductor muscle complex. Surgical treatment of laryngeal dystonia is generally reserved for patients who are refractory to BTX treatment; however, it can be a useful tool in the treatment of mixed SD.

REFERENCES

1. Titze IR, Lemke J, Montequin D. Populations in the U.S. workforce who rely on voice as a primary tool of trade: a preliminary report. *J Voice*. 1997;11(3):254–259.
2. Smith E, Gray SD, Dove H, Kirchner L, Heras H. Frequency and effects of teachers' voice problems. *J Voice*. 1997;11(1):81–87.
3. Russell A, Oates J, Greenwood KM. Prevalence of voice problems in teachers. *J Voice*. 1998;12(4):467–479.
4. Chen SH, Chiang SC, Chung YM, Hsiao LC, Hsiao TY. Risk factors and effects of voice problems for teachers. *J Voice*. 2010;24(2):183–190, quiz 191–182.
5. Cantor Cutiva LC, Vogel I, Burdorf A. Voice disorders in teachers and their associations with work-related factors: a systematic review. *J Commun Disord*. 2013;46(2):143–155.
6. Urrutikoetxea A, Ispizua A, Matellanes F. [Vocal pathology in teachers: a videolaryngostroboscopic study in 1046 teachers]. *Rev Laryngol Otol Rhinol (Bord)*. 1995; 116(4):255–262.
7. Tavares EL, Martins RH. Vocal evaluation in teachers with or without symptoms. *J Voice*. 2007;21(4):407–414.
8. Cohen SM, Kim J, Roy N, Asche C, Courey M. Prevalence and causes of dysphonia in a large treatment-seeking population. *Laryngoscope*. 2012;122(2):343–348.
9. Rees CJ, Henderson AH, Belafsky PC. Postviral vagal neuropathy. *Ann Otol Rhinol Laryngol*. 2009;118(4):247–252.
10. Van Houtte E, Van Lierde K, Claeys S. Pathophysiology and treatment of muscle tension dysphonia: a review of the current knowledge. *J Voice*. 2011;25(2):202–207.
11. Ruotsalainen J, Sellman J, Lehto L, Verbeek J. Systematic review of the treatment of functional dysphonia and prevention of voice disorders. *Otolaryngol Head Neck Surg*. 2008;138(5):557–565.
12. Schweinfurth JM, Billante M, Courey MS. Risk factors and demographics in patients with spasmodic dysphonia. *Laryngoscope*. 2002;112(2):220–223.
13. Blitzer A, Brin MF, Stewart CF. Botulinum toxin management of spasmodic dysphonia (laryngeal dystonia): a 12-year experience in more than 900 patients. *Laryngoscope*. 2015;125(8):1751–1757.
14. Hirano M. *Clinical Examination of the Voice*. New York NY: Springer; 1981.
15. Rosen CA, Lee AS, Osborne J, Zullo T, Murry T. Development and validation of the voice handicap index-10. *Laryngoscope*. 2004;114(9):1549–1556.
16. Belafsky PC, Postma GN, Koufman JA. Validity and reliability of the reflux symptom index (RSI). *J Voice*. 2002; 16(2):274–277.
17. Sataloff RT, Spiegel JR, Hawkshaw MJ. Strobovideolaryngoscopy: results and clinical value. *Ann Otol Rhinol Laryngol*. 1991;100(9 pt 1):725–727.
18. Blitzer A, Brin MF, Stewart CF. Botulinum toxin management of spasmodic dysphonia (laryngeal dystonia): a 12-year experience in more than 900 patients. *Laryngoscope*. 1998;108(10):1435–1441.

19. Blitzer A, Brin MF, Stewart C, Aviv JE, Fahn S. Abductor laryngeal dystonia: a series treated with botulinum toxin. *Laryngoscope*. 1992;102(2):163–167.

20. Aronson AE, Hartman DE. Adductor spastic dysphonia as a sign of essential (voice) tremor. *J Speech Hear Dis*. 1981; 46(1):52–58.

21. Blitzer A, Lovelace RE, Brin MF, Fahn S, Fink ME. Electromyographic findings in focal laryngeal dystonia (spastic dysphonia). *Ann Otol Rhinol Laryngol*. 1985;94(6 Pt 1): 591–594.

22. Chitkara A, Meyer T, Keidar A, Blitzer A. Singer's dystonia: first report of a variant of spasmodic dysphonia. *Ann Otol Rhinol Laryngol*. 2006;115(2):89–92.

23. Payne S, Tisch S, Cole I, Brake H, Rough J, Darveniza P. The clinical spectrum of laryngeal dystonia includes dystonic cough: observations of a large series. *Movement Dis*. 2014;29(6):729–735.

24. Brin MF, Blitzer A, Fahn S, Gould W, Lovelace RE. Adductor laryngeal dystonia (spastic dysphonia): treatment with local injections of botulinum toxin (Botox). *Movement Dis*. 1989;4(4):287–296.

25. Kirke DN, Frucht SJ, Simonyan K. Alcohol responsiveness in laryngeal dystonia: a survey study. *J Neurol*. 2015; 262(6):1548–1556.

26. Sama A, Carding PN, Price S, Kelly P, Wilson JA. The clinical features of functional dysphonia. *Laryngoscope*. 2001;111(3):458–463.

27. Young N, Blitzer A. Management of supraglottic squeeze in adductor spasmodic dysphonia: a new technique. *Laryngoscope*. 2007;117(11):2082–2084.

28. Roy N, Mauszycki SC, Merrill RM, Gouse M, Smith ME. Toward improved differential diagnosis of adductor spasmodic dysphonia and muscle tension dysphonia. *Folia Phoniatr Logop*. 2007;59(2):83–90.

29. Heman-Ackah YD, Joglekar SS, Caroline M, et al. The prevalence of undiagnosed thyroid disease in patients with symptomatic vocal fold paresis. *J Voice*. 2011;25(4): 496–500.

30. Verdolini K, Rosen C, Branski R. Special Interest Division 3. *Voice and Voice Disorders. American Speech-Language-Hearing Association*. Classification Manual for Voice Disorders–I. Mahwah, NJ: Lawrence Erlbaum Associates Inc; 2006.

31. da Cunha Pereira G, de Oliveira Lemos I, Dalbosco Gadenz C, Cassol M. Effects of voice therapy on muscle tension dysphonia: a systematic literature review. *J Voice*. 2017.

32. Troung DD, Rontal M, Rolnick M, Aronson AE, Mistura K. Double–blind controlled study of botulinum toxin in adductor spasmodic dysphonia. *Laryngoscope*. 1991;101 (6 Pt 1):630–634.

33. Pacheco PC, Karatayli-Ozgursoy S, Best S, Hillel A, Akst L. False vocal cord botulinum toxin injection for refractory muscle tension dysphonia: our experience with seven patients. *Clin Otolaryngol*. 2015;40(1):60–64.

34. Pani N, Kumar Rath S. Regional & topical anaesthesia of upper airways. *Ind J Anaesthes*. 2009;53(6):641–648.

35. Novakovic D, Waters HH, D'Elia JB, Blitzer A. Botulinum toxin treatment of adductor spasmodic dysphonia: longitudinal functional outcomes. *Laryngoscope*. 2011;121 (3):606–612.

36. Tisch SH, Brake HM, Law M, Cole IE, Darveniza P. Spasmodic dysphonia: clinical features and effects of botulinum toxin therapy in 169 patients—an Australian experience. *Journal of Clinical Neuroscience*. 2003;10(4):434–438.

37. Belafsky PC, Postma GN, Reulbach TR, Holland BW, Koufman JA. Muscle tension dysphonia as a sign of underlying glottal insufficiency. *Otolaryngol Head Neck Surg*. 2002;127(5):448–451.

38. Kupfer RA, Merati AL, Sulica L. Medialization laryngoplasty for odynophonia. *JAMA Otolaryngol Head Neck Surg*. 2015;141(6):556–561.

39. Blitzer A, Brin MF, Fahn S, Lovelace RE. Clinical and laboratory characteristics of focal laryngeal dystonia: study of 110 cases. *Laryngoscope*. 1988;98(6 Pt 1):636–640.

40. Ludlow CL, Naunton RF, Terada S, Anderson BJ. Successful treatment of selected cases of abductor spasmodic dysphonia using botulinum toxin injection. *Otolaryngol Head Neck Surg*. 1991;104(6):849–855.

41. Meleca RJ, Hogikyan ND, Bastian RW. A comparison of methods of botulinum toxin injection for abductory spasmodic dysphonia. *Otolaryngol Head Neck Surg*. 1997;117 (5):487–492.

42. Blitzer A. Spasmodic dysphonia and botulinum toxin: experience from the largest treatment series. *European J Neurol*. 2010;17 (suppl 1):28–30.

43. Dedo HH. Recurrent laryngeal nerve section for spastic dysphonia. *Ann Otol Rhinol Laryngol*. 1976;85(4 Pt 1):451–459.

44. Aronson AE, De Santo LW. Adductor spastic dysphonia: three years after recurrent laryngeal nerve resection. *Laryngoscope*. 1983;93(1):1–8.

45. Berke GS, Blackwell KE, Gerratt BR, Verneil A, Jackson KS, Sercarz JA. Selective laryngeal adductor denervation—reinnervation: a new surgical treatment for adductor spasmodic dysphonia. *Ann Otol Rhinol Laryngol*. 1999; 108(3):227–231.

46. Isshiki N, Tsuji DH, Yamamoto Y, Iizuka Y. Midline lateralization thyroplasty for adductor spasmodic dysphonia. *Ann Otol Rhinol Laryngol*. 2000;109(2):187–193.

47. Isshiki N, Sanuki T. Surgical tips for type II thyroplasty for adductor spasmodic dysphonia: modified technique after reviewing unsatisfactory cases. *Acta Otolaryngol*. 2010;130(2):275–280.

48. Chan SW, Baxter M, Oates J, Yorston A. Long-term results of type II thyroplasty for adductor spasmodic dysphonia. *Laryngoscope*. 2004;114(9):1604–1608.

49. Su CY, Lai CC, Wu PY, Huang HH. Transoral laser ventricular fold resection and thyroarytenoid myoneurectomy for adductor spasmodic dysphonia: long-term outcome. *Laryngoscope*. 2010;120(2):313–318.

50. Stong BC, DelGaudio JM, Hapner ER, Johns MM, 3rd. Safety of simultaneous bilateral botulinum toxin injections for abductor spasmodic dysphonia. *Arch Otolaryngol Head Neck Surg*. 2005;131(9):793–795.

CHAPTER 33

Dysphonia in the Elderly

Hagit Shoffel-Havakuk and Michael M. Johns III

INTRODUCTION

The definition of old age is not consistent, and the chronological age that correlates with old age diverges through history and between cultures. Similarly, the definition of old age is constantly adjusting to the rise in life expectancy. Most developed countries set the age of 60 to 65 for retirement, yet different societies may consider old age anywhere from 50 to 70 years. Nevertheless, gerontologists have recognized that most people in their 60s and early 70s are still fit and active; however, after the age of 75 years most people will become increasingly frail; hence, there are several subdivisions of older age that distinguish between the younger old population and the older old population.

The world population has continued to grow in the past century, and on top of that, due to the rise in life expectancy, the world population is also aging. The number of individuals over the age of 60 is expected to more than double by 2050, from 841 million in 2013 to over 2 billion by 2050.[1] The estimated incidence of vocal disorders in the older population is 12–35%.[2-4] As a result, we can anticipate a rise in the number of older patients seeking medical attention for vocal conditions. In the older population, vocal complaints may impact patients' quality of life (QOL), particularly when a patient is already struggling with communication issues. Thirteen percent of these patients would note a marked reduction in QOL due to dysphonia.[5] The etiologies for geriatric voice dysfunction are various and commonly multifactorial. This chapter discusses in a systematic manner the clinical approach for investigation and management of dysphonia in the elderly.

CASE PRESENTATION

A 76-year-old retired male presents with 6-month history of voice complaints. Onset of symptoms was gradual over the past 2 years; however, they deteriorated significantly in the past 6 months. He struggles to sing in church, which is an activity he used to enjoy very much. He finds it difficult to be heard and understood in noisy environments and over the phone. He excludes any swallowing problems, shortness of breath, or heartburn. He does have occasional dry cough that often exacerbates with vocal effort. His son noticed a gradual change in his pitch, he now speaks in a higher pitch than he used to.

Social: Non-smoker, mild alcohol consumption on social events. Retired for 10 years, before that he used to work as a high school teacher.

Past medical history: Hypercholesterolemia.

Medications: Simvastatin, aspirin.

No known allergies.

INITIAL ASSESSMENT

History

Standard history includes nature of symptoms, triggers and moderators, onset of symptoms, associated complaints (eg, cough, shortness of breath, difficulty swallowing), and previous and current therapies. Red flag symptoms include otalgia, bleeding, pain, weight loss, dyspnea, dysphagia, and aspiration. Review of systems, past medical and surgical history, social history (eg, smoking, alcohol) and medications.

Examination

A complete head and neck examination; red flag findings include thyroid or neck mass, any cranial or other nerve palsies, any neurological signs and signs of dyspnea. Palpation of the neck should include laryngeal structure and position as well as muscle strain.

Voice Evaluation

Voice evaluation while speaking and during vocal tasks (eg, sustained phonation, scales, voice projection) in order to characterize voice quality and dysphonia. Assessment of: overall dysphonia severity, roughness, breathiness, strain, pitch, and loudness. Special considerations should also be given to neurological disorders such as vocal tremor.

Endoscopy and Videostroboscopy

Pharyngo-laryngeal endoscopy allows for general visualization of the larynx and exclusion of laryngeal and pharyngeal lesions. This exam can also provide information regarding laryngeal sensation, muscle strength and symmetry, paresis or paralysis, spasms, tremor, and functional disorders.

Rigid transoral laryngoscopy can also provide general visualization of the larynx, with improved detailed visualization of laryngeal mucosal lesions.

Videostroboscopy: A detailed videostroboscopy using phonation in various pitches, soft and loud, and with repetitive tasks (alternating /i/-sniff) can provide diagnosis in the majority of the cases.

copy demonstrated atrophy of laryngeal structures and thin stretched vocal folds with prominent appearance of the vocal processes. On phonation there was an evident bowing of the membranous vocal folds with spindle shaped glottic gap.

Working Diagnosis

Bilateral vocal fold atrophy.

Further Investigation

Possible useful tools for voice evaluation and assessment of response to therapy: voice related QOL or handicap questionnaires, acoustic analysis, voice aerodynamics, perceptual evaluation of voice (CAPE-V).

Management

Following reassurance and consulting the patient with his condition/working diagnosis, treatment options were offered. Since the patient admitted he would not be able to follow conservative management with voice therapy, he chose to undergo awake endoscopic bilateral injection laryngoplasty using temporary injectable material (Cymetra). He had a very good response with increased projection and vocal endurance and a decrease in his pitch. By the end of the first year after the procedure, he began to experience his original symptoms, as the Cymetra had already resorbed. He was given the option of repeat injection laryngoplasty with longer-acting material (calcium hydroxyapatite) versus bilateral type I thyroplasties. He chose to undergo bilateral thyroplasties, which were performed in the standard fashion. At the post-operative follow-up the patient reported improvement of his symptoms with increased projection and vocal endurance.

SCENARIO 1

Findings

High pitch breathy voice (speaking fundamental frequency of 138 Hz) with reduced volume. Videostrobos-

SCENARIO 2

Findings

Significant breathiness with speech dyspnea, low volume, high pitched and unstable voice. Decreased maximum phonation time. Videostroboscopy demonstrates immobility of the left vocal fold with both phonation and respiration. Compared with the right, the left vocal fold appeared bowed, foreshortened, and atrophied. On phonation there was an evident hyperactivity of the right hemilarynx, with spindle shaped glottic gap, and asymmetric mucosal waves.

Working Diagnosis

Unilateral vocal fold paralysis (left).

Further Investigation

Since there was no initiating event, a complete workup searching for the etiology of the paralysis is warranted. In such cases, imaging of the vagal nerve route from the brain to the mediastinum is mandatory. Both computerized tomography (CT) scan and magnetic resonance imaging (MRI) of the brain may be appropriate. Yet, brain MRI is superior to CT and should be preferred when CNS lesions are suspected. For the mediastinum some may advocate routine chest radiography (CXR); however, CXR cannot demonstrate the neck, and CT scan is superior in detecting the etiology. In general, a contrast CT scan or MRI from the skull base to the upper chest can be adequate.

The role of laryngeal electromyography (EMG) is a subject of debate. When performed in a window period between 1 to 6 months after the onset paralysis, laryngeal EMG can help in predicting prognosis for recovery. Laryngeal EMG can be also useful in cases where the diagnosis of paralysis is in doubt and should be distinguished from other causes for immobility.

Management

After consulting the patient with his condition/working diagnosis, treatment options were offered. Complete workup did not reveal etiology for the paralysis, and it was therefore considered idiopathic. The patient chose to undergo awake left vocal fold injection laryngoplasty using temporary short-term injectable material (Cymetra) that will reabsorb in case the vocal fold mobility recovers. The patient had a very good response, his breathiness resolved, with better voice projection and vocal endurance.

Findings

Additional history: Voice significantly worsened in the recent 3 weeks. The patient has asthma and uses inhaled steroids daily.

Physical examination: Strained, effortful, and stiff voice. Videostroboscopy demonstrates bilateral inflamed membranous vocal folds, with extensive whitish plaques.

Working Diagnosis

Fungal laryngitis.

Further Investigation

In most cases empirical anti-fungal therapy is sufficient, and no further investigation is required. In cases of atypical appearance, resistant or refractory disease culture might be needed. When the diagnosis is in doubt, or when dysplasia or malignancy is suspected, tissue sample for biopsy should be obtained.

Management

After consulting the patient with his condition/working diagnosis, the patient was given oral anti-fungal treatment (fluconazole). On his next follow-up visit 2 weeks later, the patient's voice became softer and less effortful. Videostroboscopy demonstrated resolution of the inflammation and the whitish plaques.

DISCUSSION AND LITERATURE REVIEW

The estimated incidence of vocal disorders in the elderly is on the rise,[1–4] with a significant impact on patients' functionality and QOL.[5] Simultaneously, there is a global rise in the demand for rejuvenating medicine to improve functionality and appearance in the older population for multiple aspects of life, including voice.

The etiologies for geriatric voice dysfunction are various and may be multifactorial; these include: vocal fold atrophy, neurologic conditions, decreased lung capacity, laryngeal lesions, inflammatory or infectious disorders, and vocal fold paralysis/paresis.[2] When working up a geriatric patient with vocal symptoms, it is of paramount importance to first exclude any systemic or central nervous system condition that may initially present with vocal symptoms; these include: stroke, tremor, Parkinson's disease, and amyotrophic lateral sclerosis (ALS).

atrophy, result in reduced vocal fold bulk and the classic bowed membranous vocal fold appearance.

During aging, laryngeal cartilages may ossify, and the larynx may descend into the neck, which may impact vocal resonance.[7] As with other joints in the body, the articular surfaces of the cricoarytenoid joints may demonstrate breakdowns and decreased range of motion with aging.[14,15] Commonly, laryngeal mucus production is reduced and of higher viscosity; this may result in impaired lubrication and affect the ease of vibration.[16]

PRESBYPHONIA

Presbyphonia, or age-related dysphonia, is a diagnosis given only after a thorough examination and investigation have excluded other pathologies. Presbyphonia represents voice symptoms related to the aging process of several organ systems. The normal aging of the lungs, the generator of voice production, leads to a decrease in chest wall compliance, pulmonary elastic recoil, and respiratory muscle strength. By the age of 60, the respiratory compliance is reduced by 20% from the expected values at the age of 20.[6] Therefore, it becomes more difficult to produce subglottal pressure and to power voice.[7] The neuromusculature of the larynx is also prone to aging effects. Human cadaveric studies of the recurrent laryngeal nerve demonstrate loss of myelin and reduced number of axons with degeneration of the remaining axons.[8] The neuromuscular junction demonstrates reduction in axonal terminal area and an increase in unoccupied post-synaptic acetycholine receptors, similarly to that of denervated thyroarytenoid muscle.[9] The laryngeal muscles themselves demonstrate reduction in the number of type I (slow-twitch) fibers, with compensatory hypertrophy of the remaining fibers. There is also an age-related increase in type 1 and 2 myosin heavy-chain isoforms,[10] similar to muscle remodeling following denervation-reinnervation. In general, the thyroarytenoid muscle becomes weaker, slower, and more fatigable with age.[11]

Within the lamina propria, collagen normally forms a "wicker-basket" appearance, providing tension and elasticity. With aging, collagen becomes more abundant and disorganized throughout the different layers of the lamina propria. Disorganized collagen along with a decrease in hyaluronic acid and elastin[12,13] result in loss of the viscoelastic properties. These changes in the lamina propria, combined with thyroarytenoid muscle

HISTORY AND EXAMINATION

As with any patient encounter, a complete patient medical history is essential. It is important to learn about the level of vocal use, both historically and currently, and how much the vocal disability affects the patient's life. This can help to gauge the amount of trauma endured and to identify the level of voice necessary for functional daily activities. Diet and use of tobacco and alcohol are also key pieces of information in the puzzle. Investigating the vocal complaints should include: duration of symptoms, onset (sudden/gradual), aggravating or relieving factors, voice fatigability, stability, clarity, and ability to project. Aside from voice complaints, it is necessary to investigate about other symptoms that might be related to laryngeal disorders, such as: heartburn, globus sensation, cough, dyspnea, and dysphagia.

The physical examination starts with voice evaluation while speaking and during vocal tasks (eg, sustained phonation, scales, voice projection) in order to characterize the quality of dysphonia. Characteristically, patients with presbyphonia would demonstrate changes in their range and pitch (women's voices often become lower pitched initially and gradually higher pitched, men's voices become high pitched) as well as reduced loudness. Importantly, a complete neurologic and head and neck exam should not be omitted, since other causes for dysphonia in the elderly should be ruled out first.

The most important part of the clinic visit, however, is good imaging of the larynx, via videostroboscopy. Although not mandatory, when neurologic pathology (eg, paralysis/paresis, tremor) is suspected, a naso-laryngeal flexible videostroboscopic exam is preferred, while when a mucosal lesion is suspected, transoral videostroboscopic exam via rigid telescope is preferred. The classic characteristics of presbyphonia on videostroboscopy are demonstrated in Figures 33–1

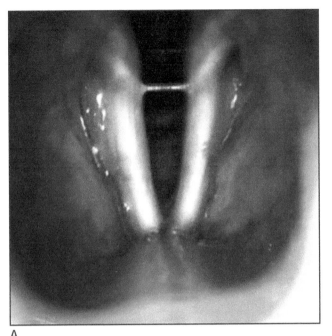 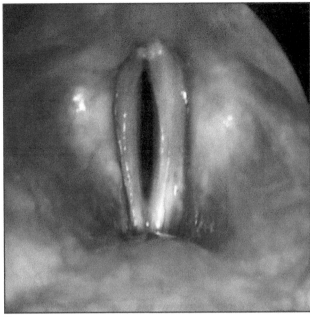

A   B

Figure 33–1. Characteristic exam findings of presbylarynx demonstrated by laryngoscopy. (A) The glottis during respiration with increased ventricular visibility, atrophy of structures, exposed vocal ligaments, and prominent appearance of the vocal processes. (B) The glottis during phonation demonstrates bowing and spindle-shaped glottic gap.

and 33–2. Figure 33–1A illustrates the glottis during respiration with increased ventricular visibility, atrophy of structures, exposed vocal ligaments couture, and prominent appearance of the vocal processes. Figure 33–1B of the glottis during phonation reveals vocal fold bowing and spindle-shaped glottic gap. These important exam findings are characteristic for presbylaryngis.[7,17,18] The increased glottal gap seen in these patients does not necessarily correlate with the severity of the dysphonia, most likely due to the compensatory mechanisms. Further videostroboscopy features of presbyphonia include: irregular or aperiodic vibration, asymmetric mucosal wave, and increased amplitude.[7] Analyzing the acoustic properties of voice in these patients may reveal breathiness, decreased loudness, reduced maximum phonation time (MPT), increased jitter and shimmer, and increased fundamental frequency (F_0) in men and decreased F_0 in women.[19]

As a diagnosis of exclusion, the practitioner must rule out other causes for dysphonia first. Table 33–1 provides a list of possible causes for dysphonia in the aging population, including neurologic disorders, vocal fold lesions, and reduced lung function. The clinical

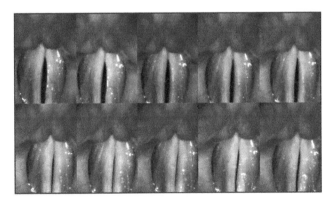

Figure 33–2. Stroboscopic montage, serial images from videostroboscopy of a patient with age related vocal fold atrophy (presbylarynx).

workup should exclude these listed etiologies before establishing the diagnosis of presbyphonia. Table 33–2 provides a summary of the clinical presentation and characteristic of presbyphonia and age-related vocal fold atrophy.

Table 33–1. Common Causes for Vocal Symptoms in Geriatric Patients

Benign mucosal lesions of the vocal folds
– Scar, sulcus, fibrous mass, cyst, polyp, nodules, granuloma, Reinke's edema
Recurrent respiratory papillomatosis
Premalignant lesions of the vocal folds
– Keratosis, dysplasia (mild, moderate, severe)
Malignant glottic lesions
– Carcinoma in situ (CIS), invasive squamous cell carcinoma (SCC)
Malignancy of the larynx or pharynx originating outside of the glottis (may affect voice)
Vocal fold paralysis/paresis
– various etiologies, may be traumatic/post-surgery, neoplastic, medical disease related, or idiopathic
Infectious laryngitis
– Viral, fungal, bacterial
Systemic and inflammatory conditions of the larynx
– Such as: amyloidosis, rheumatoid arthritis, sarcoidosis,
Neurologic conditions
– Stroke, Parkinson's disease, amyotrophic lateral sclerosis (ALS)
– Tremor and dystonia
– Essential tremor
– Spasmodic dysphonia
Impaired pulmonary function (various etiologies)
Xerostomia
– medication induced, age related, Sjogren's syndrome
Muscle tension dysphonia (MTD)
Laryngopharyngeal reflux related

TREATMENT FOR PRESBYPHONIA

Rejuvenation of the aging voice is feasible. A multidisciplinary approach with a laryngologist and a speech and language pathologist is the key. For determining the optimal approach, one must examine factors such as severity of dysfunction, patient's desires, comorbidities, as well as cooperation and compliance with the different intervention modalities. One of the most important measures the practitioner should provide the patient is reassurance. Presbyphonic patients are often referred due to voice changes with concern for malignancy. Many of these patients may be satisfied by reassurance alone and would not require any further intervention, since they still have a serviceable voice.

Table 33–2. Summary of the Clinical Characteristic of Presbyphonia

Vocal Symptoms
Voice fatigability
Increased breathiness
Voice instability
Difficulty in voice projection
Acoustic Features
Reduced loudness
Reduced maximum phonation time
Increased F_0 in men
Decreased F_0 in women
Increased jitter
Increased shimmer
Videostroboscopic Exam
Vocal fold bowing
Prominent vocal processes
Exposed vocal ligament contour
Increased ventricular visibility
Spindle-shaped glottal gap
Irregular/aperiodic vibration
Asymmetric mucosal wave
Abnormal amplitude
No evidence of vocal folds' mucosal or neurological pathology

Targeted Voice Therapy

The next step would be to consider conservative management, which may be highly effective in a subset group of these patients. The most effective conservative measure is targeted voice therapy. This therapy should focus on phonatory and respiratory strengthening and increasing neuromuscular coordination, which are needed to overcome age-related changes. The therapist should first educate the patients about their condition, resonant voice production, optimal vocal postures, and standard vocal function exercises. Therapy requires multiple sessions, but, more importantly, it requires patients' compliance to practice the exercises outside of the formal therapy sessions. Voice therapy alone has been demonstrated to be highly efficient in improving voice quality of life in presbyphonic

patients, with a mean improvement in VRQOL score of 19.21 after roughly four sessions within 5 months.[20] Sauder et al showed vocal function exercises (VFEs) can improve functional and perceptual voice measures, and demonstrate reduction in VHI.[21] These exercises strengthen and rebalance the laryngeal musculature and therefore improve vocal fold adduction.

Phonation resistance training exercise (PhoRTE) is another novel therapy program for presbyphonia. It is modeled after Lee Silverman Voice Therapy (LSVT) and consists of four exercises: loud maximum sustained phonation on /a/; ascending and descending pitch glides on /a/; shouting specific word phrases with a loud high voice; and shouting those same phrases with a low authoritative voice. The goal of these exercises is to target the degenerative and age-related changes of the respiratory system and larynx. While both VFE and PhoRTE demonstrate improvement on VRQOL scores, only the PhoRTE group demonstrates an improvement in perceived phonatory effort.[22]

For patients with a more severe dysphonia or those who failed voice therapy or cannot comply with voice therapy sessions (eg, due to traveling distance), operative intervention may be advised. In general, the surgical techniques for the treatment of presbyphonia were originally developed for treating unilateral vocal fold paralysis, and were later adopted for the treatment of glottic insufficiency caused by other etiologies.

Augmentation with Injection Laryngoplasty

Vocal fold augmentation via injection laryngoplasty repairs glottic insufficiency by augmenting the paraglottic space and medializing the vocal fold. Postma and colleagues demonstrated that this intervention can be useful in treating glottal insufficiency caused by bilateral vocal fold atrophy.[23] There are several injectable materials available (eg, collagen materials, hyaluronic acid, calcium hydroxyapatite), all of them temporary, with variable intervals for absorption. Injection laryngoplasty can be performed in the awake patient setting via percutaneous or transoral techniques. This spares the complications of general anesthesia, saves operating room related time and expenses and allows for immediate feedback by the patient's voice. Figure 33–3 demonstrates selected images from videostroboscopy of a patient with presbyphonia before and after bilateral augmentation with awake injection laryngoplasty.

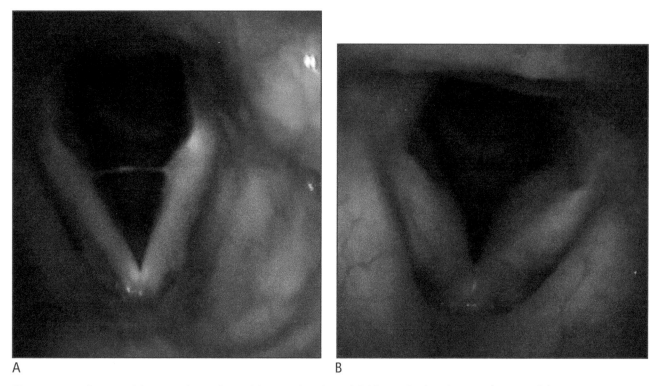

A   B

Figure 33–3. Laryngeal images of a patient with age related vocal fold atrophy (presbylarynx), before (A) and 1 month after (B) successful vocal fold augmentation via injection laryngoplasty with Cymetra.

Augmentation with Fat Injection

The consistency and viscosity of fat are considered ideal for vocal fold augmentation,[24] which can be particularly useful in cases of tissue defect related to scarring, sulci, or atrophy. Moreover, there are stem cells within the implanted adipose tissue; however, their effects on vocal folds' vitality is unknown.[25] Although long term benefits of fat injection were reported,[26,27] the long-term durability of the adipose injected implant is still a subject of debate, and therefore it is commonly considered a temporary solution. Fat injection for glottic insufficiency caused by vocal fold atrophy demonstrated improvement in functional and perceptual voice parameters, as well as in videostroboscopy reported measures.[28]

Nevertheless, the major relative disadvantage of vocal fold augmentation with fat injection is that adipose tissue harvesting and injection is commonly performed under general anesthesia. This is a major limiting factor, especially when treating geriatric patients with comorbidities.

Bilateral Medialization Laryngoplasty (Durable Implants)

Laryngeal framework surgery (LFS) is aimed to restore vocal function by restructuring the larynx without operating the vocal folds themselves. Medialization laryngoplasty or type I thyroplasty is the most commonly performed LFS. Medialization laryngoplasty offers a durable treatment option for glottic insufficiency from various etiologies, including age related vocal fold atrophy. In medialization laryngoplasty, the vocal fold is medialized by an implant inserted through a window in the thyroid cartilage into the paraglottic space, by an open transcervical approach. The commonly used implants for bilateral vocal fold atrophy are the hand-carved Silastic and the polytetrafluoroethylene ribbon (Gore-Tex). The procedure is performed in the operating room, under sedation and local anesthesia, with an indwelling flexible nasolaryngoscope. The bilateral implants' size and position within the paraglottic spaces on each side are tailored to the individual. The vocal folds' position and the patient's voice serve as immediate intraoperative feedback to optimize results.[29] Although extremely rare, medialization laryngoplasty has reported complications, including implant extrusion and inflammatory reaction.[30]

SUMMARY

Vocal complaints in the elderly are common, and may be related to various etiologies, including: systemic or neurologic conditions, impaired pulmonary function, benign or malignant laryngeal lesions, inflammatory or infectious conditions, and vocal fold paralysis/paresis. Presbyphonia is a diagnosis of exclusion which represents voice symptoms related to normal degenerative aging changes in several organ systems, primarily respiratory and laryngeal. When indicated, several efficient treatment options can be offered: targeted voice therapy or bilateral vocal fold augmentation/medialization by injection augmentation, fat injection, or medialization laryngoplasty.

REFERENCES

1. United Nations, Department of Economic and Social Affairs, Population Division. *World Population Ageing 2013.* 2013:1–111.
2. Davids T, Klein AM, Johns MM. Current dysphonia trends in patients over the age of 65: is vocal atrophy becoming more prevalent? *Laryngoscope.* 2012;122(2):332–335.
3. Roy N, Stemple J, Merrill RM, Thomas L. Epidemiology of voice disorders in the elderly: preliminary findings. *Laryngoscope.* 2007;117(4):628–633.
4. Turley R, Cohen S. Impact of voice and swallowing problems in the elderly. *Otolaryngol Head Neck Surg.* 2009;140(1):33–36.
5. Golub JS, Chen P-H, Otto KJ, Hapner E, Johns MM. Prevalence of perceived dysphonia in a geriatric population. *J Am Geriatr Soc.* 2006;54(11):1736–1739.
6. Janssens J-P. Aging of the respiratory system: impact on pulmonary function tests and adaptation to exertion. *Clin Chest Med.* 2005;26(3):469–84· vi–vii.
7. Johns MM, Arviso LC, Ramadan F. Challenges and opportunities in the management of the aging voice. *Otolaryngol Head Neck Surg.* 2011;145(1):1–6.
8. Nakai T, Goto N, Moriyama H, Shiraishi N, Nonaka N. The human recurrent laryngeal nerve during the aging process. *Okajimas Folia Anat Jpn.* 2000;76(6):363–367.
9. Connor NP, Suzuki T, Lee K, Sewall GK, Heisey DM. Neuromuscular junction changes in aged rat thyroarytenoid muscle. *Ann Otol Rhinol Laryngol.* 2002;111(7 pt 1):579–586.
10. Malmgren LT, Fisher PJ, Bookman LM, Uno T. Age-related changes in muscle fiber types in the human thyroarytenoid muscle: an immunohistochemical and stereological study using confocal laser scanning microscopy. *Otolaryngol Head Neck Surg.* 1999;121(4):441–451.
11. McMullen CA, Andrade FH. Contractile dysfunction and altered metabolic profile of the aging rat thyroarytenoid muscle. *J Appl Physiol.* 2006;100(2):602–608.
12. Madruga de Melo EC, Lemos M, Aragão Ximenes Filho J, Sennes LU, Nascimento Saldiva PH, Tsuji DH. Distribution of collagen in the lamina propria of the human vocal fold. *Laryngoscope.* 2003;113(12):2187–2191.
13. Sato K, Hirano M, Nakashima T. Age-related changes of collagenous fibers in the human vocal fold mucosa. *Ann Otol Rhinol Laryngol.* 2002;111(1):15–20.
14. Dedivitis RA, Abrahão M, de Jesus Simões M, Mora OA, Cervantes O. Cricoarytenoid joint: histological changes during aging. *Sao Paulo Med J.* 2001;119(2):89–90.
15. Paulsen F, Kimpel M, Lockemann U, Tillmann B. Effects of ageing on the insertion zones of the human vocal fold. *J Anat.* 2000;196 (pt 1):41–54.
16. Sato K, Hirano M. Age-related changes in the human laryngeal glands. *Ann Otol Rhinol Laryngol.* 1998;107(6):525–529.
17. Honjo I, Isshiki N. Laryngoscopic and voice characteristics of aged persons. *Arch Otolaryngol.* 1980;106(3):149–150.
18. Pontes P, Brasolotto A, Behlau M. Glottic characteristics and voice complaint in the elderly. *J Voice.* 2005;19(1):84–94.
19. Verdonck-de Leeuw IM, Mahieu HF. Vocal aging and the impact on daily life: a longitudinal study. *J Voice.* 2004; 18(2):193–202.
20. Berg EE, Hapner E, Klein A, Johns MM. Voice therapy improves quality of life in age-related dysphonia: a case-control study. *J Voice.* 2008;22(1):70–74.
21. Sauder C, Roy N, Tanner K, Houtz DR, Smith ME. Vocal function exercises for presbylaryngis: a multidimensional assessment of treatment outcomes. *Ann Otol Rhinol Laryngol.* 2010;119(7):460–467.
22. Ziegler A, Abbott KV, Johns M, Klein A, Hapner ER. Preliminary data on two voice therapy interventions in the treatment of presbyphonia. *Laryngoscope.* 2013.
23. Postma GN, Blalock PD, Koufman JA. Bilateral medialization laryngoplasty. *Laryngoscope.* 1998;108(10):1429–1434.
24. Chan RW, Titze IR. Viscosities of implantable biomaterials in vocal fold augmentation surgery. *Laryngoscope.* 1998;108(5):725–731.
25. Fraser JK, Wulur I, Alfonso Z, Hedrick MH. Fat tissue: an underappreciated source of stem cells for biotechnology. *Trends Biotechnol.* 2006;24(4):150–154.
26. Umeno H, Chitose S, Sato K, Ueda Y, Nakashima T. Long-term postoperative vocal function after thyroplasty type I and fat injection laryngoplasty. *Ann Otol Rhinol Laryngol.* 2012;121(3):185–191.

27. Benninger MS, Hanick AL, Nowacki AS. Augmentation autologous adipose injections in the larynx. *Ann Otol Rhinol Laryngol.* 2016;125(1):25–30.

28. Hsiung MW, Woo P, Minasian A, Schaefer Mojica J. Fat augmentation for glottic insufficiency. *Laryngoscope.* 2000; 110(6):1026–1033.

29. Zeitels SM, Mauri M, Dailey SH. Medialization laryngoplasty with Gore-Tex for voice restoration secondary to glottal incompetence: indications and observations. *Ann Otol Rhinol Laryngol.* 2003;112(2):180–184.

30. Rosen CA. Complications of phonosurgery: results of a national survey. *Laryngoscope.* 1998;108(11 Pt 1):1697–1703.

CHAPTER 34

Functional (Adaptive) Dysphonia: Considerations in Evaluation and Treatment

Rebecca Leonard

INTRODUCTION

The term "functional dysphonia" has historically referred to voice that is perceived as abnormal in the absence of organic pathology. The implication is that voice production has been altered such that the output is considered aberrant by the speaker and/or listener. Other descriptions of this type of disorder may refer to specific vocal behaviors responsible for the changes in quality, for example, "ventricular dysphonia," "anterior-posterior squeezing," or more broadly, "muscle tension dysphonia."[1,2] A variant of functional disorders, "psychogenic dysphonia," is considered a consequence of psychologic stressors affecting the patient and, again, occurring in the absence of actual physical pathology.

Many variables, of course, can contribute to abnormal voice quality. Some may arise from the demands of a particular environment or situation—for example, a need for excessive loudness or prolonged speaking (situation-specific). Such behaviors are often described as "hyperfunctional" or "phonotraumatic"[3] and can, eventually, in some cases, result in tissue pathology. Voice perceived as unusual, even abnormal, may also simply reflect a speaker's unique personality (speaker-specific), and may or may not result in pathology. Not surprisingly, it is when changes in vocal function or output significantly affect the speaker or perhaps, in the case of a child, become apparent and of concern to a parent or other adult that the laryngologist and voice clinician are likely to become involved.

In our own experience, the assumption that a diagnosis of "functional dysphonia" is *not* associated with pathology can be misleading. Voice disorders can be diagnosed as "functional" when, in fact, underlying pathology that is either subtle or difficult to identify is present. Pathology can certainly be a consequence of inappropriate vocal practices, but such behaviors may also arise in response to pathology not necessarily associated with voice use, such as granuloma. In either situation, if the pathology is not identified, the disorder may be mislabeled as "functional." In other instances, our impression has been that organic pathology did exist at one time and subsequently resolved, but with continued dysphonia. A patient who begins to use effortful phonatory practices in response to a vocal fold paresis, for example, and who continues to use these behaviors even when it appears the paresis has resolved typifies this type of dysphonia. In short, if the term "functional" causes a clinician charged with managing a patient's dysphonia to assume that actual, organic "pathology" is not a factor in the disorder, successful management may be prolonged or not achieved.

For these reasons, we have elected to use the term "adaptive dysphonia" for the general group of disorders typically referred to as "functional." The term "adaptive" suggests that voice has changed in response to some stressor, physiologic or psychologic or both, in the patient's life. Altered voice quality, in essence, represents the speaker's adaptation to an aversive event. The term doesn't rule out the possibility that tissue pathology may be, currently, or may have been, in the past, a factor in the dysphonia. As noted, if pathology is present, it can represent a *consequence* of inappropriate vocal practices, or alternatively, a *cause* of altered behaviors. Pathology can also be masked, perhaps by hyperphonatory practices, or can be sufficiently subtle that its detection is difficult. In other situations, vocal practices may be excessive or inappropriate but with no evidence of organic pathology, past or present. Voice change may reflect, in such a case, an adaptive response to psychological stressors.

In short, diagnosis and treatment of disorders considered "functional" can be perplexing. Careful history-taking and imaging of the larynx during a variety of voicing and non-voicing tasks can be critical to accurate diagnosis. In the remainder of this chapter, we will present, briefly, cases of patients diagnosed with "functional dysphonia" and referred for voice evaluation/treatment. Hopefully, the examples presented will illustrate some of the difficulties and pitfalls involved in evaluating and treating so-called functional dysphonias.

CASE 1

Initial Presentation

The patient is a 67-year-old female with a 9-month history of voice change. She describes her voice as being effortful to produce, and notes that she runs out of air quickly during speaking. She was evaluated by an otolaryngologist several months ago and subsequently diagnosed with spasmodic dysphonia (SD). Since then, she has been attending a local SD support group. A member of the group who is undergoing treatment at our clinic suggested she be seen and further evaluated at our institution to discuss potential treatment options.

Head, Eyes, Ears, Nose, Throat (HEENT) Evaluation

History and laryngeal exam are completed by an experienced laryngologist. The patient's history is not significant for variables likely to produce laryngeal pathology, e.g., previous intubation/surgery, viral illness, excessive, or inappropriate voice use. The patient does report occasional reflux symptoms (no evidence of tissue change related to these is identified on laryngeal exam). Her blood pressure is mildly elevated and controlled with medication. During her initial exam, the larynx is found to be within normal limits in

structure and function. No evidence of tissue pathology is observed. Vocal behaviors observed are consistent with a diagnosis of spasmodic dysphonia, that is, hyper-adductive behaviors involving both the true and false vocal folds. The physician report describes these as present on sustained sound, and more apparent during connected speech. The patient is next seen in voice clinic for a complete voice evaluation, including treatment probing to determine the likely potential of behavioral intervention for her dysphonia.

Voice Clinic Evaluation

Phonoscopic/Phonatory Function Evaluation

During a flexible endoscopic exam, the patient is asked to engage in a variety of voicing and non-voicing tasks (we typically refer to this exam as a "phonoscopic" exam; performed with flexible endoscopy, it mimics voice samples/voicing tasks collected during a voice, or phonatory function, evaluation). Audio recordings of voice during a similar set of tasks are also obtained (a brief sample is included in Audio 1. *Case 1pre*). Consistent with the laryngologist's previous report, voice was typically produced with excessive laryngeal adduction interspersed with brief instances of relatively normal laryngeal behavior and voice. The hyperadductive behavior appeared to begin with the true vocal folds, followed quickly by false fold adduction. In some instances, voice was precluded by excessive adduction. Of particular note, the patient's voice during soft whisper, with no actual voicing, did not differ substantially from voice produced during conversation. That is, it was still quite typical of adductor spasmodic dysphonia, with intermittent instances of hyperadduction and strained, whispered voice quality. In our experience, patients with adductor spasmodic dysphonia may be quite fluent during speaking tasks that don't require voicing.

Patient History

The patient is a recently retired social worker. She has thoroughly enjoyed her work and, in fact, would have remained employed except for her husband's health problems. He experiences fluctuations in blood pressure, including precipitous drops in pressure that have caused him to fall. He is currently recovering from a wrist fracture experienced during one of these episodes. The patient is obviously concerned about her husband and notes that, in the last few years, this concern has become a significant source of stress in her life. She is hopeful that, having retired, she will be able to monitor him more closely and perhaps prevent these incidents.

Of additional significance in this patient's history is an upcoming court case that will require her testimony. The case involves a local landlady who has been charged with the homicides of a number of her elderly, sometimes infirm, male tenants. According to court records, the woman drugged these men and then stole their social security checks and other monies. Reportedly, the crimes escalated from theft to murder from drug overdoses, with seven bodies eventually discovered buried in the boarding house owner's backyard (and two others suspected). The landlady continued to receive the victims' checks for months, and sometimes years, after their demise.

Of particular significance, it was only when the disappearance of one of her clients, a mentally disabled man, was noted by the patient, and when her suspicion was further aroused by finding that the boarding house was unlicensed, and when these concerns were then brought to the attention of local authorities that the crimes were discovered. The notoriety associated with the murders and the subsequent court case was significant, receiving even national attention. The patient's testimony in the upcoming trial was crucial, and would take place in a highly publicized venue. Interestingly, when asked if she thought this experience, and the stress associated with it, could be related to her dysphonia, the patient said she had considered this but that her understanding was that spasmodic dysphonia was an organic disease affecting the nervous system, that is, not a result of stress.

It was explained to the patient that, indeed, while some of her vocal symptoms were consistent with adductor spasmodic dysphonia, others were not. It was suggested to her that a brief period of treatment probing to explore the potential for voice change without medical/surgical interventions recommended for SD may be of value. She was also asked to consider possible counseling for the significant stressors in her life. In our opinion, these were pronounced, and might be reduced with professional intervention. Though she agreed to a trial of voice therapy, the patient was less amenable to counseling, at least at this time.

Voice Therapy/Treatment Probing

Our goal for this exercise was to determine, initially for very structured utterances, whether vocal output that was normal, without characteristics of spasmodic dysphonia or hyperfunctional behaviors, could be elicited.

To this end, the patient was first instructed in tidal breathing. When this was satisfactorily achieved, she was asked to simply produce the nasal sound, /m/, on tidal exhalation. Initially, the sound was of very short duration, with an emphasis on lightly superimposing, or "tapping," the sound on exhaled air. This task was completed successfully after a few trials, and the patient was then asked to prolong the sound, but only for the duration of a tidal exhalation. This process was gradually expanded, for example, to the sustained vowel sounds "ee . . . ah . . . oo," again produced on tidal exhalation. Once the patient could manage this and similar tasks with consistent success, the probing process was elaborated so that speaking tasks became longer, and then more complex, combining both voiced and voiceless speech sounds. Emphasis continued to be directed to sustained respiratory behaviors that provided excellent support for phonatory behavior. Typical of behavioral therapies, tasks became more true-to-life—for example, answering questions posed by the clinician and then engaging in simple conversational exercises, as long as speech continued to be fluent and relatively effortlessly produced. If a task was too difficult, the strategy was to return to the last successful exercise and then continue forward as possible. Once fluent speech was maintained in the clinical situation, emphasis was on generalizing strategies to other situations, and other speakers, and in non-clinical environments. This included attempts to simulate the question-and-answer type of situation likely to occur in her scheduled courtroom testimony. For this exercise, actual questions that would subsequently be posed to the patient were attempted. The strategy appeared useful not only as a simulation of the courtroom situation, but also as a means of thinking about, and practicing, possible answers to the questions ultimately asked. A sample of the patient's conversational speech shortly before the termination of therapy is presented in Audio 2. *Case 1post*. It should be noted that the patient was able to complete her trial testimony in excellent fashion, and reported continued normal voice production long after her initial evaluations and treatment (she was followed yearly in our center for 5 years).

Case 1 Synopsis

In summary, the voice disorder experienced by the patient in Case 1 was in some important ways typical of a "functional" disorder. Certainly, after multiple and careful exams with excellent equipment and experienced clinicians, there was no readily identifiable evidence of tissue pathology underlying the dysphonia.

And both history and treatment probing suggested that psychologic stressors were likely associated with the onset of the disorder. However, correct diagnosis was complicated by the striking similarity of the patient's voice to those characteristic of spasmodic dysphonia. In this case, it was our clinic's experience with SD, and the decision to engage in a period of treatment probing/voice therapy, that was likely most helpful to a successful resolution of the dysphonia. Of further note, the patient was offered counseling, but declined to pursue this option. In our experience, this has been true of most patients with adaptive dysphonia related to psychological stressors. And in the majority of these cases, successful resolution of the dysphonia was achieved with voice therapy alone. We have, however, continued to discuss the option of professional counseling when it appears indicated, and to encourage it strongly when the need seems, from our perspective, imperative.

CASE 2

Initial Presentation

The patient is a 63-year-old male with a 6-month history of dysphonia and aphonia. He is a rancher who owns and manages a number of ranches. His voice change was first noted in late summer, worsened over the next few months, and has progressed to the point where speaking, even in a whisper, is difficult. Shortly after his voice began to change, he was evaluated by an otolaryngologist. According to the report from this examination, the true vocal folds were mobile and otherwise within normal limits, as were other structures observed; however, the false folds were used for speaking. He was diagnosed as having a "functional" dysphonia and was referred for voice therapy. The patient notes that he has been extremely busy with the harvest season and is just now able to follow up with the voice therapy referral. He does note that his voice has worsened in the intervening period. At the time of this visit, he is largely aphonic, with voice produced as effortful whisper.

Voice Clinic Evaluation

Phonoscopic/Phonatory Function Evaluation

Laryngeal imaging is performed with rigid endoscopy and stroboscopy, as well as flexible endoscopy. The false folds are constricted even at rest. The impression is that the true vocal folds are mobile; however, good visualization is generally precluded by activity of the supraglottic structures. In addition, coughing and gagging are frequent during much of the initial exam. Typical views of the larynx are presented in Case 2, Figures 34–1 and 34–2. At this point, strategies designed to elicit a more complete view of the true vocal folds are attempted. These include pairing exhalation with relaxation, allowing better visualization of the airway under the false vocal folds, and when this is achieved, asking the patient to produce a very brief "ee" at a rather high (but not forced) fundamental frequency. The patient is also asked to pair the brief utterances with relaxation, making no attempt to control exhalation, but simply letting out "all the air" as sound is produced. After some practice, he is able to generate voice that, while still dysphonic, involves the true vocal folds. In Case 2, Figures 34–1 and 34–2 and Video 34–1, the true folds can be seen in an adducted position

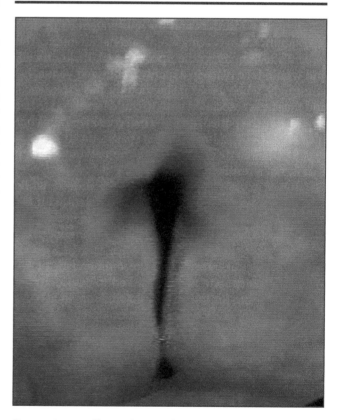

Figure 34–1. Photomicrograph of the appearance of the larynx during production of sustained vowel sound with hyperadduction of the false vocal folds and occlusion of the true vocal folds.

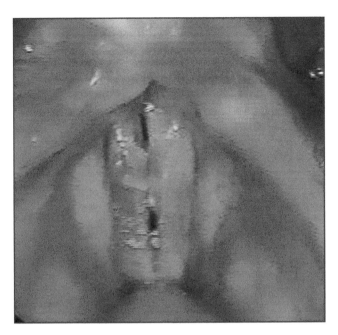

Figure 34–2. Photomicrograph demonstrating appearance of free edge of the true vocal folds following treatment probing designed to relax false folds. Tissue pathology is apparent now, on the free edge of the true vocal folds (edema, irregularity, and mucus).

during voicing, and abducted during inspiration. It is apparent that pathology is present on the true folds.

Patient History

Substantial portions of the history were provided by the patient's wife due to his difficulty speaking. His first indications of problems were a "tickling sensation" in his throat, which prompted coughing or throat clearing, and "roughness" in his voice. He also noted that his voice deteriorated markedly from early to late in the day. He had experienced no previous voice difficulties, other than those associated with an occasional cold. He was a non-smoker and reported no surgeries or medical conditions likely to affect the larynx.

Further questioning revealed a number of variables possibly related to his dysphonia. As noted, he was a rancher whose days during the harvest season (late summer through fall) began early in the morning and continued late into the evening, seven days a week. Dinner was eaten late at night, immediately before bedtime. Voice use during this time was particularly heavy and involved a great deal of talking outdoors, often over noise generated by farm machinery.

Speaking typically took place at a distance of several yards from employees, in orchards, fields and feeding lots. These environments were described as dusty and had sometimes been sprayed with agricultural chemicals. The patient also noted that harvest periods were typically quite stressful times for him, particularly so this year, as a consequence of weather conditions and economic concerns related to his business. He employed many workers, and felt responsible for their well-being as well as his family's.

Voice Therapy/Treatment

The patient was rather quickly able to use the true vocal folds for speech when exhalation was paired with relaxation and when utterances were restricted to three or four syllables per breath. Though the dysphonia persisted, he described the effort associated with speaking as markedly reduced. Added to these strategies, the patient was instructed to pause at the end of each exhalation prior to inspiration and, following instruction, to maintain comfortable frequency and intensity levels. The primary treatment recommendation was to return to the referring otolaryngologist for management of his laryngeal pathology. This physician was contacted and provided with materials from our evaluation; an appointment in his office was scheduled for the same week.

Additional recommendations were based on the likelihood that voice use, coughing and throat clearing, and possible extraesophageal reflux and exposure to airway irritants may, to varying extents, be both causative and/or exacerbating factors in the patient's dysphonia. The patient was counseled regarding each of these factors and the potential relationship of each to his condition. Other goals, discussed at length, included (1) minimal voice use, and using voice as it had been produced during treatment probing; (2) elimination, to the extent possible, of excessive and/or abusive vocal behaviors, e.g., coughing, throat clearing; (3) a conservative reflux protocol, e.g., no food intake 3 hours prior to bedtime, sleeping with the head of the bed elevated); (4) attention to improved vocal hygiene and hydration; and (5) wearing a mask when in dusty or chemically affected environments. Both the patient and his wife demonstrated good understanding of these objectives and the need for adherence to them, as well as the importance of returning to the referring otolaryngologist. The patient (who lived 3–4 hours from our site) was also scheduled to return to us in 4 to 6 weeks to reevaluate voice and, depending on progress, to consider other behavioral treatment options.

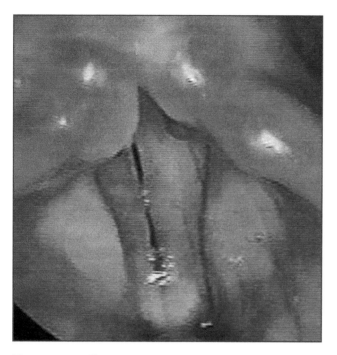

Figure 34–3. Photomicrograph of larynx following treatment. Pathology previously identified in Figure 34–2 appears significantly reduced with resolution of supraglottic constriction, reduced mucus, and smoother free edge of the vocal fold.

The status of the larynx at his follow-up visit is illustrated in Case 2, Figure 34–3 and in Video 34–2. The patient reported that he had been compliant with our previous recommendations, and had been taking reflux medications as prescribed by the otolaryngologist, who had also recommended taking a biopsy of the pathology, which was declined by the patient pending (briefly) results of conservative strategies. It is apparent in the figures that the tissue pathology previously identified has substantially resolved; all measures of vocal function, as well as voice quality, had also significantly improved. He continued to be followed by the referring otolaryngologist.

Case 2 Synopsis

This patient is of particular interest for a number of reasons. First, when he was initially examined by an otolaryngologist, he was found to use the false vocal folds for speaking, with no underlying tissue pathology identified. "Functional" dysphonia was diagnosed, and he was referred to our center for voice therapy.

Unfortunately, circumstances delayed this follow-up for several weeks. When it did take place, voice was still produced by the false vocal folds, which were constricted even at rest. Our impression, in fact, was that they were somewhat edematous, which exacerbated visualization. The underlying pathology was masked by the behavior, and possibly the size, of the false vocal folds. The severity of the dysphonia and the report that his voice had worsened since his initial evaluation were important in considering the possibility that there was, indeed, existing pathology, and for engaging in treatment probing that would relax the false folds sufficiently to observe underlying structures. This dysphonia, which we would term "adaptive," likely reflects the patient's response to, at least, both excessive vocal demands and noxious environmental stimuli. Eventually, it may have also reflected his response to the presence of pathology. Fortunately, tissue pathology resolved, as did the dysphonia. It is important for clinicians to remember, again, that a diagnosis of "functional" dysphonia may not necessarily mean that no pathology is present and, further, to recognize that, in some cases, tissue pathology may be masked by hyperfunctional vocal practices, which appeared to be the case in this situation. We would add, also, that having a male patient of this age, with no previous history of voice disorder, present with a functional dysphonia would be unusual in our practice.

CASE 3

Initial Presentation

The patient is a 9-year old girl with voice described as soft, "muffled," and very difficult to hear. Her parents indicate that she has "always sounded this way" but that her voice has become more of a problem since she entered school. Teachers and classmates have difficulty hearing and understanding her. She was recently evaluated by an otolaryngologist who reported that her true vocal folds were normal in appearance and function, and that her false vocal folds were used for phonation. "Functional dysphonia" was diagnosed, and she was referred for voice therapy. The school speech-language pathologist attempted voice therapy, but with no change in voice quality. The child was subsequently referred to our clinic for further evaluation and consideration of possible treatment strategies.

Phonoscopic/Phonatory Function Evaluation

The larynx is examined with rigid endoscopy and stroboscopy. A clip of this examination is presented in Case 3, Videos 34–3 and 34–4. In Video 34–3, the exam is presented at normal speed; in the second (Video 34–4), the playback is in slow motion. In the first clip, the impression is that the true vocal folds adduct at the initiation of phonation but that the false folds quickly constrict, partially obscuring the underlying true folds. As described, voice is soft and indistinct. When played back at a slower speed, it is apparent that there is a supraglottic web of tissue, arising anteriorly between the true and false vocal folds. As the true folds adduct, the web appears to move posteriorly, and is then obscured by the constriction of the false folds. The nature and origin of the supraglottic web is only generalized from the study, but the impression is that it in some way draws the ventricular folds to the midline during phonation. If so, this may well explain the voice quality reported, and appreciated by us, as well.

The phonatory function evaluation was of interest in that the 9-year-old's fundamental frequency was 223 Hz (range 215–405 Hz), which would be consistent with voice produced with the true vocal folds, though possibly somewhat low for her age. She was also able to sustain sound for 12 seconds, again, within normal limits for her age (and small size). In contrast to these relatively normal values, her glottal resistance during a syllable repetition task averaged over 400 dynes/cm/sec, which is substantially elevated. Measures of frequency (jitter) and amplitude (shimmer) perturbation on sustained sounds at "comfortable" fundamental frequencies were also elevated.

Patient History

Early medical records are not available, and information presented here is provided by the parents. According to their report, their daughter was born 3 months prematurely and, shortly after birth, was placed on a ventilator for 1 month. The parents don't believe ventilation involved intubation, but are not positive. During her infancy, she was frequently hospitalized for pneumonias and respiratory syncytial virus (RSV). She underwent a tonsillectomy at 3 years of age, and tympanoplasty at age 5 years. When she began school, she was placed in a special education classroom; however, she is currently doing well and is likely to transition to a mainstream classroom in the next year. As noted, her parents describe voice quality as essentially unchanged since birth, that is, very soft and "muffled."

Treatment

The patient returned to the referring physician for consideration of surgery or other treatment for the supraglottic web identified. The recommendation was for surgical excision of the web, depending on results of direct visualization of the structures involved. However, questions regarding type of surgery (laser or other), as well as the timing of a procedure, were unanswered at the time of our last contact with the patient. Now aware of the problem, the school speech-language pathologist and teachers were making every effort to facilitate the child's classroom experience, e.g., sitting in front of the room, providing amplification when appropriate.

Case 3 Synopsis

Several features of this case are of interest. First, a "functional" voice disorder, i.e., a voice disorder with no organic etiology, present from infancy, is improbable. Such a diagnosis should raise the question of whether pathology is present and just subtle, or masked by hyperfunctional behaviors, or whether earlier pathology subsequently resolved, but with persistent dysphonia. This child's history was suggestive of one of these possibilities. When the endoscopic clip is played back at the slower speed, certainly, the somewhat subtle supraglottic web is more easily appreciated. Another question concerns the origin of the pathology noted, that is, was it related to prematurity, or to early ventilation? Similarly, the possible cause or effect relationship between the supraglottic web identified and the respiratory difficulties reported at birth is intriguing. Early medical records, of course, may have clarified some of these issues.

Also of interest are results of phonatory function testing. As noted, these were in some ways consistent with voice produced with the true vocal folds, but with significant resistance, a combination that seems to fit well with the imaging evidence. The other variable of interest is the parents' report that their daughter's voice had "sounded this way" since she began vocalizing. They knew that it was not "normal" but had grown quite accustomed to it, made accommodations necessary to understand their daughter's soft, indistinct voice, and just assumed it was related in some way to her premature birth. It was only when the child was in school and having significant difficulty being understood by others that the problem became significant.

SUMMARY

The three cases presented here illustrate important considerations pertinent to patients with so-called functional dysphonias. It is, of course, true that some patients do present with no identifiable organic pathology to explain their dysphonia. In our experience, however, patients with a functional diagnosis may actually have pathology that is subtle or masked by hyperfunctional behaviors. History may also suggest a previous pathology that resolved, but with persistent dysphonia. Our preferred term for this category of disorders, as noted, is "adaptive" dysphonia, that is, a voice disorder that has arisen due to an aversive circumstance, e.g., psychological stressor, excessive or inappropriate use, present or past organic pathology. The term does not rule out organic etiology, and does, in our opinion, stress the importance of seeking the aversive source of a dysphonia, be it psychological, behavioral, or organic. Careful history-taking, imaging studies, and phonatory function analyses, as well as treatment probing to explore potential for improved voice, are, in our experience, critical to successful management.

REFERENCES

1. Aronson AE. *Clinical Voice Disorders: An Interdisciplinary Approach* (3rd ed). New York, NY: Thieme; 1990.
2. Verdolini K, Hess MM, Titze IR, Bierhals W, Gross M. Investigation of vocal fold impact stress in human subjects. *J Voice*. 1999;13(2):184–202.
3. Colton R, Caspar J, Leonard R. *Understanding Voice Problems: A Physiological Perspective for Diagnosis and Treatment* (4th ed). Philadelphia, PA: Lippincott, Williams & Wilkins: 2011.

CHAPTER 35

Episodic Laryngeal Breathing Disorders

Andrée-Anne Leclerc and Clark A. Rosen

INTRODUCTION

The diagnosis and treatment of a patient with episodic laryngeal breathing disorder (ELBD) can be a challenge. When reviewing the literature, it is obvious that there are many different terms used to describe the same pathology, as well as different pathology named with the same term. This lack of consensus results in difficulty in comparing and using data from different studies. Paradoxical vocal fold movement disorder (PVFMD), episodic laryngeal breathing disorder, vocal fold dysfunction, irritable larynx syndrome, Munchausen stridor, and more than 80 other terms can be found.[1] ELBD represents a rather heterogeneous group of pathologies that have a variety of etiologies, risk factors, and prognoses. ELBD can be first divided into two broad groups: PVFMD and dystonia. We use the term PVFMD to include disorders with adduction of vocal folds during respiration, with or without an identifiable trigger. PVFMD does not include abnormal vocal fold motion due to primary or secondary laryngeal dystonia.[1] As the term PVFMD is only a description of the symptoms (paradoxical movement), the etiology should be added to the term (ie, exercise induced PVFMD, reflux induced PVFMD, functional PVFMD).

The exact prevalence of PVFMD in the general population is unknown. A prevalence of 2.5% was reported in a group of patients in an asthma clinic.[2] Regardless of the underlying etiology, more than 80% of patients with abnormal vocal fold movement during inspiration are initially misdiagnosed[3] and it takes an average of 4.8 years before they have the right diagnosis.[4]

CASE PRESENTATION

A 25-year-old woman presents with inspiratory stridor of sudden onset for a couple of weeks. More than 6 years ago, she was diagnosed with reflux induced PVFMD that has improved with medical treatment for reflux and a Nissen fundoplication afterward. She now complains of heartburn that started 6 weeks ago. She feels that her gastroesophageal reflux (GERD) symptoms are back.

Medical history: Reflux induced PVFMD. GERD. Anemia. Chronic pain syndrome. Asthma. Gastroparesis. Lactose intolerant.

Surgical history: Nissen fundoplication. Gastrojejunostomy.

Medication: Salmeterol/fluticasone inhaled. Albuterol. Ipratropium. Montelukast. Ranitidine.

Social: No tobacco. No alcohol. No drugs.

Work: Chemist

INITIAL ASSESSMENT

History

Shortness of breath is the principal symptom in virtually all patients. Common associated primary or secondary symptoms are wheezing (36%), inspiratory stridor

(28%), chest tightness (25%), cough (25%), change in voice (12%), and choking sensation.[5,6] Some patients may also report dysphagia due to the difficulty in coordinating breathing and swallowing.[7] Depending on the severity of the airway obstruction, the symptoms can be mild to severe. Incorrect diagnosis of asthma in patients with PVFMD or dystonia often lead to escalating asthma treatment. Patients with a high risk of having PVFMD rather than asthma are usually young patients with shortness of breath, no criteria of asthma, and poor response to treatment.[8] It is also important to ask about potential triggers for respiratory distress and their time relationship with the beginning of symptoms. Known triggers are exercise, recent viral upper respiratory infection, GERD, laryngopharyngeal reflux (LPRD), postnasal drip (PND), allergies, tobacco, fumes, chemicals, cold air, sudden temperature changes, and stress.[1,3,9,10] To find possible secondary (or organic) etiologies, a review of neurologic symptoms, movement disorder symptoms, focal dystonia, tremor, cranial nerve impairment, and recent changes in medication can be helpful. There is also a known association between PVFMD and anxiety, stress, or factitious illness.[1] Thus, it can be relevant to ask questions about previous psychological disorder. Unfortunately, there is no consensus on diagnosis criteria for PVFMD, thus it is often a diagnosis of exclusion.[1]

Examination

Breathing patterns should be closely observed. If an episode of respiratory distress is not witnessed in the clinic, it can be helpful to ask the patient to film an episode of respiratory distress and bring it to the next appointment. The oximetry will be normal the vast majority of the time, even with persistent respiratory distress. Still, hypoxemia can occur during an acute episode[11] and this can be the sign of an organic etiology (secondary dystonia). Patients with PVFMD usually have a normal voice[7] but can also have a reduced maximum phonation time, reduced phonation range, and elevated jitter and shimmer measures.[5]

Endoscopy

Flexible transnasal laryngoscopy has a double purpose: visualization of vocal fold movement during breathing and exclusion of other causes of laryngeal obstruction. During respiratory distress, vocal fold adduction is essential to make the diagnosis of PVFMD[12] and should always be present during a respiratory distress episode (100%).[11] If the patient is asymptomatic during the laryngoscopy, an abnormal adduction can still be seen 60% of the time. Normal abduction of the vocal folds should also be seen at some point. It can sometimes be difficult to correlate the movement of the vocal folds with the respiratory cycle during laryngoscopy, and the help of a second person can be necessary. In some patients, the abnormal adduction of the vocal folds can also be present during the exhalation or can be accompanied by an abnormal motion of the false vocal folds.[13] Powell et al reported 32% combined glottic and supraglottic adduction, and 14% supraglottic adduction alone in adolescents with exercise induced laryngeal obstruction.[14] A normal laryngoscopic exam does not rule out PVFMD because of the intermittent nature of this pathology. In that case, trying to elicit symptoms with fast breathing, sniffing, coughing, physical exertion, or a known trigger can be trialed.[5] The differential diagnosis of respiratory distress is broad and endoscopic evaluation should help exclude most of them. The differential diagnosis includes asthma, infectious etiologies (croup, epiglottitis, etc), angioedema, aerodigestive foreign body, laryngeal or tracheal mass, laryngeal or tracheal stenosis, bilateral vocal fold paralysis, interarytenoid web, cricoarytenoid fixation, etc. Asthma is a common differential diagnosis that cannot be ruled out with laryngoscopy. As asthma is a more common diagnosis than PVFMD, most patients will have already been evaluated and treated without success for asthma before their evaluation in laryngology.

CASE: INITIAL EVALUATION

An inspiratory stridor is easily heard but her voice is near normal. Flexible laryngoscopy demonstrates severe vocal fold adduction during inspiration, and normal vocal fold abduction is demonstrated during a cough and a laugh.

Flexible Laryngoscopy

Initial evaluation (Video 35–1, see companion website).

Diagnosis

Reflux induced PVFMD.

Investigations

None. She will see her gastroenterologist to improve GERD treatment.

Management

Bilateral botulinum toxin A injection to reduce stridor and respiratory distress. Proton pump inhibitor (PPI) therapy (omeprazole 40 mg PO) increased to twice a day and ranitidine 300 mg PO QHS is added to her medication. Strict lifestyle and dietary modification for GERD is encouraged.

Discussion

In this scenario, the patient is already known for reflux induced PVFMD. She had a successful management of her GERD in the past that subsequently improved her PVFMD symptoms. Now she has respiratory distress with a positive laryngoscopy for PVFMD. She is already treated for GERD and little improvement is expected with further escalation of her reflux treatment. For this reason, bilateral botulinum toxin A injection is added to the treatment to help improve her condition until she sees her gastroenterologist.

DIFFERENTIAL DIAGNOSIS OF ABNORMAL VOCAL FOLD MOTION DURING RESPIRATION (TABLE 35–1)

PVFMD was originally described as a psychological disorder only, without a physical component.[15] We now know that there are different types of PVFMD, including inducible PVFMD (believed to have primarily a physical component) and PVFMD with psychological components. Inducible PVFMD is a large category, and therefore it is important to identify the possible or definite trigger(s). Even if exercise induced PVFMD is a subcategory of inducible PVFMD, the epidemiology and symptoms are different from the other forms of inducible PVFMD. For this reason, exercise induced PVFMD is often considered a separate category. PVFMDs with a psychological aspect can be further defined as a conversion disorder (functional PVFMD) or as malingering. According to Forrest et al, only 7% of psychological

PVFMDs (called primary PVCMD in their paper) is caused by malingering.[3] Patients who intentionally produce paradoxical movement of their vocal folds often do it for external gain. Malingering can be suspected when there is medicolegal issues, history of antisocial personality disorder, lack of cooperation during evaluation and treatment, and discrepancy between patient complaints and physical examination.[3]

Abnormal vocal fold movement during inspiration can also be a sign of primary or secondary laryngeal dystonia. Respiratory laryngeal dystonia is an involuntary contraction of adductor laryngeal muscles during inspiration, with presumably a different physiopathology than PVFMD. It can be hard to differentiate primary dystonia from PVFMD but contrary to PVFMD, primary dystonia will not respond well to speech therapy, and botulinum toxin A will be the first-line treatment. Dystonia can also be a manifestation of other diseases that affect the cortex, the brainstem, and the upper and lower motor neurons or the muscles. Scientific literature presents multiple case reports of diseases and conditions that have caused respiratory laryngeal dystonia. Finally, dystonia can also be secondary to medication and is often caused by extra-pyramidal symptoms from antipsychotics. First-generation antipsychotics are more likely to cause laryngeal dystonia but it has also been reported with second generation antipsychotics.[16] Symptoms will manifest in the first few days after starting or increasing the medication (50% will develop laryngeal dystonia in less than 48 hours and 90% in less than 5 days).[17] Additionally, propofol[18] and prochlorperazine[19] have been reported to cause laryngeal respiratory dystonia.

MANAGEMENT OF PATIENTS WITH ABNORMAL VOCAL FOLD MOTION DURING RESPIRATION

Treatment choice should be based on the etiology as well as the severity of the symptoms. For some patients with mild symptoms, reassurance and a few sessions of voice/therapy will be enough. For moderate symptoms, more comprehensive voice therapy and sometimes psychotherapy can be useful. Patients with functional PVFMD will usually respond well to voice therapy and psychotherapy, and escalation to more aggressive treatment will rarely be necessary. If a trigger is found for induced PVFMD, it should be treated or avoided.

Table 35–1. Differential Diagnosis of Abnormal Vocal Fold Motion During Respiration

Paradoxical vocal fold motion	Inducible	LPR / GERD
		Exercise
		Allergy
		Odors/perfumes
		Other
	Functional	
	Malingering	
Primary dystonia	Respiratory laryngeal dystonia	
Secondary dystonia	Brainstem	Arnold–Chiari
		Arachnoid cyst
		Cerebral aqueductal stenosis
	Cortical and motor neuron diseases	Amyotrophic lateral sclerosis
		Cerebral vascular event
		Medullary infarction
		Multiple sclerosis
		Myasthenia gravis
		Neurosyphilis
	Movement disorder	Parkinson's disease
		Progressive supranuclear palsy
		Multiple system atrophy (Shy–Drager)
		Lubag syndrome
	Pharmaceuticals	First-generation antipsychotics
		Second-generation antipsychotics
		Propofol
		Prochlorperazine
	Xeroderma pigmentosum	

Patients with refractory or severe PVFMD, patients with laryngeal respiratory dystonia, or patients with secondary dystonia are more likely to need pharmacological or surgical treatment. Botulinum toxin A injection can be used if conventional treatment fails. Grillone et al published the effect of bilateral botulinum toxin A injection in the thyroarytenoid muscles of nine patients with refractory PVFMD.[20] After the injection, all patients had improvement of their stridor for an average of 13.8 weeks. Breathy voice and mild choking with liquids was found in 56% of those patients and lasted between 1 and 6 weeks. Other possible side effects are hoarseness and pain at the injection site (1%).[7] There is no consensus in literature regarding the dose and muscles to inject. Woisard et al suggests starting with a dose of 4 U for the first injection, and they report that this dose can be enough to have good benefits.[21] Age and gender does not seem to have an influence on the dose needed.[22]

During acute episodes, heliox (80% helium, 20% oxygen) inhalation with or without non-invasive positive pressure ventilation can help patients recover.[23] Benzodiazepines and ketamine are also reported to decrease symptoms of functional PVFMD. It is important to keep in mind that, with benzodiazepines, there is a potential risk of respiratory drive suppression and, with ketamine, of laryngospasm. Both should only be used in the presence of a physician with the ability to manage difficult airways and with the appropriate equipment accessible.[23] Finally, a small number of patients will still have desaturation after those interventions and will need a tracheostomy to relieve their symptoms. Surgical management is usually a last option for patients with severe, refractory symptoms.

CASE: 6 MONTHS LATER

The botulinum toxin A injection improved her symptoms initially without any voice or respiratory issues. Her gastroenterologists confirmed a relapse of her GERD and she underwent a surgical procedure to facilitate gastric emptying. Since the surgery, she has a significant improvement of her symptoms. Flexible laryngoscopy does not show paradoxical movement during the appointment.

Diagnosis

Improved reflux induced PVFMD.

Management

Observation.

CASE: 1 YEAR LATER

In the last year, she had three recurrences of stridor associated with gastric obstruction. Those three times, she had botulinum toxin A injections to relieve her symptoms and gastrointestinal surgery to relieve the obstruction. She is now hospitalized for nausea, intolerance of oral diet, and gastrointestinal obstruction that did not improve with surgery. She is also having recurrence of PVFMD with stridor. She did not get better with a bilateral botulinum toxin A injection.

Flexible Laryngoscopy

 Exacerbation (Video 35–2, see companion website).

Diagnosis

Severe reflux induced PVFMD.

Management

Tracheostomy.

Discussion

In the past, her PVFMD had always resolved with the treatment of her gastrointestinal disease. She is now hospitalized with a gastrointestinal obstruction that did not improve with surgery and a severe respiratory distress. She responded well to botulinum toxin A injections in the past but unfortunately, on this occasion she still reports respiratory distress 10 days after botulinum toxin injection. In this case, the next step to improve her distress was a tracheostomy. Her symptoms were greatly improved with the tracheostomy. It took 4 months to control her gastrointestinal disease after the tracheostomy. When she is having gastrointestinal disease or reflux recurrences, she has recurrences of PVFMD with severe stridor if she has her tracheostomy tube plugged. Her symptoms are easily relieved when she removes the cap. She is not a candidate for decannulation.

Flexible Laryngoscopy–Tracheostomy (Video 35–3, see companion website)

In the presence of gastric acid, alginates precipitate, forming a gel. Alginate-based raft-forming formulations usually contain sodium or potassium bicarbonate; in the presence of gastric acid, the bicarbonate is converted to carbon dioxide, which becomes entrapped within the gel precipitate, converting it into a foam which floats on the surface of the gastric contents, much like a raft on water.

FUNCTIONAL PVFMD

Functional PVFMD is often categorized as a conversion disorder, defined as a deficit in voluntary motor or sensory function with symptoms that are not intentionally produced.[3,12,24-26] Functional PVFMD can manifest without other psychological disorders (29%[3] to 50%[27]) or with other comorbid conditions: other conversion disorder (12%), anxiety disorder (11%), personality disorder (6%), depression (4%), psychosomatic disorder (2%), factitious disorder (2%), or somatization disorder (1%).[28] Unlike malingering, patients with functional PVFMD do not create their symptoms intentionally and they are not seeking external gain. This form of PVFMD is most often seen in young women[3,27] and can be preceded by an upper respiratory tract infection[12] or a stressful event.[29] Kuppersmith et al also reports it more commonly among health care professionals.[27] Symptoms are similar to other forms of PVFMD and dystonia.

Patients identified with functional PVFMD may be frustrated because of previous misdiagnosis or unnecessary medication or interventions. Some patients could also have been confronted about faking their disease. Thus, it is important to educate the patient about what we know of this disease and the normal role of the larynx during breathing. Reassurance about the benign aspect of the disease can also provide relief to the patient. Voice therapy is the first line of treatment for functional PVFMD with breathing techniques to interrupt the abnormal respiratory pattern, such as nasal inspiration with pursed-lip exhalation[23] and therapies that increase laryngeal control and awareness during breathing.[3] Psychotherapy can also be a good additional treatment for some patients. Guglani et al recently reviewed the literature on psychological interventions for functional PVFMD and concluded that even if there is a lack of data on efficiency of the different treatment options, they can still be beneficial when used according to the specific needs of each patient. Psychotherapy, behavioral therapy, and hypnotherapy were described only in small studies and case reports, with little information on outcomes.[30] Patients with functional PVFMD will sometimes benefit from a trial botulinum toxin A injection if they do not respond to speech therapy.[3] More invasive and morbid interventions are almost never needed for this category of patients.[3] Another aspect of voice therapy is to provide patients with biofeedback by allowing them to see their larynx via flexible laryngoscopy and letting them see the positive and negative results of various laryngeal and neck behaviors.

INDUCIBLE PVFMD

Inducible PVFMD, also called irritable larynx syndrome,[31] laryngeal hyperresponsiveness,[32] or inducible laryngeal obstruction,[33] is a PVFMD resulting from a defined triggering stimulus. Inducible PVFMD is believed to be caused by a chronic noxious exposure which leads to a neural or epithelial injury, to accumulation of inflammatory mediators and then to neuronal changes (molecular, cellular, and/or synaptic changes).[34] Those neuronal changes alter laryngeal sensory function and the larynx develops a chronic hyper-excitable state. Subsequent exposure to stimuli can then trigger PVFMD. This hyper-responsiveness can also be seen in other diseases. Morrison et al studied 195 patients (90% of women) with inducible PVFMD and reported the prevalence of other central sensitivity syndrome. They reported concomitant diagnosis of irritable bowel syndrome (54%), chronic headaches (49%), chronic fatigue syndrome (42%), multiple chemical sensitivity (35%), fibromyalgia (28%), and temporomandibular joint disorder (17%).[31]

Among possible triggers, GERD was reported to have a prevalence of between 18%[35] and 21%,[32] but Forrest et al have determined that as many as 90% of patients with inducible PVFMD have GERD.[3] Chronic exposure to acid reflux can alter one's laryngeal sensory function and change the threshold for laryngeal closure when exposed to subsequent acid reflux events or to other irritants. Acute exposure to acid reflux can also trigger laryngospasm during inspiration via activation of chemoreceptors and stimulation of the superior laryngeal nerve.[5,34] Viral infections may also be the initial insult that triggers hypersensitivity.[31] Up to 30% of patients have a history of recent viral infection before developing inducible PVFMD.[3] Work-related triggers such as cleaning agents, anhydrides, isocyanates, formaldehyde, fumes, or dye[34] can also induce PVFMD, even if the patient has been working in the same environment for many years before developing symptoms. Symptoms are often dose dependent, and onset will be almost immediately after exposure.[34] Patients will present with inspiratory dyspnea, dysphonia, chronic cough, globus sensation, and throat clearing. Dyspnea can also be seen during expiration in inducible PVFMD.[32] A detailed timeline of symptoms is particularly important for inducible PVFMD.

Clinical evaluation of those patients should be able to demonstrate vocal fold adduction triggered by an external stimulus. A standard transnasal laryngoscopic evaluation should be done first and then followed by a provocation challenge. It is beneficial to have a standardized protocol for provocation challenge[3] to ensure reproducibility and efficiency. A specific causative agent can be used if the patient is able to identify one. Alternatively, generic irritants can also be used: perfume, hand sanitizer, or cleaning solution.[34] Changes should be seen almost immediately after exposure. It is usually easier to perform a provocation challenge in a controlled environment (eg, hospital) with a physician and speech language pathologist present to monitor and reassure the patient during the test.[34] The speech-language pathologist can also use this time to teach different respiratory-laryngeal control techniques to the patient. Patients should also be monitored with a pulse oximeter during the test to ensure safety as well as help confirm the diagnosis of PVFMD (other diagnoses should be considered if there is a desaturation during the test).[3]

Treatment of induced PVFMD should always start with education on the disease and on different respiratory and laryngeal control techniques. If a specific trigger is identified, avoidance of this irritant should be the next step. If it is not possible to avoid it completely, increasing ventilation in the environment or the use of personal protective equipment may decrease exposure. If there is no specific irritant found in the patient history, treatment of other potential triggers like dehydration, GERD, or post-nasal drainage can be tried for a short period of time, and continued depending on the response.[3,5,34] In refractory cases, botulinum toxin A may be an option depending on the severity of the symptoms.

EXERCISE INDUCED PVFMD

The prevalence of exercise induced PVFMD in the general population is not known but the prevalence in adolescents was reported to be up to 7%.[36,37] It seems to be more frequent in adolescent athletes, especially with winter sports, swimming, handball, basketball, and soccer.[38] Unlike functional PVFMD, the difference of prevalence between gender is not as obvious for exercise induced PVFMD,[37] with an equal prevalence between men and women.

There is little evidence on the physiopathology of exercise induced PVFMD but Roksund et al reported an aerodynamic hypothesis and a hyper-responsive hypothesis.[38] The aerodynamic hypothesis is based on the normal increased negative pressure during inspiration. When associated with an abnormally poor support of the laryngeal structures from posterior arytenoid muscle and arytenoids, laryngeal structures become medialized during inspiration. The hyper-responsive hypothesis is based on a change of threshold for induction of the laryngeal closure reflex, a natural reflex loop that closes the laryngeal introitus to protect the lower respiratory tract. In patients with lower thresholds for stimulation, hyperventilation during physical activity could trigger abnormal laryngeal closure.

Symptoms are often associated with high-intensity sprinting activities[3] rather than longer low-intensity activities. Dyspnea is present in all patients and half of them will also have hoarse voice or stridor. Rundell et al also reported a higher prevalence of inspiratory stridor during outdoor activities.[39] They can also present with respiratory distress, throat or chest pain, prolonged inspiration, hyperventilation attacks, and panic reaction.[37] In this case, PVFMD is not related to psychological factors and it is the respiratory distress that triggers a panic reaction. Lightheadedness and paresthesia are possible manifestations of exercise induced PVFMD, but hypoxia and cyanosis are uncommon and should prompt searching for another diagnosis.[40] Asthma and exercise induced bronchoconstriction are the most common differential diagnoses for exercise induced PVFMD. Because asthma is a frequent disease and is often diagnosed based on symptoms only, exercise induced PVFMD is frequently misdiagnosed as asthma and patient are treated with inappropriate medication.[38,40] Up to 85% of patients diagnosed with exercise induced PVFMD have been treated for asthma in the past and 64% reported no improvement of symptoms with the treatment.[41] In asthmatic patients, dyspnea is present during expiration, starts gradually within 3 to 15 minutes after high-intensity exercise, and resolves in minutes to hours. In patients with exercise induced PVFMD, dyspnea is present at inspiration, starts abruptly during or shortly after high intensity exercise (less than 3 minutes) and resolves in seconds.[38] An incorrect diagnosis of asthma leads to increased use of corticosteroids (and increased risk of corticosteroid side effects), avoidance of physical activity or poor athletic performance, and overuse of medical care. Still, coexistence of asthma and PVFMD is possible and is reported to be present 30% to 56% of the time.[29,37,42] A PVFMD Screening Questionnaire has been developed and validated by Ye et al to try to differentiate PVFMD from asthma.[29] They used questions from the Dyspnea Index[43] mixed with other questions developed specifically for their study. Then, they selected 15 questions from it and chose a 4-point Likert scale for the final questionnaire. With a sensitivity of 85% and specificity of 73%, their PVFMD Screening Questionnaire was able to differentiate asthma from PVFMD (but not asthma from PVFMD with asthma). This questionnaire does not replace laryngoscopic evaluation but can guide referrals in laryngology. Pulmonary function tests with methacholine challenge test are routinely used in the evaluation of asthma and should be advocated as the gold standard to make the diagnosis of asthma to prevent the overdiagnosis in the face of PVFMD. Roksund et al report a literature review on exercise induced PVFMD and conclude that those same tests are not useful to confirm or reject the diagnosis of exercise induced PVFMD because asthma and exercise induced PVFMD are not mutually exclusive and because there is a low sensitivity, repeatability, and interrater analysis agreement of the flow-volume loop. In exercise induced PVFMD, the flow-volume loop is often reported to be flat during inspiration but inadequate instruction or suboptimal effort can mimic extrathoracic limitations and give a false positive result.[38]

Laboratory provocation challenge with visualization of laryngeal structures during exercise is the gold standard to diagnose exercise induced PVFMD. Visualization after exercise is easier to do but increases false negative results given that exercise induced PVFMD symptoms are at their peak during exercise. A normal laryngeal response to exercise has been described by Beaty et al and includes a complete opening of the larynx with anterior rotation of the epiglottis toward the base of tongue, stretching of the aryepiglottic folds, and contraction of the posterior cricoid muscles, ahead of the diaphragm.[44] During a continuous laryngoscopy exercise test, laryngeal movements are observed and analyzed at rest, during exercise, at peak exercise, and during the recovery phase. The exercise used can be cycling, rowing, or stair climbing, but treadmill running is probably the best to reach adequate intensity to replicate symptoms in young adults.[38] Cardiopulmonary data including ECG, flow-volume loop, and minute ventilation are measured, with video recording of the upper part of the body and sound tracks also obtained during the test. Subsequently, vocal fold adduction and medial rotation of aryepiglottic folds during the breathing cycle and during different phases of exercise can be analyzed. A scoring system has been developed and validated by Maat et al to analyze laryngeal movement during inspiration.[45] Adduction is scored from 0 to 3 at two moments (moderate exercise and peak effort) and at two levels (glottal and supraglottic). The total of those four scores is used to classify patients into three groups (score: 0–2, 3–4, ≥5). Studies show that there is a correlation between this score and the patient's symptoms[45] and that normal patients are asymptomatic during this test.[46] Instead of using exercise, eucapnic voluntary hyperventilation has also been used to trigger PVFMD symptoms. Patients inhale air with 5% CO_2 to induce laryngeal obstruction.

Christensen et al compared this trigger with exercise and found that patients reported the same symptoms with both methods.[47]

There is little evidence on treatment options for exercise induced PVFMD. What we know and don't know about the pathology and the treatment options should be thoroughly discussed with the patient before coming up with a shared decision. Many patients will change their lifestyle to avoid respiratory symptoms and, depending on the kind of activity that triggers their PVFMD, some will completely stop the offending activity. Biofeedback,[48] inspiratory muscle training,[49,50] and psychotherapy[37] have been reported as treatment options for exercise induced PVFMD. Therapeutic laryngoscopy during exercise, a therapy where the patient does high-intensity exercise during laryngoscopic examination and receives specific instructions regarding maneuvers to maximize laryngeal aperture, has also been described and was well tolerated by patients.[51] The clinical effectiveness of this technique has not been studied yet. Laryngeal control therapy, which focuses on increasing awareness of the opening of glottal structures, has been reported effective in 88% of patients after two sessions.[52] With regard to pharmacological treatment, inhaled ipratropium bromide can be used right before exercise to prevent symptoms of PVFMD.[53] Botulinum toxin A can also be used in patients with refractory symptoms. Finally, endoscopic supraglottoplasty (aryepiglottic folds incision and partial removal of the mucosa around the upper parts of the tubercles)[54] has also been reported as an effective treatment for some very specific patients with supraglottic obstruction. Decision to undertake a surgical treatment should be based on laryngoscopic evaluation during exercise. Patients reported improvement of their symptoms but there were no statistically significant changes in their objective respiratory measurements.[55]

RESPIRATORY LARYNGEAL DYSTONIA

Primary focal dystonia is an involuntary and counterproductive muscular contraction of a muscle or group of muscles.[7] The pathophysiology is not well understood but seems to involve an abnormal basal ganglia function with imbalance between excitation and inhibition signals.[56] Primary focal dystonia usually starts during adulthood.[57] There is a familial history of dystonia in 12% of patients.[57] The site of onset for primary focal dystonia has been reported to be the larynx in 19%. Nine percent to 16% of them developed other sites of dystonia (torticollis, oromandibular dystonia, blepharospasm, tongue dystonia, upper and lower extremity dystonia).[20,57,58] Primary laryngeal dystonia included adductor spasmodic dysphonia, abductor spasmodic dysphonia, mixed spasmodic dysphonia, and respiratory laryngeal dystonia. Tremor laryngeal dystonia[59] and laryngeal dystonia gravidarum[60] have also been included in this group by some authors. Of those, only the respiratory laryngeal dystonia will present with respiratory distress and stridor.

Patients with respiratory laryngeal dystonia will have acute onset of symptoms and persistent stridor, with relief of symptoms during sleeping and improvement during phonation.[7,61] Symptoms may worsen during stress or exercise.[20] Due to constant respiratory effort, patients will sometimes report tiredness during the day that can interfere with work. Most of the time, there will be no associated desaturation with respiratory distress episodes, but life-threatening events are also possible with severe acute dystonia.

There is no cure for primary laryngeal dystonia. Speech therapy for this category of patient is less effective than for patients with PVFMD. Yet, speech therapy, psychotherapy, and biofeedback can be partially beneficial and can also help to differentiate primary dystonia from PVFMD.[7] Botulinum toxin A is the treatment of choice for these patients. Other options are benzodiazepines, anticholinergic medications, and dopamine blocking agents, but as mentioned previously, they should be used with caution and are not as effective as botulinum toxin A. If treatments are not effective, tracheostomy may be the last resort.

SUMMARY

ELBD is a heterogeneous group of diseases all characterized by at least an abnormal movement of the vocal folds during respiration with a sensation of respiratory distress. When a diagnosis of PVFMD is made, practitioners should attach the suspected trigger or etiology to the diagnosis. Flexible laryngeal examination should always be done to rule out other pathologies and to see the pattern of abnormal movement. There are multiple possible triggers for ELBD, and finding the trigger for each patient will help choose the appropriate treatment. Patients with functional PVFMD will have a good response to speech therapy and sometimes to psychotherapy. Patients with identifiable triggers will have a better response when they can avoid

this specific trigger. Finally, patients with dystonia will most of the time need botulinum toxin A to improve.

REFERENCES

1. Shembel AC, Sandage MJ, Verdolini Abbott K. Episodic laryngeal breathing disorders: literature review and proposal of preliminary theoretical framework. *J Voice*. 2017;31:125.e127–125.e116.
2. Ciccolella DE, Brennan KJ, Borbely B. Identification of vocal cord dysfunction (VCD) and other diagnoses in patients admitted to an innercity university hospital asthma center. *J Respir Crit Care Med*. 1997;155.
3. Forrest LA, Husein T, Husein O. Paradoxical vocal cord motion: classification and treatment. *Laryngoscope*. 2012; 122:844–853.
4. Hicks M, Brugman SM, Katial R. Vocal cord dysfunction/paradoxical vocal fold motion. *Prim Care*. 2008;35:81–103.
5. Franca MC. Differential diagnosis in paradoxical vocal fold movement (PVFMD): an interdisciplinary task. *Internat J Pediatr Otorhinolaryngol*. 2014;78:2169–2173.
6. Morris MJ, Christopher KL. Diagnostic criteria for the classification of vocal cord dysfunction. *Chest*. 2010;138: 1213–1223.
7. Grillone GA, Chan T. Laryngeal dystonia. *Otolaryngol Clin North Am*. 2006;39:87–100.
8. Li RC, Singh U, Windom HP, Gorman S, Bernstein JA. Clinical associations in the diagnosis of vocal cord dysfunction. *Ann Allergy Asthma Immunol*. 2016;117:354–358.
9. Munoz X, Roger A, De la Rosa D, Morell F, Cruz MJ. Occupational vocal cord dysfunction due to exposure to wood dust and xerographic toner. *Scand J Work Environ Health*. 2007;33:153–158.
10. Tonini S, Dellabianca A, Costa C, Lanfranco A, Scafa F, Candura SM. Irritant vocal cord dysfunction and occupational bronchial asthma: differential diagnosis in a health care worker. *Intern J Occ Med Environ Health*. 2009; 22:401–406.
11. Fretzayas A, Moustaki M, Loukou I, Douros K. Differentiating vocal cord dysfunction from asthma. *J Asthma Allergy*. 2017;10:277–283.
12. Maschka DA, Bauman NM, McCray PB Jr, Hoffman HT, Karnell MP, Smith RJ. A classification scheme for paradoxical vocal cord motion. *Laryngoscope*. 1997;107:1429–1435.
13. Weinberger M, Doshi D. Vocal cord dysfunction: a functional cause of respiratory distress. *Breathe*. 2017;13:15–21.
14. Powell DM, Karanfilov BI, Beechler KB, Treole K, Trudeau MD, Forrest LA. Paradoxical vocal cord dysfunction in juveniles. *Arch Otolaryngology Head Neck Surg*. 2000;126:29–34.
15. Patterson R, Schatz M, Horton M. Munchausen's stridor: non-organic laryngeal obstruction. *Clin Allergy*. 1974;4: 307–310.

16. Tsai CS, Lee Y, Chang YY, Lin PY. Ziprasidone-induced tardive laryngeal dystonia: a case report. *Gen Hosp Psych.* 2008;30:277–279.

17. Collins N, Sager J. Acute laryngeal dystonia associated with asenapine use: a case report. *J Clinical Psychopharm.* 2017;37:738–739.

18. Steckelberg RC, Tsiang D, Pettijohn K, Mendelsohn A, Hoffman N. Acute vocal fold dystonic reaction to propofol: a case report. *Am J Otolaryng.* 2015;36:303–305.

19. Freudenreich O. Atypical laryngeal dystonia caused by an antiemetic. *Am Fam Phys.* 2004;69:1623.

20. Grillone GA, Blitzer A, Brin MF, Annino DJ Jr, Saint-Hilaire MH. Treatment of adductor laryngeal breathing dystonia with botulinum toxin type A. *Laryngoscope.* 1994; 104:30–32.

21. Woisard V, Liu X, Bes MC, Simonetta-Moreau M. Botulinum toxin injection in laryngeal dyspnea. *Euro Arch Otorhinolaryngol.* 2017;274:909–917.

22. Vasconcelos S, Birkent H, Sardesai MG, Merati AL, Hillel AD. Influence of age and gender on dose and effectiveness of botulinum toxin for laryngeal dystonia. *Laryngoscope.* 2009;119:2004–2007.

23 Denipah N, Dominguez CM, Kraai EP, Kraai TL, Leos P, Braude D. Acute management of paradoxical vocal fold motion (vocal cord dysfunction). *Ann Emerg Med.* 2017; 69:18–23.

24. Ramirez J, Leon I, Rivera LM. Episodic laryngeal dyskinesia. Clinical and psychiatric characterization. *Chest.* 1986;90:716–721.

25. Appelblatt NH, Baker SR. Functional upper airway obstruction. A new syndrome. *Arch Otolaryngol.* 1981;107: 305–306.

26. Husein OF, Husein TN, Gardner R, et al. Formal psychological testing in patients with paradoxical vocal fold dysfunction. *Laryngoscope.* 2008;118:740–747.

27. Kuppersmith R, Rosen DS, Wiatrak BJ. Functional stridor in adolescents. *J Adol Health.* 1993;14:166–171.

28. Leo RJ, Konakanchi R. Psychogenic respiratory distress: a case of paradoxical vocal cord dysfunction and literature review. *Prim Care Companion J Clin Psychiatry.* 1999;1:39–46.

29. Ye J, Nouraei M, Holguin F, Gillespie AI. The ability of patient-symptom questionnaires to differentiate pvfmd from asthma. *J Voice.* 2017;31:382.e381–382.

30. Guglani L, Atkinson S, Hosanagar A, Guglani L. A systematic review of psychological interventions for adult and pediatric patients with vocal cord dysfunction. *Front Pediatr.* 2014;2:82.

31. Morrison M, Rammage L, Emami AJ. The irritable larynx syndrome. *J Voice.* 1999; 13:447–455.

32. Morrison M, Rammage L. The irritable larynx syndrome as a central sensitivity syndrome. *Canadian J Speech-Lang Path Audiol.* 2010;34:8.

33. Christensen PM, Heimdal JH, Christopher KL, et al. ERS/ELS/ACCP 2013 international consensus conference nomenclature on inducible laryngeal obstructions. *Euro Resp Rev.* 2015;24:445–450.

34. Anderson JA. Work-associated irritable larynx syndrome. *Curr Opin Allergy Clin Immunol.* 2015;15:150–155.

35. Shepherd MW, Curtis C, Long S, Sr, Phillips G, Ogbogu PU. Atopic characteristics of patients with vocal cord dysfunction. *Ann Allergy, Asthma Immunol.* 2017; 118:228–230.

36. Johansson H, Norlander K, Berglund L, et al. Prevalence of exercise-induced bronchoconstriction and exercise-induced laryngeal obstruction in a general adolescent population. *Thorax.* 2015;70:57–63.

37. Liyanagedera S, McLeod R, Elhassan HA. Exercise induced laryngeal obstruction: a review of diagnosis and management. *Eur Arch Otorhinolaryngol.* 2017; 274: 1781–1789.

38. Roksund OD, Heimdal JH, Clemm H, Vollsaeter M, Halvorsen T. Exercise inducible laryngeal obstruction: diagnostics and management. *Paed Resp Rev.* 2017;21:86–94.

39. Rundell KW, Spiering BA. Inspiratory stridor in elite athletes. *Chest.* 2003;123:468–474.

40. Olin JT, Clary MS, Deardorff EH, et al. Inducible laryngeal obstruction during exercise: moving beyond vocal cords with new insights. *Phys Sports Med.* 2015;43:13–21.

41. Roksund OD, Maat RC, Heimdal JH, Olofsson J, Skadberg BT, Halvorsen T. Exercise induced dyspnea in the young. Larynx as the bottleneck of the airways. *Resp Med.* 2009; 103:1911–1918.

42. Low K, Ruane L, Uddin N, et al. Abnormal vocal cord movement in patients with and without airway obstruction and asthma symptoms. *Clin Exper Allergy.* 2017;47: 200–207.

43. Gartner-Schmidt JL, Shembel AC, Zullo TG, Rosen CA. Development and validation of the Dyspnea Index (DI): a severity index for upper airway-related dyspnea. *J Voice.* 2014; 28:775–782.

44. Beaty MM, Wilson JS, Smith RJ. Laryngeal motion during exercise. *Laryngoscope.* 1999;109:136–139.

45. Maat RC, Roksund OD, Halvorsen T, et al. Audiovisual assessment of exercise-induced laryngeal obstruction: reliability and validity of observations. *Euro Arch Otorhinolaryngol.* 2009;266:1929–1936.

46. Tervonen H, Niskanen MM, Sovijarvi AR, Hakulinen AS, Vilkman EA, Aaltonen LM. Fiberoptic videolaryngoscopy during bicycle ergometry: a diagnostic tool for exercise-induced vocal cord dysfunction. *Laryngoscope.* 2009;119:1776–1780.

47. Christensen PM, Rasmussen N. Eucapnic voluntary hyperventilation in diagnosing exercise-induced laryngeal obstructions. *Eur Arch Otorhinolaryngol.* 2013;270: 3107–3113.

48. Rhodes RK. Diagnosing vocal cord dysfunction in young athletes. *J Am Academy Nurse Prac.* 2008;20:608–613.

49. Mathers-Schmidt BA, Brilla LR. Inspiratory muscle training in exercise-induced paradoxical vocal fold motion. *J Voice.* 2005;19:635–644.

50. Ruddy BH, Davenport P, Baylor J, Lehman J, Baker S, Sapienza C. Inspiratory muscle strength training with

behavioral therapy in a case of a rower with presumed exercise-induced paradoxical vocal-fold dysfunction. *Int J Ped Otorhinolaryngol.* 2004;68:1327–1332.

51. Olin JT, Deardorff EH, Fan EM, et al. Therapeutic laryngoscopy during exercise: a novel non-surgical therapy for refractory EILO. *Ped Pulmonol.* 2017; 52:813–819.

52. Chiang T, Marcinow AM, deSilva BW, Ence BN, Lindsey SE, Forrest LA. Exercise-induced paradoxical vocal fold motion disorder: diagnosis and management. *Laryngoscope.* 2013;123:727–731.

52. Weinberger M, Abu-Hasan M. Pseudo-asthma: when cough, wheezing, and dyspnea are not asthma. *Pediatrics.* 2007;120:855–864.

54. Maat RC, Roksund OD, Olofsson J, Halvorsen T, Skadberg BT, Heimdal JH. Surgical treatment of exercise-induced laryngeal dysfunction. *Eur Arch Otorhinolaryngol.* 2007; 264:401–407.

55. Maat RC, Hilland M, Roksund OD, et al. Exercise-induced laryngeal obstruction: natural history and effect of surgical treatment. *Eur Arch Otorhinolaryngol.* 2011; 268:1485–1492.

56. Simonyan K, Cho H, Hamzehei Sichani A, Rubien-Thomas E, Hallett M. The direct basal ganglia pathway is hyperfunctional in focal dystonia. *Brain.* 2017;140: 3179–3190.

57. Weiss EM, Hershey T, Karimi M, et al. Relative risk of spread of symptoms among the focal onset primary dystonias. *Move Dis.* 2006;21:1175–1181.

58. Blitzer A, Brin MF, Stewart CF. Botulinum toxin management of spasmodic dysphonia (laryngeal dystonia): a 12–year experience in more than 900 patients. *Laryngoscope.* 2015;125:1751–1757.

59. Hillel AD. The study of laryngeal muscle activity in normal human subjects and in patients with laryngeal dystonia using multiple fine–wire electromyography. *Laryngoscope.* 2001;111:1–47.

60. Ankola A, Sulica L, Murry T. Laryngeal dystonia gravidarum: sudden onset of adductor spasmodic dysphonia in pregnancy. *Laryngoscope.* 2013;123:3127–3130.

61. Zwirner P, Dressler D, Kruse E. Spasmodic laryngeal dyspnea: a rare manifestation of laryngeal dystonia. *Eur Arch Otorhinolaryngol.* 1997;254:242–245.

.

CHAPTER 36

Exercise-Induced Laryngeal Obstruction

Emil Schwarz Walsted, Andrew J. Kinshuck, and James H. Hull

CASE DESCRIPTION

The patient is a 16-year-old woman who is referred with unexplained exertional breathlessness. Her symptoms first started when she was 14 years old and only present during sport. Specifically, she describes a rapid onset of breathing difficulty with an inability to get a "satisfying breath" and a burning sensation in her throat during vigorous exercise. Her symptoms develop most often in the context of competitive sport and rapidly abate on exercise cessation; i.e., taking less than 5 minutes to resolve. She reports the presence of a coexisting "whistling" sound that develops during more severe episodes. On direct questioning, this sound occurs almost exclusively on inspiration.

Her symptoms had worsened in the year prior to presentation and were impacting her ability to train and compete successfully in her chosen sport. She had no other significant past medical history; however, at the time of referral, she had been diagnosed with asthma and was treated with inhaled medication for some time prior to referral, with no symptomatic benefit. She denied symptoms of gastroesophageal reflux or nasal disease.

Her referring center arranged initial baseline investigations, revealing a normal chest radiograph, electrocardiogram, and basic hematological profile (eg, full blood count and inflammatory markers). Baseline physiological testing, including spirometry with peak inspiratory flow, was normal. She also completed a methacholine bronchoprovocation test to determine if she had lower airway hyperreactivity, and this was negative.

She proceeded to a continuous laryngoscopy during exercise (CLE) test (example of test given in Figure 36–1). During the CLE test, exercise intensity was increased on the ergometer until she developed her typical symptoms. At this point she developed evidence of exercise-induced laryngeal obstruction (EILO), at least, grade 2 (ie, moderate) in severity with closure of the laryngeal inlet. This closure was predominantly manifest by inward rotation of the supraglottic (arytenoid) structures (Figure 36–2). She scored her symptom as 7/10 in severity, with 10 representing the maximum severity of closure. Her SpO_2 was reduced during exercise to 93%. She discontinued exercise and her symptoms resolved, entirely, in under 5 minutes.

Her diagnosis was discussed in a session with her CLE video reviewed. She was then discussed at a dedicated multidisciplinary team meeting (with speech and language therapy, laryngologist, physiotherapist, and a respiratory physician present) and initially referred for physiotherapy for breathing technique work.

A bubble echocardiogram revealed a patent foramen ovale (PFO). Antireflux treatment and anticholinergic inhaled therapy (ie, Atrovent 20 mcg II puffs, 15 minutes pre-exercise) was prescribed. She was also trained with an inspiratory muscle training device. Despite having at least five therapy sessions, her symptoms remained refractory to treatment and she was referred for consideration of surgical intervention, i.e., supraglottoplasty. She returned for a post-surgery CLE and reported that her symptoms had improved significantly.

DISCUSSION POINTS (LIST)

1. Describe the diagnostic workup for exercise-associated breathing problems arising from the larynx.
2. Understand the impact and epidemiology of EILO.
3. Describe the role and place of surgical intervention in the treatment algorithm for EILO.

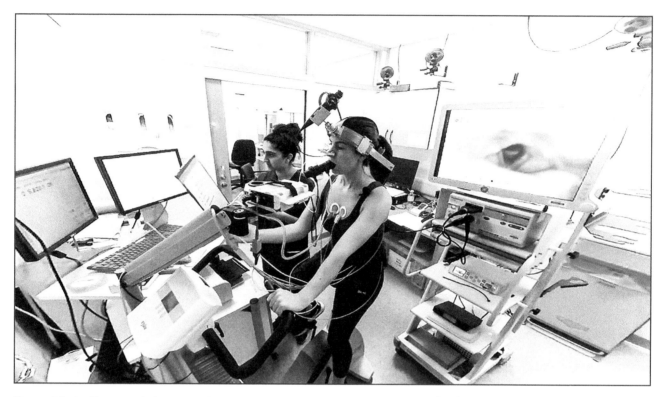

Figure 36–1. Photograph demonstrating continuous laryngoscopy during exercise (CLE) test setup.

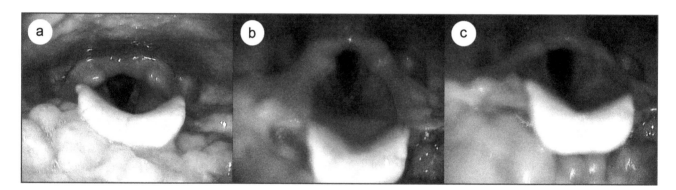

Figure 36–2. Endoscopic photomicrographs taken during CLE demonstrating (A) larynx at commencement of exercise, (B) larynx with medial movement of aryepiglottic folds and overlying corniculate cartilages as exercise effort increases, and (C) larynx demonstrating additional anteroposterior contraction with approximation of epiglottis toward posterior interarytenoid region.

| CASE RESOLUTION | DIAGNOSTIC APPROACH |

Initial Evaluation

The clinical presentation for this patient is classical for EILO. Most patients present in early adolescence and the condition appears to be most common in young females between 12 and 16 years old.[1] It is currently not clear why EILO is more common in females; however, this may relate to anatomical differences or developmental changes in the larynx.[2,3] In Scandinavian countries, it is estimated that EILO affects between 5% and 7% of all adolescents,[4,5] and this value is likely to be higher in competitive athletes.[6] To date, the epidemiology of EILO has not been evaluated in countries other than Denmark, Sweden, and Norway, and has only been evaluated in adolescents and young adults.

Individuals with EILO most often present with symptoms that are confined to athletic activity, and initial presentation is usually temporally associated with an increase in training load or certain competitive events. Respiratory work of breathing is increased in individuals with EILO, likely due to an increased airway resistance and a correspondingly decreased airway patency at the level of the larynx.[7] It is most often reported by individuals partaking in endurance-type sport (runners, cyclists, rowing) but has now been reported by athletic individuals partaking in a wide range of activities (including swimming, tennis, etc.).[8–10]

Several studies have now demonstrated poor diagnostic precision of a clinically based (ie, based on history and physical examination [H&P]) or questionnaire-based approach to diagnosis. This may relate to some of the non-specific clinical features and symptoms present in this condition but is also likely due to the overlap with manifestations from other airway-centric clinical conditions, e.g., asthma. Indeed, the vast majority of individuals with EILO have been initially treated for asthma prior to diagnosis. Features that help differentiate exercise-induced bronchoconstriction (EIB) from EILO are shown in Table 36–1. It is also important to note that EILO and EIB can, and often do, coexist in the same individual and this may confound diagnostic accuracy.[4,6] There are typically no abnormal findings on physical examination. Indeed, given that this is an exercise-related phenomenon, office-based clinical assessment (ie, with the individual at rest) is thus typically unrewarding diagnostically. Likewise, resting lung function testing (eg, spirometry with flow-volume loop assessment of inspiratory flow) or bronchoprovocation testing[11] does not reliably detect the condition.[12]

The gold standard test, and the only way to establish the diagnosis of EILO in a robust fashion, is the CLE test. This test involves placement of a flexible laryngoscope and then fixation with specialist headgear to secure the camera and allow continuous video recording of the laryngeal aperture. The transient nature of EILO and the fact that the condition predominantly

Table 36–1. The Continuous Laryngoscopy During Exercise (CLE) Test

	Exercise-Induced Laryngeal Obstruction (EILO)	Exercise-Induced Bronchoconstriction (EIB)
Onset	• Sudden onset within seconds during high intensity exercise • Warm-up does not affect symptom severity	• Gradual onset within 5 minutes of terminating exercise • Warm-up can attenuate symptom severity
Symptom localization	• Throat or upper chest	• Chest
Symptom quality	• Inspiratory only • High-pitch or wheezing sound on inspiration • Throat tightness • Cough during exercise	• Inspiratory and expiratory • Chest tightness • Cough following exercise cessation
Post exercise duration	Under 10 minutes	Approximately 30 minutes
Response to inhalers	Little to none	Symptom resolution

develops during peak exercise means that EILO can only be reliably diagnosed using direct laryngoscopy performed continuously during exercise. This test was first described in and became more widely utilized following a seminal methodological publication in 2006.[13] There is now a body of evidence outlining the excellent safety profile of this test and the fact that the test can be safely utilized in children as young as 10 years of age.[14] More recent work has outlined the versatility of the test, describing CLE application during rowing[15] and in the aquatic environment.[16] Despite this progress there remains an urgent need for a robust scoring system to classify the severity of EILO, and at the current time the most widely employed system utilizes grade scoring, with a severity score from 0 (normal) to 3 (severe closure) assessed at the glottic and supraglottic level, respectively.[9] Most clinicians classify a score ≥2 as supportive of a diagnosis in the context of coexisting typical symptoms. Unfortunately, the inter- and intra-rater reliability of this approach is at best only moderate,[17] and truly objective methods of assessment are urgently needed.[1]

COMORBIDIDITIES

The most common comorbid condition encountered is asthma. Indeed, in one study of young athletes, it was revealed that EILO was seen in 11% of subjects with EIB.[4] The reason for the coexistence of EIB and EILO has yet to be determined but may relate to common pathways of inflammation or environmental interactions at the airway surface. It is important that EIB is detected and treated, in order that an athlete will benefit from EILO therapy; and indeed the coexistence of EILO is often a key reason young individuals may have exercise "treatment-refractory" symptoms. A comprehensive clinical assessment should also include evaluation of the presence of gastroesophageal reflux and sino-nasal disease. Again, it is important that these comorbididities be treated to facilitate normal laryngeal function.

MANAGEMENT

The approach to treatment should be conducted in the context of a multidisciplinary approach, with involvement of therapists (eg, physiotherapy, speech and language therapy, and health psychology), an otorhinolaryngologist, and a respiratory physician. An important initial step is to discuss the condition with

the patients and review the CLE images. This often enlightens the individual to the condition and is central to providing patient-centric care. Recent work has extended this discussion to demonstrate the benefits of a biofeedback session, whereby a subject visualizes laryngeal movement with initiation of techniques to facilitate laryngeal abduction.[18] Indeed, several unique breathing strategies have recently been described to aid laryngeal patency during strenuous exercise.[19] Strategies to improve physical conditioning are also likely to be important, and further work is needed to establish the place and efficacy of inspiratory muscle training. Thereafter, if this conservative approach fails, then surgical intervention may be warranted in carefully selected cases with a predominantly supraglottic form of the condition.

PROCEDURAL STRATEGIES

The surgical approach to supraglottic EILO represents an adaptation of the surgical technique historically performed for laryngomalacia.[20] The technique was first popularized for EILO by Maat and colleagues in 2007.[9] A number of centers have now published surgical outcomes detailing the short-term effect of supraglottoplasty as a treatment for EILO (Table 36–2).

Table 36–2. Studies Reporting Surgical Outcomes from Supraglottoplasty

Author	Year	Surgically Treated Cases
Smith et al[20]	1995	1
Bent et al[22]	1996	2
Bjørnsdóttir et al[10]	2000	2
Chemery et al[23]	2002	1
Maat et al[9]	2007	10
Richter et al[24]	2008	3
Maat et al[25]	2011	23
Norlander et al[26]	2015	15
Mehlum et al[27]	2016	17
Hilland et al[21] (conference abstract)	*2017*	*(66)*
Clemm et al, 2018[28]	2018	1
Total number of surgically treated cases		**75**

The studies overall report a substantial improvement in symptoms and laryngeal patency in most subjects, although a few individuals had little or no change. Currently, there are no data available on long-term (>5 years) effect and complication rates, although anecdotal evidence of postoperative complications such as unilateral recurrent laryngeal nerve palsy or reoperation have been reported.[21]

The procedure entails removal of part of the aryepiglottic structures which impede on the airway when the epiglottis is pressed anteriorly by increased ventilation. The extent of the surgical resection is guided by the preoperative CLE. The operation "supraglottoplasty" is performed under general anesthesia in suspension laryngoscopy. A Lindholm laryngoscope is preferable as it allows a wide view of the larynx and especially the arytenoids. A tubeless ventilation field is necessary to allow mobilization of the supraglottic structures. Supraglottic jet ventilation is not always possible with the Lindholm scope and therefore a transglottic jetting catheter such as Hunsaker (Medtronic) is used (shown in Figure 36–3A). The Hunsaker catheter is extremely fire resistant, although standard laser precautions should be taken.

Once the patient is under suspension laryngoscopy and jet ventilated, the operating microscope is used with an attached CO_2 laser. The AcuBlade™ (Lumenis) is a laser scanning system which is particularly useful for this operation as it allows for a predetermined incision length, shape, and penetration depth. The aryepiglottic folds are first divided with the laser as shown in Figure 36–3B-E; a video of the procedure is also available in the online supplementary material (Video 36–2). A slight arc to the laser is created using the AcuBlade. An adrenaline soaked neuropatty is placed over the vocal fold and jetting catheter as shown in Figure 36–3C-E. This is a precaution to prevent collateral laser damage to the true vocal cord and avoid the potential risk of an airway fire. Once the aryepiglottic fold has been divided, the cuneiform and corniculate cartilages can be fully mobilized. Traction is applied to the tissue using micro-cupped forceps or Bouchayer forceps as shown in Figure 36–3E-G. This allows for dissection posteriorly and anteriorly without causing any injury to the underlying vocal fold. Once the cuneiform, corniculate, and overlying mucosa has been excised, a small area of the superior arytenoid cartilage is exposed as shown in Figure 36–3H. The procedure is

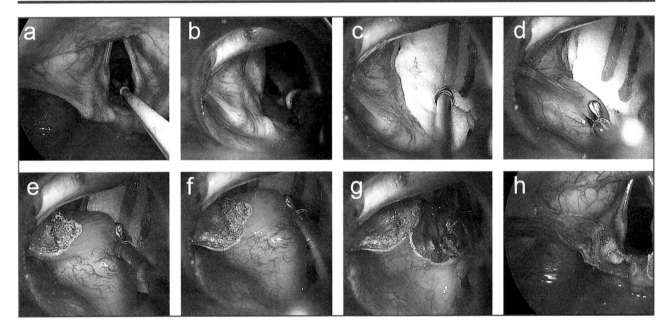

Figure 36–3. Series of endoscopic images demonstrating the key aspects of supraglottoplasty. (A) Larynx with Hunsaker jet ventilation needle in situ. Green subglottic basket seen in trachea. (B) Further view of Hunsaker needle in place and left arytenoid complex and overlying corniculate beneath mucosa. (C–E) An adrenaline soaked neuropatty is placed over the vocal fold and jetting catheter as shown. This is a precaution to prevent collateral laser damage to the true vocal cord and avoid the potential risk of an airway fire. (E–G) Traction is applied to the tissue using micro-cupped forceps or Bouchayer forceps and the aryepiglottic fold is divided and the cuneiform and corniculate cartilages can be fully mobilized and removed. (H) Once the cuneiform, corniculate, and overlying mucosa have been excised, a small area of the superior arytenoid cartilage is exposed as shown.

performed as a day case and simple analgesia is normally adequate. The patients are advised strict voice rest for 72 hours to reduce edema. A short course of postoperative broad-spectrum antibiotics is also routinely prescribed due to the small area of exposed cartilage. Other potential adverse effects from the surgery include dental injury, bleeding, and laser damage to the vocal folds effecting voice. Although there are no clear contraindications to the surgery, it does require the patient to be medically fit for a general anesthesia and normal coagulation. Suspension laryngoscopy can be challenging in certain patients (eg, with prominent teeth, retrognathia); however, the Dedo–Pilling laryngoscope can be used in such cases.

INDICATIONS

The procedure targets supraglottic closure only, but the indications for supraglottoplasty remain unclear. Some centers will only consider surgery in patients with severe degree of supraglottic obstruction, and with no apparent glottic closure. It is, however, not known if moderate degrees of supraglottic closure should be considered an indication for surgery and the subjectivity of the current scoring system adds to this uncertainty. Likewise, the importance of the presence of concurrent glottic closure is also unclear; some centers approach this by making an assessment of whether glottic closure is likely secondary to supraglottic closure or rather the primary mechanism of obstruction, amplifying supraglottic closure.

DISCUSSION POINTS (ADDRESSED)

1. Describe the diagnostic workup for exercise-associated laryngeal problems.

   - The diagnostic gold standard is continuous visualization of the larynx during exercise. This can be applied using a variety of exercise modalities and protocols; ideally the patient's symptoms should be fully reproduced.
   - Respiratory symptoms can guide investigations but have poor diagnostic precision.

   - The presence of comorbidities such as asthma, GERD, and nasal disease should be considered and managed.
   - A multidisciplinary approach is essential for optimal patient care.

2. Understand the impact and epidemiology of EILO.

   - EILO is seen more frequently in females and usually in physically active individuals.
   - Patients typically present in adolescence or as young adults.
   - The prevalence in Scandinavian countries is thought to be 5 to 7% of adolescents or young adults.
   - Often patients with EILO have been treated for asthma for years before a diagnosis of EILO is finally established.
   - Asthma and EILO can coexist, often with an ambiguous symptom presentation.

3. Describe the role and place of surgical intervention in the treatment algorithm for EILO.

   - Before considering surgery for EILO, any comorbidities must be properly investigated and managed.
   - Appropriate first-line treatments are non-invasive. No solid evidence exists to back one approach over the other, but several options are available: speech and language therapy, respiratory physiotherapy, anticholinergic inhalers, and inspiratory muscle training. When choosing an intervention, it is likely beneficial to consider the individual patient's specific problems, motivation, and adherence.
   - Surgical treatment for EILO can be beneficial, but there is currently a limited dataset supporting its efficacy; less than 100 cases in total have been published in scientific literature at the time of writing. There are no long-term follow-up data and given the small number of procedures described in the literature, the risk of potential complications is unclear. This acknowledged, the procedure has been life-changing and resolved breathing problems in many of the cases published to date.
   - Special consideration should be given before performing surgery in patients who are in puberty or younger. It is unknown if respiratory problems can resolve with time, i.e., as the larynx grows.

REFERENCES

1. Halvorsen T, Walsted ES, Bucca C, et al. Inducible laryngeal obstruction (ILO): an official joint European Respiratory Society and European Laryngological Society Statement. *Eur Respir J* [Internet]. 2017;(50). Available from: https://doi.org/10.1183/13993003.02221-2016
2. Wysocki J, Kielska E, Orszulak P, Reymond J. Measurements of pre- and postpubertal human larynx: a cadaver study. *Surg Radiol Anat.* 2008;30(3):191–199.
3. Castelli WA, Ramirez PC, Nasjleti CE. Linear growth study of the pharyngeal cavity. *J Dent Res.* 1973;52(6):1245–1248.
4. Johansson H, Norlander K, Berglund L, et al. Prevalence of exercise-induced bronchoconstriction and exercise-induced laryngeal obstruction in a general adolescent population. *Thorax.* 2015;70(1):57–63.
5. Christensen PM, Thomsen SF, Rasmussen N, Backer V. Exercise-induced laryngeal obstructions: prevalence and symptoms in the general public. *Eur Arch Otorhinolaryngol.* 2011;268(9):1313–1319.
6. Nielsen EW, Hull JH, Backer V. High prevalence of exercise-induced laryngeal obstruction in athletes. *Med Sci Sports Exerc.* 2013;45(11):2030–2035.
7. Walsted ES, Faisal A, Jolley CJ, et al. Increased respiratory neural drive and work of breathing in exercise-induced laryngeal obstruction. *J Appl Physiol.* 2017; jap.00691.2017.
8. Hseu A, Sandler M, Ericson D, Ayele N, Kawai K, Nuss R. Paradoxical vocal fold motion in children presenting with exercise induced dyspnea. *Int J Pediatr Otorhinolaryngol.* 2016;90:165–169.
9. Maat RC, Roksund OD, Olofsson J, Halvorsen T, Skadberg BT, Heimdal J-H. Surgical treatment of exercise-induced laryngeal dysfunction. *Eur Arch Otorhinolaryngol.* 2007;264(4):401–407.
10. Björnsdóttir US, Gudmundsson K, Hjartarson H, Bröndbo K, Magnússon B, Juliusson S. Exercise-induced laryngochalasia: an imitator of exercise-induced bronchospasm. *Ann Allerg Asthm Immunol.* 2000;85(5):387–391. Available from: http://linkinghub.elsevier.com/retrieve/pii/S1081120610625525
11. Walsted ES, Hull JH, Sverrild A, Porsbjerg C, Backer V. Bronchial provocation testing does not detect exercise-induced laryngeal obstruction. *J Asthma.* 2017;54(1):77–83.
12. Christensen PM, Maltbæk N, Jørgensen IM, Nielsen KG. Can flow-volume loops be used to diagnose exercise induced laryngeal obstructions? A comparison study examining the accuracy and inter-rater agreement of flow volume loops as a diagnostic tool. *Prim Care Respir J.* 2013;22(3):306–311.
13. Heimdal J-H, Roksund OD, Halvorsen T, Skadberg BT, Olofsson J. Continuous laryngoscopy exercise test: a method for visualizing laryngeal dysfunction during exercise. *Laryngoscope.* 2006;116(1):52–57.
14. Hilland M, Roksund OD, Sandvik L, et al. Congenital laryngomalacia is related to exercise-induced laryngeal obstruction in adolescence. *Arch Dis Child.* 2016;101(5):443–448.
15. Panchasara B, Nelson C, Niven R, Ward S, Hull JH. Lesson of the month: rowing-induced laryngeal obstruction: a novel cause of exertional dyspnoea: characterised by direct laryngoscopy. *Thorax.* 2015;70(1):95–97.
16. Walsted ES, Swanton LL, van van Someren K, et al. Laryngoscopy during swimming: a novel diagnostic technique to characterize swimming- induced laryngeal obstruction. *Laryngoscope.* 2017;127(10):2298–2301.
17. Walsted ES, Hull JH, Hvedstrup J, Maat RC, Backer V. Validity and reliability of grade scoring in the diagnosis of exercise-induced laryngeal obstruction. *ERJ Open Research.* 2017;3(3):00070–2017.
18. Olin JT, Deardorff EH, Fan EM, et al. Therapeutic laryngoscopy during exercise: a novel non-surgical therapy for refractory EILO. *Pediatr Pulmonol.* 2016;24:445.
19. Johnston KL, Bradford H, Hodges H, Moore CM, Nauman E, Olin JT. The Olin EILOBI breathing techniques: description and initial case series of novel respiratory retraining strategies for athletes with exercise-induced laryngeal obstruction. *J Voice.* 2018;32(6):698–704.
20. Smith RJH, Kramer M, Bauman NM, Smits WL, Bent JP, Ahrens RC. Exercise-induced laryngomalacia. *Ann Otol Rhinol Laryngol.* 1995;104(7):537–541.
21. Hilland M, Engesæter I, Sandnes A, et al. Postoperative complications after surgical treatment for exercised induced laryngeal obstruction: 3660 Board #107 June 3 800 AM–930 AM. *Medi Sci Sports Exer.* 2017;49 N2 -(5S).
22. Bent JP, Miller DA, Kim JW, Bauman NM, Wilson JS, Smith RJH. Pediatric exercise-induced laryngomalacia. *Ann Otol Rhinol Laryngol.* 1996;105(3):169–175.
23. Chemery L, Le Clech G, Delaval P, Carré F, Gogibu J, Dassonville J. [Exercise-induced laryngomalacia]. France; 2002 Oct;19(5 pt 1):641–643.
24. Richter GT, Rutter MJ, deAlarcon A, Orvidas LJ, Thompson DM. Late-onset laryngomalacia: a variant of disease. *Arch Otolaryngol Head Neck Surg.* 2008;134(1):75–80. Available from: http://archotol.jamanetwork.com/article.aspx?doi=10.1001/archoto.2007.17
25. Maat RC, Hilland M, Roksund OD, et al. Exercise-induced laryngeal obstruction: natural history and effect of surgical treatment. *Eur Arch Otorhinolaryngol.* 2011;268(10):1485–1492.
26. Norlander K, Johansson H, Jansson C, Nordvall L, Nordang L. Surgical treatment is effective in severe cases of exercise-induced laryngeal obstruction: a follow-up study. *Acta Otolaryngol.* 2015;135(11):1152–1159.
27. Mehlum CS, Walsted ES, Godballe C, Backer V. Supraglottoplasty as treatment of exercise induced laryngeal obstruction (EILO). *Eur Arch Otorhinolaryngol.* 2016;273(4):945–951.
28. Clemm HSH, Sandnes A, Vollsæter M, et al. The heterogeneity of exercise induced laryngeal obstruction. *Am J Respir Crit Care Med.* 2018 Feb 1;rccm.201708–1646IM.

CHAPTER 37

Inducible Laryngeal Obstruction

Julia Selby and James H. Hull

INTRODUCTION

The human larynx has a central role in airway protection, swallowing, and phonation. In some individuals, the larynx appears to have become hyperreactive and exhibits a heightened and unwarranted tendency toward inappropriate closure or "dysfunction," resulting in respiratory distress and upper airway discomfort.[1] The seminal report of "vocal cord dysfunction" (VCD) appeared in the *New England Journal of Medicine* in 1983, with the description of paradoxical laryngeal closure causing unexplained dyspnea and wheeze in a small cohort of patients, without an apparent structural or neurological cause.[2]

Since this time, a great number of terms have been proposed to describe this laryngeal dysfunction, including paradoxical vocal fold movement (PVFM) and laryngochalasia (Table 37–1). To date, respiratory physicians and allergists have favored the term VCD, whereas otolaryngologists and speech and language therapists (SLTs) have preferred PVFM. All terms refer to the similar clinical phenomenon of inappropriate glottic closure and, classically, vocal cord adduction occurring on the inspiratory phase of the breathing cycle.

A multidisciplinary task force was established at the ERS/ELS/ACCP 2013 International Consensus Conference, with representatives from the European Respiratory Society (ERS), the European Laryngological Society (ELS), and the American College of Chest Physicians (ACCP). This expert collaboration identified "inducible laryngeal obstruction" (ILO) as the most appropriate term to describe paradoxical adduction of the vocal folds, in response to an external stimulus and resulting in respiratory difficulties.[3] This chapter describes a typical case of ILO, highlighting clinical features and current practice in diagnosis and treatment.

Table 37–1. Terminology Used to Describe Laryngeal Closure

First Author; year	Term
Patterson; 1974	Munchausen stridor
Dailey; 1976	Pseudoasthma
Cormier; 1980	Nonorganic upper airway obstruction
Appelblatt; 1981	Functional upper airway obstruction
Downing; 1982	Factitious asthma
Collett; 1983	Spasmodic croup
Rodenstein; 1983	Emotional laryngeal wheezing
Barnes; 1986	Psychogenic upper airway obstruction
Ramirez; 1986	Episodic laryngeal dyskinesia
Liistro; 1990	Exercise-induced laryngospasm
Pitchenik; 1991	Functional laryngeal obstruction
Lund; 1993	Hysterical stridor
Smith; 1993	Functional laryngeal stridor
Gallivan; 1996	Episodic paroxysmal laryngospasm
Morrison; 1999	Irritable larynx syndrome
Patel; 2004	Paradoxical vocal fold motion
Morris; 2010	Periodic occurrence of laryngeal obstruction

The patient is a 40-year-old female referred to our upper airway clinic, with a 2-year history of episodic throat tightness, difficulty breathing, and voice loss. On arrival, she was wearing a mask over her mouth and nose to protect herself from environmental stimuli that had triggered her symptoms in the past, such as perfumes, cleaning products, and car fumes. She had attended her local accident and emergency (A&E) department 23 times during the last 2 years and was hospitalized on three occasions, having lost consciousness with sudden upper airway closure. She lost her job as a care home assessor due to repeated sickness absence and had become socially isolated, confining herself to her home in order to avoid the likelihood of having an attack. At the time of referral, she only left her home to visit her son and her mother, whose homes were free of perfumes and chemicals, and to attend medical appointments, always covering her mouth and nose away from her home environment. She had been given a diagnosis of asthma 15 years previously, but asthma treatment and local speech and language therapy had been unsuccessful in reducing her upper airway symptoms.

1. Understand the epidemiology and potential mechanisms underlying the development of ILO
2. Describe the assessment and diagnosis of ILO
3. Describe the treatment approach for ILO

Epidemiology

There is considerable variation in the reported epidemiology of ILO, depending on the diagnostic criteria employed. To date, much of the data available in this area are based on case reports and small case series. Further work is needed to prospectively evaluate key epidemiological data, such as prevalence, incidence, age, and gender distribution of ILO in the general population using robust diagnostic methodologies. However, one of the largest series, by Newman et al,[4] described 95 adults (84% female) hospitalized with

laryngeal symptoms, with an average age of 39 years. In an evaluation of VCD in a 2010 review (n=1587), there was approximately a 2:1 female predominance, 71% were adults, and the remaining 29% were predominantly adolescents.[5] The patient reported above reflects this finding.

Mechanisms

Laryngeal closure may occur at either the glottic (ie, vocal cord/fold adduction), or supraglottic level (ie, arytenoid and aryepiglottic infolding) and indeed at both levels simultaneously in some individuals. Airflow through the larynx is compromised as a result, creating audible turbulence with added respiratory sounds and nociceptive sensations of throat tightness or constriction, often accompanied by changes in voice quality.

The pathophysiological mechanisms underlying the development of ILO remains to be determined; however, several hypotheses have been put forward, including heightened upper airway hyperreactivity with irritation from postnasal drip and acid reflux, neural control deficits, anatomical and mechanical considerations in the larynx, and psychological attributes.[1] Given the many sophisticated roles of the larynx, it seems unlikely that ILO could be explained by a single cause, and clinical experience supports the likely combination of causative factors. Furthermore, there may be differences in pathogenesis between exercise-induced laryngeal obstruction (EILO; see Chapter 36) and ILO triggered by other stimuli. Certainly, in the case of EILO, this condition develops under states of heightened airflow and it is likely that the laryngeal inlet closes under the pressure changes that can develop in susceptible individuals.[6]

Upper Airway Hyperreactivity

The concept of laryngeal hypersensitivity is becoming increasingly well recognized as an important underlying and associated feature in laryngeal dysfunction and may act to account for the symptom complex/spectrum that is encountered.[7] Many patients with ILO also have chronic refractory cough (ie, minimally productive cough that has been present for over 8 weeks despite logical approach to treatment), globus sensation, discomfort on swallowing, and voice changes.[8] The larynx may become sensitized through a precipitating event, such as an upper respiratory tract infection, and further

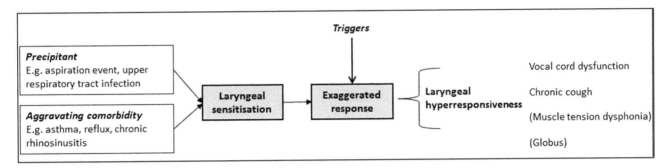

Figure 37–1. Potential mechanisms underpinning development of laryngeal hyperresponsiveness and ILO. Reproduced with permission from Hull JH et al AJRCCM 2016.[1]

aggravated through comorbid irritants, such as acidic and non-acidic reflux and postnasal drip, such that the glottal closure reflex becomes heightened and an engrained pattern of hyperresponsiveness ensues (Figure 37–1). Anecdotally, proton pump inhibitors have improved reflux but not VCD. Environmental factors, such as temperature, may be involved in the etiology of ILO, potentially acting to enhance laryngeal sensitivity.

Interestingly, the patient described above denied respiratory tract infection at the time of onset of her symptoms and did not report postnasal drip or acid reflux, but these are common findings in many upper airway patients. Other important considerations include the presence of coexisting asthma or lower airway hyperreactivity.

Laryngeal involvement in respiration, swallowing, and airway protection is achieved through fine neural control mechanisms. The hypothesis behind "reflex-associated VCD" is that direct stimulation of sensory nerve endings in the respiratory tract may induce a protective reflex, triggering laryngeal closure. Mechanical or chemical stimulation of the supraglottic mucosa or direct stimulation of the superior laryngeal nerve may activate the laryngeal adductor reflex to protect the airway from aspiration or asphyxiation. It has also been postulated that autonomic dysregulation may play a role in the development of laryngeal dysfunction.

Psychological Factors

Psychological factors may be relevant in ILO. Specifically, in a sample of 171 cases with "paradoxical vocal cord motion" (PVCM), only 7% did not have a psychiatric diagnosis. Some authors have claimed that ILO represents the physical manifestation of underlying psychological problems, while others focus on the relevance of behavioral health factors, such as stress reactivity, perfectionistic tendencies, poor self-efficacy, and weak internal locus of control, in the generation of paradoxical movement. In the early stages of treatment, our patient showed very little belief in her ability to get better and an external locus of control, as discussed in more detail below. Other authors argue that psychological factors may result from rather than cause ILO symptoms, viewing anxiety and panic as appropriate behavioral responses to severe or perceived respiratory distress.

ASSESSMENT AND DIAGNOSIS

Clinical Assessment

Case History

In addition to standard questions on medical and social background, it is essential to gain a detailed description of the patient's symptoms and typical attacks, in order to separate the relative contributions of the upper and lower airway and achieve a correct diagnosis. Some patients with upper airway dysfunction may also have coexisting asthma that requires optimization. Relevant inquiry should be made into triggering agents; the localization of any tightness or wheeze; whether the breathing difficulty is on inspiration, expiration, or both; the time course of attacks, including recovery; and the presence of any additional upper airway and laryngeal symptoms, such as globus sensation, voice changes, or swallowing problems. A model of joint working with an upper airway specialist SLT can be beneficial in gaining a comprehensive profile of upper airway function and in interpreting the relevance of subjective sensations around swallowing and voicing, for example.

The most common triggers of laryngeal obstruction are irritants, emotional stress, and exercise. A broad range of irritants have been described in case reports and case series, including odors, sleep, stress, cold air, gastrolaryngeal reflux, environmental and occupational exposures, wood dust, and chemicals.[9] The mechanism of irritation remains unclear, but may result from a direct response to the irritant stimulus itself (eg, via mucosal inflammatory reactions), or to altered reflex sensitivity. Negative anticipation may be present on the basis of past irritant exposure, thereby magnifying upper airway symptoms through increased anxiety and disrupted breathing patterns.

The described patient's history was typical of classical ILO. She experienced recurrent attacks of throat tightness, dyspnea, wheeze, and prolonged voice changes in response to perfumes, smoke, cleaning products, car fumes, temperature changes, and foggy weather. She reported more difficulty getting air in than out and described her vocal cords as "breathing the wrong way." She believed that her larynx had become irritated and sensitized through repeated exposure to cleaning agents in her work as a care home assessor, creating compatible upper airway symptoms of tightness, hoarseness, and wheeze.

There are several published symptom questionnaires which may be helpful in detecting and characterizing ILO and underlying laryngeal hypersensitivity, but these have yet to be comprehensively validated. Additional questionnaires may be used to gain information about anxiety, mood, and health-related quality of life, as well as visual analogue scales to rate breathlessness, voice changes, throat discomfort, swallowing difficulties, and cough frequency on the day of assessment and through the course of treatment.

Diagnostic Tests

Lung Function Tests

One of the most commonly used tests of pulmonary function in the diagnosis of ILO is flow-volume measurement with spirometry. Patients with ILO typically have a normal flow-volume loop while asymptomatic; however, during an attack, a variable extrathoracic obstruction pattern can be present, with attenuation in

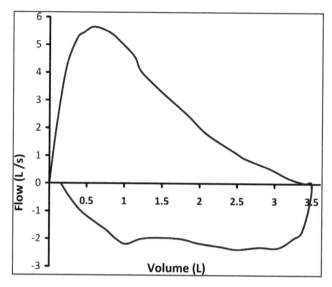

Figure 37–2. Truncated inspiratory loop on a flow-volume curve from spirometry, indicative of extrathoracic obstruction (ie, glottic narrowing).

the inspiratory flow compared with expiratory flow (Figure 37–2).

Spirometry in this context has poor diagnostic precision. There are several causes of a blunted or truncated inspiratory flow-volume curve, including inadequate instruction, suboptimal effort, and inability to perform the procedure, as was the case with this patient.[10] The physical and ventilatory effort involved in performing the first maneuver elicited an immediate inspiratory and expiratory wheeze and a highly variable voice quality, which raised the suspicion of a hyperreactive upper airway. Further lung function tests would not have been possible for this patient and we proceeded with laryngoscopy, as described below.

Other diseases such as diaphragm weakness, fixed large airway obstruction, and any cause of reduced lung compliance also affect spirometric findings. It is not surprising, therefore, that the diagnostic precision of spirometric assessment of ILO is poor. Furthermore, although respiratory physicians tend to agree which flow-volume loops signified ILO, this was not predictive of laryngoscopic diagnosis. Thus, ILO remains difficult to diagnose with either spirometry or flow-volume loops. If ILO is suspected, it is essential to proceed with laryngoscopy, even in the presence of normal flow-volume loop patterns, particularly as laryngeal examination is the only means of differentiating supraglottic from glottic ILO, a distinction that is fundamental to appropriate and effective management.

Use of Surrogate "Inducers"

Substitute (surrogate) methods have been used to elicit ILO. Specifically, the use of methacholine, mannitol, and histamine as laryngeal provocation agents has been studied, using standard bronchoprovocation test methodologies, but with focus on the inspiratory component of the flow-volume loop on spirometric measurements. Patients with laryngoscopic evidence of ILO may have ILO during methacholine challenge, as well as with saline placebo. Overall it is believed that bronchoprovocation testing is actually of little help in differentiating ILO from asthma, and indeed the two conditions may coexist.[11]

Computed tomography has been reported to identify ILO in a cohort of patients with difficult-to-treat asthma.[12] Limitations of this technique include the absence of documentation of a symptomatic spontaneous or provoked episode during testing, the need for supine positioning, and a brief data acquisition window, due to concerns about radiation exposure.

Laryngoscopy

The gold standard means for diagnosing ILO is laryngoscopy, in order to demonstrate vocal cord adduction on inspiration, which can only be captured through visualization, when a patient is symptomatic.[5] Classically, the vocal cord configuration in ILO is documented as being closed anteriorly during inspiration with the presence of a posterior chink (Figure 37–3). This configuration is actually rarely seen in its classical form,

however, and other laryngeal structures may play a role in generating laryngeal closure and wheeze. The degree of airway obstruction varies from mild to severe, but there is currently no validated scoring system to differentiate normal from abnormal findings, and ratings remain highly subjective. Attempts to quantify degree of laryngeal obstruction include measurement of the anterior glottic angle and laryngeal anteroposterior diameter. The exact location of obstruction within the larynx should be documented, with the timing of events noted in cases of obstruction at more than one level, along with an indication of mode and speed of recovery.

Laryngoscopic examination of the patient reported here, who became symptomatic during spirometry, revealed narrowing along the length of the glottis on inspiration with visible medial compression of the false vocal folds and a generalized reduction in the anterior-posterior dimension. A diagnosis of ILO was made. She was able to generate only a breathy voice quality with incomplete adduction on phonation. Her vocal folds abducted well with a sniff, but resumed a narrowed position on return to her default breathing pattern.

Other accompanying laryngeal findings should be recorded and treated, with onward referral to an otolaryngologist where necessary. In a study of 30 patients with PVFM, for example, sixteen patients had laryngeal findings suggestive of gastro-esophageal reflex disease, 12% had laryngoscopic findings of chronic laryngitis, and 33% had additional findings, including laryngomalacia, vocal fold motion impairment, sulcus vocalis, nodules, and subglottic stenosis.

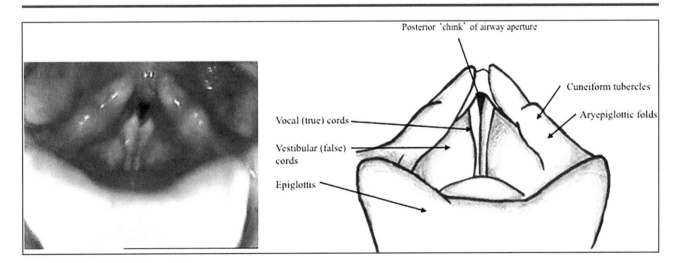

Figure 37–3. Appearance of the larynx in "classical" inducible laryngeal obstruction.

Continuous Laryngoscopy During Provocation

This patient became symptomatic in clinic with spirometry, and ILO was confirmed with immediate laryngoscopic examination. However, if the specific trigger for laryngeal closure is not present during the laryngoscopic examination, the larynx may be unresponsive, and crucial diagnostic behavior may be missed. Continuous Laryngoscopy during Exercise (CLE) is now established as the gold standard diagnostic test for EILO and use of continuous laryngoscopy during other forms of provocation (CLP) is now becoming more widespread. Continuous monitoring negates repeated passage of the nasendoscope and improves diagnostic accuracy by documenting the presence or absence of paradoxical movement.

CLP procedures have yet to be standardized across specialist centers in the UK and differences exist around use of a sealed provocation booth, placement of the endoscope on specialist headgear to allow the patient to move independently from the examining clinician, and specific components of the test protocol.

In our clinic, patients are invited to bring self-selected provocation agents to elicit their typical symptoms. After completion of paperwork (ie, symptom checklist and consent form), nursing observations, and spirometry, where appropriate, the flexible nasendoscope is passed without anesthetic and secured on specialist headgear (Figure 37–4). Patients enter a sealed provocation booth, where they are exposed to the agents they have selected, unable to see their larynx on the endoscopy monitor. On elicitation of upper airway symptoms, the specialist SLT initiates laryngeal control strategies with visual biofeedback. The test ends when the patient's typical symptoms have been generated or when exposure exceeds the point of previous symptom provocation.

Summary of Diagnosis of the Patient

The case history described was suggestive of ILO, comprising sudden episodes of breathlessness, wheeze, and changes to the voice. The patient became immediately symptomatic during the initial consultation in our clinic, when attempting spirometry. Laryngoscopy confirmed glottic narrowing on inspiration and a diagnosis of ILO was made. Table 37–2 summarizes the components required to reach an accurate diagnosis.

Table 37–2. Summary of Diagnostic Approach in ILO

Evaluation	Finding/Report
Clinical Assessment	
History	Typically dyspnea, throat tightness/closure, chest tightness, globus, audible wheeze (Insp>Exp). Time course of symptoms varies (see Figure 37–1), but typically periodic and precipitated by trigger. May persist throughout day and limit activities of daily living.
Triggers	Classical triggers include non-specific irritants (eg perfumes or scents) and exercise.
Diagnostic Tests	
Direct visualization/laryngoscopy/CLP	Adduction of vocal cords during inspiration, or both inspiration and expiration. The classical description of "posterior chinking" is rarely seen. Up to 30% vocal cord movement on passive respiration is normal. Therefore 50% closure of cords deemed abnormal. Findings may be intermittent and require provocation with typical trigger.
Lung function tests	Truncation of inspiratory loop on spirometry. Other findings described but non-specific and sensitive.

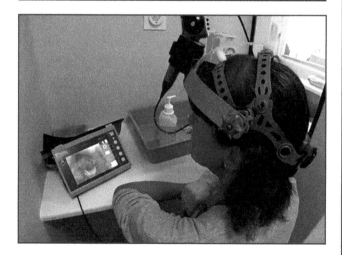

Figure 37–4. Demonstration by the first author of flexible nasendoscope placement for continuous laryngoscopy during provocation test.

TREATMENT

General Approach

There are currently no published randomized controlled treatment trials of ILO.[10] The ability to conduct treatment studies has been restricted by the confusion surrounding the definition of the condition and by insufficient details on diagnostic procedures and outcome measure used, thereby challenging the homogeneity of any subject group. Furthermore, as outlined above, patients with ILO may present with other overlapping manifestations of hypersensitivity, necessitating an individualized rather than standardized treatment program.

Relevant to all patients with ILO, however, is a multidisciplinary team (MDT) approach to management. The symptoms of patients with ILO bridge the disciplines of respiratory medicine, otolaryngology, speech and language therapy, physiotherapy, and clinical psychology and the benefits to patients of receiving centralized, coordinated care should not be underestimated. Joint working can be highly effective in improving patients' understanding of their condition, particularly at the time of diagnosis, and in reinforcing treatment plans. In addition, a weekly MDT meeting is advisable to review laryngeal images, facilitate prompt onward referrals, and reach a consensus on treatment of complex cases, for example.

Medical Treatment

Although not required for the patient in this case study, it is essential to eliminate any potential irritation to the larynx from postnasal drip, allergic rhinitis, and/or acid reflux. Anti-reflux therapy has been reported to be beneficial in reducing laryngeal symptoms of ILO by some, but not all, authors. Interpretation of the results is compounded by differences in treatment protocols.

Benzodiazepines have also been shown to be effective in terminating acute symptoms of ILO, through sedation and muscle relaxation, but normal oxygen saturation must be confirmed and hypercapnea excluded before administering these drugs. Other studies have indicated that daily low-dose amitriptyline may improve ILO, but it has been used in conjunction with other therapy approaches and the nature of the treatment effect is poorly defined as a result.

Therapy Approaches

Speech and Language Therapy

Speech and language therapy plays a central role in the management of ILO. It is crucial, however, that therapy is delivered by a clinician with in-depth knowledge of the larynx and significant experience in treating voice, breathing, and ENT disorders. The various components of an SLT approach are presented in Table 37–3.

Table 37–3. Components of Speech and Language Therapy in the Treatment of ILO

Area	Component
Reassurance & engagement	Place symptoms in context
	Rationale for SLT
	Outline therapy process
Explanation/ education	Normal laryngeal function and patient's symptoms
	Biofeedback using endoscopy
	Identification of triggers
	Throat versus chest symptoms
Upper airway lubrication	Hydration (minimal caffeine and alcohol)
	Management of acid reflux, postnasal drip
	Steam inhalation
	Reduce mouth breathing
Eliminating upper body & laryngeal strain	Awareness of habitual technique
	Posture, alignment, neck and shoulder exercises
	Breathing technique
	Voice, swallow & laugh technique
Laryngeal & cough control strategies	Sniff/sniff and blow
	Pursed lip blowing
	Secret yawn
	Deconstriction
Psychological	Sense of well-being, past/current emotional upset.
	Attitude toward self and symptoms, acceptance
	Realistic goals and expectations
	Pacing and general self-care
	Facilitating change, cost-benefit approach

The patient presented above developed an upper airway wheeze and marked voice changes on performing spirometry, and a diagnosis of ILO was made using laryngoscopy. She began working immediately, on the day of attendance, with the specialist SLT on acute alleviation strategies to release laryngeal constriction. Such laryngeal control strategies, also known as rescue strategies, are essential in giving patients confidence in overcoming their symptoms and in reducing fear of attacks. Sniffing, nasal flow, and pursed lip blowing are most commonly used to release the paradoxical movement of the vocal cords and maintain an adequately open glottis during inhalation. Additional exercises were used to restore this patient's normal voice quality. Although her symptoms were successfully brought under control with behavioral techniques, she found it hard to take a new diagnosis of ILO on board, having attributed her symptoms to asthma for many years, and could not accept that she had a central role to play in her recovery. Adequate time must be spent with the patient explaining the diagnosis of ILO and redirecting beliefs toward a mindset of recovery, based on an effective set of laryngeal control exercises that leads to increased confidence and empowerment. This sense of internal control and confidence may need to be reinforced over several therapy sessions, as was the case with the patient above, whose self-talk reflected a strong external locus of control and who referred to her voice as "having a mind of its own."

Although CLP was not required diagnostically for this patient because she had become symptomatic in clinic, its use in progressing therapy was invaluable. Despite being able to settle ongoing symptoms very effectively during therapy sessions with the therapist's support, she reported lack of control between sessions, especially with very strong, unexpected exposure to irritant smells. With the nasendoscope in situ, the patient was guided through her strategies pre-exposure for confidence and on provocation with strong smells. She found the visual evidence of her ability to control vocal cord movement transformational. She subsequently began a graded exposure and desensitization program at home and reported an increasing sense of reassurance and control over her symptoms.

In addition to acute alleviation strategies, it is important to ensure good hydration and upper airway lubrication and to identify and release any day-to-day ingrained tension in and around the laryngeal area, which may increase the likelihood of upper airway attacks. Tension can be reduced using classic deconstriction exercises from voice therapy, such as the silent giggle or yawn, to increase the sensation of space in the throat, and using more general tensing, stretching, and release maneuvers for the neck and shoulders.

Many patients with ILO present with dysphonia and cough, both of which must be addressed to eliminate traumatic behavior that results in further strain on the vocal cords and larynx. Therapy to normalize voice quality must be tailored according to an individual's specific vocal presentation and technique, but typically includes abdominal breath support, deconstriction, forward resonance, flow phonation, as well as any necessary modifications to pitch and loudness. Treatment for chronic cough consists of promoting understanding of cough generation and the negative impact of repeated coughing, early identification of cough triggers, implementation of cough control strategies, vocal hygiene, and collaborative working toward an increased sense of control.

Physiotherapy

This patient's symptoms were focused on the larynx and SLT was the treatment of choice for her. Specialist respiratory physiotherapy, however, is indicated in cases of exercise-related obstruction and when symptoms may be exacerbated by a breathing pattern disorder. Assessment focuses on breathing pattern, channel, flow, rate, and rhythm and on signs of air hunger. Joint physiotherapist-SLT assessment can be highly effective in cases of complex or unusual breathing patterns.

Inspiratory Muscle Training

Inspiratory muscle training (IMT) has been used to treat patients with EILO,[13] based on the relation between the diaphragm and the posterior crico-arytenoid muscle (PCA), which is the main abductor of the vocal folds. When diaphragm stimulation is increased through increased resistance, PCA activity increases in a coordinated manner and increases glottal area, resulting in less turbulent airflow through the larynx. A potential concern is that enhancing the ability of the diaphragm and inspiratory accessory muscles to generate increased flow can be counterproductive if the constriction is centered in the larynx, particularly at a supraglottic level. However, IMT may be valuable when response to standard respiratory retraining techniques has been poorer than expected or with patients who find it hard to break ingrained, automatic apical breathing patterns and engage the diaphragm during an acute attack, for example.

Clinical Psychology

Several authors have reported successful treatment of ILO with psychotherapy, often in conjunction with speech and language therapy. Leaving aside the lack of agreement over the role of psychological factors in the mechanism of ILO, many patients exhibit altered mood, increased anxiety, additional life stresses, and reduced self-esteem as a result of their symptoms. Input from a clinical psychologist, preferably within an MDT framework, can be very effective in enhancing treatment outcomes.

Several joint SLT and clinical psychology sessions were carried out with the patient in this case study. There was an indication of underlying psychological distress from the profile of prolonged and repeated voice loss that did not normalize on resolution of the breathing symptoms. Joint working between the SLT and clinical psychologist facilitated disclosure of unresolved trauma from a past relationship and an explanation of how this may have resulted in laryngeal symptoms, difficulty in regulating emotions, and poor self-efficacy in achieving symptom control. The concurrent use of cognitive-behavioral therapy in conjunction with direct SLT techniques was highly effective in challenging negative thoughts, reducing muscle tension, and limiting avoidance.

Other Treatments

Continuous positive airway pressure (CPAP) has been reported to be effective in overcoming glottic narrowing on inhalation by creating a favorable pressure gradient, and on exhalation by reducing expiratory flow rate.

Heliox is a mixture of helium and oxygen with a density nearly six times lower than atmospheric air and its inhalation generates significantly lower turbulence, lower overall airway resistance, and increased flow rate. Heliox has been used effectively to relieve symptoms of ILO, possibly by reducing the work of breathing. However, heliox is not readily available in most hospitals and certainly not in general practices, and its use in the treatment of ILO is impractical and unrealistic for most patients.

There are a few reports of the use of botulinum toxin injections in the vocal folds to treat ILO, but the results are equivocal with some cases showing complete resolution and others no improvement at all. There is insufficient evidence to date from which we can draw conclusions on the safety, efficacy, and long-term outcomes of botulinum toxin injections. Temporary side effects of dysphonia and dysphagia would likely render this treatment option unsuitable and undesirable for many patients.

Long-Term Management/Patient Outcome

There is clearly a wide variation in the duration of care for patients with ILO. The patient in this report had a total of 16 sessions of speech and language therapy over 18 months, with joint sessions and consultant clinic review scheduled as necessary. Sessions were held less frequently toward the end of the episode of care, to encourage independence in applying control techniques and resuming pre-morbid activities. The patient had no hospital attendances during her therapy, gradually became less housebound, and has been free of upper airway symptoms since discharge. While the duration of care will be determined by specific details of each individual case and to some extent by service provision, it is wise in all cases to be alert to lack of progress and to discuss this as a multidisciplinary team, in order to address ongoing perpetuating factors. It is also prudent not to discharge patients before there is a mutual confidence in the patient's symptom control, to prevent recurrence and avoid the potential loss of faith in the diagnosis of ILO and the effectiveness of treatment.

Discussion Points

1. Understand the epidemiology and potential mechanisms underlying the development of ILO

   - adult female dominant condition
   - laryngeal hyperresponsiveness and psychological factors are most likely mechanisms

2. Describe the assessment and diagnosis of ILO

   - detailed case history around symptoms, nature of attacks, and triggers
   - separate upper from lower airway symptoms, using lung function tests
   - confirm presence of paradoxical movement on inspiration with CLP or laryngoscopy

3. Describe the treatment approach for ILO

   - multidisciplinary
   - medical/pharmacological management of laryngeal irritants
   - therapy-focused, typically SLT, with clear focus on increasing patient confidence in controlling symptoms

REFERENCES

1. Hull J, Backer V, Gibson P, Fowler S. Laryngeal dysfunction: assessment and management for the clinician. *Am J Respir Crit Care Med*. 2016;194;1062–1072.
2. Christopher K, Wood R, Eckert R, et al. Vocal-cord dysfunction presenting as asthma. *N Engl J Med*. 1983;308: 1566–1570.
3. Christensen P, Heimdal, J, Christopher K, et al. ERS/ELS/ACCP 2013 international consensus conference nomenclature on inducible laryngeal obstructions. *Eur Respir Rev*. 2015;24:445–450.
4. Newman K, Mason U, Schmaling K. Clinical features of vocal cord dysfunction. *Am J Respir Crit Care Med*. 1995; 152:1382–1386.
5. Morris M, Christopher K. Diagnostic criteria for the classification of vocal cord dysfunction. *Chest*. 2010;138: 1213–1223.
6. Røksund O, Maat R, Heimdal J, et al. Exercise induced dyspnea in the young. Larynx as the bottleneck of the airways. *Respir Med*. 2009;103:1911–1918.
7. Hull J, Menon A. Laryngeal hypersensitivity in chronic cough. *Pulm Pharmacol Ther*. 2015;35:111–116.
8. Vertigan A, Theodoros D, Gibson P, Winkworth A. Voice and upper airway symptoms in people with chronic cough and paradoxical vocal fold movement. *J Voice*. 2007;21:361–383.
9. Perkner J, Fennelly K, Balkissoon R, et al. Irritant-associated vocal cord dysfunction. *J Occ Envir Med.*. 1998;40:136–143.
10. Halvorsen T, Walsted E, Bucca C, et al. Inducible laryngeal obstruction: an official joint European Respiratory Society and European Laryngological Society statement. *Eur Respir J*. 2017;50.
11. Walsted E, Hull J, Sverrild A, Porsbjerg C, Backer V. Bronchial provocation testing does not detect exercise-induced laryngeal obstruction. *J Asthma*. 2017;54:77–83.
12. Holmes P, Lau K, Crossett M, et al. Diagnosis of vocal cord dysfunction in asthma with high resolution dynamic volume computerized tomography of the larynx. *Respirology*. 2009;14:1106–1113.
13. Clemm H, Sandnes A, Vollsæter M, et al. The heterogeneity of exercise induced laryngeal obstruction. *Am J Respir Crit Care Med*. 2018.

CHAPTER 38

Treatment of Idiopathic Subglottic Stenosis During Pregnancy

Robert J. Morrison and Alexander Gelbard

A 37-year-old gravida 1, para 0 female at 26 weeks gestation presents to clinic. She reports progressive dyspnea with exertion over the past 8 months. Her symptoms are severe enough that she cannot climb a flight of stairs without requiring 10 minutes of rest. She had empirically been diagnosed with and treated for asthma, without alleviation of her symptoms by bronchodilators. She has no history of dermatologic, renal, cardiac, rheumatologic, or autoimmune conditions and no history of endotracheal intubation or tracheal injury. Her family history is negative for autoimmune conditions. She denies symptoms of gastroesophageal reflux disease. However, she has noted an acceleration in the severity of her breathing symptoms and "noisy breathing" over the course of her pregnancy.

Her physical exam shows no otologic pathology or nasal deformity. She has no thyromegaly or cervical neck adenopathy. She does demonstrate audible inspiratory stridor. Her vocal quality is normal and she is able to speak in complete sentences, but she demonstrates increased work of breathing while ambulating to the exam room. In-office flexible fiberoptic laryngoscopy demonstrates normal mobility of the vocal folds but cicatricial scarring of the subglottis with 80% narrowing of the subglottic lumen (Figure 38–1).

Subsequent laboratory studies reveal negative titers to cytoplasmic antineutrophil cytoplasmic antibodies (cANCAs), myeloperoxidase (MPO), and proteinase

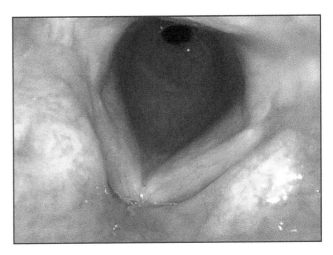

Figure 38–1. In-office flexible fiberoptic laryngoscopy at the level of the glottis, demonstrating full mobility of the bilateral true vocal folds, and cicatricial circumferential stricture with associated hyperemic mucosa in the subglottis.

3 (PR3), consistent with a diagnosis of idiopathic subglottic stenosis (iSGS). She has evidence of occult inflammation with a significantly elevated high-sensitivity c-reactive protein (6.3 mg/L, >1 is abnormally elevated) with a normal erythrocyte sedimentation rate (19 mm/h) and normal red cell distribution width (13.8%, >14% elevated).

CASE RESOLUTION

Initial Evaluation: Physical Examination, Complementary Tests, and Functional Status

Assessment

The clinical presentation of a caucasian adult female with slowly progressive inspiratory stridor is classic for iSGS, an enigmatic extrathoracic inflammatory process involving the lower larynx and upper trachea. Demographically, the disease almost exclusively affects middle aged females of European descent (regardless of the geographic area studied).[1] Given the observed natural history of disease, it has been hypothesized that a sex-linked genetic or hormonal driver of the disease process may exist.[2] Recent studies have provided evidence for associated bacterial pathogens such as Mycobacterium species and aberrant interleukin-17A inflammatory pathway activation.[3-4] Alternative hypotheses have been proposed, including anatomic predisposition of the smaller female subglottis, gastric reflux, mechanical trauma (ie, "telescoping" of the cricoid and first tracheal ring), or immunoglobulin (Ig) G4–related fibrosis.[5-7] However, these concepts await empiric confirmation. Interestingly, there are several case reports of iSGS diagnosed and managed during pregnancy.[7-11] However, the contribution of the hormonal and physiologic changes of pregnancy to the tempo of disease progression in iSGS has not been studied and remains unknown.

Examination begins with an assessment of the patient's ability to maintain adequate ventilation to support physiologic demands and determination of the severity of airway compromise. Subjective impressions of a patient's general well-being are crucial and can be derived from the overall level of alertness, response to the surrounding environment, and interaction with the examiner. The ability to speak in complete sentences, ambulate up a flight of stairs, or walk to the clinic speaks powerfully about the degree of clinical ventilation impairment.

In patients presenting with ventilation impairment exceeding their physiologic demands, speaking in one-word sentences, substernal retractions, tachypnea, and air hunger (the feeling of not enough oxygen) are suggestive of the need for emergent airway stabilization. Stridor is the most common presenting sign of extrathoracic airway obstruction in adults and warrants prompt investigation. Stridor occurs when the laminar flow through the extrathoracic airway is disrupted by a narrowing or partial obstruction, creating a Venturi effect (the acceleration of flow observed through a narrowed segment of a tube). The resulting turbulence and vibration of the airway during inspiration are perceived as stridor on physical examination.

Our approach includes a multidimensional evaluation of every patient referred for iSGS, regardless of pregnancy status. Each patient receives validated questionnaires assessing severity of dyspnea symptoms, functional status, and quality of life.[12] We then perform a comprehensive physical exam, paying particular attention to otologic and nasal evaluation, where pathology is suggestive of underlying granulomatosis with polyangitis (GPA). Nearly all surgeons utilize flexible fiberoptic laryngoscopy in clinic to assess vocal fold mobility and screen for posterior glottic involvement, as well as to characterize the degree of inflammation in the glottis and subglottis.

Many authors also advocate for in-office flexible tracheobronchscopy after further anesthetization of the laryngopharynx to more thoroughly assess the subglottis and trachea. In lieu of in-office fiberoptic examination, cross-section computed tomography (CT) imaging with virtual reconstruction and virtual endoscopy has been shown to have a high sensitivity and specificity with comparison to intraoperative findings in the non-gravid patient.[13] The addition of both inspiratory and expiratory sequences (ie, dynamic CT) can provide additional information regarding tracheal structure affected by malacia. With the proliferation of CT access, soft tissue radiographs have largely fallen out of favor. The role of ultrasound or magnetic resonance imaging remains largely relegated to research.

Endoscopic examination in the operating room with flexible, rigid, or telescopic tracheobronchoscopy remains the gold standard for evaluation of laryngotracheal stenosis due to its ability not just to quantify severity of luminal obstruction, but also accurately define the length and location of the stenosis. There are two grading systems most commonly employed when assessing laryngotracheal stenosis. The Cotton–Myer classification is the most widely known staging system and classifies the stenosis by degree of luminal obstruction.[14] Alternatively, the McCaffrey classification system characterizes the stenosis by the length and degree of involvement of the glottis.[15] Limited reports in adults suggest the McCaffrey stage may offer greater precision than the Cotton–Myer stage in predicting overall outcome in laryngotracheal stenosis.[16]

LABORATORIES

We perform screening for pro-inflammatory and auto-immune conditions which may contribute to underlying inflammation and scar in all newly diagnosed iSGS patients. We routinely obtain cANCA titers to assess for GPA, the most common other non-iatrogenic cause of subglottic stenosis. We will also obtain high sensitivity C-reactive protein (hsCRP) quantification to screen for active systemic inflammation and monitor response to therapy. Many authors also advocate obtaining screening antinuclear antibody (ANA) and rheumatoid factor (RF) titers as well as quantification of angiotensin conversion enzyme (ACE) level to assess for other autoimmune causes of laryngotracheal stenosis, as well as IgG subclass to assess for an IgG4-related fibrosis.[17] However, the standard practice of what markers to obtain and their diagnostic utility remains unclear.[18]

DIAGNOSTIC STUDIES

We obtain baseline pulmonary function testing (PFTs) on all patients with iSGS. It offers a rapid, minimally invasive, and inexpensive objective measurement from which subsequent interventions or clinical changes can be compared. When the flow volume loops are compared, Nouraei et al have found the expiratory disproportion index (EDI) useful for screening laryngotracheal stenosis from PFT, with a value >50% suspicious for underlying laryngotracheal stenosis.[19] The patient had a depressed peak expiratory flow (PEF) (51% predicted) with EDI of 73% predicted, with a normal diffusion capacity (DCLO), suggesting normal alveolar/capillary gas exchange and extrathoracic airway obstruction (Figure 38–2). Inexpensive portable peak flow meters are also routinely employed to objectively follow airflow through time.

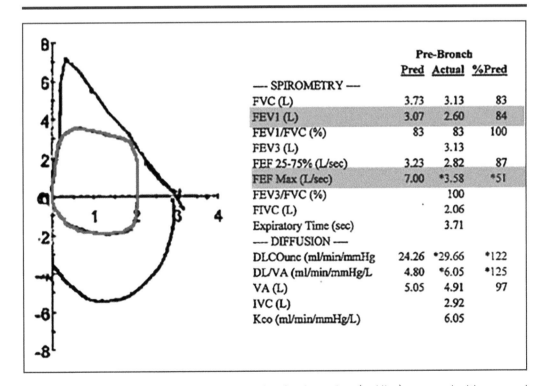

Figure 38–2. Baseline pulmonary function testing for the patient (*red line*) compared with age- and sex-matched normal flow-volume loop (*black line*). The patient demonstrated a first second forced expiratory volume (FEV1) of 84% predicted, peak expiratory flow (PEF) of 51% predicted, and an expiratory disproportion index (EDI) [(FEV1/PEFR)*100] of 73%.

Some authors advocate for routine study for gastroesophageal reflux disease with pH probe or impedance probe testing, even in the absence of symptoms.[17] Reflux disease is a known common comorbidity in the general population, and there is suggestion that it may exacerbate the degree or severity of recurrent scarring.[20] However, we typically reserve formal gastroenterology consultation for patients reporting symptomatic gastroesophageal reflux.

COMORBIDITIES

Airway obstruction in pregnancy is a unique clinical scenario, as the surgeon must minimize risk to both the patient and the fetus. To date, there are only six reported cases of management of iSGS in pregnancy in the literature. Much like the underlying disorder in general, a lack of consensus exists on management in pregnancy.[1] However, it is clear that a failure to adequately recognize the severity of the condition and make appropriate management decisions ahead of time can result in a catastrophic "cannot intubate, cannot ventilate" scenario, particularly if the mother experiences peripartum issues and requires emergent operative intervention.[9]

Physiologic changes in the pregnant patient make perioperative management of laryngotracheal stenosis more harrowing for both the mother and fetus. Primarily, maternal anesthesia poses risks to the fetus via intraoperative hypoxia, alterations in uterine blood flow, and fetal exposure to placental passage of systemic maternal medications.

Additionally, a gravid female experiences a 20% increase in oxygen consumption and a 20% decrease in pulmonary functional residual capacity, both of which contribute to the rapid decrease in maternal PaO_2 that is observed even during brief apnea. Increased chest wall diameter, breast enlargement, and weight gain from pregnancy all serve to decrease chest wall compliance and decrease effectiveness of passive ventilatory strategies such as jet ventilation. Weight gain may make exposure of the larynx and trachea via operative laryngoscopy more difficult. Uterine blood flow is not autonomically regulated, making placental blood flow more sensitive to use of vasoactive medications.

Concerns about the effect of anesthesia on the developing human fetus are both well founded and long standing.[21] All anesthetic drugs affect cell signaling, mitosis, and DNA synthesis, which are central to cellular differentiation and organogenesis. Yet despite years of animal studies and observational studies in humans, no anesthetic drug has been shown to be clearly dangerous to the human fetus and there is no optimal anesthetic technique. It is known that non-obstetric surgery is a significant risk for induction of preterm labor in the pregnant patient. In a study by Visser et al of pregnant patients undergoing abdominal surgery during pregnancy, preterm labor occurred in 26% of the second-trimester patients and 82% of the third-trimester patients.[22] While there is debate whether the phenomenon is due to anesthetic exposure or the physiologic stress response of non-obstetric surgery, the risk remains an important consideration in the decision for surgical intervention. It is estimated that up to 2% of pregnant women will require general anesthesia for non-obstetric surgery during their pregnancy.[23] This can be accomplished safely for mother and fetus but requires experienced clinicians and coordination between obstetrics, anesthesia, and surgeons.

SUPPORT SYSTEM

The patient was married with a supportive spouse and family, but she was newly diagnosed and wishing to learn more about her condition. In addition to counseling received in her clinic visitation, the patient was encouraged to visit the website for the North American Airway Collaborative (https://www.noacc.net), where there is information for support groups as well as patient-specific information materials on diagnosis, symptom management, and treatment.[24]

MEDICAL DECISION MAKING AND PATIENT PREFERENCES

We had a discussion of the therapeutic options for subglottic stenosis, and the alterations to this algorithm in pregnancy.

Subglottic stenosis is traditionally thought of as a surgical disease, most commonly employing operative endoscopic endotracheal examination and intervention. However, there has been limited early evidence suggesting that in-office corticosteroid injection into the subglottic scar may therapeutically arrest progression of stenosis in some patients with iSGS.[25,26] Patients receive submucosal administration of triamcinolone, dexamethasone, methylprednisolone, or solumedrol directly in the stenosis (there are no established differences between reagents). This is repeated three to five times (at

3-week intervals) at which time patients are transitioned into clinical surveillance. Systemic and inhaled steroids (both nasal and pulmonary) have an established track record in pregnancy (particularly as asthmatic patients) and are widely regarded as safe in pregnancy.

However, progressive airway obstruction despite medical management or patient inability to tolerate in-office transcutaneous corticosteroid injection necessitates operative intervention. A variety of techniques have been described, including cold or laser incision, ablation, or resection of tissue often combined with rigid or balloon dilation. Operative endoscopic treatment of subglottic stenosis has been successfully performed in pregnancy, with numerable techniques.[8,11,27] While endoscopic treatment almost inevitably results in recurrence of disease,[1] many patients have a prolonged asymptomatic interval between treatments (thereby providing an adequate airway through the remainder of pregnancy). There is evidence that concurrent injection of corticosteroid into the operating room may extend the interdilation interval.[28] Mitomycin C, an alkylating agent, has been topically applied by some authors to prevent fibroblast proliferation and recurrent scar. However, efficacy data for mitomycin is conflicting and the potential teratogenic effects make it contraindicated in pregnancy.[29]

Alternatively, placement of a tracheostomy under local anesthesia provides a secure airway without requiring systemic reagents that cross the placenta or imparting the same risks of maternal hypoxia.[8] However, many patients find the psychological impact of tracheostomy prohibitive to this treatment approach, and tracheostomy may complicate future airway reconstructive procedures should they become necessary.

Open airway reconstruction, either with resection of the affected segment via cricotracheal resection or with expansion of the affected area via laryngotracheoplasty, have both been described as definitive operations in the non-gravid patient. There is a high rate of success, in particular, with patients with iSGS via cricotracheal resection with primary thyrotracheal anastomosis.[30] While morbidity and mortality of the procedure are low, anastomotic complications can often be catastrophic, and there is a predictable lowering of pitch of the voice in women resulting in a masculine quality which is often seen as prohibitive to the surgery in this patient population. As a result, most surgeons advocate reserving open airway reconstruction for patients with recurrent disease that is refractory to endoscopic treatment, or at the point that the quality of life of repeated endoscopic treatments is prohibitive. To date, there is no published case of cricotracheal resection being performed during pregnancy, though Naqvi et al described successful tracheal resection with primary anastomosis in a 28 weeks gestational age pregnant patient with intubation-related tracheal stenosis refractory to endoscopic management.

While the patient was functionally impacted by the degree of her stenosis, she expressed a strong preference to avoid tracheostomy due to perceived negative impacts on her quality of life. As such, this was considered only as a last resort in the event of disease progression not responsive to other therapeutic interventions. Additionally, the risk of open segmental resection with re-anastamosis was felt to be prohibitive by the treatment team when less-invasive, established alternative options existed. She ultimately elected to undergo endoscopic management of her stenosis, with radial incision, balloon dilation, and corticosteroid injection.

PROCEDURAL STRATEGIES

Indications

In general, indication for intervention in iSGS depends on the patient's preferences, clinical assessment of the degree of physiologic ventilatory impairment, and a discussion of the risks and benefits of the varied treatment approaches. Objective criteria for intervention have yet to be established. This patient was sufficiently symptomatic with exertion to require surgical intervention. As an additional concern, her subglottis was felt to be sufficiently restricted that endotracheal intubation would be difficult in the event she would require emergency operative intervention during the peripartum or immediate postpartum period of her pregnancy.

Contraindications

No absolute contraindications to endoscopic treatment were identified. In particular, the patient had no underlying pulmonary or cardiovascular disease which would preclude successfully navigating bag mask ventilation and general anesthesia. We perform routine examination of interincisor mouth opening, neck mobility, and tongue and palate position (Mallampati score) in all patients in clinic prior to proceeding with endoscopic operative treatment, in order to assess for risk factors which might result in inability to expose the larynx and tracheobronchial complex using rigid instrumentation in the operating room. Our patient was noted to have normal neck mobility with no evidence of trismus and normal tongue and palate position.

Team Experience

Perioperative management of laryngotracheal stenosis requires careful communication between surgeon and anesthesiologist to maintain spontaneous ventilation on induction until ability to bag mask ventilate the patient is confirmed. A variety of airway management techniques may need to be employed to safely navigate the patient through the perioperative period, including endotracheal intubation, supraglottic or subglottic jet ventilation, rigid bronschosopy, or emergent tracheotomy. As such, we suggest that patients with iSGS are managed within the context of a multidisciplinary team familiar with surgical procedures used to treat the condition.

TECHNIQUES AND RESULTS

Anesthesia and Perioperative Care

The patient's pregnancy introduces several conflicting factors regarding typical perioperative management of patients with iSGS undergoing endoscopic treatment. While the baseline risk for venous thromboembolism during endolaryngeal and endotracheal procedures is unknown, pregnancy is also a significant risk factor for deep venous thromboembolism (VTE) and pulmonary embolism, with this being the leading cause of maternal death in the United States.[23] We recommend routine use of perioperative pneumatic stockings. We also routinely administer 10 mg of intravenous dexamethasone to temporize laryngeal edema in the postoperative period, which may be exacerbated by pregnancy.

Fetal and uterine monitoring during surgery is often possible using an electronic fetal heart rate monitor or by Doppler ultrasound, and allows early detection of factors which lead to fetal distress which may manifest with fetal bradycardia, tachycardia, or repetitive decelerations. We recommend consultation with colleagues in obstetrics, such that personnel appropriately trained in fetal heart rate interpretation can be available perioperatively.

The patient is typically placed supine on the operating table with the head of the patient facing the surgical team rotated 180 degrees from the anesthesia machine. However, fully supine positioning in pregnant patients beyond 18 to 20 weeks gestation may result in aortocaval compression and cardiovascular compromise. As such, it is recommended that the patient be positioned with a 15 degree left lateral tilt or with a wedge under the right hip.

Due to decreased vital capacity in the pregnant patient, there is decreased respiratory reserve and increased propensity to desaturation during periods of apnea. We recommend preoxygenation with 100% oxygen for 3 to 5 minutes prior to induction of anesthesia. The surgical team and anesthesiologist should discuss the airway management plan in detail prior to administration of any medications. We routinely induce using propofol to maintain spontaneous ventilation while the surgical team verifies the ability to bag mask ventilate the patient. Following successful bag mask ventilation, neuromuscular blockage is performed to aid in exposure while laryngoscopy is performed. Resultantly, the surgical team is the first to instrument the airway.

Once the larynx is exposed and the stenosis is visualized, supraglottic or subglottic jet ventilation is attempted, with the anesthesiologist controlling the ventilatory frequency. If jet ventilation results in sufficient ventilation and oxygenation, the entirety of the procedure can be done in this manner. However, in pregnancy there is decreased chest wall compliance and displacement of the diaphragm by the gravid uterus, which may result in insufficient ability to ventilate the patient in this manner. If jet ventilation is inadequate, we prefer to perform the procedure under intermittent apnea utilizing a 4.0 uncuffed endotracheal tube (ETT) placed via the suspended laryngoscope. After the stenosis has been sufficiently expanded, intermittent apnea can also be performed via intermittent endotracheal intubation with a larger cuffed ETT, during which the operative laryngoscope can remain in place.

Pregnant women are at increased risk for gastric acid aspiration with anesthetic induction or unconscious sedation. While it is not advisable to perform rapid sequence induction during endolaryngeal and endotracheal procedures due to the initial need to avoid paralytic, the patient must be closely monitored for evidence of refluxate. Gastric aspiration using an orogastric suction catheter may be beneficial to prevent refluxate during emergence.

Pregnancy is associated with decreased anesthetic requirements due to decrease in minimum alveolar concentration of inhalational anesthetic. As previously noted, uterine blood flow is not autonomically regulated and is more sensitive to vasoactive drug use. Pregnant women also have decreased concentrations of plasma cholinesterase and decreased hepatic blood flow, which may lead to alterations in the onset and duration of neuromuscular blocking agents. As such, neuromuscular blockage and depth of anesthesia are closely monitored and repeat doses of neuromuscular blocker may need to be administered.

Following the procedure, 4% lidocaine is applied to the vocal cords to prevent laryngospasm, and the laryngoscope is removed. The patient is allowed to emerge from anesthesia while bag mask ventilation is performed. Alternatively, a small microlaryngeal endotracheal tube can be placed and the patient allowed to emerge prior to extubation. Reversal agents such as glycopyrrolate should be used sparingly, as the corresponding increases in acetylcholine may lead to uterine contractions.

Patients are monitored in the postoperative recovery ward and are often kept overnight to ensure that no laryngeal or subglottic edema occurs. This also affords a longer opportunity for fetal monitoring.

Instrumentation and Operative Technique

We routinely place tape and moist eye pads on the eyes to protect from corneal injury, and place a tooth guard over the maxillary dentition to protect from dental injury. Following induction of anesthesia and verification of bag mask ventilation, the larynx was exposed using a rigid laryngoscope. We prefer the adult Dedo laryngoscope as it provides adequate working room for use of the operating microscope and two-handed surgery when necessary yet is small enough to obtain adequate endolaryngeal exposure in most patients. The laryngoscope was atraumatically inserted into the pharynx, then used to displace the tongue to the left, allowing visualization of the supraglottic larynx with the laryngoscope placed within the right glossotonsillar sulcus. The laryngoscope was then used to lift the epiglottis and advanced to the level of the glottis, such that it is partially splaying the true vocal folds, allowing visualization of the subglottis and trachea. After the larynx and subglottis were adequately exposed, the laryngoscope was suspended to a Mayo stand affixed to the operative table. Supraglottic jet ventilation was then instituted by placing a jet ventilation needle into the suction port of the laryngoscope. We also placed an endotracheal tube into the pharynx adjacent to the laryngoscope to instill 100% oxygen, which we have found to be helpful for preventing progressive desaturation with jet ventilation.

We initially performed telescopic laryngoscopy and bronchoscopy using a 0 degree rigid endoscope to photodocument the stenosis and perform measurements of the diameter and length of stenosis. The patient was verified to have a 1.0 cm length stenosis with an airway lumen measuring 4-by-5 mm (Figure 38–3A-C). There was no evidence of multilevel stenosis or dynamic airway collapse. A small right angle ball probe instrument is helpful to assess the areas of greatest overhang of the stenosis, and which areas are most amenable to radial incision. We typically perform between two and four radial incisions through the stenosis depending on the character of the stenosis, with care taken to preserve mucosa between the incisions. We prefer to use an endolaryngeal sickle blade for incisions, though some authors advocate use of the CO_2 laser with a pattern generator. In the event of laser use, close communication with the anesthesiologist and minimizing oxygen levels is essential to prevent risk of airway fire. We routinely perform a biopsy of the subglottis at the time of intervention for pathologic analysis and microbial culture.

Following radial incisions, the stenosis is injected submucosally with 1 mL of triamcinolone (40 mg/mL) using a Xomed laryngotracheal injector with an endoscope for guidance. Once sufficient steroid is administered, we pass a Boston Scientific Pulmonary Balloon Dilator across the stenosis and inflate to 6 atm of pressure to provide radial expansion of the segment. In general, we attempt to maintain dilation for approximately 30 seconds to allow for appropriate stretching of the stenosis, though duration of dilation is often limited by the patient's pulmonary reserve. Airway patency was then noted to be restored such that the subglottis could readily accept a cuffed 6.0 endotracheal tube for intubation (Figure 38–3D-E). The procedure lasted 20 minutes, after which the patient was allowed to emerge from anesthesia under bag mask ventilation and was transferred to the postanesthesia care unit for ongoing monitoring.

Results and Post-Procedure Management

With endoscopic interventions, small gains of the radius of the airway can often result in significant symptomatic improvement for the patient in accordance with Poiseuille's law, where airway resistance is proportional to the radius of the airway to the fourth

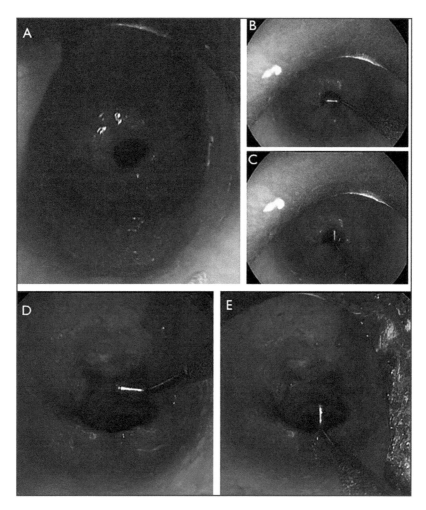

Figure 38–3. Telescopic bronchoscopy demonstrating the cicatricial stenosis involving the subglottis immediately below the true vocal folds (A). Initial measurements with a 5 mm probe showed a 4 mm × 5 mm airway (B and C). Results after endoscopic treatment show a 11 × 10 mm airway caliber (D and E). The stenosis was treated with cold sharp radial incisions into the stenosis, following by submucosal injection of triamcinolone (40 mg/mL) and dilation with a Boston Scientific Pulmonary Balloon Dilator.

power. The patient was observed overnight with no evidence of dyspnea or stridor. Fetal heart tones remained normal throughout her hospitalization. At this point she was deemed appropriate for discharge. We typically visit with the patient in the clinic 4 to 6 weeks following the first endoscopic treatment to ensure stability of symptoms and for surveillance laryngoscopy and PFT assessment.

Some authors advocate for empiric use of postoperative proton pump inhibitor therapy after endoscopic treatment, due to the described association between gastroesophgeal reflux and laryngotracheal stenosis.[20] There is also suggestion that empiric use of inhaled corticosteroids and anti-inflammatory antibiotics such as trimethoprim-sulbactam (Bactrim) and azithromycin may also delay interdilation interval.[28,31] We routinely prescribe anti-reflux treatment, an inhaled corticosteroid, and anti-inflammatory azithromycin in our iSGS patients during the first postoperative month. However, in the setting of pregnancy, we allow the patient to discuss these medication recommendations with their obstetrics provider and formulate a comprehensive perioperative treatment plan.

Therapeutic Alternatives

The patient did well symptomatically for several weeks but one month following her procedure returned to clinic with recurrent exertional dyspnea. She was noted to have recurrent inspiratory stridor but demonstrated no extremis or evidence of labored breathing. Flexible fiberoptic laryngoscopy was performed which demonstrated interval worsening of her stenosis with 75% restriction in airway caliber and a moderate amount of inflammation within the mucosa overlying the lesion (Figure 38–4A). In-office PFTs demonstrated a PEF of 49% predicted.

We had an extensive discussion about tracheotomy performed under local anesthesia, which was felt to provide her the safest means of respiration through the remainder of her pregnancy and delivery.

However, the patient remained resistant to tracheostomy and felt it would further compromise her quality of life. We also discussed repeat endolaryngeal operative treatment with incision and dilation of the stenosis with concurrent corticosteroid injection. However, she had significant reservations about repeated anesthetic exposure and risk of preterm labor, given that she was now 30 weeks gestational age and in her third trimester of pregnancy. Given the rapid recurrence of the patient's disease process and her desire to avoid tracheotomy or repeated anesthetic, we elected to proceed with a trial of serial intralesional steroid injections in the office.

Technical Considerations

The patient underwent injection of triamcinolone (40 mg/mL) via a cricothyroid approach using flexible fiberoptic laryngoscopic guidance. The procedure is performed by the surgeon with an assistant, with one person controlling the flexible fiberoptic laryngoscope and the other performing the injection. The nose is initially anesthetized with a topical decongestant and

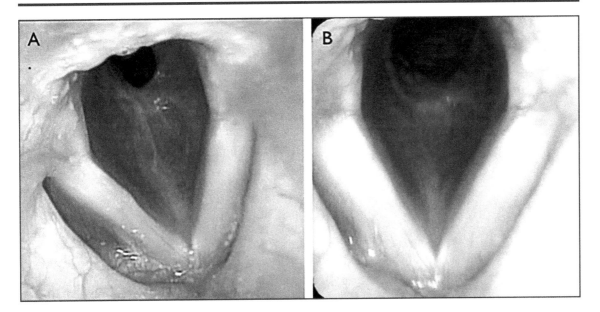

Figure 38–4. In-office flexible fiberoptic laryngoscopy at the level of the glottis, demonstrating full mobility of the bilateral true vocal folds, and recurrent cicatricial stricture with associated hyperemic mucosa in the subglottis (A). Improved airway caliber following 3 intralesional corticosteroid injections spaced 4 weeks apart (B). Corresponding peak expiratory flow rate (PEF) changed from 49% predicted to 72% predicted over this interval. (Photo provided by Dr. Bridget Hopewell MD)

anesthetic allowing passage of the endoscope. The cricoid cartilage is palpated on the anterior neck and 1% lidocaine is injected into the skin and soft tissue overlying the cricothyroid membrane. The needle is then used to puncture the cricothyroid membrane and additional 2% lidocaine is injected to provide laryngotracheal anesthesia. Prior to injection the syringe is drawn back demonstrating air to ensure the end of the needle is within the tracheal lumen. The patient should be counseled that she will cough as a result, and should be provided a towel or tissue to expectorate into.

The flexible laryngoscope is then introduced via the nose and used to visualize the larynx, with the images projected onto a monitor to allow both members of the team to view the procedure. Following transtracheal injection of lidocaine, the patient can tolerate the endoscope being advanced to the level of the glottis to fully visualize the subglottis. The corticosteroid is drawn into a 1 to 3 mL syringe on a 27-gauge needle and is administered through the cricothyroid membrane into the subglottis via the area of skin previously anesthetized until the end of the needle is seen on the monitor. Corticosteroid is then injected submucosally into several quadrants of the stenosis and the needle and endoscope are withdrawn.

Injection can alternatively be performed using a flexible 27-gauge needle through the working channel of a flexible endoscope which could potentially obviate the need for transtracheal injection of lidocaine. In this situation, 4% lidocaine is dripped directly onto the larynx during sustained phonation via the working channel of the endoscope. This allows sufficient topical anesthesia to allow tracheoscopy, at which time the flexible needle can be passed through the working channel of the endoscope and injection performed.

The patient is instructed to avoid eating or drinking for 1 hour or until the topical anesthesia has abated. She is counseled to expect a small amount of blood-streaking in sputum for 24 hours and that there may be some worsening of dyspnea for 24 to 48 hours due to mass effect of the injectable liquid restricting diameter of the stenosis until full absorption into the tissues occurs.

Clinical Surveillance

The patient received a total of three awake in-office corticosteroid injections separated by 4 weeks, with her last injection occurring at 38 weeks gestation. Pulmonary function testing was performed at each appointment, with improvement of her PEF from 49% predicted to 72% predicted after her last injection (Figure 38–4B). The patient noted improvement of symptoms following her second injection, with an arrest of exertional dyspnea. Most importantly, her airway caliber was felt to be sufficient to accept a small microlaryngeal endotracheal tube without difficulty should the need arise.

At 39 weeks gestation, the patient had spontaneous onset of labor with an uncomplicated delivery of a healthy baby boy. She had no significant peripartum issues with dyspnea or hypoxia; however, our service was aware of her admission and available to offer guidance and assistance with airway management should the need have arisen.

She continues to visit in our clinic for routine surveillance every 6 months. Objective testing shows her stenosis has worsened slightly (with a drop in PEF% to 65% predicted) but she has remained relatively asymptomatic and has not required repeat treatment in the 11 months since her uncomplicated delivery.

REFERENCES

1. Gelbard A, Donovan DT, Ongkasuwan J, et al. Disease homogeneity and treatment heterogeneity in idiopathic subglottic stenosis. *Laryngoscope*. 2016;126(6):1390–1396.
2. Dedo HH, Catten MD. Idiopathic progressive subglottic stenosis: findings and treatment in 52 patients. *Ann Otol Rhinol Laryngol*. 2001;110(4):305–311.
3. Gelbard A, Katsantonis NG, Mizuta M, et al. Molecular analysis of idiopathic subglottic stenosis for Mycobacterium species. *Laryngoscope*. 2017;127(1):179–185.
4. Gelbard A, Katsantonis NG, Mizuta M, et al. Idiopathic subglottic stenosis is associated with activation of the inflammatory IL-17A/IL-23 axis. *Laryngoscope*. 2016;126(11):E356–E361.
5. Damrose EJ. On the development of idiopathic subglottic stenosis. *Med Hypotheses*. 2008;71:122–125.
6. Blumin JH, Johnston N. Evidence of extraesophageal reflux in idiopathic subglottic stenosis. *Laryngoscope*. 2011;121:1266–1273.
7. Kobraei EM, Song TH, Mathisen DJ, Deshpande V, Mark EJ. Immunoglobulin G4-related disease presenting as an obstructing tracheal mass:consideration of surgical indications. *Ann Thorac Surg*. 2013;96:e91–e93.
8. Darjani HRJ, Parsa T, Pirzeh A, Heydarnazhad. Idiopathic subglottic stenosis in a pregnant woman: successful treatment with dilatation and Nd:YAG laser ablation. *Taffanos*. 2007;6(4):58–62.
9. Karippacheril JG, Goneppanavar U, Prabhu M, Revappa KB. Idiopathic subglottic stenosis in pregnancy: a deceptive laryngoscopic view. *Indian J Anaesth*. 2011;55(5):521–523.

10. Kuczkowski KM, Benumof JL. Subglottic tracheal stenosis in pregnancy: anaesthetic implications. *Anaesth Intensive Care*. 2003;31:576–577.

11. Scholz A, Srinivas K, Stacey MRW, Clyburn P. Subgottic stenosis in pregnancy. *Br J Anaesth*. 2008;100(3):385–388.

12. Nouraei SA, Nouraei SM, Randhawa PS, et al. Sensitivty and responsiveness of the Medical Research Council dyspnoea scale to the presence and treatment of adult laryngotracheal stenosis. *Clin Otolaryngol*. 2008;33:575–580.

13. Morshed K, Trojanowska A, Szymanski M, et al. Evaluation of tracheal stenosis: comparison between computed tomography virtual tracheobronchoscopy with multiplanar reformatting, flexible tracheofiberoscopy and intra-operative findings. *Eur Arch Otorhinolaryngol*. 2011;268(4):591–597.

14. Myer CM, O'Conner DM, Cotton RT. Proposed grading system for subglottic stenosis based on endotracheal tube sizes. *Ann Otol Rhinol Laryngol*. 1994;103:319–323.

15. McCaffrey TV. Classification of laryngotracheal stenosis. *Laryngoscope*. 1992;102:1335–1340.

16. Gelbard A, Francis DO, Sandulache VC, Simmons JC, Donovan DT, Ongkasuwan J. Causes and consequences of adult laryngotracheal stenosis. *Laryngoscope*. 2015; 125(5):1137–1143.

17. Wang H, Weight CD, Wain JC, Ott HC, Mathisen DJ. Idiopathic subglottic stenosis: factors affecting outcome after single-stage repair. *Ann Thorac Surg*. 2015;100(5): 1804–1811.

18. Gnagi SH, Howard BE, Anderson C, Lott DG. Idiopathic subglottic and tracheal stenosis: a survey of the patient experience. *Ann Otol Rhinol Laryngol*. 2015;124(9):734–739.

19. Mouraei SA, Nouraei SM, Patel A, et al. Diagnosis of laryngotracheal stenosis from routine pulmonary physiology using the expiratory disproportion index. *Laryngoscope*. 2013;123(12):3099–3104.

20. Blumin JH, Johnston N. Evidence of extraesophageal reflux in idiopathic subglottic stenosis. *Laryngoscope*. 2001; 121:1266–1273.

21. Rosen MA. Management of anesthesia for the pregnant surgical patient. *Anesthesia*. 1999;91(4):1159–1163.

22. Visser BC, Glasgow RE, Mulvihill KK, Muhilvill SJ. Safety and timing of nonobstetric abdominal surgery in pregnancy. *Dig Surg*. 2001;18(5):409–417.

23. Chang J, Elam-Evans LD, Berg CJ, et al. Pregnancy-related mortality surveillance—United States, 1991–1999. *MMWR Surveill Summ*. 2003;52(2):1–8.

24. North American Airway Collaborative. North American Airway Collaborative. https://noaac.net/.

25. Franco RA, Husain I, Reder L, Paddle P. Awake serial intralesional steroid injections without surgery as a novel targeted treatment for idiopathic subglottic stenosis. *Laryngoscope*. 2017 Oct 8. doi: 10.1002/lary.26874 [Epub ahead of print]

26. Hoffman MR, Coughlin AE, Dailey SH. Serial office-based steroid injections for treatment of idiopathic subglottic stenosis. *Laryngoscope*. 2017 Jun 5. doi: 10.1002 /lary,26682 [Epub ahead of print]

27. Andrews BT, Graham SM, Ross AF, et al. Technique, utility, and safety of awake tracheoplasty using combined laser and balloon dilation. *Laryngoscope*. 2007;117(12): 2159–2162.

28. Shabani S, Hoffman MR, Brand WT, Dailey SH. Endoscopic management of idiopathic subglottic stenosis: factors affecting inter-dilational interval. *Ann Otol Rhinol Laryngol*. 2017;126(2):96–102.

29. Hartnick CJ, Hartley BEJ, Lacy PD, et al. Topical mitomycin application after laryngotracheal reconstruction: a randomized, double-blind, placebo-controlled trial. *Arch Otolaryngol Head Neck Surg*. 2001;127(10):1260–1264.

30. Grillo HC, Mathisen DJ, Wain JC. Laryngotracheal resection and reconstruction for subglottic stenosis. *Ann Thorac Surg*. 1992;53(1):54–63.

31. Maldonado F, Loiselle A, DePew ZS, et al. Idiopathic subglottic stenosis: an evolving therapeutic algorithm. *Laryngoscope*. 2014;124(2):498–503.

CHAPTER 39

Intubation–Related Tracheal Stenosis

S. A. Reza Nouraei

INTRODUCTION

Laryngotracheal stenosis is an umbrella description which encompasses a heterogeneous group of uncommon conditions that cause abnormal narrowing of the central airways from the supraglottic larynx to the main bronchi (Figure 39–1).[1] The main symptoms of adult laryngotracheal stenosis are exertional dyspnea, effort intolerance, voice change, chronic cough and mucus, and, in a proportion of patients, added respiratory sounds. These sounds may resemble and, without a high index of clinical suspicion, can be readily mistaken for lower airway wheeze.[2] The diagnosis of laryngotracheal stenosis, being a very uncommon cause of a very common clinical presentation, is often delayed and patients are frequently mislabeled diagnostically as "resistant asthmatics" and are treated incorrectly, in many cases for prolonged periods.[3,4]

Laryngotracheal stenosis has been described since antiquity and its most common historical causes were infections and trauma.[5] Iatrogenic laryngotracheal stenosis as a complication of tracheostomy insertion was recognized in the late 1800s.[6] Laryngotracheal stenosis as a complication of translaryngeal intubation became increasingly prevalent from the middle of the twentieth century as a corollary of the birth and growth of intensive care medicine, which, at its inception and core, involved changing the management of acute respiratory failure from external negative-pressure iron-lung ventilation (Figure 39–2) to endotracheal intubation and positive-pressure ventilation.[7–9] Despite significant advances in intensive care airway management, in the design of the tubes, in the meticulous attention that is being paid to their management, and in the earlier switch from translaryngeal to transtracheal ventila-

tion,[10,11] intubation and tracheostomy-related airway strictures remain the most common causes of laryngotracheal stenosis.

Other historical trends, which are beyond the scope of this chapter, have also influenced laryngotracheal stenosis disease patterns. As one example, introduction of systemic immune suppression in the 1980s and 1990s transformed the prognosis of patients with vasculitis from months to decades,[12,13] and as a result, airway strictures, which are a long-term complication of avascular mucosal and cartilage necrosis, emerged as a disease entity.[14] It occurs in approximately 15% of patients with granulomatosis with polyangiitis and now follows intubation-related strictures as the second most common cause of benign adult laryngotracheal stenosis.[1]

CASE PRESENTATION

A 49-year-old lady was admitted under the care of respiratory medicine with a working diagnosis of infective exacerbation of long-standing "difficult" asthma. She had been born uneventfully but had an emergency tracheostomy at 6 months of age for diphtheria and was successfully decannulated just before the age of 1 year. She was labeled a "wheezer" as a baby and toddler and a "difficult asthmatic" throughout childhood and adult life. She had numerous hospital admissions for "asthma attacks" in the decades that followed her tracheostomy decannulation.

On that particular admission, recognition of acute voice change by the medical team precipitated an otolaryngology consult for laryngeal evaluation. This resulted in the reevaluation of airway symptoms as

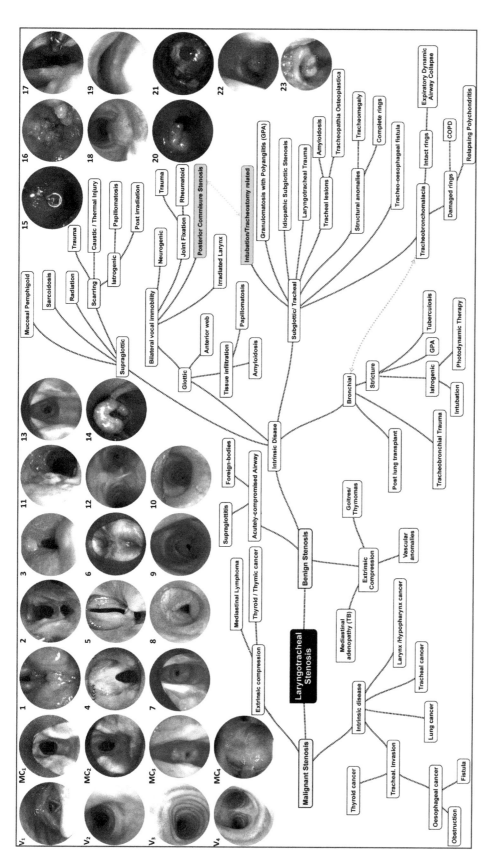

Figure 39–1. Different causes of laryngotracheal stenosis. V$_{1-4}$ shows the standard airway views of the larynx, subglottis, trachea, and the carina. MC$_{1-4}$ show different Myer-Cotton grades: MC$_1$ (<50%), MC$_2$ (51–70%), MC$_3$ (71–99%) and MC$_4$ (no lumen). Images 1–23 shows some of the different subtypes of laryngotracheal stenosis; 1–2: acute inflammatory laryngeal stenosis; 3: acute inflammatory tracheal stenosis; 4: Anterior glottic web; 5: bilateral vocal fold immobility due to incomplete posterior commissure stenosis; 6: bilateral vocal fold immobility due to complete posterior commissure stenosis; 7: cicatricial tracheal stenosis; 8: lambdoid tracheal deformity; 9: cicatricial tracheal stenosis due to tracheostomy stoma; 10: cicatricial tracheal stenosis due to granulomatosis with polyangiitis; 12: bronchial stenosis due to granulomatosis with polyangiitis; 13: idiopathic subglottic stenosis; 14: laryngeal sarcoidosis; 15: tracheal amyloidosis; 16: recurrent respiratory papillomatosis; 17: chondrosarcoma of the cricoid cartilage; 18: tracheomalacia with normal tracheal rings (expiratory dynamic airway collapse –EDAC–); 19: tracheomalacia with abnormal tracheal rings; 20: benign tracheal tumor; 21: adenoid cystic carcinoma of the trachea; 22: squamous cell carcinoma of the trachea; 23: acute airway compromise due to laryngeal squamous cell carcinoma.

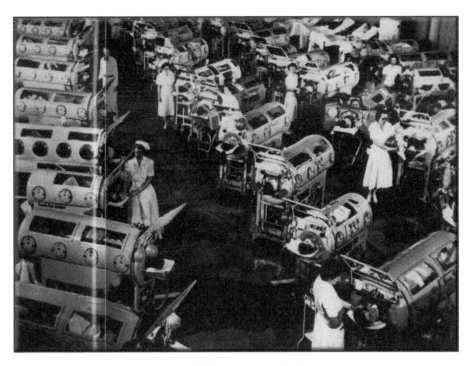

Figure 39–2. Negative-pressure ventilation using the iron lung.

being more consistent with upper airway pathology, and the resulting computed tomography scan showed "a narrowing of the trachea. . . . This is quite focal extending over a vertical length of 5 mm. The trachea is narrowed to a minimal size of 9 × 15 mm. The appearance is that of scarring rather than of a soft tissue mass narrowing the trachea. The level of this narrowing is 15 mm below the cricoid cartilage." A microlaryngoscopy and tracheoscopy was then performed and confirmed the diagnosis of an isolated lambdoid-pattern tracheal stenosis.[15] She was offered a tracheal resection but declined. She was subsequently lost to follow-up of the local services and presented 10 years later, having had recurrent chest and throat infections and a refractory cough in the intervening years. She again declined the option of an open tracheal resection and did not present for regular follow-up upon discharge. Approximately 10 years later, aged 69, she presented to respiratory physicians with acute respiratory failure during an acute lower respiratory tract infection. She had been becoming increasingly effort intolerant, with worsening chronic cough and difficulties with expectoration of pulmonary secretions. She had no known cardiovascular morbidities.

On this occasion she had an in-office flexible laryngoscopy and tracheoscopy which confirmed the presence of a lambdoid-pattern tracheal stenosis[15] with normal distal trachea and no evidence of malacic disease (Figure 39–3). She also had a maximum-effort flow-volume loop and whole-body plethysmography which showed an extrathoracic pattern of upper airway obstruction, normal lung volumes, and increased respiratory resistance (Figure 39–4).

The option of an endoscopic resection tracheoplasty[16] had at this time become available within the unit and she elected for this course of treatment. The procedure was successfully undertaken (Figure 39–5 and Video 39–1). This led to normalization of her postoperative flow-volume loops (Figure 39–6), but somewhat surprisingly, she subjectively remained breathless and did not feel that she had derived any significant benefit from her surgery. She underwent an airway-focused cardiopulmonary exercise test (CPET) according to a protocol developed in partnership with the New Zealand Sleep and Respiratory Institute (www.nzrsi.co.nz) to evaluate the upper airway. She was able to exercise for 4.07 minutes and had a peak oxygen consumption of 22.5 mL/kg/min, which was 82% of her

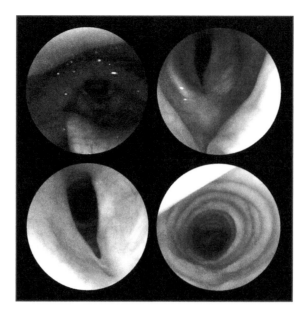

Figure 39–3. Four-shot flexible endoscopic views of the larynx, subglottis, trachea, and the carina showing a lambdoid-pattern tracheal stenosis.

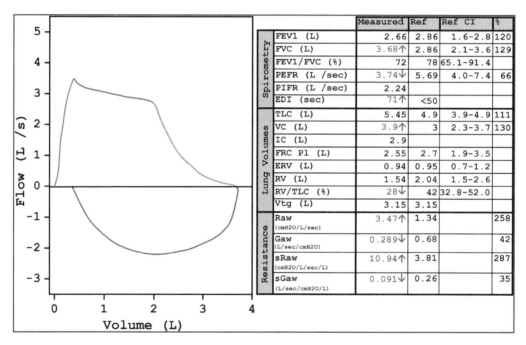

		Measured	Ref	Ref CI	%
Spirometry	FEV1 (L)	2.66	2.86	1.6-2.8	120
	FVC (L)	3.68↑	2.86	2.1-3.6	129
	FEV1/FVC (%)	72	78	65.1-91.4	
	PEFR (L /sec)	3.74↓	5.69	4.0-7.4	66
	PIFR (L /sec)	2.24			
	EDI (sec)	71↑	<50		
Lung Volumes	TLC (L)	5.45	4.9	3.9-4.9	111
	VC (L)	3.9↑	3	2.3-3.7	130
	IC (L)	2.9			
	FRC Pl (L)	2.55	2.7	1.9-3.5	
	ERV (L)	0.94	0.95	0.7-1.2	
	RV (L)	1.54	2.04	1.5-2.6	
	RV/TLC (%)	28↓	42	32.8-52.0	
	Vtg (L)	3.15	3.15		
Resistance	Raw (cmH2O/L/sec)	3.47↑	1.34		258
	Gaw (L/sec/cmH2O)	0.289↓	0.68		42
	sRaw (cmH2O/L/sec/L)	10.94↑	3.81		287
	sGaw (L/sec/cmH2O/L)	0.091↓	0.26		35

Figure 39–4. Maximum-effort flow-volume loop and whole-body plethysmography prior to airway surgery. The blue portion of the loop is a maximum-effort expiration from full lung volume. The red component of the flow-volume loop shows expiratory flow limitation due to the presence of the stenosis. The green component of the loop shows the phenomenon of expiratory flow limitation which continues until full expiration, at which point a maximum-effort breath (gray line) is taken back to full lung volume. Spirometry shows normal forced expiratory volume in one second (FEV1), increased forced vital capacity (FVC), reduced peak expiratory and peak inspiratory flow rates (PEFR and PIFR), and an increased Expiratory Disproportion Index (EDI). Whole-body plethysmography showed normal lung volumes (total lung capacity [TLC], vital capacity [VC], inspiratory capacity [IC], functional residual capacity [FRC], expiratory reserve volume [ERV], residual volume [RV], and thoracic gas volume [Vtg]). The airway resistance was significantly increased (Raw) and admittance (Gaw).

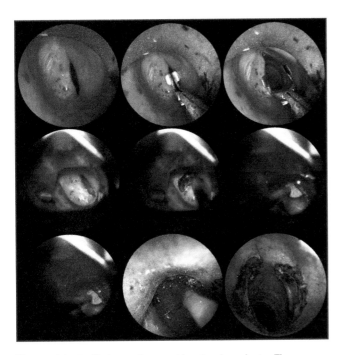

Figure 39–5. Endoscopic resection tracheoplasty. The operation involves laser resection of herniated tracheal ring down to tracheal adventitia to allow wound contracture to proceed cranio-caudally. It is important to maintain both anterior and posterior mucosal bridges.

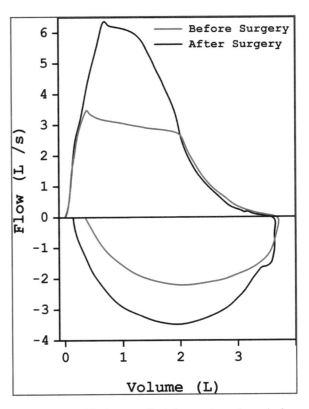

Figure 39–6. Maximum-effort flow-volume loops before and one week after endoscopic resection tracheoplasty showing significant improvements in both inspiratory and expiratory flow rates.

predicted value. There were no desaturations and no cardiac ischemia. She reached a peak exercise power of 138 watts and stopped due to a combination of breathlessness and leg fatigue. She had a Borg dyspnea score of 0 at the start of the exercise and 9 at the end. She was able to raise her minute ventilation in response to increased exercise power and did not have a major fall in the expired partial pressure of oxygen, nor a major rise in the expired partial pressure of carbon dioxide (Figure 39–7). Her exercise flow-volume loops, performed by asking her to perform full inspirations at different exercise powers (Figure 39–8), showed an abnormal persistent breathing pattern, characterized by a failure to increase both the respiratory rate and per-breath flow rate in response to increased exercise demand, but instead taking deeper and slower breaths in order to increase minute ventilation. The signal for the change in breathing pattern was reaching expiratory flow maxima (Figure 39–8-5). She closely approached but did not reach the inspiratory flow maxima (Figure 39–8-8). She underwent a period of respiratory rehabilitation which led to resolution of her dyspnea symptoms and she remains asymptomatic over 1 year later.

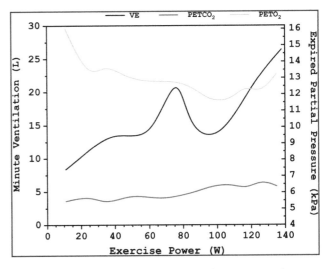

Figure 39–7. Airway-focused cardiopulmonary exercise test showing increases in minute ventilation, and expired partial pressures of oxygen and carbon dioxide. Supplied courtesy of Dr Andrew Veale at the New Zealand Respiratory and Sleep Institute.

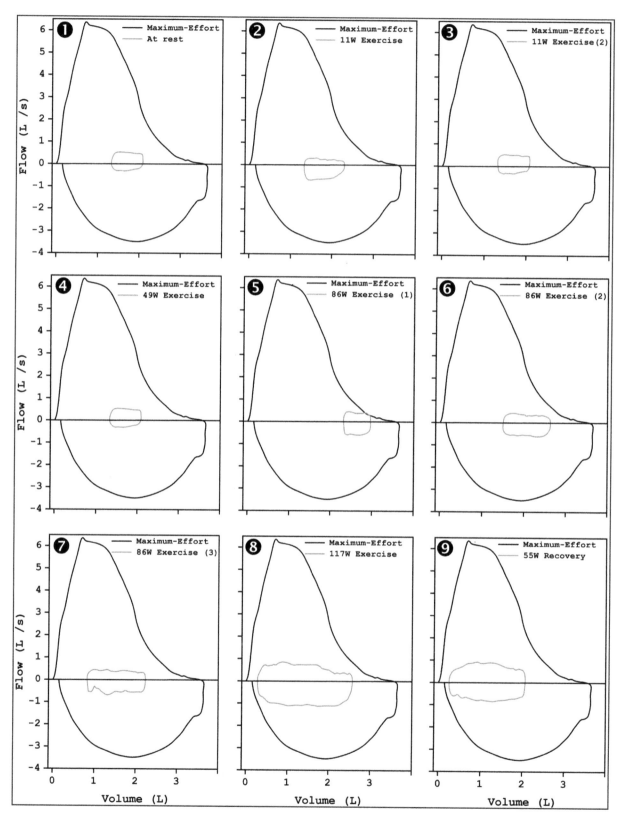

Figure 39-8. Exercise flow-volume loops constructed within the maximum-effort flow-volume loop envelope showing an abnormal pattern of breathing consisting of failure to raise ventilatory flow rate in response to increased exercise demand. Supplied courtesy of Dr Andrew Veale at the New Zealand Respiratory and Sleep Institute.

DISCUSSION

Recognition and management of airway stenosis may have a marked impact on quality of life and it is important for a multidisciplinary approach (respiratory, otolaryngology, radiology, gastroenterology, speech pathology, physiotherapy) to be employed to ensure that a correct diagnosis (and therefore appropriate management plan) is reached.

Incidence of Intubation-Related Laryngotracheal Stenosis

Adult intubation-related laryngotracheal stenosis is estimated to occur in 1 in 204,000 adults per year.[17] However, this number relates to patients who presented for treatment, and it is further estimated that as many as 80% of patients with this condition may actually remain undiagnosed.[18]

Pathophysiology of Intubation-Related Laryngotracheal Stenosis

This condition is a response to injury caused by the presence of a translaryngeal or a transtracheal ventilatory conduit and, as such, the locations and patterns of stenosis are specific and consistent (Figure 39–9). It may also arise in the context of particular systemic diseases or where there is significant extra-esophageal reflux combined with airway instrumentation. A detailed description of normal and abnormal mucosal wound healing at a cellular level is beyond the scope of this chapter and has been provided by Sandhu and Nouraei.[1]

Diagnostic Evaluation of Intubation-Related Laryngotracheal Stenosis

Correct diagnosis will enable specific targeted treatment and is the key to patient symptom relief.

Clinical History

In addition to a comprehensive general medical history, an airway history aims to answer a number of specific questions:

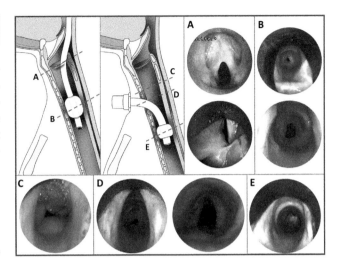

Figure 39–9. Patterns and locations of intubation-related laryngotracheal stenosis. (A) Translaryngeal intubation can cause anterior or posterior commissure stenosis which are among the most complex of all airway injuries to treat; tracheal stenosis can be caused by endotracheal tube cuff or tip (B), tracheostomy stoma (C and D), or tracheostomy tube cuff (E).

How Have the Symptoms Evolved? There is no period of intubation time below which a significant airway injury is improbable, nor is there a period of intubation time above which such an injury becomes inevitable. Particular attention must therefore be paid to ascertaining a detailed history of surgical and critical care intubations, including, as was the case in the patient presented, events during early years of life. A significant mechanical obstruction, once established, will very likely have respiratory manifestations, but these manifestations will often have been attributed, sometimes for many decades,[3] to other conditions like asthma or post critical care bronchopulmonary morbidity.

As such, a detailed respiratory history preceding identification of laryngotracheal stenosis must be sought. One exception to this, which must be borne in mind, is development of new symptoms in a male patient with a history of neonatal intubation, at or around puberty due to what is a complex interaction between pre-existing but hitherto asymptomatic anatomic anomalies and the laryngeal growth spurt. In cases of relatively recent intubation events, the length of time from extubation to the onset of airway symptoms must be sought. It can take up to one year from extubation for maturation of an airway injury into a symptomatic stenosis but most patients with significant stenoses become symptomatic within 3 months. Breathlessness is not a symptom that is primarily evaluated by laryngologists, and, as such, most tracheostomy-free breathless patients are referred with established diagnoses. An important exception to this, although not directly related to intubation-related laryngotracheal stenosis, is development of airway strictures in patients with granulomatosis with polyangiitis[19] who are under otolaryngologist follow-up for nasal and sinus symptoms. To avoid potentially life-threatening diagnostic delays,[4] new-onset dyspnea should be inquired about in the otolaryngological follow-up of vasculitis patients and appropriate investigations ordered.

What Are the Risk Factors for Intubation-Related Laryngotracheal Stenosis?

There are a wide range of risk factors which influence occurrence of intubation-related laryngotracheal stenosis (Figure 39–10). An effort must be made to obtain details of the intubation event preceding development of the stenosis and particular attention must be paid to agitation and problems with sedation during intubation,[20] persistent hypotension, use of inotropes, presence of immune suppression, endotracheal tube size selection, and time from endotracheal to tracheostomy ventilation.

With regard to tube size selection in particular, it is important to recognize that height and sex exert identical influence on adult trachea size[21,22] and yet, in many cases, endotracheal tube size selection in adults is based on patient sex and not height and sex. As such, and particularly in relation to posterior glottic injury,[23] an over-sized endotracheal tube may be a specific and iatrogenic etiological factor.

What Is the Likelihood of the Presence of a Different Airway Pathology?

There are diagnostic pitfalls that may lead to misattribution of an airway stenosis as being intubation related. An airway stenosis may develop as a complication of a vasculitic process, principally granulomatosis with polyangiitis,[19] or *de novo* in idiopathic subglottic stenosis.[24] Stenosis progression may cause increasing but misattributed respiratory morbidity and precipitate respiratory failure, the treatment of which may then require endotracheal intubation or tracheostomy tube placement. A careful clinical history of vasculitis, which should be ascertained in all patients,

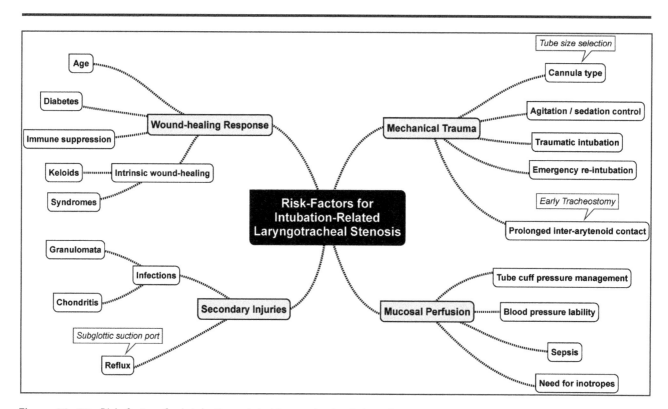

Figure 39–10. Risk-factors for intubation-related laryngotracheal stenosis.

if necessary using a formal symptoms inventory instrument like the Birmingham Vasculitis Activity Score,[25] and a precise understanding of the evolution of symptoms should reduce the likelihood of diagnostic misattribution. This pitfall may also be avoided by paying close attention to the precise stenosis geometry. The subglottis is not the narrowest part of the adult airway and only a small minority of long-term intubation-related airway injuries occur in the true subglottis.[26] By contrast, both vasculitis-related and idiopathic stenoses frequently, although not exclusively, occur in the true subglottis, and the endoscopic appearance of the stenosis (see Figure 39–1) can provide significant clues about the underlying etiology.

What Are the Current Symptoms and Disability Levels? A laryngotracheal stenosis impacts multiple domains of patient symptom and often has a profound impact on well-being. The four principal symptom domains are *dyspnea, voice, swallowing*, and *cough*. Two additional domains—of airway and independence—also influence the patient's overall quality of life. The ADV-CSI score (Table 39–1) provides a disease-specific symptoms inventory and complications grading systems both for initial evaluation and for outcomes assessment.[27]

What Are Patient Expectations and Prognostic Considerations in Determining Management Strategies? The aim of laryngotracheal reconstructive surgery is to restore an airway lumen that can support the ventilatory demands of the patient while minimizing collateral injury to the voice and swallowing mechanisms. This aim is achievable in most patients who have intubation-related laryngotracheal stenosis, and indeed in many cases, this can be achieved using only minimally invasive surgical techniques.[28,29] However, patients with extensive injuries, those with significant concurrent laryngeal and tracheal injuries, and patients with laryngeal stenosis who have borderline pretreatment swallow safety may need to be maintained with long-term luminal stents or a long-term tracheostomy. Likewise, in patients who have long-term neurological injury whose respiratory demands are likely to remain minimal in the long term, performing major open cervicomediastinal surgery, while technically feasible, may not serve the best holistic interests of the patient, and treatment goal may need to shift toward creating an airway that will likely remain safe during intercurrent episodes of lower respiratory tract infection. The appropriate treatment goals and approach are frequently nuanced and should, in all cases, be a shared decision between the patient and the airway team.

Clinical Examination

Thorough evaluation is always warranted by the surgeon, even if the patient has been reviewed by other services.

General Examination. The most common clinical scenarios in which intubation-related laryngotracheal stenosis is encountered are a chronically breathless or tracheostomy-dependent patient with an established diagnosis, a failed or difficult critical care extubation/decannulation, and an acute clinical presentation with respiratory decompensation. In the acute settings, clinical examination follows standard intermediate and advanced life-support protocols. Management of an acutely compromised airway is discussed elsewhere in this volume. General examination aims to ascertain the degree of respiratory effort through assessing for tracheal tug, use of accessory respiratory muscles, chest recession, and stridor. Stridor should be elicited by asking the patient to take deep breaths through an open mouth while the neck is auscultated. Whether the stridor is inspiratory, expiratory, or biphasic should be documented. Oxygen saturation on room air needs to be measured. The patient should be examined for peripheral stigmata of abnormal scarring like keloid and hypertrophic scars, presence of syndromes associated with abnormal scarring like Turner's or Noonan's, connective tissue disorders like joint hypermobility associated with Ehlers–Danlos syndrome, and immune-related conditions like sarcoid nodules, saddle-nose deformity of granulomatosis with polyangiitis, and lobule-sparing ear inflammation of relapsing polychondritis.

Laryngotracheoscopy. Historically, airway assessment required an examination under general anesthesia using suspension laryngoscopy, and for some conditions, specifically for bilateral vocal fold immobility when palpation of the cricoarytenoid joints is required, this remains a minimum standard of care. For most tracheal conditions, however, an office-based laryngotracheoscopy is readily feasible. Key pharyngeal findings to document are presence of scars and hypopharyngeal secretions which can be a sign of abnormal swallowing. Stigmata of pharyngolaryngeal reflux, including inflammation of the respiratory mucosa within the postnasal space, cobblestoning of the posterior

Table 39-1. The ADV-CSI System and Classification of Airway Stenosis and Complications

Please indicate which of the five responses below best describes your level of breathlessness over the past two weeks. (only one response out of the five available options below).

Dyspnoea
1. I get short of breath only on strenuous exercise.
2. I get short of breath when hurrying on the level or climbing up a slight hill.
3. I walk slower than people of the same age on the level because of breathlessness, or have to stop for breath when walking at my own pace on the level.
4. I stop for breath after walking 100 yards or after a few minutes on the level.
5. I am too breathless to leave the house

Please indicate which of the five responses below best describes your voice over the past two weeks (only one response out of the five available options below).

Voice
1. I have had no problems with my voice
2. I have had some problems with my voice, for example the quality of my voice may vary throughout the day, or I have difficulty being heard in loud environments
3. I struggle to make my voice heard, particularly in loud environments
4. Despite my best efforts, I can only produce a weak voice/whisper and have difficulty being heard in a normal conversation/on the phone
5. I have no voice

Please indicate which of the five responses below best describes your voice over the past two weeks (only one response out of the five available options below). If you have had any episodes of being unable to breathe/having to go to hospital because of mucous plugs or crusting please since the last time you took this test, choose option 5.

Cough / Mucus
1. I have had no problems with coughing or with mucous in my airway or throat.
2. I do have a fairly regular cough and/or need to clear mucus, but it does not bother me.
3. I do have a bothersome problem with cough and/or mucus. For example:
   • Problems with cough/needing to clear mucus causes me physical pain/discomfort (eg rib/throat pain).
   • Problems with cough/needing to clear mucus has an impact on my social life.
4. I have a significant problem with coughing and/or mucus. For example:
   • I regularly have to clear clumps or mucus/crust from my throat/airway.
   • I have experienced at least one episode of my airway "blocking" due to mucous/crust which I had to clear with coughing/nebulising.
   • I have needed to see a doctor regarding my cough / mucous symptoms.
5. Since the last time I answered these questions, I have needed to call an ambulance / attend hospital in an emergency due to my airway blocking off with "mucous plugging" / "airway crusting."

Please indicate which of the five responses below best describes your use of devices (eg humidifiers or nebulisers) for your airway over the past two weeks (only one response out of the five available options below).

Independence
1. I have not needed to use any devices (eg nebuliser or humidifier) for my airway.
2. I have needed to humidify my airway (either by steam inhalation or by use of a humidifier), and/or use a saline nebuliser. I have not needed to do this more than 2-3 times a week.
3. I have needed to use a nebuliser or humidify my airway one or more times a day.
4. I have an internal airway stent in place.
5. I have a tracheostomy or a T-tube in place.

Table 39-1. (*continued*)

Please indicate which of the five responses below best describes your swallowing over the past two weeks (only one response out of the five available options below).

Swallowing
1. I have been able to eat and drink normally.
2. I have been able to eat a normal diet but with some difficulty. For example:
   - I have occasionally had to cough to clear my throat
   - I find some foods more difficult than others to swallow
   - It takes me longer to finish a meal than it does people around me
   - I sometimes cough when I drink liquids quickly
3. I have had significant swallowing difficulties. For example:
   - I cough to clear my throat, or do a double-swallow during most meals
   - I tend to eat soft or pureed foods, that are easier to swallow.
   - It takes me much longer to finish a meal than most people
   - Drinking fluids, frequently makes me cough.
4. My swallowing is a serious problem / is seriously abnormal. For example:
   - My diet consists almost entirely of semi-liquid / liquidized foods
   - I need to take a significant amount of the fluids I drink, as thickened fluids
   - I take regular dietary supplements -or- I receive a proportion of my diet through a stomach tube (PEG).
5. I am unable to swallow. I take all of my nutrition through a stomach tube (PEG).

Please indicate which of the five responses below best describes your overall sense of health and well-being over the past two weeks (only one response out of the five available options below).

Overall Health
In general, I would say that my health is:.
1. Excellent
2. Very good.
3. Good.
4. Fair.
5. Poor.

Modified Myer-Cotton grading system
Grade 0.   No or minimal (<10%) discernible stenosis
Grade 1.   Discernible obstruction between 10 and 50%
Grade 2.   Obstruction between 51 and 70%
Grade 3.   Obstruction between 71 and 99%
Grade 4.   No discernible lumen

Dindo-Clavien classification of complications.
Grade 1.   Any deviation from the normal postoperative course without the need for pharmacological intervention 1 or surgical, endoscopic, or radiological interventions.
Grade 2.   Required pharmacological treatment with drugs other than such allowed for grade 1 complications. Blood transfusion and total parenteral nutrition are also included.
Grade 3.   Requiring surgical, radiological, or endoscopic interventions.
Grade 4.   Life-threatening complications (including Central Nervous System complications) 2 requiring intermediate or intensive care management.
Grade 5.   Death of a patient.

[1.] Allowed therapeutic regimens are: drugs as antiemetics, antipyretics, analgesics, diuretics, electrolytes, and physiotherapy. This grade also includes wound infections opened at the bedside.
[2.] Brain haemorrhage, ischaemic stroke, subarachnoid haemorrhage but excluding transient ischaemic attack.

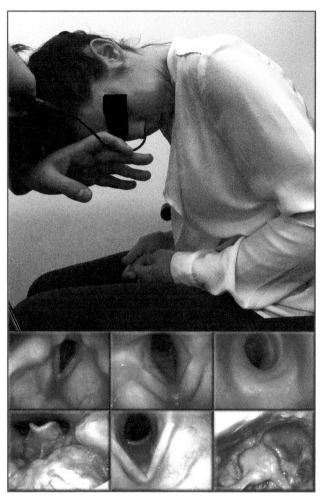

Figure 39–11. The laryngeal distraction maneuver is accomplished by asking the patient to move forward and bend in the upper back, to put his or her chin down onto the chest and to look to the side. In this position, the larynx and trachea are brought into the bird's-eye view of the endoscope and the epiglottis is pulled anteriorly. With careful maneuver it is possible to obtain full views of the subglottis without needing to administer anesthesia. The same position, when combined with a trumpet Valsalva maneuver, allows for visualization of the posterior cricoid region and the upper esophageal sphincter.

pharyngeal wall, post-cricoid and inter-arytenoid edema, and glottic pseudosulcus should be ascertained and documented. The larynx should be examined for gross movement and a stroboscopic assessment of vocal vibrations should be performed.

The subglottis and proximal trachea can be examined without the need for topical anesthesia by per-

forming a Laryngeal Distraction Maneuver (LDM) (Figure 39–11). This brings the glottic inlet and the trachea into bird's-eye view of the endoscope. The patient is asked to take slow and deep breaths in order to demonstrate the subglottis and the trachea. The same position, if instead of deep inspiration is accompanied by a trumpet Valsalva maneuver, opens and demonstrates the post-cricoid space.[30] Full tracheal examination can readily be performed by instillation of 3 to 5 mL of 2% lidocaine across the laryngeal vestibule and lumen. This can be administered through a mucosal atomization device (Figure 39–12), through the working channel of a laryngoscope, or through a thyrohyoid or cricothyroid injection. This procedure is safe to perform in the clinic but as with all airway interventions, full resuscitation facilities and personnel, and oxygen, must be available. A note of caution is performing this procedure in patients with laryngospasm, secondary breathing-pattern disorders, or high anxiety. In these patients, temporary inability to sense airflow through the larynx or trachea may cause claustrophobia and precipitate either laryngospasm or poorly controlled hyperventilation, which may then worsen airflow across a stricture. If a tracheoscopy is performed, then four standard views (see Figure 39–1$_{V1-4}$) should, as a minimum, be documented, and in patients with granulomatosis with polyangiitis or previous tuberculosis, the left and right main bronchi should also be visualized. These assessments may be readily performed using a standard flexible laryngoscope with video recording functionality.

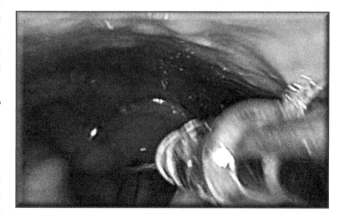

Figure 39–12. Use of a mucosal atomization device (MAD) to anesthetize the larynx and trachea to allow in-office laryngotracheoscopy.

Investigations

Supplementary investigations can provide stratification and prognostic assistance.

Blood Tests. All patients should undergo a complete blood count, basic blood biochemistry, and thyroid function tests. Inflammatory markers including erythrocyte sedimentation rate and c-reactive protein should be measured. An immune screen including angiotensin converting enzyme (ACE), anti-nuclear cytoplasmic antibody (ANCA) including myeloperoxidase (MPO) and proteinase 3 (PR3),[31] and rheumatoid factor (RF) titers should be measured as screening for systemic inflammation and vasculitis. In very specialist contexts other tests like matrilin assays for relapsing polychondritis[32] may be considered.

Flow Physiology. All patients should undergo a maximum-effort flow-volume loop[33] at each visit to the airway unit (Figure 39–13) and should be supplied with a flow meter to measure at least peak expiratory flow at regular intervals (Figure 39–14).

Effort Physiology. Cardiopulmonary exercise testing (CPET)[34] should become a routine test for evaluating laryngotracheal stenosis. It has proven utility in differentiating between causes of dyspnea.[35] It can also, as shown in the case presented, identify breathing-pattern disorders and may come to find particular utility in reducing the likelihood of secondary breathing pattern disorders developing in patients with recurrent disease processes like idiopathic subglottic stenosis, or in patients with chronic marginal laryngeal airways. Other tests like the six-minute walk test[36] or shuttle test[37] may also provide information about effort intolerance but they provide significantly less information compared with CPET.

Cross-sectional Imaging. Cross-sectional imaging and in particular, computed tomography of the neck and chest, has historically been used to establish the diagnosis of laryngotracheal stenosis. Imaging can now be reconstructed to provide 3-dimensional lumen views (Figure 39–15), and efforts are being made to investigate flow dynamics within reconstructed lumen geometries.[38] In practice, most patients continue to undergo

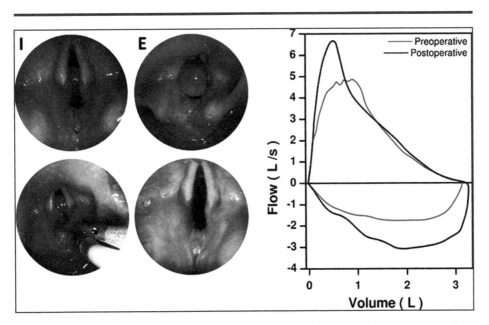

Figure 39–13. Maximum-effort flow-volume loops before and after treatment of an obstructive intubation granuloma arising from the medical surface of the left arytenoid cartilage. Features of note are improvement in the inspiratory portion of the loop, increase in peak expiratory flow and "sharpening" of the "expiratory peak."

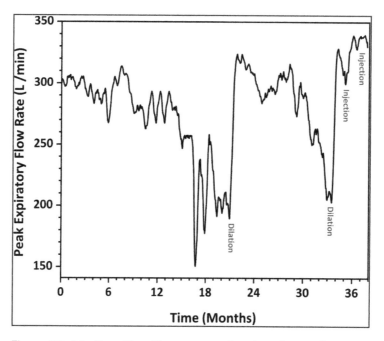

Figure 39–14. Biweekly rolling average of peak expiratory flow rates of one patient with idiopathic subglottic stenosis, measured daily for over 3 years, following treatment of idiopathic subglottic stenosis with endoscopic laryngotracheoplasty with biological inhibition. Changes in peak flow rate clearly identify initial and subsequent treatment failures.

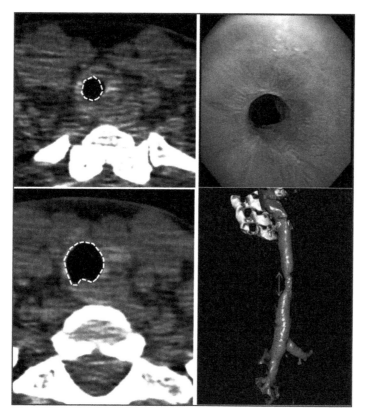

Figure 39–15. Computed tomography and 3-dimensional airway lumen reconstruction views from CT scans. The endoscopic image corresponds to the point of maximum narrowing of the stenosis.

CT scanning or are referred with cross-sectional imaging already performed. Cross-sectional imaging is useful in evaluating extraluminal causes of airway stenosis like vascular anomalies or compressive adenopathy. It also provides a useful screen of the lung tissue. It provides no information about mucosal status and in particular, presence of acute inflammatory stenoses, and as such, it does not by itself provide an adequate airway assessment and must, in all cases, be supplemented by direct visualization of the endoluminal mucosal surfaces.

Voice Analysis. Patients should undergo objective voice analysis. As a minimum, this should include perceptual voice assessment which may be performed using GRBAS or CAPE-V systems, and phonation time. Aerodynamic measures including transglottic flow rates and derived subglottic pressure may also provide insights. Strong consideration should be given to performing electroglottographic analysis of connected speech in all patients.[39,40]

Tests for Reflux. There should be a low threshold for requesting 24-hour pH and impedance monitoring,

especially for patients who are being considered for open laryngotracheal surgery.

Swallowing Function Tests. All patients who are being considered for open airway surgery, and all patients who are being considered for endoscopic surgery to the larynx, should undergo swallow function testing. A videofluoroscopic swallowing study (VFSS) is the preoperative investigation of choice and a minimum standard of care, while functional endoscopic evaluation of swallowing (FEES) may be preferred for monitoring swallowing safety following airway surgery.

Tissue Biopsy. Diagnosis of airway obstruction secondary to intubation-related laryngotracheal stenosis does not require histological confirmation. However, biopsies are useful in establishing diagnoses other than intubation-related stenosis, including vasculitis,[19] non-caseating granulomata in sarcoidosis,[41] Mickulicz cells in rhinoscleroma,[42] apple green birefringence with polarized light examination in amyloidosis,[43] immunofluorescence studies in mucosal pemphigoid,[44] and different tumor pathologies. At present, the differentiation between acute inflammatory and mature fibrotic stenoses is endoscopic (Figure 39–16) but it is likely

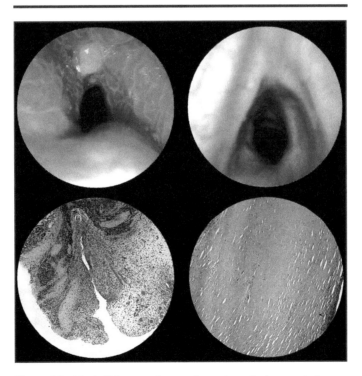

Figure 39–16. Left images show endoscopic and microscopic images of acute inflammatory airway stenosis. Right images show endoscopic and microscopic images of a mature fibrotic airway stenosis.

that as novel therapeutic approaches become available and scar tissue modulation becomes more tailored to the underlying abnormalities of the scar formation pathways,[45] the role of biopsies to guide personalized treatment approaches will increase.

Management of Intubation-Related Laryngotracheal Stenosis

Extent of pathology and underlying etiology will help determine effective management strategies.

Acute Inflammatory Obstructions Versus Mature Fibrotic Strictures. The prime consideration in managing adult intubation-related laryngotracheal stenosis is whether the lesion is acute and inflammatory or chronic and fibrotic (Figure 39–17).[29] Acute inflammatory lesions almost invariably respond to treatment with intralesional depot corticosteroids, judicious laser treatment, controlled radial dilation, and regular follow-up with repeat procedures to manage the evolution of the scarring process.

Laryngeal Versus Tracheal Stenosis. The next consideration is the exact location and pattern of the stenosis, what specific structures have been damaged, and whether or not the stenosis involves the larynx. Management of intubation-related bilateral vocal fold immobility continues to evolve. Vocal cordotomy or a partial arytenoidectomy are minimally invasive procedures but ones that can be associated with voice morbidity, airway violation of food and fluid, and a recurrence rate.[46–49] A laryngotracheal reconstruction, consisting of a laryngofissure, posterior cricoid split, and placement of a T-shaped costal cartilage graft has been the mainstay reconstructive approach for managing interarytenoid scarring,[1] and transoral approaches for performing the same procedure have also been described.[50] The larynx, however, is a dynamic structure and laryngeal movements regulate the respiratory time-constant.[51] As such, static procedures at best offer a very partial solution to managing laryngeal stenosis due to posterior commissure scarring. Moreover, placing a costal cartilage graft necessarily leads to healing by secondary intention and over a period of months to a few years, a combination of ongoing scar contracture and graft resorption leads to stenosis recurrence in a significant proportion of cases.

The use of local post-cricoid flaps for posterior glottic wound closure combined with intra-articular cricoarytenoid joint surgery represents a major paradigm shift from static glottic widening toward laryngeal remobilization and restoration of respiratory and phonatory laryngeal movements. The cricoarytenoid joint is unusual in that it can remain viable for up to 17 years after denervation[52] and in cases of joint ankylosis, careful intra-articular division of adhesions or partial excision of the joint may restore laryngeal mobility. In this context, a comparison may be drawn between mobility of an abnormal cricoarytenoid joint and a Girdlestone hip.[53] The principal approach for achieving laryngeal remobilization is through the use of the post-cricoid flap combined with intra-articular joint remobilization.[54] This operation may be performed endoscopically in many cases or, in cases of damaged cricoid cartilage or unfavorable transoral access, may be performed as a combined glottic reconstruction via a laryngofissure combined with costal cartilage grafting that is placed under a post-cricoid mucosal flap for primary mucosal wound closure (Figures 39–18 and 39–19).[55]

Tracheal Stenosis Configuration. There are a number of classification systems for laryngotracheal stenosis and the best known is the Myer–Cotton grade (see Figure 39–1M$_{C1-4}$). This system characterizes the degree of cross-sectional obstruction as being less than 50%, between 51% and 70%, between 71% and 99%, and 100%. It was devised for pediatric airway surgery where the subglottis is the narrowest part of the airway and the severity of subglottic injury is reflected in the degree of cross-sectional narrowing.[56] As such, in children, the degree of cross-sectional impairment provides information about disease prognosis. This is not the case in adults, where in practice, although the degree of cross-sectional obstruction is often documented, it does not provide the same prognostic information compared with pediatric cases. Figure 39–20 provides a framework for identifying and documenting individual components of a global approach to airway assessment. Specific injuries may be managed using specific procedures. For example, an isolated cricoid injury can be managed with a hyoid-on-sternohyoid flap[57] or a cricotracheal resection[58] using the trachea to reconstruct the anterior cricoid arch. A lambdoid deformity may be managed using endoscopic resection tracheoplasty,[16] as demonstrated in the case presented. Structural tracheal collapse, if resectable, should be managed with tracheal resection,[59,60] and unresectable lengths may be reconstructed with augmentation tracheoplasty[61,62] or maintained with long-term stents. In selected cases, an injury may heal in a favorable position around a long-term soft silicon tracheal stent. There are very few, if any, indications for circumferential tracheal replacement for

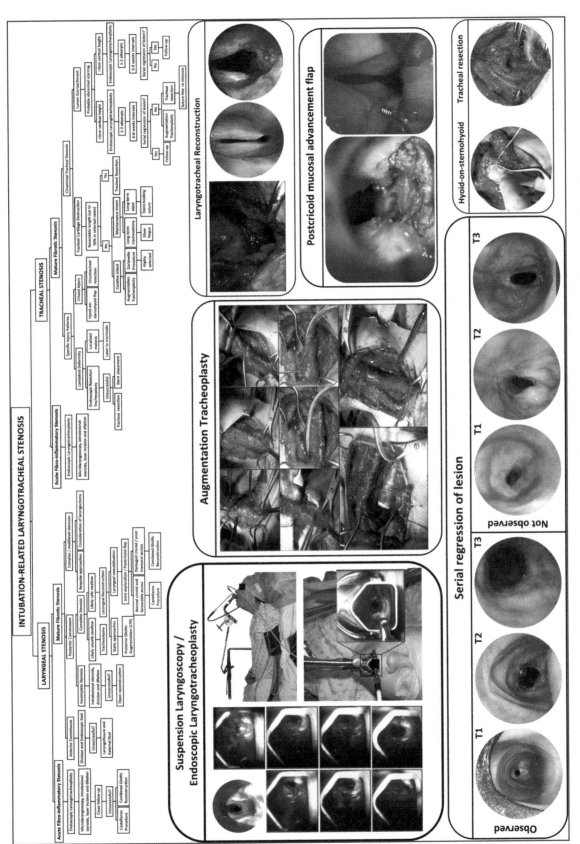

Figure 39–17. A decision tree and images of key surgical procedures used for managing intubation-related laryngotracheal stenosis.

415

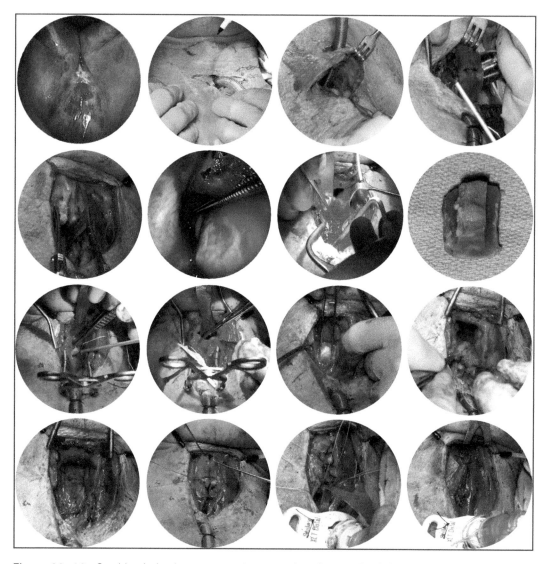

Figure 39–18. Combined glottic reconstruction procedure for treating bilateral vocal fold immobility due to interarytenoid scarring in the presence of poor transoral access and/or injury to the cricoid cartilage, precluding transoral reconstructive laryngeal microsurgery.

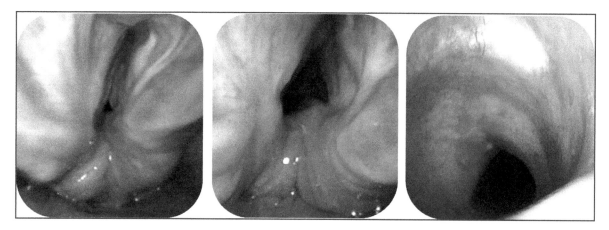

Figure 39–19. Outcome of combined glottic reconstruction four months after treatment, showing restoration of laryngeal mobility, lowering of post-cricoid height, and healed tracheostomy scar.

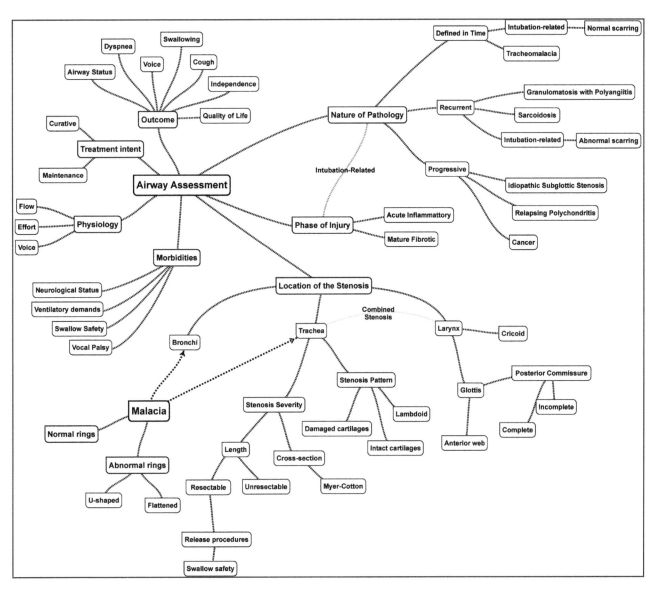

Figure 39–20. A framework for outcomes documentation in laryngotracheal stenosis.

benign intubation-related laryngotracheal stenosis and in particular, the bar for considering tracheal transplantation for this condition should be set extraordinarily high indeed. In that highly unusual scenario where any form of circumferential tracheal replacement for benign intubation-related laryngotracheal stenosis is contemplated, an autologous replacement using the Dartevelle[63] or Olias[77] procedures should be considered.

Structural Collapse Versus Lamina Propria Fibrosis. Patients with lumen-encroaching strictures within a normal cartilaginous framework warrant special conside-

ration. An interesting trend has been the change in dominant pattern of intubation-related tracheal stenosis from a combined mucosal and cartilaginous injury that is associated with the collapse of the tracheal structure, to a lamina propria disease characterized by formation of a lumen-encroaching cicatrix within a largely intact tracheal cartilaginous framework (Figure 39–21). This may be a corollary of greater awareness of airway injuries by intensive care clinicians and as a result, better care of endotracheal tubes and earlier switch to tracheostomy. In this context, if a stenosis still develops, and particularly an injury that does not involve

418

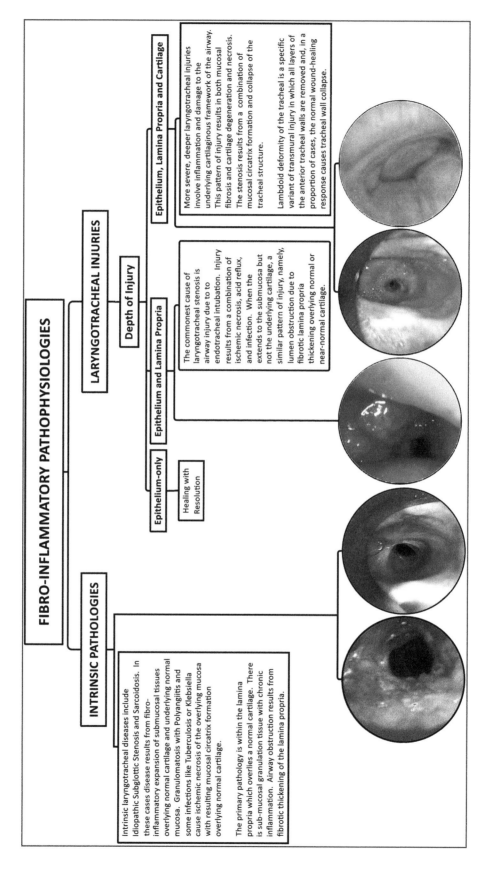

FIBRO-INFLAMMATORY PATHOPHYSIOLOGIES

INTRINSIC PATHOLOGIES

Intrinsic laryngotracheal diseases include Idiopathic Subglottic Stenosis and Sarcoidosis. In these cases disease results from fibro-inflammatory expansion of submucosal tissues overlying normal cartilage and underlying normal mucosa. Granulomatosis with Polyangiitis and some infections like Tuberculosis or Klebsiella cause ischemic necrosis of the overlying mucosa with resulting mucosal circatrix formation overlying normal cartilage.

The primary pathology is within the lamina propria which overlies a normal cartilage. There is sub-mucosal granulation tissue with chronic inflammation. Airway obstruction results from fibrotic thickening of the lamina propria.

LARYNGOTRACHEAL INJURIES

Depth of Injury

Epithelium-only

Healing with Resolution

Epithelium and Lamina Propria

The commonest cause of laryngotracheal stenosis is airway injury due to endotracheal intubation. Injury results from a combination of ischemic necrosis, acid reflux, and infection. When the extends to the submucosa but not the underlying cartilage, a similar pattern of injury, namely, lumen obstruction due to fibrotic lamina propria thickening overlying normal or near-normal cartilage.

Epithelium, Lamina Propria and Cartilage

More severe, deeper laryngotracheal injuries involve inflammation and damage to the underlying cartilaginous framework of the airway. This pattern of injury results in both mucosal fibrosis and cartilage degeneration and necrosis. The stenosis results from a combination of mucosal circatrix formation and collapse of the tracheal structure.

Lambdoid deformity of the tracheal is a specific variant of transmural injury in which all layers of the anterior tracheal walls are removed and, in a proportion of cases, the normal wound-healing response causes tracheal wall collapse.

Figure 39–21. Pathophysiology of laryngotracheal stenosis as a function of depth of injury.

cartilage, it is likely to be a manifestation of abnormal wound-healing response rather than an iatrogenic complication per se. As such, a tracheal resection is more likely to cause suture-line restenosis and recurrence. These patients are initially managed with planned and staged endoscopic laryngotracheoplasty (see Figure 39–17) and are observed for "serial regression of lesion." This is attempted using the standard "endoscopic laryngotracheoplasty" procedure, which consists of suspension laryngoscopy using a Dedo–Pilling laryngoscope, intralesional injection of 60 to 80 mg of methylprednisolone acetate, cruciate laser incision at 5 watts continuous CO_2 laser setting, and stenosis dilation using a controlled radial expansion balloon. Mitomycin C[64] is generally not used due to its association with significant post-procedure pain and risk of acute airway crusting. If serial regression of lesion does not occur, then augmentation tracheoplasty, which aims both to introduce new tissue and to break the circumferential scar, is considered. Use of antimetabolite therapy for highly selected cases of rapidly recurrent laryngotracheal stenosis[65] is favorably but cautiously considered. The recent year has seen an increase in modulating fibrosis using existing novel agents and existing medications in this new indication,[66,67] and as genomic[68] and transcriptomic analyses provide increasingly patient-tailored targets for modulating recurrent scar formation, it is likely that the role of novel agents and existing agents in novel indications will increase.

Treatment Intent and Shared Decision Making

A prosthesis-free airway capable of meeting the ventilatory demands of the patient, accompanied by normal voice and swallowing functions, is the goal of laryngotracheal reconstructive surgery. This goal is achievable in the majority of patients, and indeed for many patients it can be achieved using only minimally invasive surgical techniques. The main considerations relate to the stenosis configuration, patients' general fitness to undergo surgery, and, when laryngeal surgery is considered, safety of swallowing and risk of aspiration (see Figure 39–20).

In some cases, like the patient presented, this can be achieved with a single endoscopic procedure lasting less than an hour. In other cases, definitive airway treatment may require more extensive open cervico-mediastinal surgery, with the ultimate expectation being long-term restoration of the airway without the need for ongoing maintenance treatments. However, not all patients and not all stenoses lend themselves to curative treatment. For example, patients with post-radiation laryngeal ste-

nosis and patients with complex stenoses involving both the larynx and trachea may not be reconstructable. Caution must be exercised over blinkered or narrow decision making—once the patient and the surgeon have resolved to keep out a tracheostomy at all cost, with each maintenance procedure, the decision to consider either a tracheostomy or a laryngectomy becomes progressively more difficult to revisit, and target fixation may cause major patient harm.

Repeated hospital admissions for stenosis dilation and airway maintenance can reinforce the sick role, and dysfunctional breathing as a consequence of fluctuations in a patient's ability to breathe consistently can rapidly develop. This can lead to significant physical and psychological morbidity and repeated emergency hospital admissions. Moreover, living with a chronically marginal airway places the patient at ongoing risk of acute-on-chronic respiratory failure, particularly during episodes of intercurrent respiratory infections, and this may ultimately prove fatal. In addition, endoscopic treatment for intubation-related laryngotracheal stenosis is less cost-effective than open surgery,[69] and this will be particularly the case when treatment turns to an open-ended approach of multiple and repeated hospital admissions for secondary dysfunctional breathing principally to avoid a stent or a tracheostomy.

Professor Isaac Eliachar described the technique of a permanent tubeless tracheostomy for non-reconstructable laryngotracheal stenoses.[70] A further option is the use of a Silver Negus tracheostomy,[71] which may reduce the morbidity associated with tracheostomy maintenance. A long-term tracheostomy and an intraluminal airway stent are doubtless associated with reductions in the patient's quality of life and are to be avoided if possible. However, if deemed necessary, they must not be seen as treatment failures by either the patient or the surgeon and their use should be considered early for selected patients.

Outcomes Assessment

Assessing what management pathways provide the best outcomes is difficult in airway stenosis, as quantifiable measures do not always equate to patient-rated success.

Pathology–Based Stratification. The primary consideration in relation to outcomes and what constitutes treatment success in laryngotracheal stenosis is the nature of the underlying pathology. For example, idiopathic subglottic stenosis is a progressive fibromatosis with a high expectation of recurrence following endoscopic treatment.[24] A lambdoid tracheal deformity, on the other hand, is a structural stenosis caused by contracture of the anterior tracheal wall following removal of a tracheostomy in the context of otherwise normal wound healing.[16] The expectation following endoscopic treatment is therefore full and permanent resolution of the condition. Stenosis recurrence following treatment of a lambdoid tracheal deformity therefore constitutes a true treatment failure, whereas stenosis recurrence after endoscopic treatment of idiopathic subglottic stenosis is expected. As such, even though both conditions cause laryngotracheal stenosis, the appropriate statistical methodology for studying these two conditions varies, being actuarial analysis for lambdoid tracheal deformity and intervention-free interval for idiopathic subglottic stenosis.

Defining Treatment Success. Decannulation rate has been used to measure treatment success. However, in contemporary practice, many stenosis patients do not receive tracheostomies, and decannulation rate alone, in the absence of information about functional outcomes, does not provide a picture of treatment success that is even remotely adequate. There is a pyramid of outcomes which, at the lowest level, involve impact of surgery on stenosis anatomy. The next set of outcomes are physiological and measure the impact of the presence and treatment of the stenosis on flow limitation and effort tolerance. Toward this, minimum clinically important difference (MCID) values for flow-volume loops have been calculated.[72] As demonstrated in the case presented, the relationship between anatomy, physiology, and symptoms is not always clear-cut and since ultimately intubation-related laryngotracheal stenosis is a benign condition, what matters is the extent to which treatment leads to improvements in the patient's symptoms and quality of life, that is, **efficacy** of treatment. **Durability** of treatment defines how long these improvements last, and **patient safety** assesses both incidence of general and disease-specific complications, and duration of time a patient is exposed to risk (Figure 39–22). For example, a patient with idiopathic subglottic stenosis may be treated with serial endoscopic treatments, including serial in-office steroid injections. This treatment approach has good efficacy, short durability, and low risk in terms of exposure to major complications of open surgery. It does, however, have a higher risk of exposing the patient to dysfunctional breathing in the longer term and to proximal stenosis migration and glottic fixation. A cricotracheal resection has over 90% long-term cure rate but it does expose the patient to complications of ma-

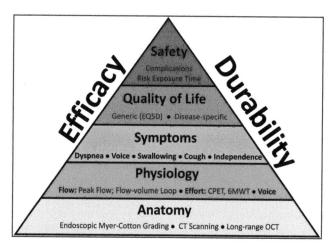

Figure 39–22. The outcomes assessment pyramid for laryngotracheal stenosis.

jor surgery and places the patient at risk of permanent voice morbidity. An endoscopic laryngotracheoplasty with biological inhibition may likewise achieve long-term disease remission,[73] but exposes the patient to significant long-term risk of chronic cough and mucus. The shared decision on surgical approach is informed by a multitude of factors related to upfront and long-term risks, morbidities associated with different domains affected by the disease and its treatment, and the array of outcomes tools used to measure treatment success and compare different approaches need to comprehensively assess the different domains that are affected by the disease and its treatment. A holistic approach to outcomes assessment in laryngotracheal stenosis depends on the integration and communication of the different types and probabilities of expected risk and benefit in the context of a shared decision-making process with the patient, and while excellent research is now being performed in this area,[69,74] a significant body of work remains to be done.

Outcomes Assessment Instruments. As discussed above, outcomes assessment in laryngotracheal stenosis is an area that is undergoing rapid evolution at this time. Table 39–2 provides the range of outcomes assessment instruments that are currently deployed at the Robert White Centre for Airway Voice and Swallowing.

Prevention

A full discussion of the risk factors for the occurrence of intubation-related laryngotracheal stenosis and the

Table 39–2. Outcomes Assessment Instruments for Laryngotracheal Stenosis

	When Assessed	Instruments Used
Anatomy		
Distance from glottis	Every visit	
Cross-section of the stenosis	Every visit	
Physiology		
Voice	Every visit	GRBAS
	Every Visit	Electroglottogram
Flow	Every visit	Peak expiratory flow
		Flow-volume loop
Effort	Major treatments	Cardiopulmonary Exercise
Symptoms	Every visit	ADV-CSI Instrument
	Major treatments	VHI10
		EAT10
		CCQ
		HCQ
Quality of life	Major treatments	EQ5D

strategies deployed to reduce its incidence are beyond the scope of this chapter. The use of high-volume low-pressure endotracheal cuffs and careful monitoring of endotracheal cuff pressures during critical illness are now near-universal practices within modern intensive care medicine. Use of tubes which contain a subglottic suction port to reduce tracheal exposure to digestive enzymes is also becoming standard of care. While traumatic intubation, particularly in the settings of cardiopulmonary resuscitation, cannot always be prevented, good attention to sedation technique and management of agitation may reduce ongoing trauma. Hemodynamic instability and in particular prolonged hypotension reduce tracheal perfusion pressure and need to be carefully managed. Paying close attention to endotracheal tube selection and in particular taking account of patient height as well as sex in choosing the most appropriate tube size may be particularly helpful in reducing inter-arytenoid trauma.

A particularly pertinent consideration for the airway surgeon is the timing of switch from endotracheal tube to tracheostomy. A tracheal stenosis, if it develops, can be successfully managed in the overwhelming majority of cases and as demonstrated in this case and previously published,[16] lambdoid tracheal deformity which is a specific complication of tracheostomy placement is particularly amenable to treatment. By contrast, a mature interarytenoid scar causing bilateral vocal fold immobility is one of the most complex airway injuries to manage. While development of endoscopic and open laryngeal remobilization procedures is beginning to change the poor outcome of this injury, prevention remains far more desirable. Interarytenoid scarring exclusively occurs in translaryngeal intubation. Interestingly, patient height is an independent risk-factor for the development of this injury,[23] and this reinforces the notion of a height-inappropriate, abnormally large endotracheal tube causing inter-arytenoid ulceration and stenosis formation. There is an expanding literature on the relative merits of early vs late tracheostomy within the broader intensive care context, but from an airway surgical perspective, an early tracheostomy, in the sole context of preventing a laryngeal injury, even at the expense of a higher risk of tracheal injury, is a desirable strategy.

Screening for Intubation-Related Laryngotracheal Stenosis

Intubation-related laryngotracheal stenosis fulfills the World Health Organization criteria (Table 39–3) as a condition that should be screened for.[75] Its identification and treatment is wholly consistent with guidelines issued by the National Institute of Health and Care Excellence for rehabilitating adults following critical illness (CG83).[76] An important factor to consider, however, is the numbers needed to treat. At or shortly

Table 39–3. Wilson and Junger Criteria for Screening Programs

• The condition sought should be an important health problem.
• There should be an accepted treatment for patients with recognized disease.
• Facilities for diagnosis and treatment should be available.
• There should be a recognizable latent or early symptomatic stage.
• There should be a suitable test or examination.
• The test should be acceptable to the population.
• The natural history of the condition, including development from latent to declared disease, should be adequately understood.
• There should be an agreed policy on whom to treat as patients.
• The cost of case-finding (including diagnosis and treatment of patients diagnosed) should be economically balanced in relation to possible expenditure on medical care as a whole.
• Case-finding should be a continuing process and not a "once and for all" project.

following extubation, almost half of all patients have evidence of significant laryngotracheal injury, and yet fewer than 10% of these patients go on to develop significant long-term laryngotracheal stenosis.[26] As such, acute intervention for every laryngotracheal injury would lead to significant overtreatment.

One possible and pragmatic approach is to perform at least a laryngoscopy on every patient within 48 hours of extubation (Figure 39–23). This can be done by the critical care team in partnership with the laryngologist. All patients with post-extubation stridor should be further assessed and if necessary treated. Among patients who are minimally symptomatic, patients with laryngeal injury, and in particular patients with inter-arytenoid ulceration should be acutely treated to reduce the likelihood of progression to bilateral vocal fold immobility due to inter-arytenoid scarring. Patients with evidence of significant but asymptomatic tracheal injury should be followed up with office tracheoscopy and flow-volume loops and only treated if they develop airway symptoms. All critical care follow-up clinics should have access to flow-volume loop testing and ideally to office laryngotracheoscopy. There is a clear progression in the natural history of intubation-related laryngotracheal stenosis from readily treatable acute fibro-inflammatory lesion

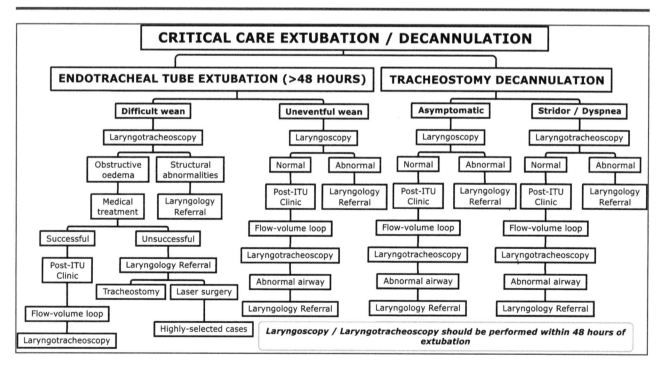

Figure 39–23. An approach for screening for intubation-related laryngotracheal stenosis.

to mature fibrotic scars that can be much harder to treat. While occurrence of an airway stenosis is multifactorial and by no means per se evidence of poor care, failure to identify and arrange for early intervention for an evolving stenosis would be more difficult to justify, and in particular all effort must be made to identify and treat laryngeal injuries early.

SUMMARY

Intubation and tracheostomy-related injuries and strictures are the most common cause of adult laryngotracheal stenosis. Injuries follow specific anatomic patterns and demonstrate temporal evolution from acute fibro-inflammatory lesions toward mature fibrotic strictures that are more difficult to treat. Injury prevention is critical and increasing attention to airway care during critical illness has reduced the incidence of this injury. Different patterns of injury are treatable with a small number of tailored surgical approaches, and strong consideration should be given to screening all patients following intubation and mechanical ventilation in order to identify and treat lesions early in order to prevent progression to mature fibrotic strictures.

REFERENCES

1. Sandhu GS, Nouraei SAR, eds. *Laryngeal and Tracheobronchial Stenosis*. San Diego, CA: Plural Publishing; 2015.
2. Mark EJ, Meng F, Kradin RL, Mathisen DJ, Matsubara O. Idiopathic tracheal stenosis: a clinicopathologic study of 63 cases and comparison of the pathology with chondromalacia. *Am J Surg Pathol*. 2008;32:1138–1143.
3. Galvin IF, Shepherd DRT, Gibbons JRP. Tracheal stenosis caused by congenital vascular ring anomaly misinterpreted as asthma for 45 years. *Thorac Cardiovasc Surg*. 1990;38:42–44.
4. Nunn AC, Nouraei SA, George PJ, Sandhu GS, Nouraei SA. Not always asthma: clinical and legal consequences of delayed diagnosis of laryngotracheal stenosis. *Case Rep Otolaryngol*. 2014;2014:325048.
5. Ryland F. *A Treatise on the Diseases and Injuries of the Larynx and Trachea*. London, UK: Longman, Rees, Orme, Brown, Green and Co; 1837.
6. Colles CJ. I. On stenosis of the trachea after tracheotomy for croup and diphtheria. *Ann Surg*. 1886;3(6):499–507.
7. Berthelsen PG, Cronqvist M. The first intensive care unit in the world: Copenhagen 1953. *Acta Anaesthesiol Scand*. 2003;47(10):1190–1195.
8. Ibsen B. Bulbar poliomyelitis and its treatment from the anaesthetist's viewpoint. *Arch Belg Med Soc*. 1954;12(4-5):13641.
9. Trubuhovich RV. August 26th 1952 at Copenhagen: 'Bjørn Ibsen's Day'; a significant event for Anaesthesia. *Acta Anaesthesiol Scand*. 2004;48(3):27–27.
10. Dayal VS, el Masri W. Tracheostomy in intensive care setting. *Laryngoscope*. 1986;96(1):58–60.
11. Sugerman HJ, Wolfe L, Pasquale MD, et al. Multicenter, randomized, prospective trial of early tracheostomy. *J Trauma*. 1997;43(5):741–747.
12. Hoffman G, Kerr G, Leavitt R, et al. Wegener granulomatosis: an analysis of 158 patients. *Ann Intern Med*. 1992;116:488–498.
13. Fauci A, Haynes B, Katz P, Wolff S. Wegener's granulomatosis: prospective clinical and therapeutic experience with 85 patients for 21 years. *Ann Intern Med*. 1983; 98:76–85.
14. Lebovics RS, Hoffman GS, Leavitt RY, et al. The management of subglottic stenosis in patients with Wegener's granulomatosis. *Laryngoscope*. 1992;102:1341–1345.
15. Nouraei SAR, Kapoor KV, Nouraei SM, Ghufoor K, Howard DJ, Sandhu GS. Results of endoscopic tracheoplasty for treating tracheostomy-related airway stenosis. *Clin Otolaryngol*. 2007;32:471–475.
16. Nouraei SA, Sandhu GS. Outcome of endoscopic resection tracheoplasty for treating lambdoid tracheal stomal stenosis. *Laryngoscope*. 2013;123(7):1735–1741.
17. Nouraei SAR, Ma E, Patel A, Howard DJ, Sandhu GS. Estimating the population incidence of adult post-intubation laryngotracheal stenosis. *Clin Otolaryngol*. 2007; 32:411–412.
18. Nouraei S, Battson R, Koury E, Sandhu G, Patel A. Adult post-intubation laryngotracheal stenosis: an underestimated complication of intensive care? *J Intensive Care Soc*. 2009;10:229.
19. Gluth MB, Shinners PA, Kasperbauer JL. Subglottic stenosis associated with Wegener's granulomatosis. *Laryngoscope*. 2003;113(8):1304–1307.
20. Thomas R, Kumar EV, Kameswaran M, et al. Post intubation laryngeal sequelae in an intensive care unit. *J Laryngol Otol*. 1995;109(4):313–316.
21. Karmakar A, Pate MB, Solowski NL, Postma GN, Weinberger PM. Tracheal size variability is associated with sex: implications for endotracheal tube selection. *Ann Otol Rhinol Laryngol*. 2015;124(2):132–136.
22. Tai A, Corke C, Joynt GM, Griffith J, Lunn D, Tong P. A comparative study of tracheal diameter in Caucasian and Chinese patients. *Anaesth Intensive Care*. 2016;44(6):719–723.
23. Katsantonis NG, Kabagambe EK, Wootten CT, Ely EW, Francis DO, Gelbard A. Height is an independent risk factor for postintubation laryngeal injury. *Laryngoscope*. 2018;128(12):2811–2814.
24. Nouraei SA, Sandhu GS. Outcome of a multimodality approach to the management of idiopathic subglottic stenosis. *Laryngoscope*. 2013;123(10):2474–2484.

25. Suppiah R, Mukhtyar C, Flossmann O, et al. A cross-sectional study of the Birmingham Vasculitis Activity Score version 3 in systemic vasculitis. *Rheumatology (Oxford)*. 2011;50:899–905.

26. Esteller-Moré E, Ibañez J, Matiñó E, Ademà JM, Nolla M, Quer IM. Prognostic factors in laryngotracheal injury following intubation and/or tracheotomy in ICU patients. *Eur Arch Otorhinolaryngol*. 2005;262(11):880–883.

27. Nouraei SAR, Heathcote KJ. A patient-centred multidomain instrument for improving the clarity of outcomes reporting and documentation in complex airway surgery. *Clin Otolaryngol*. 2018;43(6):1634–1639.

28. Nouraei SAR. Outcome of endoscopic treatment of adult postintubation tracheal stenosis. *Laryngoscope*. 2007;117:1073–1079.

29. Nouraei S, Singh A, Patel A, Ferguson C, Howard D, Sandhu G. Early endoscopic treatment of acute inflammatory airway lesions improves the outcome of postintubation airway stenosis. *Laryngoscope*. 2006;116:1417–1421.

30. Sakai A, Okami K, Sugimoto R, et al. A new technique to expose the hypopharyngeal space: the modified Killian's method. *Auris Nasus Larynx*. 2014;41(2):207–210.

31. Watts RA, Robson J. Introduction, epidemiology and classification of vasculitis. *Best Pract Res Clin Rheumatol*. 2018;32(1):3–20.

32. Hansson AS, Holmdahl R. Cartilage-specific autoimmunity in animal models and clinical aspects in patients—focus on relapsing polychondritis. *Arthritis Res*. 2002;4(5):296–301.

33. Hyatt RE. Evaluation of major airway lesions using the flow-volume loop. *Ann Otol Rhinol Laryngol*. 1975;84(5 pt 1):635–642.

34. Mezzani A. Cardiopulmonary exercise testing: basics of methodology and measurements. *Ann Am Thorac Soc*. 2017;14(suppl 1):S3–S11.

35. Guazzi M, Bandera F, Ozemek C, Systrom D, Arena R. Cardiopulmonary exercise testing: what is its value? *J Am Coll Cardiol*. 2017;70(13):1618–1636.

36. Brown AW, Nathan SD. The value and application of the 6-minute-walk test in idiopathic pulmonary fibrosis. *Ann Am Thorac Soc*. 2018;15(1):3–10.

37. Hill K, Ng C, Wootton SL, et al. The minimal detectable difference for endurance shuttle walk test performance in people with COPD on completion of a program of high-intensity ground-based walking. *Respir Med*. 2019;146:18–22.

38. Cheng T, Carpenter D, Cohen S, Witsell D, Frank-Ito DO. Investigating the effects of laryngotracheal stenosis on upper airway aerodynamics. *Laryngoscope*. 2018;128(4):E141–E149.

39. Dejonckere PH, Lebacq J. Acoustic, perceptual, aerodynamic and anatomical correlations in voice pathology. *ORL*. 1996;58:326–332.

40. Hirano M. *Clinical Examination of Voice*. Springer; 1981.

41. Polychronopoulos VS, Prakash UBS. Airway involvement in sarcoidosis. *Chest*. 2009;136(5):1371–1380.

42. Verma G, Kanawaty D, Hyland R. Rhinoscleroma causing upper airway obstruction. *Can Respir J*. 2005;12(1):43–45.

43. Ginat DT, Schulte J, Portugal L, Cipriani NA. Laryngotracheal involvement in systemic light chain amyloidosis. *Head Neck Pathol*. 2018;12(1):127–130.

44. Maglie R, Borgi A, Caproni M, Antiga E. Indirect immunofluorescence in mucous membrane pemphigoid: which substrate should be used? *Br J Dermatol*. 2019;180:1266-1267.

45. Luo YH, Ouyang PB, Tian J, Guo XJ, Duan XC. Rosiglitazone inhibits TGF-beta 1 induced activation of human Tenon fibroblasts via p38 signal pathway. *PLoS One*. 2014;9(8):e105796.

46. Al-Fattah HA, Hamza A, Gaafar A, Tantawy A. Partial laser arytenoidectomy in the management of bilateral vocal fold immobility: a modification based on functional anatomical study of the cricoarytenoid joint. *Otolaryngol Head Neck Surg*. 2006;134:294–301.

47. Aubry K, Leboulanger N, Harris R, Genty E, Denoyelle F, Garabedian E-N. Laser arytenoidectomy in the management of bilateral vocal cord paralysis in children. *Int J Pediatr Otorhinolaryngol*. 2010;74(5):451–455.

48. Riffat F, Palme CE, Veivers D. Endoscopic treatment of glottic stenosis: a report on the safety and efficacy of CO_2 laser. *J Laryngol Otol*. 2011:1–3.

49. Yilmaz T, Suslu N, Atay G, Ozer S, Gunaydin RO, Bajin MD. Comparison of voice and swallowing parameters after endoscopic total and partial arytenoidectomy for bilateral abductor vocal fold paralysis: a randomized trial. *JAMA Otolaryngol Head Neck Surg*. 2013;139(7):712–718.

50. Yawn RJ, Daniero JJ, Gelbard A, Wootten CT. Novel application of the Sonopet for endoscopic posterior split and cartilage graft laryngoplasty. *Laryngoscope*. 2016;126(4):941–944.

51. Brancatisano TP, Dodd DS, Engel LA. Respiratory activity of posterior cricoarytenoid muscle and vocal cords in humans. *J Appl Physiol Respir Environ Exerc Physiol*. 1984;57(4):1143–1149.

52. Gacek M, Gacek RR. Cricoarytenoid joint mobility after chronic vocal cord paralysis. *Laryngoscope*. 1996;106(12 Pt 1):1528–1530.

53. Vincenten CM, Den Oudsten BL, Bos PK, Bolder SBT, Gosens T. Quality of life and health status after Girdlestone resection arthroplasty in patients with an infected total hip prosthesis. *J Bone Jt Infect*. 2019;4(1):10–15.

54. Atallah I, Mk M, Al Omari A, Righini CA, Castellanos PF. Cricoarytenoid joint ankylosis: classification and transoral laser microsurgical treatment. *J Voice*. 2018.

55. Nouraei SAR, Dorman EB, Vokes DE. Management of posterior glottic stenosis using the combined glottic reconstruction procedure. *Clin Otolaryngol*. 2018;43(5):1415–1418.

56. Myer C, O'Connor D, Cotton R. Proposed grading system for subglottic stenosis based on endotracheal tube sizes. *Ann Otol Rhinol Laryngol*. 1994;103:319–323.

57. Burstein FD, Canalis R, Ward PH. Composite hyoid-sternohyoid interposition graft revisited: UCLA experience 1974-1984. *Laryngoscope*. 1986;96(5):516–520.

58. Laccourreye O, Brasnu D, Seckin S, Hans S, Biacabe B, Laccourreye H. Cricotracheal anastomosis for assisted ventilation-induced stenosis. *Arch Otolaryngol Head Neck Surg.* 1997;123(10):1074–1077.

59. Wilson RS. Tracheal resection In: Marshall BE, Longnecker DE, Fairley HB, eds, *Anesthesia for Thoracic Procedures.* Boston, MA: Blackwell Scientific; 1988:415–432.

60. Johnson VA, Sanders RJ, Altshuler JH, Cooper DR. Tracheal resection with end-to-end anastomosis. *Rocky Mt Med J.* 1970;67(12):45–48.

61. Eliachar I. The rotary door flap: a breakthrough in laryngotracheal reconstruction. *Ear Nose Throat J.* 1992;71: 584–586.

62. Nouraei SAR, Nouraei SM, Sandison A, Howard DJ, Sandhu GS. The prefabricated sternohyoid myocartilagenous flap: a reconstructive option for treating recalcitrant adult laryngotracheal stenosis. *Laryngoscope.* 2008; 118(4):687–691.

63. Fabre D, Kolb F, Fadel E, et al. Successful tracheal replacement in humans using autologous tissues: an 8-year experience. *Ann Thorac Surg.* 2013;96(4):1146–1155.

64. Whited CW, Dailey SH. Is mitomycin C useful as an adjuvant therapy in endoscopic treatment of laryngotracheal stenosis? *Laryngoscope.* 2015;125(10):2243–2244.

65. Rosow DE, Ahmed J. Initial experience with low-dose methotrexate as an adjuvant treatment for rapidly recurrent nonvasculitic laryngotracheal stenosis. *JAMA Otolaryngol Head Neck Surg.* 2017;143(2):125–130.

66. Ekinci A, Koc S, Erdogan AS, Kesici H. Profilactic role of simvastatin and mitomycin C in tracheal stenosis after tracheal damage: study in rats. *Int J Pediatr Otorhinolaryngol.* 2018;105:79–84.

67. Namba DR, Ma G, Samad I, et al. Rapamycin inhibits human laryngotracheal stenosis-derived fibroblast proliferation, metabolism, and function in vitro. *Otolaryngol Head Neck Surg.* 2015;152(5):881–888.

68. Anis MM, Zhao Z, Khurana J, Krynetskiy E, Soliman AM. Translational genomics of acquired laryngotracheal stenosis. *Laryngoscope.* 2014;124(5):E175–E179.

69. Yin LX, Padula WV, Gadkaree S, et al. Health care costs and cost-effectiveness in laryngotracheal stenosis. *Otolaryngol Head Neck Surg.* 2018:194599818815068.

70. Eliachar I, Levine SC, Tucker HM. A modified technique for tubeless tracheostomy. *Otolaryngol Head Neck Surg.* 1986;94:548–552.

71. Tzifa KT, Jeynes PJ, Shehab ZP, Proops DW. Cosmetic tracheostomy locket: an attempt to improve the aesthetic component of tracheostomy tubes. *J Laryngol Otol.* 2000;114(10):777–778.

72. Nouraei SM, Franco RA, Dowdall JR, et al. Physiology-based minimum clinically important difference thresholds in adult laryngotracheal stenosis. *Laryngoscope.* 2014; 124(10):2313–2320.

73. Carpenter PS, Pierce JL, Smith ME. Outcomes after cricotracheal resection for idiopathic subglottic stenosis. *Laryngoscope.* 2018;128(10):2268–2272.

74. Naunheim MR, Paddle PM, Husain I, Wangchalabovorn P, Rosario D, Franco RA, Jr. Quality-of-life metrics correlate with disease severity in idiopathic subglottic stenosis. *Laryngoscope.* 2018.

75. Wilson JMG, Jungner G. *Principles and Practice of Screening for Disease.* Geneva, Switzerland: World Health Organization; 1968.

76. *Rehabilitation after Critical Illness in Adults (CG83).* Manchester, UK: National Institute of Health and Care Excellence.

77. Olias, J., Millán, G., da Costa, D. Circumferential tracheal reconstruction for the functional treatment of airway compromise. *Laryngoscope.* 2005; 115: 159–161.

CHAPTER 40

Rare Complications of Percutaneous Tracheostomies

Aphrodite Iacovidou and Taranjit Singh Tatla

INTRODUCTION

Percutaneous tracheostomies have become key interventional procedures for intensive care and anesthesia physicians since their introduction in 1985.[1] These have been aimed at patients requiring prolonged intubation on the intensive care unit (ICU) and the presumed benefits include reduction of anesthetic and sedative drug requirements, greater comfort for patients through removal of endotracheal tubes (allowing communication and potential for swallow), reduction in anatomical dead space for improved weaning off of mechanical ventilation, and endotracheal toileting of secretions in patients with pneumonia.[2] The TracMan study did not show any significant difference in morbidity and mortality following early versus late ICU tracheostomy, recommending each individual case be considered independently.[2]

As with open surgical tracheostomy, there is the potential for complications. A number of systematic reviews and meta-analyses comparing percutaneous with open tracheostomy in the ICU environment illustrate shorter procedure time and reduced stoma inflammation and infection rates; however, no difference is reported in bleeding risk, rates of subcutaneous emphysema, false track formation, desaturation episodes, and pneumothorax. Complications do seem to be related to training grade of operator, where the procedure was performed, and difference between percutaneous

methods.[3,4] Other important considerations for preventing complications are patient and tube-specific factors, as well as the embedding of organizational systems for delivery of quality multidisciplinary aftercare (stoma/trachea/tube monitoring) in the acute through to more medium and long-term tracheostomy patients.[5] Beyond the ICU, patients may pass between the ICU and hospital wards, between the hospital and community localities (home, nursing home, etc), and back and forth between multiple hospitals and superspecialist care environments if not co-located. The importance of close inter/multidisciplinary working, handover, and communication is critical, including patient-specific and tube-specific information. A multidisciplinary team approach is demonstrated to improve tracheostomy care outcomes.[6,7] Cautions and relative contraindications for percutaneous tracheostomy do exist and are subject to operator experience and clinical judgment. These can be found in Table 40–1 as adopted from the Standards and Guidelines of Tracheostomy Care as published by the Council of the Intensive Care Society and the Association of Anaesthetists of Great Britain and Ireland.[8,9]

Complications associated with percutaneous tracheostomy can be divided into immediate (peri-procedure), intermediate (<7 days), and late (>7 days). These can be serious and sometimes fatal, and the utmost effort should be made to limit them. A summary of these can be seen in Table 40–2 as adopted from Tatla and Fitzgerald.[5]

Table 40-1. Cautions and Relative Contraindications for Percutaneous Tracheostomy

Airway Emergency—Obstruction	
Difficult anatomy	Morbid obesity with short neck
	Limited neck movement
	Traumatic cervical spine injury—suspected or otherwise
	Aberrant blood vessels
	Enlarged thyroid gland or pathology
	Tracheal pathology
Moderate coagulopathy	Prothrombin time or activated partial thromboplastin time greater than 1.5 times the reference range
	Platelet count less than 50,000/mcL
Potential instability	Patients unable to tolerate cardiovascular or respiratory changes
Significant gas exchange problems: eg, PEEP > 10 cm H_2O or FiO_2 greater than 0.6	
Evidence of infection in the soft tissue of the neck	
Age less than 12 years old	

Table 40-2. Summary of Percutaneous Tracheostomy Complications

Immediate/early complications (intraoperative/perioperative)	Air embolism
	Haemorrhage (primary or secondary)
	Pneumothorax (especially in children)
	Subcutaneous emphysema
	Recurrent laryngeal nerve injury
	Posterior tracheal injury (tracheoesophageal fistula)
	Tube/airway blockage
	Tube displacement/migration
	Tracheitis/peristomal skin infection
Intermediate complications	Infection/peristomal granulation tissue formation
	Tracheitis and tracheal granulation
	Tube/airway blockage
	Tube displacement/migration
	Hemorrhage (trachea-innominate artery fistula)
	Tracheoesophageal fistula
Late-stage complications	Tracheocutaneous fistula or poor scar (following decannulation)
	Tracheal or subglottic stenosis
	Tracheomalacia

CASE BASED SCENARIOS/DISCUSSION

Case Scenario 1

Background

An 18-year-old otherwise fit and healthy young man was admitted through the Accident and Emergency (A&E) department with a traumatic leg stabbing, resulting in significant hemorrhage. On arrival via private transport, he was in pulseless electrical activity (PEA) arrest and had cardiopulmonary resuscitation for 24 minutes. He was intubated and transferred to theatre for control of bleeding by the vascular surgical team, where he underwent repair of the right superficial femoral artery, right popliteal artery, and fasciotomy. Postoperatively, he returned to ICU where he remained intubated for 4 days. CT scan of head confirmed left frontal lobe ischemia with no cerebral edema.

Timeline

Day 5: Successfully extubated for a short period of time, after which he deteriorated rapidly with seizures and decorticate posturing. He was reintubated on the day and plans were made for percutaneous dilatational tracheostomy (PDT).

Day 6: PDT was performed in ICU, with two consultant intensivists, one training-grade registrar, and an ICU nurse present. Flexible bronchoscopy was used to initially visualize tracheal needle entry and air aspiration prior to guide-wire insertion (as per Seldinger technique) without difficulty. It was documented that subsequent dilatational steps prior to tracheotomy tube insertion were met with resistance due to "tough" skin. A scalpel was therefore used to formally make a skin incision at point of skin entry, and with manipulation during further dilatational steps, a size 7.5 Portex blue-line cuffed tracheostomy was inserted. A second repeat bronchoscopy at this point showed the tracheostomy tube sitting intratracheal within the lumen and no other abnormalities. The tracheostomy cuff was inflated and the airway circuit completed with attachment to a mechanical ventilator.

On the same day, there was a sudden oxygen desaturation with difficulties ventilating, so an urgent portable chest x-ray (CXR) was performed confirming a large right-sided pneumothorax (Figure 40–1).

This was decompressed with thoracocentesis and Seldinger technique for insertion of a chest drain. However, oxygen levels remained poor with pCO_2 9.8 kPa and continued large right pneumothorax, despite a bubbling first chest drain. A second chest drain was then felt necessary and inserted; oxygen saturations subsequently improved. On the same day, CT neck and thorax was performed, demonstrating a large posterior tracheal laceration measuring 4 cm, adjacent to the inflated tracheostomy cuff in situ. The balloon appeared expanded outside the boundaries of the trachea, extending through the defect. Extensive mediastinal air was noted, bilateral basal lung consolidation accompanying a large right-sided pneumothorax, despite appropriate position of the two surgical drains. See Figures 40–2A-D (lung settings).

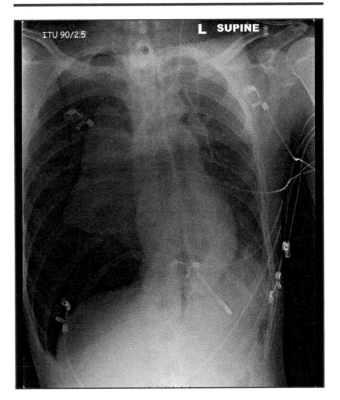

Figure 40–1. Post PDT CXR illustrating large right-sided tension pneumothorax.

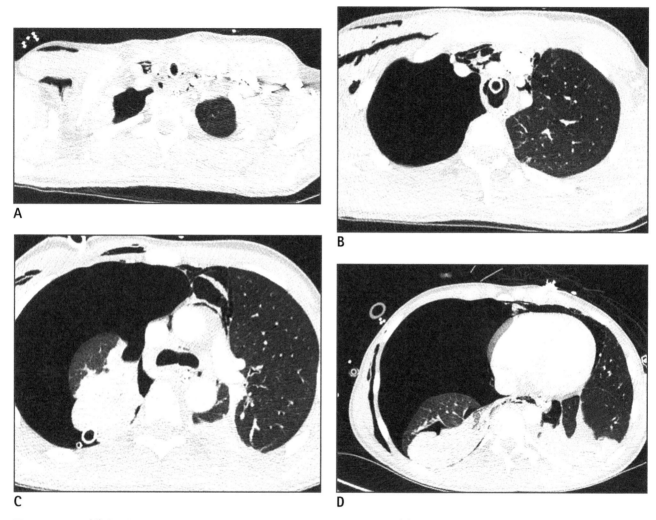

Figure 40–2. (A) Axial view of CT neck and thorax at upper tracheal level. (B) Axial view of CT thorax at mid tracheal level. (C) Axial view of CT thorax at level of carina. (D) Axial view of CT thorax at lower lobes.

Day 9: He was discussed with the thoracic surgical team at the neighboring regional unit (10 miles away) and was transferred across for same-day rigid bronchoscopy. The traumatic tracheal defect was seen posterolaterally and an 18 × 60 mm expandable covered stent inserted. The stent was intubated proximally with a size 8.0 Tracheo® twist (OD 11.0 mm) tracheostomy tube and the patient repatriated back to the parent ICU. The patient continued to be fed through a nasogastric tube.

Day 17: While he made a good recovery on ICU, he had a further episode of significant desaturation. Portable CXR was arranged and confirmed distal migration of the tracheal stent

down to the level of the carina and right main bronchus (Figure 40–3A). He was transferred urgently to theatre by the ENT team for rigid bronchoscopy and stent retrieval (Figure 40–3B).

At rigid bronchoscopy (rigid 0⁰ Hopkins rod endoscopic visualization with jet ventilation through lumen of tracheal stent) the tracheal defect appeared to have healed and so the stent was removed, leaving the tracheostomy tube in situ. He was decannulated successfully on day 37, with no further airway or chest-related issues. He required ongoing neurological care and discharge to the regional rehabilitation unit for his cerebral hypoxic injury, including a feeding gastrostomy while swallow remained unsafe.

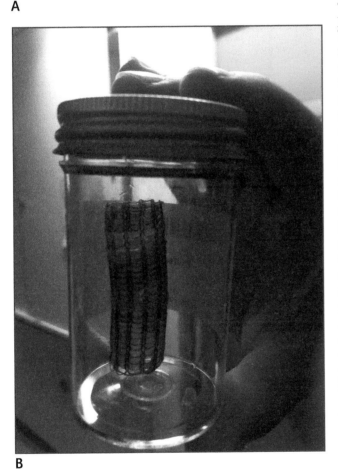

A

B

Figure 40–3. (A) Migrated tracheal stent into right main bronchus. (B) Removed 18 × 60 mm covered bronchial stent.

Considerations from Case Scenario 1

This interesting case illustrates the acute development and subsequent management of a rare complication associated with PDT insertion in an otherwise fit, young male patient. In this case, there were no issues with regard to risk factors in the patient (ie, obesity, distorted or anomalous neck anatomy, etc). It is most probable that the complication resulted directly as a consequence of the dilatational technique employed and sequence of steps performed with the PDT kit.

Flexible bronchoscopic view of the tracheal lumen is recommended as an important adjunct to the PDT technique to ensure both correct tracheal entry of the guide wire and positioning of the tracheostomy tube once inserted. This guideline was followed with experience and competency among the operating team. The lumen was not, however, visualized uninterrupted through the procedure when the difficulty in dilatational steps was encountered with "tough" skin. This would be essential for the operator to be satisfied a posterior tracheal wall injury (particularly perforation of the soft, non-cartilaginous trachealis muscle) did not result. It is also the manufacturer's guideline with the PDT kit employed that a small 2 to 2.5-cm horizontal skin incision be made at the very outset when skin has been prepped and landmarks palpated, below the level of the cricoid ring. This step was performed out of sequence and only once dilatational difficulties had been encountered during the later steps. As in this example, younger male patients will generally have thicker skin and a more elastic tracheal framework (compared with the elderly, for example, in whom skin is often less tough and tracheal rings more calcified and less elastic). The resistance and haptic sensory feedback for the operator during the initial puncture and dilatational task would be very different in these two circumstances. Neither the assistant intensivist performing the flexible bronchoscopy nor the assisting intensive treatment unit (ITU) nurse and observing trainee ICU registrar would receive this sensory feedback. The need for reliance upon endoscopic visualization, throughout all the steps of the invasive procedure (from beginning to end), is therefore self-justifying. Not only should this be an endoscopic view that the assistant intensivist has through the eyepiece him/herself, it should be a view that all members of the team share on a portable camera screen linked to the endoscope. Single-use, disposable endoscopes incorporating light source, integrated complementary metal-oxide semiconductor (CMOS) camera chips, suction and irrigation ports, as well as an interfacing digital display screen are now affordable and readily available for such clinical use. Recent National Institute for Health and Care Excellence (NICE) medical technologies advisory committee guidance recommends that such equipment be routinely employed in the National Health Service (NHS), where standard nasendoscopes are not available for difficult airway management (Figure 40–4 Ambuscope).[10]

Currently, there appear to be no national or other consensus guidelines to set standards and explicitly advise on bronchoscopy protocol during PDT insertion. It is highly likely that considerable force was used during dilatation and tracheostomy tube insertion, in the face of resistance encountered, resulting in a posterior tracheal wall perforation and tear. The vigilance and rapidity in instigating urgent investigations, including portable CXR and CT neck/chest, allowed early recognition and address of the tension pneumothorax. Although this is a rare complication of PDT insertion, it is life threatening and should be considered in the early differential when patients desaturate shortly after the procedure. Prompt, atraumatic chest drain insertion (Seldinger technique) followed, allowing stabilization of the patient prior to considering a definitive management plan for the perforation. The patient was transferred out to the regional thoracic center for rigid bronchoscopic evaluation and tracheal stent insertion across the site of injury. This allowed an important period of stability and time for the traumatic injury to heal through conservative measures.

Distal migration of tracheal stents is considered a not uncommon complication.[5] Early specialist airway support from appropriate ENT experts, interventional pulmonologists, and/or thoracic surgery colleagues ensures that complications with T-tubes and tracheal stents too are minimized and addressed readily and successfully. Long-term management of such stents is complex and requires an ongoing specialist airway multidisciplinary team approach to care.

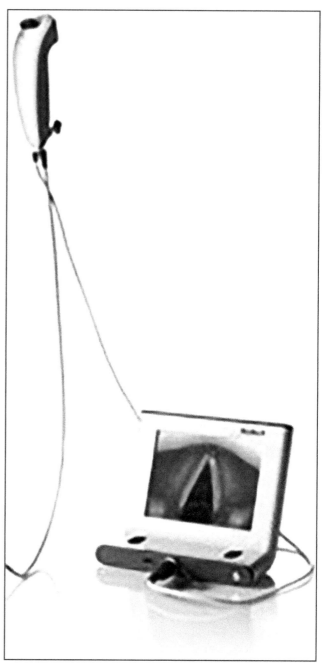

Figure 40–4. Ambu® aScope™ 2 and Monitor (Image reproduced with permission courtesy of Ambu A/S; see http://www.ambu.com).

Case Scenario 2

Background

A 21-year-old Indian student, previously fit and healthy, was admitted through A&E with confusion, sepsis, and signs of meningitis (increased intracranial pressure, reduced Glasgow Coma Score). He was intubated and ventilated and following CT scan of the head and lumbar puncture was treated for a left thalamic lesion and tuberculous meningitis. He was transferred to the regional neighboring neurosurgical unit (13 miles distance), where he underwent craniotomy, washout, external ventricular drain for hydrocephalus, and then treatment with appropriate high dose intravenous antibiotics.

Day 8: Neurosurgical ICU anticipated a prolonged stay and weaning and so organized a PDT on their unit. No difficulties, incidents, or complications were documented or communicated from the ICU to the downstream multidisciplinary tracheostomy team.

Day 14: As he was recovering from his neurological insult (notable right-sided facial nerve weakness), ENT flexible nasendoscopic evaluation of the larynx confirmed initially bilateral vocal cord palsy which appeared to improve subsequently, mirroring his neurological improvement. This allowed safe decannulation of tracheostomy in coming weeks. Percutaneous endoscopic gastrostomy (PEG) tube insertion was, however, required for ongoing feeding needs during rehabilitation.

Week 11: He was transferred across to the regional rehabilitation unit, requiring handover and ongoing input from the Speech and Language Team. He had two episodes of pneumonia which were attributed to poor swallow and possible aspiration prior to transfer.

Week 21: A formal videofluoroscopy swallow (VFS) test was performed to assess oral/oropharyngeal stages of swallow and advise on function and strategy to avoid further risks of aspiration pneumonia. This noted a small tracheoesophageal fistula (TEF), which was felt by the local radiologist as the likely cause of his chest infections. He was kept strictly nil by mouth and referred to the local ENT specialist swallow clinic for further evaluation.

Week 31: At ENT consultant review the patient was noted to have a persistent unilateral vocal cord abductor weakness, although this was incomplete. He had started oral intake against medical advice and had remained well in preceding weeks. He reported no cough and had been without chest infection. He was therefore allowed to "risk feed" while imaging was formally reviewed at the regional Integrated Care of Swallow Multidisciplinary Team (ICOS MDT) meeting.

Week 50: VFS imaging was reviewed at the ICOS MDT meeting and was considered suboptimal. Arrangements were therefore made for a repeat VFS examination at the specialist unit (St Mark's Hospital, London), involving higher resolution

digital video (Figure 40–5). This confirmed a fine fistula tract (Video 40–1 and Video 40–2).

Week 52 until discharge at Week 70: The patient continued to voluntarily swallow both liquids and solids without restriction. He reported no coughing, choking, or chest infections while he remained within the rehabilitation unit up until his discharge and repatriation to his home country. Surgical options were discussed, including minimally invasive endoscopic approaches to repair of the small TEF. However, on the balance of risks, including notable resolution of vocal cord paresis, a conservative management strategy was adopted in discussion with the patient—surgery to remain a future treatment option if required on return to India.

Considerations from Case Scenario 2

The care of this patient extended across several geographical boundaries of care, as well as a number of specialties and teams. He required multidisciplinary management, appropriate communication, and handover of care between hospitals and health care staff. The priorities for handover information (verbal and in written documentation) appear to have related to the underlying life-threatening neurological insult and infection. Information related to the tracheostomy appears to have been an "add-on," commenting on dates that the PDT was performed, dates that patient was decannulated, and simply a single line statement to say "no issues with tube insertion or subsequent management" at the neurosurgical unit. In trying to determine the type of PDT technique/kit used, whether flexible bronchoscope guidance was used as adjunct, and whether or not any subtle difficulties were encountered during the ITU intervention (ie, "tough skin"), the authors have had to try and gain access to in-patient paper records from the neighboring unit and the practicalities of this have been difficult and time consuming.

It is possible that the small TEF resulted as a consequence of the PDT guide wire perforating to produce the posterior tracheoesophageal wall defect at the time of the initial procedure (akin to the production of a tracheoesophageal primary puncture to allow valve insertion and surgical voice restoration following laryngectomy). Alternatively, trauma could have resulted from initial needle puncture attempts performed without flexible bronchoscopic visualization. Without viewing the operator's notes, it is difficult to say more.

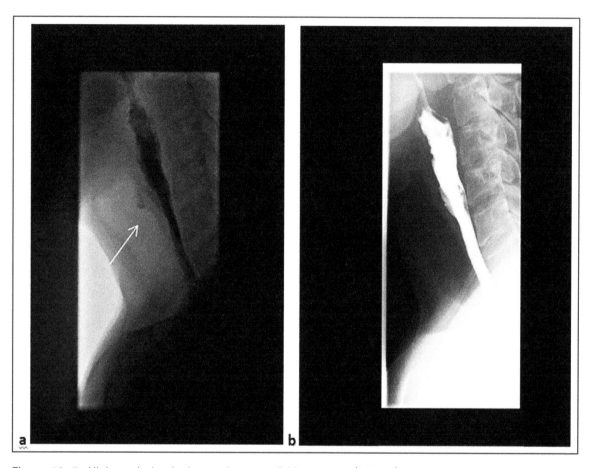

Figure 40–5. High resolution barium and water-soluble contrast (iohexol) video swallow test. Water soluble contrast is seen to penetrate anteriorly at the level of C5/C6 vertebra (just below the cricoid) with a very fine and short fistula tract seen (A). Interestingly, this is not seen when the thicker barium contrast was used (B), but was seen again when water soluble contrast was repeated.

Theoretically, such an issue may also result from pressure erosion in the area between an inflated tracheostomy balloon cuff and the nasogastric tube.[3]

A multidisciplinary team approach (SLT interaction between radiologists at the rehab unit, prompting onward ENT specialist referral and assessment) helped identify and explore the issue further, although with significant delays in system processes and sharing of DICOM data from VFS recordings. A picture archiving and communication system (PACS) for such data, as well as for functional endoscopic evaluation of swallow (FEES), has been proposed locally to help support further multidisciplinary integrated service developments for swallow dysfunction.

Benign acquired TEF can result as a complication of tracheostomy tube insertion technique, a complication

of pressure erosion from the tube or cuff itself, as well from erosion caused by endotracheal tubes or tracheal stents that may or may not have migrated.[5] Management of such TEF may involve minimally invasive and open surgical approaches to close the fistula, depending on size, position, and functional impact/morbidity (frequency and severity of aspiration, coughing, chest infections, etc). Minimally invasive approaches are advocated by some, including endoscope-assisted siting of Montgomery T-tubes, which is particularly attractive for patients who are otherwise poor surgical candidates.[11] Operations are described involving single-stage repair (simple division and closure of the fistula or two-layer mucosal closure of the esophagus and trachea, interposed with a sternocleidomastoid muscle flap as well as tracheal resection to approach esophageal repair.[12,13] This is usually contemplated after a period of conservative management when a patient is no longer mechanical ventilator dependent. To buy time, to allow safe lung ventilation without pneumothorax/pneumomediastinum, and to prevent overspill of esophago-gastric contents into the bronchial tree, a cuffed endotracheal or tracheostomy tube is kept in place with cuff distal to the TEF. For larger TEF, a draining gastrostomy and separate feeding jejunostomy tube are often inserted pending formal repair. In this particular patient, the TEF was more obvious on high resolution VFS when taking a thin fluid bolus, as opposed to thick fluid or solids. The tracheal penetration seen is similar to laryngectomy patients who have leaking speaking valves in place for voicing through a vibratory pharyngeal segment. The small aspiration events are often clinically insignificant and infrequent in these situations, allowing a non-interventional and "watch and wait" strategy to be entertained, with or without dietary modification through support of speech therapist and dietetics team members.

Case Scenario 3

Background

A 28-year-old lady with a known hypoxic brain injury presented from her nursing home to A&E with an acute and significant bleed from around her long-term adjustable flange tracheostomy tube. Four years previously she had suffered from an anaphylactic reaction during a spinal epidural for obstetric delivery, resulting in hypoxic brain injury and persistent vegetative state. Review of hospital records confirmed an uneventful surgical tracheostomy was performed at the time of the insult, while being treated on ICU, due to relative contraindications to PDT (raised body mass index [BMI] with short, fat neck and possible coagulopathy).

Since the initial injury, she had been cared for in an approved nursing home for tracheostomy, gastrostomy, and general nursing care. Although the local nursing home staff looked after her daily tracheostomy tube and stoma care (dressing changes, cuff pressure management, inner tube cleaning, suctioning, nebulizer, and humidification), regular monthly tube changes were all performed by tracheostomy-skilled specialist nursing staff in the hospital ENT outpatient department. During these 4 years, she required multiple and repeated hospitalizations for pneumonias and tube blockages resulting from increased and altered tracheobronchial secretions, tracheitis, and observed tracheal granulations.

Day 0: She was resuscitated aggressively and transferred for an urgent CT angiogram and theatre. Her scan did not identify a specific named vessel causing this hemorrhage. She received 4 units of red blood cells, 2 pools of platelets, 2 units of fresh frozen plasma, and inotropic support. Unfortunately, despite best efforts she succumbed to her airway major hemorrhage within 4 hours of admission. Her post mortem reported trachea and bronchi containing fresh, partially clotted blood, with hemorrhage tracking in to the peritracheal soft tissues on the right side of the neck. It was concluded that a major neck vessel fistulation had resulted, most likely due to long-term tracheostomy tube pressure necrosis, resulting in a catastrophic and terminal airway bleed.

Considerations from Case Scenario 3

The 2014 National Confidential Enquiry into Patient Outcome and Death (NCEPOD) report "On the Right Trach?" summarized data from a compulsory 3-month NHS audit of all tracheostomy insertions performed in England and Wales.[14] This showed emphatically that obesity (raised BMI) was associated with increased risk for tube complications (obstruction and displacement in particular) and that greater awareness was required in such high risk patients, requiring increased multidisciplinary vigilance for impending minor, major, repeat, and catastrophic complications; these in turn resulted in higher patient morbidity and mortality.

Tube type and size are important considerations, the exact choice determined by any of multiple factors, including: individual and local team preferences, familiarity and availability, patient-specific issues (neck anatomy, anomaly of local vasculature, pre-tracheal soft-tissue redundancy, spine/neck curvature), tracheostomy indication, ongoing tube requirements (eg, need for inflated balloon cuff if patient ventilated, need for protecting the bronchial tree from aspirated blood or other oropharyngeal secretions, need for deep suctioning) as well as continuing changing tube requirements in light of developing complications, such as tracheal granulations, stenosis, and malacia. Regular multidisciplinary oversight, for both inpatient and outpatient management of care episodes, ideally would allow prevention, early pick-up, and appropriate remedy of evolving complications and issues, before a catastrophic event results such as tube blockage, displacement, or major hemorrhage into the lower airway. Absolutely essential are management support to ensure appropriate MDT staffing levels and equipment needs and teaching/training requirements to ensure that knowledge and competencies are up-to-date, coupled with clear and unambiguous evidence-based guidelines (where possible) for tracheostomy care (tube cleaning and change, cuff pressure monitoring, decannulation protocols etc). Multidisciplinary teams delivering such cross-cutting specialist services, as mentioned earlier, facilitate earlier decannulations and shortened hospital lengths of stay in tracheostomy patients. Where care is suboptimal, repeated hospitalizations for secretion management through chest infections, ICU/high-dependency unit (HDU) admissions, and ultimately progressive complications are inevitable. Retrospective study of this one patient's multiple hospital paper records (four files) reveals an interesting timeline and pattern of events over the preceding 4-year period, illustrated in Figure 40–6.

In this particular patient's case, from the outset on surgical tracheostomy when it was determined that she required an adjustable-length tracheostomy tube to circumnavigate anatomical limitations (short, obese neck), the subsequent development of intra-tracheal complications was predictable (ie, granulations from tip and cuff trauma, traumatic trigger for tracheitis and increased tracheobronchial secretions resulting in mucus plugging and repeat chest infections, tube blockages, tracheomalacia, etc). Furthermore, although her changing metabolic status while moribund and bed bound was accurately recorded and managed appropriately for nutritional/caloric needs by dietetics staff (her BMI was noted to fall from 30 to 26 during the same timeline), the parallel likely reduction of neck circumference was not necessarily appreciated by the MDT, with its possible impact on variable tracheostomy flange/tube position and recurrent complications.

Catastrophic airway bleeding was the ultimate cause for her death. Bleeding as a complication from tracheostomy may result from a variety of sources and is more likely to occur when coagulopathies coexist (Table 40–3).

Major airway bleeding complicating tracheostomy is very rare (trachea-innominate fistula has reported incidence of 0.1 to 1% after surgical tracheostomy and 0.35% after PDT)[15] and is usually related to chronic pressure and ulceration of the surrounding tissues. Unfortunately, in this patient there were no herald bleeds or other warning signs prior to this episode, as far as we have been able to determine from nursing home handover. Fistulation into major neck and mediastinal vessels such as the subclavian vein,[16] innominate artery,[17] and carotid vessel[18] have been previously documented.

In this lady's case, specialist interventional radiologist review of the CT angiogram confirms an aberrant right subclavian artery (aka lusoria artery) (Figure 40–7), which may or may not have been the site of vascular fistulous communication to the trachea.

The best management approach for such rare complications is preventative care (anticipation and avoidance), good tracheostomy tube oversight and aftercare, multidisciplinary team vigilance, and early specialist alert and intervention to prevent onward escalation to a catastrophic bleed or aspiration. In this case, endovascular management may have been considered and delivered successfully as reported by others.[19]

In addition to bronchoscopy adjunct to facilitate safe PDT insertion, increasingly more and more units are using point of care ultrasound scanning (USS) as a first-line, simple, and non-invasive tool.[20] USS has become more and more portable and affordable, its scope of use being limited only by the operator's introduction to it and expertise.[21] Clinical information alone (Video 40–3) may not always be sufficient to provide necessary and important anatomical detail to safeguard against tracheostomy complication. USS may allow characterization and avoidance of normal and abnormal neck vessels, recognition of potential pitfalls such as large thyroid goiters, measurement of important dimensions for pre/extra-tracheal soft-tissue and tracheal lumen width to plan more accurate tracheostomy tube sizing, as well as allow first pass and more accurate/direct tracheal needle puncture under USS guidance. This is particularly the case where PDT applications are being extended to recognized more difficult patient categories, that is, obese patients and children.[22,23]

DISCUSSION

All the above case illustrations of rare tracheostomy complications are presented on a background of increasing numbers of tracheostomies (and specifically PDTs) being performed internationally, with the rise of intensive care medicine. The NCEPOD audit demonstrated that in the NHS (England and Wales), approximately two-thirds of all tracheostomies are percutaneous and one-third surgical. The latter usually occur in the most challenging patients due to limitations in

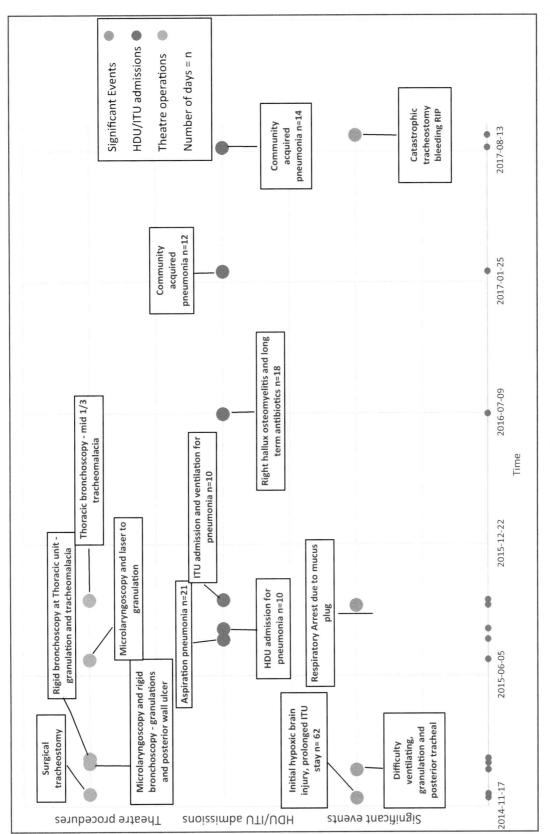

Figure 40–6. Timeline of care pathway–repeated hospitalizations, HDU/ITU admissions, lengths of stay, significant events and complications (NB repeated GP visits to nursing home and ENT outpatient department for monthly tube changes not illustrated).

437

Table 40–3. Causes of Tracheostomy-Related Hemorrhage[1]

Early Bleeding (<4 days)	Skin related bleeding (e.g. anterior jugular vein or communicating veins)
	Thyroid related bleeding (esp. if divided and edges not over-sewn)
	Related to anticoagulant or antiplatelet treatment
Late Bleeding (>4 days)	Erosion into a large artery (e.g. trachea-innominate fistula, due to pressure from inferior end of tube onto high riding innominate vessels, due to cuff or tip causing tracheal wall erosion, common carotid artery, internal jugular / innominate vein or other aberrant vasculature e.g. subclavian artery)
	Granulation tissue
	Mucosal trauma due to suction catheters, tracheostomy tube change etc.

[1] Austin Health 2016. Clinical Guideline: Tracheostomy related bleeding. URL: http://tracheostomyteam.org/data/uploads/pdf/tracheostomy_related _bleeding2016.pdf. Retrieved 3rd March 2018.

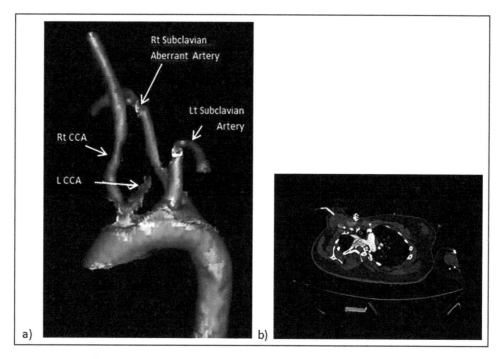

Figure 40–7. (A) Image of developmental anomaly in aberrant subclavian artery. Three-dimensional reconstruction (triple phase CT angiogram of neck and chest) showing aortic arch and aberrant route of right subclavian artery posterior to tracheal wall in mediastinum. Possible tip or cuff erosion may have contributed. No ongoing hemorrhage was noted at the time of scan; however, anatomical anomaly is identifiable and a distinct tracheal dilatation is noted at the point where the artery crosses the trachea. (B) Oblique CT axial cross-section at level of tracheostomy tube balloon cuff, compressing right subclavian aberrant artery between trachea and prevertebral tissue.

anterior neck access and cervical spine mobility, along with other patient-related factors as mentioned earlier.

Even though the surgical tracheostomy has a standardized WHO checklist requirement, this is not widely available or practiced routinely in the ICU setting, where most PDTs are performed. This is a standard that requires early adoption and systematic implementation.

The MDT approach to tracheostomy care, including oversight and management of the whole care pathway, from ICU/operating theatre to hospital wards and beyond hospital boundaries to other geographically separate units and community care localities (nursing and rehabilitation units, as well as patient's own homes), needs to be encompassed and services commissioned appropriately for integrated multidisciplinary service delivery.

Tracheostomy care passports and care bundles have been the focus of service development activity at the senior authors' host organization for the last 10 years. It has formed the basis of defining and delivering multidisciplinary tracheostomy training, evolving local processes and protocols based on evidence-based and best practice international guidelines, as well as embedding a team approach to tracheostomy care. It remains a work in progress as protocols and systems for oversight, patient safety, and governance are extended out to linked community and other care provider sites. Patients with tracheostomy are frequently moved between wards and departments within sites and often across sites and organizations; an electronic tracheostomy tube–specific passport, clearly recording the indication, circumstances, and outcome of the initial operative procedure, as well as any difficulties encountered (either at the time of the procedure or subsequently as long as the tube remains in situ), would allow necessary improvements in communication between team members. It would also allow remote oversight of patients with long-term tracheostomy tubes that are nursed outside of an acute care organization in the community, as well as improved, more efficient service structure and safer care delivery. For the long-term tracheostomy patients nursed in the community, there appear to have been very few drivers looking to influence or change the current status quo. Multidisciplinary community nursing care (often privately delivered) for tracheostomy patients is expensive, in many cases financially supported through third party insurance or medical indemnity settlements in the context of brain or spinal central nervous system injury. Impact and financial cost, however, are significant for NHS organizations, where repeated hospitalizations for chest infections and management of other tube complications ensues, burdening already stressed acute and specialist care services.

Scientific evidence-based guidance and standards are lacking for the long-term management of patients with tracheostomies in the home or other non-institutional environment, with absence of controlled studies or substantial peer reviewed research papers to guide care and practice (much of the long-term tracheostomy care standards of practice in the United States, for example, are based on extrapolations of bedside tracheostomy care performed in acute care settings).[24] Patient, family, caregiver, and system costs, as well as

other economic considerations relating to the whole patient care pathway, need visibility and oversight. Limitations for data collection, audit, and research resources in acute care organizations, as well difficulty in performing effective, controlled research studies on these patients within uncontrolled community environments, bear heavily on available intelligence.

A whole-system, integrated care approach, involving a combination of process validation (through additional but focused health-economic research) accompanied by multidisciplinary expert consensus, is necessary to standardize and improve the long-term care of tracheostomy patients. This would have global relevance to countries providing a variety of health service delivery models, public and insured.

Very few (if any) tracheostomy MDTs have matured to the point where informed (data and evidence-based), ethically and legally considered discussions can take place with family, relatives, and other interested parties, weighing up advantages and disadvantages of long-term tracheostomy (or gastrostomy) care in patients diagnosed with severe brain injury amounting to a persistent vegetative/minimally conscious state. Consensus clinical guidelines of a Royal College of Physicians multidisciplinary working party have touched upon the sensitive subject of withdrawing active tube care and exploring benefits of more palliative end-of-life supportive care options in patients with prolonged disorders of consciousness.[25]

Shared electronic patient records (without care provider boundaries) and a whole-systems digital data overview hold great promise for improving cost-effective care and decision making in this complex patient group.

Post-procedure complications including hemorrhage, pneumothorax, loss of airway, and loss of tracheal tract can be life-threatening; other complications have great impact on the patient's quality of life and could have long-term impact, increasing morbidity for these patients. The impact for these patients (some would say these are the most vulnerable and neglected patients we see) and for the health care system is large. The costs of delivering multidisciplinary care and the costs of the complex care pathways are larger still. There is much to be gained from a more seamless, integrated, opportunistic, and preventative multidisciplinary approach to care in these patients.

In all these cases, the tracheostomy MDTs were critical for anticipating and preventing complications. The wider multidisciplinary super-specialist support teams can ensure an optimized approach to imaging considerations where rare complications may result or require investigation and expert management. The wider team can also help explore or revisit end-of life supportive options. Increasingly, multidisciplinary team learning and simulation is being used for teaching anticipation of and successful management in difficult airway scenarios, as well as optimized technical performance of operative tasks such as PDT and open tracheostomy.[26] This too holds promise for sustainable reduction in complications and improving outcomes for both short- and longer-term tracheostomy patients.

REFERENCES

1. Ciaglia P, Firsching R, Syniec C. Elective percutaneous dilatational tracheostomy: a new simple bedside procedure; preliminary report. *Chest*. 1985;87(6):715–719.
2. Young D, Harrison DA, Cuthbertson BH, Rowan K, TracMan Collaborators FT. Effect of early vs late tracheostomy placement on survival in patients receiving mechanical ventilationthe tracman randomized trial. *JAMA*. 2013;309(20):2121–2129. doi:10.1001/jama.2013.5154
3. Putensen C, Theuerkauf N, Guenther U, Vargas M, Pelosi P. Percutaneous and surgical tracheostomy in critically ill adult patients: a meta-analysis. *Crit Care*. 2014;18(6):544. doi:10.1186/s13054-014-0544-7
4. Delaney A, Bagshaw SM, Nalos M. Percutaneous dilatational tracheostomy versus surgical tracheostomy in critically ill patients: a systematic review and meta-analysis. *Crit Care*. 2006;10(2):R55.
5. Tatla TS, Fitzgerald CE. Care of patients with tracheostomies, T-tubes and other airway devices. In: *Laryngeal and Tracheobronchial Stenosis*. San Diego, CA: Plural Publishing; 2014: 151–194.
6. Garrubba M, Turner T, Grievenson C. Multidisciplinary care for tracheostomy patients: a systematic review. *Crit Care*. 2009;13(6):109.
7. Speed L, Harding KE. Tracheostomy teams reduce total tracheostomy time and increase speaking valve use: a systematic review and meta-analysis. *J Crit Care*. 2013;28(2):216–210.
8. Council of the Intensive Care Society. Standards for the Care of Adult Patients with a Temporary Tracheostomy; 2014. Retrieved February 20, 2018, from http://www.theawsomecourse.co.uk/ICS/ICS%20Tracheostomy%20standards%20(2014).pdf
9. Bhandary R, Niranjan N. Tracheostomy Anaesthesia Tutorial of the Week 241. The Association of Anaesthetists of Great Britain and Ireland. Retrieved February 20, 2018, from https://www.aagbi.org/sites/default/files/241%20Tracheostomy%20.pdf
10. National Clinical Excellence. Medical Technologies Guidance MTG 14: Ambu aScope2 for Use in Unexpected Difficult Airways; July 2013. Retrieved February 27, 2018, https://www.nice.org.uk/guidance/mtg14
11. Tran et al, 2015. Minimally invasive management of tracheoesophageal fistula with T-tube. *Laryngoscope*. 2015;125:1911–1914.
12. Mathisen DJ et al. Management of acquired non-malignant tracheoesophageal fistula. *Ann Thorac Surg*. 1991;52:759–765.
13. Udagawa H et al. Management of tracheoesophageal fistula after tracheostomy. *JIBI Inkoka Tembo*. 2002;45(2):124–131.
14. National Confidential Enquiry into Patient Outcome and Death. On the Right Trach? A Review of the Care Received by Patients Who Underwent a Tracheostomy; 2014. Retrieved March 3, 2018, http://www.ncepod.org.uk/2014report1/downloads/OnTheRightTrach_Summary.pdf
15. Dempsey G, Grant C, Jones T. Percutaneous tracheostomy: a 6 yr prospective evaluation of the single tapered dilator technique. *Br J Anaesth*. 2010;105(6):782–788.
16. Desvant C et al. Tracheotomy bleeding from an unusual tracheo-arterial fistula: involvement of an aberrant right subclavian artery. *J Laryngol Otol*. 2010;124(12):1333–1336.
17. Ogawa K et al. Tracheo-brachiocephalic artery fistula after tracheostomy associated with thoracic deformity: a case report. *J Med Case Reports*. 2011;5:595.
18. Hoiting O et al. Late fatal bleeding after percutaneous dilatational tracheostomy. *Neth J Crit Care*. 2010;14(5):335–337.
19. Desvant C, Chevalier D, Mortuaire G. Tracheotomy bleeding from an unusual tracheo-arterial fistula: involvement of an aberrant right subclavian artery. *J Laryngol Otol*. 2010;124(12):1333–1336. doi:10.1017/S0022215110001362
20. Alansari M, Alotair H. Use of ultrasound guidance to improve the safety of percutaneous dilatational tracheostomy: a literature review. *Crit Care*. 2015;19(1):229.
21. Ravi PR, Vijay MN, Shouche S. Realtime ultrasound percutaneous tracheostomy in emergency setting: the glass ceiling has been broken. *Dis Mil Med*. 2017;3:7. doi: 10.1186/s40696-017-0035-x
22. Rudas et al. Traditional landmark versus ultrasound guided tracheal puncture during percutaneous dilatational tracheostomy in adult intensive care patients: a randomised controlled trial. *Crit Care*. 2014; 18(5):514.
23. Guinot et al. Ultrasound-guided percutaneous tracheostomy in critically ill obese patients. *Crit Care*. 2012;16:R40.
24. Lewarski JS. Long-term care of the patient with a tracheostomy. *Resp Care*. 2005;50(4):534–537.
25. Turner-Stokes L et al. Royal College of Physicians. Prolonged Disorders of Consciousness: National Clinical Guidelines. London, RCP; 2013. https://www.rcplondon.ac.uk/file/4050/download?token=vXQIJzgk
26. Mehta N et al. Multidisciplinary difficult airway simulation training: two-year evaluation and validation of a novel training approach at a district general hospital based in the UK. *Eur Arch Otolaryng*. 2013;270(1):211–217.

CHAPTER 41

Management of the Airway in Thyroid Disease

Jahangir Ahmed and Alasdair Mace

A 45-year-old lady felt a reduction in exercise tolerance, with mild exercise-induced dyspnea, following a protracted upper respiratory tract infection (URTI). This was resistant to a number of courses of antibiotics instigated by her family doctor. She was otherwise healthy and a non-smoker.

Following a normal chest radiograph, she was referred to a respiratory physician. As part of her respiratory work up, lung spirometry revealed an extra-thoracic obstructive pattern. A subsequent contrast enhanced computerized tomography (CT) scan demonstrated a mass lesion adjacent and inferior to and separate from the left thyroid lobe. The trachea appeared to be extensively invaded and there were multiple suspicious lymph nodes in the lateral neck spanning level 2 to 4 nodal regions (Figure 41–1). The chest was clear of disease. She was urgently referred to the head and neck team for urgent airway management.

Assessment and Perioperative Airway Management

When assessing the airway of a patient with a benign or malignant thyroid lesion, closely question the patient for clinical features suggestive of airway obstruction, namely: stridor at rest, with exertion or in certain positions, dysphonia and dyspnea, limited exercise tolerance. Concurrent vascular compression of the major veins draining the head and neck by a goiter may be

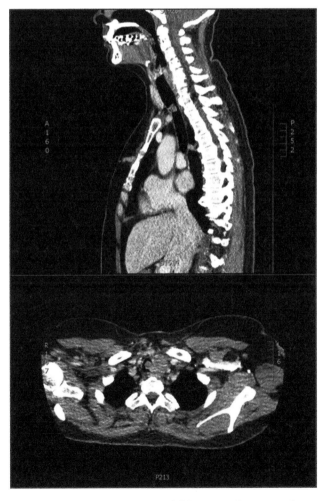

Figure 41–1. Sagittal and axial CT images demonstrating a left paratracheal lesion infiltrating the trachea at the level of the thoracic inlet.

441

exacerbated by raising the arms above the head, causing venous engorgement of the skin of the head and neck (Pemberton's sign). Such compression, if severe, may also cause laryngeal venous engorgement and edema, prompting the patient to present acutely with biphasic stridor, particularly in the presence of a superimposed URTI. Inquire directly about any swallowing difficulties. A recent change in voice and hemoptysis are worrying symptoms that may point to the underlying nature of the lesion.

Laryngoscopy is vital to confirm the anatomical position of the larynx, and exclude airway edema and vocal fold palsy. Often a view of the subglottis and proximal trachea is also obtained. Lung function testing should be performed and may aid in predicting a patient who could develop airway difficulties postoperatively, necessitating nursing in an appropriate environment.

If any of the clinical features above are present, high-resolution cross-sectional imaging is mandatory and will demonstrate tracheal deviation, narrowing, and/ or infiltration as well as staging a possible malignancy.

The patient was assessed by an ENT surgeon. In the clinic she was mildly stridulous at rest; transnasal fiberoptic endoscopy revealed restricted left-sided vocal fold abduction, but there was no phonatory gap. She had a palpable left-sided neck mass extending from neck nodal levels 2 to 4 that was discrete from a separate swelling on the upper pole of the left thyroid lobe. An ultrasound-guided fine needle biopsy was ordered and she was initially listed for a laser-assisted debulking by suspension microlaryngoscopy.

Patients with large goiters or with features of airway obstruction should be preoperatively assessed by an experienced anesthetist. Classical extra-tracheal anatomical predictors of difficult intubation such as decreased neck extension, high Mallampati scores,[1] restricted mouth opening, a short neck with a short thyromental distance, and a retrognathic mandible are significantly more likely to be associated with difficult intubation than compressive tracheal pathology.[2,3] The extents of tracheal deviation and axial caliber, or size of goiter, have not been positively correlated to the ease of intubation in a number of large case series.[4] Anatomically, the larynx and its position are usually not altered by thyroid pathology. Nevertheless, a narrow axial tracheal diameter on CT is sensitive in predicting potential postoperative airway problems.

The majority of elective intubations should therefore be able to be performed transorally by an experienced anesthetist under standard general anesthetic and paralysis. A well-lubricated relatively small caliber endotracheal tube (ETT) should be able to pass through most benign, externally compressive goiters. Nevertheless, difficulty in intubation may occur in up to 12 % of cases[4] and adjunctive methods of intubation should be available in all settings. These include awake fiberoptic intubation and the use of video-aided transoral intubation using devices such as the Glidescope©. There is currently no clear guidance as to the precise role and indication for these, and their pre-emptive use remains a matter of judgment from the attending anesthetist. Indeed, in one series, patients in whom awake fiberoptic intubation (AFOI) had failed were all subsequently successfully intubated transorally, prompting the authors in that study to recommend that all elective patients with goiter be intubated transorally as first line, provided there were no other mitigating supralaryngeal anatomical factors such as poor mouth opening.[4] Video assisted intubation may be useful in ensuring correct placement of nerve monitoring ETTs in this setting[5] and has been shown to hasten the time to intubation and reduce the number of attempts required when intubating patients with goiters.[6]

The situation with a patient who presents acutely in considerable airway distress due to compression or edema or with an infiltrating malignant tumor is different, however. In this situation anesthetic or sedation without intubation may cause catastrophic airway collapse. Here AFOI by an experienced anesthetist is often the first-line method of intubation. This should ideally be performed in the operating room, to enable a swift transition to a rigid laryngoscopic or bronchoscopic attempt at intubation by the surgeon if necessary. Many surgeons have a rigid laryngoscopic tray ready and are in attendance when intubating patients with large or retrosternal goiters. A surgical tracheostomy may be required but in the context of a patient with a large distorting goiter, this should be a last resort; an awake tracheostomy in such a patient, who has difficulty with neck extension and is unable to lie flat, is extremely challenging.

For patients with clinical or radiological tumor infiltration causing acute airway compromise, endotracheal intubation is again the first-line option but should ideally be performed following a planned surgical debulking if expertise and equipment allow. It is ideally performed via rigid suspension laryngoscopy and supraglottic jet ventilation with preceding anesthesia via a laryngeal mask airway. For patients with a large body habitus or a significant tracheal stenosis, the passage of a small caliber, basketless subglottic jetting catheter, which is laser resistant, is an effective means of ventilation. Tumor may then be biopsied and debulked with a carbon dioxide (CO_2) laser or laryngeal microdebrider prior to the safe placement under direct vision of an appropriate caliber ETT. Rigid bronchoscopic debulking is an alternative method of safely debulking the airway.

Intraoperatively, the patient had tumor infiltration of at least 1.5 cm of the length of trachea involving the second to fourth tracheal rings. This was debulked with the aid of the CO_2 laser. She was successfully extubated and her airway symptoms temporarily improved. The histology demonstrated differentiated papillary thyroid carcinoma.

Managing Thyroid Malignancy with Laryngotracheal Invasion

Although differentiated thyroid malignancy has a good prognosis overall, with over 90% 5-year survival,[7] invasive disease, which occurs in 1 to 23% of large series, signifies a much poorer prognosis.[8,9] Invasion of the laryngotracheal complex accounts for 50% of disease specific deaths.[10] Structures relevant to the airway include one or both recurrent laryngeal nerves (RLNs), trachea, and larynx as well as their enveloping muscles, including the esophagus. Invasive cancer may occur from capsular breach of the thyroid gland but also commonly from metastatic lymph nodes. Pathologically, invasive malignancies tend to be poorly differentiated, in relation to disease confined to the gland (50% versus 11.4%[11]) and, as such, are likely to be less responsive to radioactive iodine (RAI), making complete surgical clearance at the initial setting imperative for cure.

Risk factors for airway invasive thyroid malignancy include being male, elderly, and recurrent in the central compartment. Invasion may not be clinically apparent but could include classical obstructive symptoms such as stridor, exertional dyspnea, and dysphagia as well as more specific features such as dysphonia, hemoptysis, or hematemesis. The presence of a fixed mass or lymphadenopathy is also worrying. Fiberoptic endoscopic examination should be performed in all patients presenting with benign or malignant thyroid disease and may reveal an RLN palsy that is often compensated by the healthy vocal fold. These clinical features warrant urgent investigation with cross-sectional imaging with a contrast enhanced MRI and/ or CT neck and thorax to delineate invasive primary tumor and disseminated disease. CT scans should be contrast enhanced where possible to aid identification of lymphadenopathy and delineate extent of disease. Iodine mediated stunning of residual thyroid tissue is not relevant in the likely context of commencing RAI at greater than 6 weeks.

As for our patient, any patient with invasion of the laryngotracheal complex on cross-sectional imaging should undergo tracheobronchoscopy and esophagoscopy prior to definitive surgical management to enable biopsy confirmation, tumor debulking with laser or microdebrider, and in some cases temporary stenting. This should ideally be performed by a team familiar with the use of tubeless jet ventilation in suspension and significant experience in airway reconstruction. This will ensure appropriate multidisciplinary team (MDT) surgical and medical planning for optimal outcome and is vital to patient counseling.

Following discussion in the local thyroid MDT, the patient underwent a total thyroidectomy, central neck dissection. and left levels 2 to 4 selective neck dissection. The segment of trachea (in total, 3.5 cm) that was infiltrated by the large left sided metastatic deposit was resected en bloc. The remaining trachea was mobilized in the mediastinum and closed directly, end to end, with a covering distal tracheostomy. She also underwent sacrifice of the left RLN, which was invaded by tumor and not functioning preoperatively. She made good postoperative progress and a further endoscopic assessment a week later revealed a well-healed patent tracheal anastomosis and she was able to be decannulated successfully. She had no airway compromise and the right vocal fold was normally mobile on endoscopic examination, aiding full compensation of the left RLN palsy. An immediate postoperative hypocalcemia normalized with calcium supplementation that was subsequently weaned off. There was a 1.5 cm differentiated papillary thyroid carcinoma in the left upper thyroid pole on histology in association with a total of 9 of 28 lymph nodes containing metastatic papillary thyroid carcinoma. The tracheal resection specimen demonstrated papillary thyroid carcinoma with features of de-differentiation. There was no tumor at the resection margin. The final pathological staging was pT4a N1b. Following discussion at the thyroid MDT, in view of de-differentiation and lymphovascular invasion, she also underwent external beam radiotherapy (EBRT) as well as RAI.

Intraoperative management of invasion of the trachea is controversial. Shaving superficially invasive disease off the anterior tracheal wall has a much higher (possibly up to eight times) rate of local failure in comparison to segmental resection due to microscopic disease within cartilage being relatively sheltered from the effects of radiotherapy.[10] It should therefore be reserved for tumor that only abuts but does not invade the trachea.[12]

Partial resection in the form of a window should only be contemplated if less than two tracheal rings and one third of the diameter are involved.[10] Even at these limits a covering tracheostomy will often be needed and consequent intraluminal soft tissue bulge may make decannulation difficult. Larger windows in terms of width or length may be replaced with vascularized tissue such as regional or free myocutaneous flaps. With regard to the latter, the epithelial (skin) lining should prevent the formation of granulation tissue in comparison to muscle alone. Ideally this would be reconstructed over a prosthetic stent to afford structural support during healing. Circumferential microscopic involvement is often a source of recurrence, however, and it is oncologically safer to perform a segmental resection if a tension-free end-to-end anastomosis is feasible. In experienced hands the mortality for this is low (1.4% in one series[13]).

It is important to exclude risk factors detrimental to healing, such as prior radiotherapy or active inflammation, which are relative contraindications. Two to three tracheal rings or up to 6 cm in length may be resected following tracheal mobilization facilitated by release of tissue in the hilum and/or intra/suprahyoid muscle release; although the latter may interfere with swallow. Care must be taken to not injure the RLNs by dissecting close to the trachea, or to completely devascularize the trachea, especially if adjuvant EBRT is contemplated. A temporary open endoluminal silicone stent may obviate the need for a tracheostomy and reduces the chance of surgical emphysema, granulation, and tracheal stenosis. Regular saline nebulization is imperative to prevent the formation of crusts within the stent. If the trachea has been appropriately mobilized, it is usually not necessary to use a stitch from chin to chest to maintain a flexed head position as advocated by some; however, the patient should not hyperextend the neck during the first postoperative week.

Although even rarer, laryngeal invasion usually occurs through or around the posterior thyroid alae or anteriorly through the cricothyroid membrane. Laryngopharyngo-esophagoscopic assessment will determine the extent of penetration and if the hypopharynx (pyriform sinus) is not invaded it may be possible to clear disease by partial cartilaginous resection of components of the laryngeal framework. The cost of partial laryngectomy and reconstructive efforts must be balanced by the expected functional outcome, particularly in the likely context of adjuvant

EBRT. A total laryngectomy with surgical voice restoration may be a safer and more effective means of securing airway, swallow, and vocalization. Suffice it to say that such cases will need careful MDT planning and patient counseling. It is imperative that the extent of surgery required for complete resection of gross disease and thus patient outcome be decided prior to adjuvant treatment with RAI and EBRT. Further surgical intervention particularly after EBRT is fraught with a high risk of complications due to poor healing.

Our patient remains disease free in the neck with no symptoms of airway compromise and a satisfactory voice. A further treatment dose of radioiodine was, however, required for distant metastatic disease.

SCENARIO 2

A 78-year-old lady was referred to the head and neck rapid diagnostic clinic. She had felt dyspneic on minor exertion for 6 weeks previously and her husband had noticed that her breathing had become quite noisy, particularly when she lay on her back. There was no change in her voice or swallow and she hadn't noticed any neck lumps. Apart from medically controlled hypertension, she was relatively healthy.

She was mildly stridulous in the clinic but comfortable, with 98% oxygen saturation on pulse oximetry. Examination confirmed a full suprasternal neck and no other abnormal cervical lumps. Flexible nasal endoscopic examination of the larynx confirmed normal, symmetrically mobile vocal folds.

She had an ultrasound scan that revealed a 6 cm thyroid isthmic nodule. Cytology from an aspirate was graded as Thy 3F, an indeterminate follicular lesion.[14]

She underwent a contrast enhanced CT neck and chest after confirming normal thyroid and renal function. This demonstrated a thyroid goiter with retrosternal extension into the anterior mediastinum compressing the trachea at the thoracic inlet (Figure 41–2).

The Airway in Large and Retrosternal Goiters

The main indication for total thyroidectomy for a large benign goiter is to relieve compression of the tracheal airway; this is epitomized by a goiter with retrosternal extension. Persistent growth within a fixed bony

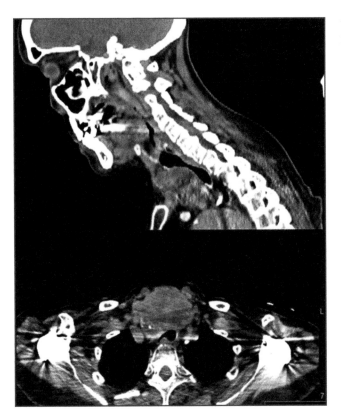

Figure 41–2. Sagittal and axial CT images demonstrating tracheal compression at the level of the thoracic inlet by a thyroid goiter with retrosternal extension into the anterior mediastinum.

thoracic inlet and thoracic cage places the intrathoracic trachea at great risk of distortion and compression.

The two commonest definitions of retrosternal goiter include growth below the plane of the thoracic inlet or goiter in which greater than 50% of its volume lies within the mediastinum. Most originate cervically with growth directed inferiorly by the straps; accordingly, their blood supplies also originate from cervical sources where they may be controlled intraoperatively. More surgically challenging are the rarer retrosternal goiters (0.2–1%) that originate from ectopic thyroid sources within the thoracic cavity which derive their circulation from the intrathoracic great vessels.[15,16] Although most goiters descend into the anterior mediastinum and will thus lie anterior to the RLNs, the 15% that descend into the posterior mediastinum displace the carotid arteries and RLNs anteriorly, placing them at significant iatrogenic risk. The surgical approach to these will usually require a thoracotomy.

Patients are often in the fifth or sixth decades at presentation, and although a significant number (up to 40%) may have been discovered incidentally, having become apparent on plain radiographic or cross-sectional imaging for other causes, closer questioning often reveals long-standing symptoms attributable to airway compression. Stable asthma and fixed exercise tolerance are common examples where one should consider imaging the thoracic inlet if the symptoms are refractory to medical treatment. Overt symptoms include gradually worsening stridor, positional (supine) or exertional dyspnea (30–90%), chronic cough, choking sensation, and dysphagia (15–60%). A patient with a larger goiter with retrosternal extension may demonstrate Pemberton's sign, as previously mentioned. As described earlier, dysphonia may indicate RLN compression or infiltration. Although rare, other structures that may be compressed and thus dysfunctional include the cervical sympathetic chain, branches of the brachial plexus, and phrenic nerve.[17] These will manifest with specific symptoms and signs, and in such cases, one should be highly vigilant for malignancy.

It is important to perform thyroid function tests prior to iodinated contrast enhanced CT to exclude subclinical hypothyroidism (in 25% of patients) as an iodine bolus in this context may induce hyperthyroidism and further thyroid swelling. A CT scan will delineate the cross-sectional diameter and position of the trachea. Some patients will tolerate an impressively narrow airway, particularly if compression has been slowly progressive. A flow-volume lung function loop is usually characteristic of a fixed cervical/intrathoracic narrowing. If preliminary cross-sectional imaging has revealed an isolated intrathoracic mass, radioiodine may confirm an ectopic goiter and distinguish it from other pathologic entities such as thymomas and neurogenic or congenital tumors.

There is continuing debate about whether all substernal goiters should be surgically excised if the patient is medically fit. Medical options are, however, relatively limited. Thyroid hormone mediated suppressive therapy is not effective[18] and the side effect profile is generally not tolerated in the elderly. A single dose of RAI may reduce the volume of large retrosternal goiters by up to 30%,[19] but radiation induced thyroiditis may temporarily enhance tracheal compression, which if already severe may need pretreatment stenting. Radiation thyroiditis may make future thyroid surgery difficult due to scarring and tissue distortion. RAI slows but does not halt continued growth,[19] the danger of which therefore remains.

Proponents of surgery argue that patients are rarely truly asymptomatic. Indeed, cross-sectional imaging will often identify a small caliber trachea in "asymptomatic" patients. The natural history is likely to be that of slow progression with inevitable worsening of airway compression. Operation at an earlier stage of goiter development may be technically easier in a younger potentially fitter patient. In addition, potentially catastrophic acute on chronic airway obstruction—for example, from hemorrhage, thyroiditis, or traumatic insult—has a reported incidence of 5 to 11%.[20,21] The incidence of carcinomatous change within goiters is 1.3 to 3.7 per 1000[22,23] and is likely to be the same in retrosternal goiters.[24] Ultrasound and cytological surveillance of potentially malignant nodules within retrosternal goiters is difficult, and this inability to exclude malignancy is another rationale for surgical excision. Complications following surgery for retrosternal goiters are, however, higher than purely cervical ones. In a large observational cohort comprising 32,777 (1153 retrosternal goiters) from multiple centers in New York State, the risk of permanent RLN damage for retrosternal goiters was 2.1% versus 0.6% in purely cervical goiters.[25] Likewise permanent hypoparathyroidism: 5.5% versus 3.5% and postoperative hemorrhage: 2.2% versus 0.9%, respectively. There was also an increased mortality rate in this study: 1.4% versus 0.1%.[23,25] Suffice it to say that retrosternal goiters should be operated on by a team with a high-volume thyroid practice with easy access to cardiothoracic surgical assistance, although the likelihood of actually requiring cardiothoracic intervention is relatively low: 2 to 15% in large series. Extracervical approaches will likely be required in ectopic intrathoracic goiters, invasive malignancy, posterior mediastinal extension, and revision cases and with extension beyond the aortic arch. where the goiter is likely to be too large to fit through the inlet.

Where a patient has clinical and/or radiological airway compression but is not medically fit enough to have major surgery or indeed refuses, bronchoscopic placement of self-retaining stents is a palliating option. These are, however, fraught with potential life-threatening complications, including blockage, displacement, and fracture.

Following discussion at the thyroid MDT, the recommendation was for total thyroidectomy. This was performed at a center with cardiothoracic surgery on site. She was intubated transorally without issue following laryngoscopy (Figure 41–3). The thyroid gland was removed transcervically with both lobes able to be delivered from within the thoracic cage via blunt finger mobilization. Both RLNs and superior laryngeal nerves were identified intraoperatively and confirmed to be functionally intact by direct nerve stimulation. The trachea was not deformed or malacic on palpation. Bilateral neck drains were placed. She was extubated uneventfully and nursed overnight on a

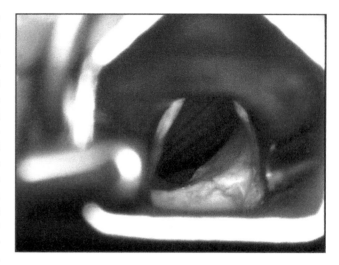

Figure 41–3. Laryngoscopic view of extrinsic compression of trachea from thyroid goiter.

high dependency unit. The postoperative parathyroid hormone and calcium levels were normal. Histologically the nodule was a follicular adenoma. At her first follow-up 2 weeks later, she was clinically much improved, with no stridor or exertional dyspnea. Fiberoptic endoscopic examination of the larynx confirmed symmetrically mobile vocal folds.

Airway Problems Post Thyroid Surgery

As for any operation but especially for thyroid surgery, emergence from endotracheally intubated general anesthesia should be smooth, with the aid of intravenous opiates to reduce cough, agitation, and laryngospasm that may contribute to acute hemodynamic swings and increased venous pressure promoting postoperative hemorrhage and its attendant complications. The surgical team should be present in the operating room until successful extubation has occurred.

Postoperative symptoms suggesting the need for reintubation may be immediate, manifest within minutes, or delayed, presenting in hours with a rapidly deteriorating airway. The most common causes are obstructive and include bilateral vocal fold paralysis, hematoma or tracheomalacia. Occasionally respiratory failure is the cause, with impaired gaseous exchange due to pulmonary edema, pneumothorax, or neuromuscular failure. Patients who require reintubation are at increased risk of needing tracheostomy and prolonged hospital stay and of mortality.[26]

Preoperative laryngoscopy will identify preexisting unilateral RLN palsy in 2 to 4% of patients in whom compensation has spontaneously occurred.[27] At least one RLN is permanently injured in a further 0 to 4% of patients, and this is positively related to surgical inexperience, revision cases, reoperation to evacuate hematoma, toxic goiters, retrosternal goiters, and malignancy, which in some cases may be planned. Routine intraoperative nerve identification and preservation significantly reduce iatrogenic RLN palsy.[28] A traumatic intubation or extubation may sublux or dislocate one or both arytenoids and should be considered if intraoperative anatomical nerve integrity is certain; laryngoscopy may demonstrate significant arytenoid edema and loss of symmetry.

Bilateral recurrent laryngeal nerve palsy will manifest with stridor immediately post extubation, sometimes exacerbated by flash pulmonary edema associated with an acute rise in negative intrathoracic pressure due to acute glottic obstruction. In some patients the airway may stabilize without the need for reintubation if the vocal folds lie in a lateralized position. A short expectant policy may therefore be prudent, but many will require reintubation and subsequent tracheostomy. If RLN integrity is not expected to recover, the caliber of the glottic airway may be improved by laser posterior cordectomy and/ or partial (medial) arytenoidectomy, perhaps as a prelude to extubation or tracheostomy decannulation. If recovery is expected, e.g., when one was sure of anatomical and functional nerve preservation, a suture lateralization technique may open the glottis, retaining an element of reversibility. In many cases, however, a tracheostomy will be required.

Compressive hematoma occurs in 1% of cases, mostly in the first 8 hours, although anticoagulated patients may present later.[29,30] Airway compression occurs largely due to venous engorgement of the larynx as a consequence of impaired venous return, which in turn is caused by hematoma trapped beneath the strap muscles. Arterial bleeds may occur from named vessels such as the cricothyroid and superior and inferior thyroid arteries due to a slipped ligature; other sources include reopened cauterized vessels or ooze from the remaining thyroid lobe or muscle edge. Often, dissatisfyingly, a source is not found during reexploration. Routine drainage does not reduce the rate of postsurgical hematoma and reoperation.[31] The neck should be visible postoperatively to ensure early detection of neck swelling and nursing staff should be vigilant for symptoms of acute airway obstruction such as stridor and dyspnea. A clip remover and stitch cutter should be at the bedside in order to swiftly evacuate the hematoma and release the tension in the neck while awaiting reintubation, definitive neck exploration, hemostasis, and postoperative drainage.

The existence of tracheomalacia in the context of large or retrosternal goiters is controversial. Classically it is defined as a reduction of the cross-sectional area of a segment of trachea by more than 50% upon inspiration.[32] Theoretically, long-standing compression by a large external mass distorts and weakens the cartilaginous structural support of the trachea, which becomes prone to collapse with negative pressure. Although the incidence has been reported to occur in up to 1.5% of benign goiters,[33] some case series failed to show any.[20] Clinically it may manifest with inspiratory stridor and progressive hypoxia unresponsive to oxygenation, although other causes of post extubation respiratory distress, including bilateral RLN palsy, glottic or subglottic trauma, and edema also present this way and should be excluded prior to making this diagnosis. A "floppy" trachea on palpation may be an intraoperative indicator, being more pronounced upon gradual withdrawal of the ETT. Indeed, slow withdrawal on extubation may demonstrate a sudden increase in ventilatory pressures, associated with an inability to pass a suction catheter beyond the ETT tip. If severe and discovered intraoperatively, consider inserting a tracheostomy tube, which not only acts as a stent but is also thought to promote fibrosis around the malacic tracheal segment, aiding subsequent decannulation.[34] Prolonged intubation for more than 48 hours has been advocated to achieve the same, where improvement in respiratory physiological parameters will guide extubation. This is unlikely to reverse long-standing structural changes, however. Intratracheal open stenting with a silicone prosthesis in the medium term is another option. If indeed a short segment is unequivocally affected, a tracheal resection may ultimately be a safer option, surgical expertise permitting.

Finally, long-standing compressive goiters may inadvertently create an auto-positive end expiratory pressure (PEEP) circuit akin to obstructing naso-oropharyngeal masses causing obstructive sleep apnea (OSA). Post-surgery, the loss of this auto-PEEP may generate negative intrathoracic pressures and induce pulmonary edema. This usually responds to continuous positive airway pressure (CPAP)/bilevel positive airway pressure (BiPAP) but may require reintubation and mechanical ventilation in the worst case scenario. If patients describe symptoms classically associated with OSA, such as nocturnal apnea, poor sleep, and daytime somnolence preoperatively, then a sleep study in conjunction with an obstructive flow-volume loop analysis may identify those patients at risk. If time and resources allow, these investigations should routinely be performed in chronically enlarged goiters. These patients should be nursed postoperatively in a high dependency environment in anticipation of respiratory compromise.

REFERENCES

1. Mallampati SR, et al. A clinical sign to predict difficult tracheal intubation: a prospective study. *Can Anaesth Soc J*. 1985;32(4):429–434.
2. Bennett AM, et al. The myth of tracheomalacia and difficult intubation in cases of retrosternal goitre. *J Laryngol Otol*. 2004;118(10):778–780.
3. Bouaggad A, et al. Prediction of difficult tracheal intubation in thyroid surgery. *Anesth Analg*. 2004:99(2):603–606, table of contents.
4. Loftus PA, et al. Risk factors for perioperative airway difficulty and evaluation of intubation approaches among patients with benign goiter. *Ann Otol Rhinol Laryngol*. 2014;123(4):279–285.
5. Kanotra SP, et al. GlideScope-assisted nerve integrity monitoring tube placement for intra-operative recurrent laryngeal nerve monitoring. *J Laryngol Otol*. 2012;126 (12):1271–1273.
6. Bensghir M, et al. [Comparison between the Airtraq, X-Lite, and direct laryngoscopes for thyroid surgery: a randomized clinical trial]. *Can J Anaesth*. 2013;60(4):377–384.
7. Haugen BR, et al. 2015 American Thyroid Association management guidelines for adult patients with thyroid nodules and differentiated thyroid cancer: the American Thyroid Association Guidelines Task Force on Thyroid Nodules and Differentiated Thyroid Cancer. *Thyroid*. 2016; 26(1):1–133.
8. McCaffrey JC, Aerodigestive tract invasion by well-differentiated thyroid carcinoma: diagnosis, management, prognosis, and biology. *Laryngoscope*. 2006;116(1):1–11.
9. Ito Y, et al. Clinical significance of extrathyroid extension to the parathyroid gland of papillary thyroid carcinoma. *Endocr J*. 2009;56(2):251–255.
10. Alon EE, Urken M. Management and prevention of laryngotracheal and oesophageal injuries in thyroid surgery. In: Miccoli P, et al, eds, *Thyroid Surgery Preventing and Managing Complications*. West Sussex, UK: John Wiley & Sons; 2013:153.
11. Tsumori T, et al. Clinicopathologic study of thyroid carcinoma infiltrating the trachea. *Cancer*. 1985;56(12):2843–2848.
12. Honings J, et al. The management of thyroid carcinoma invading the larynx or trachea. *Laryngoscope*. 2010;120(4): 682–689.
13. Gaissert HA, et al. Segmental laryngotracheal and tracheal resection for invasive thyroid carcinoma. *Ann Thorac Surg*. 2007;83(6):1952–1959.
14. Perros P, et al. Guidelines for the management of thyroid cancer. *Clin Endocrinol (Oxf)*. 2014;81(suppl 1):1–122.

15. Foroulis CN, et al. Primary intrathoracic goiter: a rare and potentially serious entity. *Thyroid*. 2009;19(3):213–218.
16. Hall TS, et al. Substernal goiter versus intrathoracic aberrant thyroid: a critical difference. *Ann Thorac Surg*. 1988; 46(6):684–685.
17. Anders HJ. Compression syndromes caused by substernal goitres. *Postgrad Med J*. 1998;74(872):327–329.
18. Shimaoka K, Sokal J. Suppressive therapy of nontoxic goiter. *Am J Med*. 1974;57(4):576–583.
19. Bonnema SJ, et al. Does radioiodine therapy have an equal effect on substernal and cervical goiter volumes? Evaluation by magnetic resonance imaging. *Thyroid*. 2002; 12(4):313–317.
20. Mackle T, Meaney J, Timon C. Tracheoesophageal compression associated with substernal goiter. Correlation of symptoms with cross-sectional imaging findings. *J Laryngol Otol*. 2007;121(4):358–361.
21. Ben Nun A, Soudack M, Best L. Retrosternal thyroid goiter: 15 years experience. *Isr Med Assoc J*. 2006;8(2):106–109.
22. Winbladh A, Jarhult J. Fate of the non-operated, nontoxic goitreiter in a defined population. *Br J Surg*. 2008; 95(3):338–343.
23. Hardy RG, et al. Management of retrosternal goiters. *Ann R Coll Surg Engl*. 2009;91(1):8–11.
24. White M, Doherty G, Gauger P. Evidence-based surgical management of substernal goiter. *World J Surg*. 2008; 32(7):1285–1300.
25. Pieracci F, Fahey T 3rd. Substernal thyroidectomy is associated with increased morbidity and mortality as compared with conventional cervical thyroidectomy. *J Am Coll Surg*. 2007;205(1):1–7.
26. Rady M, Ryan T. Perioperative predictors of extubation failure and the effect on clinical outcome after cardiac surgery. *Crit Care Med*. 1999;27(2):340–347.
27. Randolph G, Kamani D. The importance of preoperative laryngoscopy in patients undergoing thyroidectomy: voice, vocal cord function, and the preoperative detection of invasive thyroid malignancy. *Surgery*. 2006;139(3): 357–362.
28. Chiang FY, et al. Recurrent laryngeal nerve palsy after thyroidectomy with routine identification of the recurrent laryngeal nerve. *Surgery*. 2005;137(3):342–347.
29. Shaha A, Jaffe B. Practical management of post-thyroidectomy hematoma. *J Surg Oncol*. 1994;57(4):235–238.
30. Rosenbaum M, Haridas M, McHenry C. Life-threatening neck hematoma complicating thyroid and parathyroid surgery. *Am J Surg*. 2008. 195(3):339–43; discussion 343.
31. Samraj K, Gurusamy K. Wound drains following thyroid surgery. *Cochrane Database Syst Rev*. 2007(4):CD006099.
32. Jokinen K, et al. Acquired tracheobronchomalacia. *Ann Clin Res*. 1977;9(2):52–57.
33. Green WE, et al. Tracheal collapse after thyroidectomy. *Br J Surg*. 1979;66(8):554–557.
34. Moran A, Fliss D. Respiratory failure following extubation In: Miccoli P, et al, eds, *Thyroid Surgery Preventing and Managing Complications*, West Sussex, UK: John Wiley & Sons; 2013.

SECTION III
GENERAL/SYSTEMIC

CHAPTER 42

A Case of Upper Respiratory Infection, Reflux, and Persistent Cough

Anne E. Vertigan

INTRODUCTION

Cough is the most common reason for patients seeking ambulatory care.[1,2] Acute cough often resolves spontaneously or after a single dose of medical treatment. Cough persisting beyond the acute phase is known as chronic cough. The most common causes of chronic cough include smoking, lung pathology, asthma, rhinosinusitis, gastroesophageal reflux disease (GERD), obstructive sleep apnea, and eosinophilic bronchitis.[3] Medical treatment directed toward these conditions is effective in relieving cough in up to 80% of patients; however, cough can be refractory to medical management.[2] Behavioral intervention and neuromodulator therapies can be helpful in patients with refractory cough.

DEFINITION

Chronic cough is defined as a cough that lasts for longer than 8 weeks.

CASE PRESENTATION

A 47-year-old woman, FJ, presented with a 3-month history of cough following upper respiratory tract infection. The cough was dry and triggered from the throat and was occasionally so severe it led to vomit-ing. Onset occurred 3 months earlier after an upper respiratory tract infection that was associated with rhinorrhea, cough, and headache. Symptoms resolved after seven days; however, the cough has persisted. FJ has long-standing symptoms of reflux which have been worse over the last 2 years. Previous medical history includes appendectomy. She was not taking any regular medication except for occasional salbutamol without a spacer. FJ works as an accounts manager in a bank. She is married with two children.

INITIAL ASSESSMENT

FJ was examined by a respiratory physician.

History

There were no red flag symptoms such as dysphagia, hemoptysis, substantial sputum production, recurrent pneumonia, prominent dyspnea, or systemic symptoms such as fever and weight loss. She is a non-smoker. There were reflux symptoms which have worsened over the last 2 years including heartburn and burping after large meals. She reported intermittent hay fever including mild nasal itching and discharge. She has had asthma since childhood but has never undergone any formal asthma testing. There were no signs of significant emotional distress.

Examination

The patient appeared well without any obvious shortness of breath; however, there was constant coughing during the assessment. The chest radiograph was normal and the chest was clear. There was no lymphadenopathy, and heart sounds were dual and normal.

Investigations for Reflux

Twenty-four-hour ambulatory pH monitoring with a single sensor was conducted. The patient did not attend work for the duration of the test but reported she performed her other usual activities. The DeMeester score was 15.2, which is mildly elevated.

Pulmonary Function Testing with Airway Provocation Challenge

Baseline spirometry was normal. There was a 30% fall in forced inspiratory flow at 50% (FIF_{50}) following administration of 4.5% hypertonic saline but no evidence of bronchial hyperreactivity, as denoted by no significant fall in forced expiratory volume in 1 second (FEV_1).

TREATMENT

FJ was prescribed pantoprazole (40 mg once daily) and lifestyle modification for reflux. Asthma puffers were withdrawn as they were deemed unnecessary. Antihistamines were prescribed.

Follow-Up

Twelve weeks later, FJ reported a significant improvement in reflux symptoms but no improvement in cough. She continued to cough continually during the assessment. She had ceased antihistamines after 2 weeks due to drowsiness. Chronic refractory cough was diagnosed, as the cough did not respond to treatment for reflux, and possible vocal cord dysfunction (VCD) based on the results of the hypertonic saline challenge whereby a fall of more than 20 to 25% in FIF_{50} is suggestive of vocal cord dysfunction.

MANAGEMENT OPTION 1

One management option is to consider further medical investigations, including bronchoscopy, gastroscopy, esophageal manometry, chest CT, sinus CT, and allergy testing. Bronchoscopy was not selected as it has a low diagnostic yield in non-smokers with chronic cough.[4] Further investigations of gastroesophageal reflux disease including gastroscopy and esophageal manometry were considered but not thought to be a priority at this time as reflux symptoms had resolved; however, these investigations could determine the need for additional anti-reflux measures. Chest CT was not considered a priority. Similarly, sinus CT, skin prick testing, and serum immunoglobulin E were not deemed to be priorities at this time as sinonasal symptoms were not significant.

MANAGEMENT OPTION 2

Referral for speech pathology intervention: FJ was referred to a speech pathologist for behavioral management of her cough. She underwent assessment, laryngoscopy, and a course of speech pathology intervention for cough.

Speech Pathology Assessment

Presenting Symptoms

The cough is preceded by a sudden onset of throat tightness and FJ coughs to relieve this sensation. Voice is hoarse particularly in the morning. She reported taking the pantoprazole but in contrast to details of the medical assessment, denied knowledge of any lifestyle reflux strategies.

Triggers include cold air and talking.

Vocal Hygiene

Negative factors include reduced water intake (1 liter daily) and extensive vocal use, including talking over background noise when coaching children's sporting matches. Positive factors include non-smoking, minimal caffeine and alcohol intake, and nasal breathing.

Table 42–1. Questionnaire Scores

Scale	Domains Measured	Normal Range	Pre-Treatment Results	Post-Treatment Results	Minimal Clinically Important Difference
Leicester Cough Questionnaire	Cough	>19	16	18.7	1.3
Laryngeal Hypersensitivity Questionnaire	Laryngeal sensation	<17.1	14.6	16.8	1.7
Voice Handicap Index	Voice	<10	10	8	18
Hospital Anxiety & Depression Scale	Mood	<8	Anxiety 3 Depression 4	Anxiety 4 Depression 4	

Clinical Observations

There was continual forced coughing and throat clearing every 10 to 15 seconds that appeared to be triggered from the throat. Symptoms were also triggered by deep breathing and voice assessment tasks. The oral cavity was dry. The timed swallow test result was 17.0 mL/second, which is normal. There were no clinical signs of aspiration on thin fluids. Voluntary cough was normal. No respiratory difficulties were noted at rest but there was some difficulty coordinating respiration and phonation and breathing was shallow at times. Extrinsic laryngeal muscle tension was present at rest and during phonation, particularly in the thyrohyoid region.

Questionnaires

Results of symptom rating questionnaires are shown in Table 42–1. Leicester Cough Questionnaire[5] and Laryngeal Hypersensitivity Questionnaire[6] scores were in the abnormal range. The Voice Handicap Index[7] score was borderline, suggesting no significant impact of voice symptoms on quality of life. Hospital Anxiety and Depression Scale scores were normal.

Voice Assessment

The voice assessment included auditory perceptual voice analysis, voice performance testing, and acoustic voice analysis.

Auditory Perceptual Analysis

The Consensus Auditory Perceptual Evaluation (Voice) score was 11/100 for vowels, 6/100 for sentences, and 52/100 for connected speech, which indicates a moderate-severe rating. It was characterized by rough vo-

cal quality and mildly reduced pitch. These findings were not consistent with the Voice Handicap Index rating.

Maximum phonation time was 9.5 seconds, which is reduced. There was a sudden intake of air at the conclusion of this task, suggesting difficulty coordinating respiration and phonation. The prolongation time for /s/ was 12 seconds, which is also reduced. Laryngeal diadochokinesis is normal. There is no evidence of vocal fatigue. Pitch range is adequate. Loudness range is reduced.

Acoustic Voice Analysis. Acoustic voice assessment results are shown in Table 42–2. Intensity measures were outside the normal range, with difficulty achieving minimum and maximum intensity. Frequency measures

Table 42–2. Acoustic Voice Assessment Results

$SPL_{Habitual}$	55 dB SPL
SPL_{Min}	51 dB SPL
SPL_{Max}	81 dB SPL
$F_{0Connected\ speech}$	152 Hz
SDF_{0Vowel}	37 Hz
$SDF_{0Connected\ speech}$	53 Hz
F_{0Max}	576 Hz
F_{0Min}	111 Hz
Phonation frequency range	29 semitones
Harmonic to noise ratio	14.8 dB SPL

Note: SPL = sound pressure level; F_0 = fundamental frequency; SDF_0 = standard deviation of fundamental frequency; Hz = hertz.

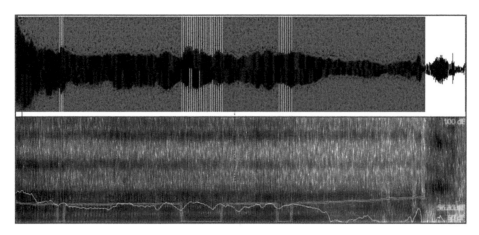

Figure 42–1. Spectrogram of sustained vowel /a/.

showed reduced fundamental frequency in connected speech, reduced stability during vowel prolongation, but adequate frequency range. Harmonic to noise ratio, an acoustic correlate of vocal quality, was below the normal range. A spectrogram of the sustained vowel /a/ (Figure 42–1) shows reduced acoustic energy, difficulty sustaining pitch, and reduced formant definition. These results were consistent with the perceptual analysis.

Laryngoscopy

Transnasal laryngoscopy revealed normal vocal fold structure. There was no erythema around the arytenoids or post cricoid region and no vocal fold edema. There was no paradoxical vocal fold movement during quiet respiration. There was a small posterior glottic chink present during phonation. Moderate medio-lateral and mild anterior-posterior constriction were present during phonation. An odor challenge triggered paradoxical vocal fold movement and cough.

Speech Pathology Intervention for Chronic Refractory Cough

Based on the results of the above assessment, a course of speech pathology intervention for chronic refractory cough was recommended. This treatment is multimodal and encompasses four main components: education, cough suppression exercises, reduction of laryngeal irritation, and psychoeducational counsel-

ing. FJ attended four therapy sessions addressing the above components.

Education

Four issues were discussed as part of the education component. First, there can be increased cough hypersensitivity at the time of an upper respiratory tract infection. In most cases this hypersensitivity spontaneously resolves within 2 to 3 weeks; however, in some cases it persists for protracted periods of time. Second, although an urge to cough may be present, the cough is not always necessary.[8] The urge to cough is present because of hyperstimulation of airway sensory nerves in the absence of material in the lungs or bronchial tubes that requires expectoration. Third, the act of coughing can exacerbate laryngeal irritation and increase the risk of laryngeal injury. Finally, it is possible to exert voluntary control over the cough. Functional MRI studies have shown increased cortical activation during reflexive and voluntary cough and during voluntary cough suppression.[9,10] Speech pathology intervention for cough exploits the capacity for voluntary control by teaching patients to respond to the urge to cough in a manner other than coughing.

Symptom Control Exercises

A relaxed breathing technique was used. This technique involved gentle nasal breathing without tension. FJ was encouraged to sit with a relaxed posture while being invited to notice any tension around the shoulder and neck region. She was also encouraged to attend to her posture when sitting by noticing whether her weight was evenly distributed between her feet and sit bones (ischial tuberosity). She was encouraged to take gentle breaths in through her nose without breath holding and without taking large breaths of air. Emphasis was placed on breathing with a regular rhythm.

The relaxed breathing technique was taught during the first therapy session. Coughing and throat clearing ceased immediately while performing the technique. FJ was encouraged to practice this technique at regular intervals throughout the day during asymptomatic periods and to use it to prevent, abort, or delay cough during symptomatic periods. A range of symptom control exercises can be used in speech pathology treatment of chronic refractory cough, and the choice of technique will be guided by the speech pathologist.

Reducing Laryngeal Irritation

Laryngeal irritation is targeted during speech pathology intervention in order to reduce stimulation of cough receptors. Strategies utilized in this case included hydration, lifestyle modification for reflux, and resonant voice therapy. Systemic hydration was targeted by increasing water intake. It is believed that fluids are absorbed by intestinal cells, transferred to the capillary network and transported around the body by the vascular system.[11] Inadequate systemic hydration can raise phonation threshold pressure.[12] More detailed information about lifestyle modification for reflux, including diet changes, raising the head of the bed, and avoiding eating 2 hours before going to sleep, was provided and time was spent explaining the rationale for this. Resonant voice therapy was commenced to reduce phonotraumatic vocal behaviors and subsequent irritation. FJ required ongoing coaching to utilize the correct technique as there was a tendency to perform the exercises with increased laryngeal tension.

Rationale and Evidence

Studies of speech pathology treatment for chronic refractory cough to date have focused entirely on patients with chronic refractory cough rather than all causes of chronic cough.

Speech pathology treatment for chronic refractory cough has been evaluated in two randomized controlled trials.[13,14] Therapy results in reduced cough frequency and severity and improved quality of life,[13,14] along with reduced cough reflex sensitivity.[15]

At Review

A review appointment was conducted following 4 weeks of speech pathology intervention for cough. Adherence to the therapy was good. There was a reduction in cough during the clinical setting. FJ reported that she still had an occasional urge to cough but was able to utilize the therapy techniques to prevent the cough from occurring. Leicester Cough Questionnaire and Laryngeal Hypersensitivity Questionnaire scores improved by more than the minimal clinically important difference for the scales and was consistent with the patient self-report of improvement (see Table 42–1). Voice quality had improved but was not consistently normal. FJ was aware of her voice quality but reported that she was not particularly bothered by her voice. FJ was discharged from speech pathology but advised that further therapy may be needed if her voice or cough became more problematic in the future.

MANAGEMENT OPTION 3: NEUROMODULATORS

Centrally acting neuromodulators used in chronic cough include gabapentin, pregabalin, morphine, amitriptyline, and baclofen. These drugs act on the heightened neural sensitization that is involved in the pathogenesis of chronic cough.[2,16] Neuromodulators may be an alternative or adjunct treatment to speech pathology intervention for cough. They may be useful for patients who prefer medication to speech pathology therapy or for those who have a partial or unsatisfactory response to such intervention.

Randomized trials of gabapentin,[17] morphine,[18] and amitriptyline[19] have shown improved cough quality of life. Gabapentin (1800 mg/day) showed reduced cough severity and cough frequency. These improvements were maintained while taking the medication but returned following withdrawal of the medication. There is no consistent effect on cough reflex sensitivity.[20] The use of neuromodulators can be limited by side effects which can be managed by dose reduction.[2] A randomized trial of combined pregabalin and speech pathology versus combined placebo medication and speech pathology showed better cough quality of life and cough severity in those receiving pregabalin but equal improvement in cough frequency and cough reflex sensitivity.[20] By combining speech pathology with pregabalin, there was no attenuation of treatment effect after withdrawal of the medication. FJ declined neuromodulator therapy as she was concerned about the potential side effects.

DIFFERENTIAL DIAGNOSIS FOR CHRONIC REFRACTORY COUGH

The differential diagnosis in this case is reflux, allergy, VCD, or idiopathic cough. There was no evidence of asthma, and asthma medication was withdrawn.

Reflux

Reflux is a normal physiological event. GERD is defined as a condition which develops when the reflux of stomach contents causes troublesome symptoms and/or complications.[21] Although there are no specific symptoms for GERD,[22] reflux in this case was diagnosed by a combination of symptoms and pH monitoring. Gastroscopy was not undertaken, hence signs of tissue damage could not be determined.

The recent American College of Chest Physicians clinical guideline on reflux cough recommends behavioral management of reflux, including diet modification to promote weight loss, elevating the head of the bed, avoiding meals within 3 hours of bedtime, and medications such as proton pump inhibitors (PPI).[23] These recommendations are summarized in Table 42–3. Although there are limited controlled data about the efficacy of anti-reflux treatment for cough.[24,25] there is some evidence demonstrating therapy efficacy in select patients.[26] In a randomized trial, high dose esomeprazole had no benefit on cough severity or quality of life in patients with cough and negative investigations for acid reflux disease.[27]

While pantoprazole appears to have been effective in relieving this patient's esophageal symptoms, it had little impact on cough. PPI therapy can be more effective for healing esophageal lesions than cough.[28] The

Table 42–3. Recommendations from the American College of Chest Physicians Guideline and Expert Panel Report on Chronic Cough Due to Gastroesophageal Reflux in Adults

Recommendation	Grade
1. Cough be managed according to a published management guideline that initially considers the most common potential etiologies as well as symptomatic gastroesophageal reflux	Ungraded consensus statement
2. Treatment of reflux-cough syndrome should include (1) diet modification to promote weight loss in overweight or obese patients; (2) head of bed elevation and avoiding meals within 3 hours of bedtime; and (3) in patients who report heartburn and regurgitation, proton pump inhibitors, H2-receptor antagonists, alginate, or antacid therapy sufficient to control these symptoms.	Grade 1C
3. In adult patients with suspected chronic cough due to reflux-cough syndrome, but without heartburn or regurgitation, PPI therapy alone is not recommended because it is unlikely to be effective in resolving the cough.	Grade 1 C
4. In adult patients with chronic cough potentially due to reflux-cough syndrome who are refractory to a 3-month trial of medical antireflux therapy and are being evaluated for surgical management (antireflux or bariatric), or in whom there is strong clinical suspicion warranting diagnostic testing for gastroesophageal reflux, esophageal manometry, and pH-metry with conventional methodology is recommended.	Grade 2C
5. In adult patients with chronic cough and a major motility disorder (eg, absent peristalsis, achalasia, distal esophageal spasm, hypercontractility) and/or normal acid exposure time in the distal esophagus, antireflux surgery is not recommended.	Grade 2C
6. In adult patients with chronic cough, adequate peristalsis, and abnormal esophageal acid exposure determined by pH-metry in whom medical therapy has failed, antireflux (or bariatric when appropriate) surgery for presumed reflux-cough syndrome is suggested.	Grade 2C

Note: Adapted from ACCP guidelines.[23]

treatment duration of PPI was over 3 months, which was thought to be an adequate time frame for the treatment of cough. It is unclear whether the lack of effectiveness was due to inadequate reflux treatment, including dose or adherence to lifestyle modifications. It is possible that non-acidic reflux could be the cause of cough. While lifestyle modification for reflux was included during the initial medical consultation, FJ was unable to recall this advice and had not implemented it. Zalvan[29] recently published retrospective data suggesting that diet modifications alone were equally effective as PPI in patients with laryngopharyngeal reflux symptoms. Effective behavioral management of reflux relies on patient adherence and adequate time needs to be invested in providing education and facilitating behavior change.

Reflux can coexist but not be a significant causal factor in cough. Smith suggests that the frequency and severity of reflux episodes are not significantly different between individuals with cough and controls but there is a temporal association between cough and reflux episodes.[30] In some cases, reflux might be a trigger rather than a cause of cough.[31] This was seen in FJ where reflux symptoms were present for 2 years in the absence of cough. It was not until an upper respiratory tract infection occurred that cough symptoms developed. It could be argued that reflux did not trigger cough until there was sufficient underlying hypersensitivity caused by the upper respiratory tract infection, and that the combination of these two factors was sufficient to trigger cough.[31]

Allergy

Formal allergy testing was not conducted. Empirical treatment of allergic rhinitis was commenced based on the patient self-report of intermittent hay fever but not continued due to side effects. The potential effect of allergy on cough in this case is difficult to determine as there was no definitive diagnosis of allergy and the treatment was poorly tolerated.

Vocal Cord Dysfunction

VCD occurs when there is involuntary and episodic closure of the vocal folds during respiration, typically inspiration, leading to cough, dyspnea, stridor, and dysphonia. The cause of VCD is unknown but it appears to be associated with chronic cough, reflux, and laryngeal hypersensitivity. There is an overlap in the symptom profile and sensitivity between patients with VCD and those with chronic refractory cough[32,33] and a significant degree of similarity in the speech pathology management of these conditions. FJ demonstrated evidence of VCD during the laryngoscopy procedure. Interestingly the VCD was only evident during odor provocation challenge and may not have been detected without this provocation challenge.

Chronic refractory cough shares many features with VCD and both may represent forms of laryngeal hypersensitivity. There is an overlap in the symptoms and voice features between the two conditions. Cough frequency and severity are similar between the two conditions.[33] There is considerable overlap in the speech pathology management of these conditions. Consideration of VCD can be helpful in individuals with chronic refractory cough who have not responded to medical treatment. Patients may complain of inspiratory dyspnea, throat tightness, a choking sensation, and being unable to inspire sufficient air.

Idiopathic or Unexplained Cough

Idiopathic or unexplained cough is said to occur when all other causes of cough have been considered and eliminated. It is a clinically significant cough that persists despite appropriate investigation and treatment.[2] An upper respiratory tract infection typically precedes cough even if it is associated with other conditions, such as GERD.[34]

MANAGEMENT

The management chosen will depend upon the results of the medical investigations. Medical intervention and assessment is essential before considering speech pathology intervention. This is necessary to rule out serious medical conditions such as cancer, and to rule out medical conditions requiring treatment such as gastroesophageal reflux disease and asthma. Furthermore, the efficacy of speech pathology management for chronic cough has only been demonstrated in patients with chronic refractory cough and not those with cough due to other causes.

1. Embarking on speech pathology management before complete medical investigations have been undertaken.
2. Adherence to speech pathology interventions. If patient compliance is poor, then this therapeutic approach will have limited benefit.
3. There is debate among clinicians as to the extent of medical investigation required and whether treatment should be provided in a stepwise or simultaneous fashion. In the case of FJ, bronchoscopy, gastroscopy, and allergy testing were not performed.

DISCUSSION

Chronic cough is a common and debilitating symptom. It has an adverse effect on quality of life, causing patients to cease employment and social activities and even speaking as talking triggers cough.[5] While medical treatment of chronic cough is effective for the majority of patients, approximately 20 to 40% of patients experience prolonged cough.[34]

Once smoking and lung pathology have been excluded, the most common causes of cough are gastroesophageal reflux disease, eosinophilic bronchitis, asthma, obstructive sleep apnea, and rhinosinusitis[3]; however, a single cause for chronic cough is unknown and treatment of associated diseases can be unsuccessful. Finding the cause of the cough is essential when cough is the result of a serious medical condition or when it is due to an associated medical condition that requires treatment; however, the cause of chronic cough will not be able to be identified in many patients.[2,34] Furthermore, while cough has been associated with the diseases described above, many individuals with these diseases do not develop a chronic cough. Cough can occur without these diseases and treatment of these conditions may be ineffective in resolving cough.

The concept of cough hypersensitivity syndrome (CHS) was recently proposed[35] to address some of the questions surrounding cough. CHS proposes that chronic cough occurs when there is a combination of underlying cough hypersensitivity and a trigger. Triggers can be environmental such as perfumes, behavioral such as talking or exercise, or intrinsic. Diseases such as GERD, asthma, and rhinosinusitis act as triggers rather than causes of the cough in an individual

with underlying cough hypersensitivity.[31] In the case of FJ, reflux would be seen as a trigger for cough episodes rather than a cause of the chronic refractory cough. The concept of CHS places more emphasis on treating cough hypersensitivity than extensive investigations to seek out the underlying cause of the cough.

CHS involves peripheral and central sensitization pathways similar to chronic pain.[36] Inflammatory mediators including mast cells and inflammatory cytokines in the upper and lower airway are likely to be the underlying mechanism for CHS.[20,37] Inflammatory processes impact nerve endings leading to peripheral sensitization. Chung[20] suggests that the site of hypersensitivity—for example, larynx, trachea, or esophagus—may differ between patients. The onset of cough following an upper respiratory tract infection is consistent with findings that rhinovirus can infect neuronal cells leading to an upregulation of transient receptor potential cation channel subfamily A member 1 (TRPA1) and transient receptor potential cation channel subfamily V member 1 (TRPV1) within 2 to 4 hours of infection[39] along with a release of nerve growth factor (NGF), interleukin (IL)-6, and IL-8.[20,38] Chung[20] proposed that CHS relating to esophageal factors may be the result of neuronal signal interference between the esophagus and airway that connects gastroesophageal reflux events and cough triggering.[20]

SUMMARY

Chronic cough is rarely serious but has a significant impact on quality of life. Medical treatment directed at the cause of cough can be effective; however, in some cases it might relieve the underlying condition but not the cough. The cause of cough cannot always be determined and in these cases symptomatic treatment using speech pathology or neuromodulators can be effective.

REFERENCES

1. Schappert S, Rechtsteiner E. Ambulatory medical care utilization estimates for 2007.*Vital Health Stat 13*, 2011: Apr(169):1–38.
2. Gibson P, Wang G, McGarvey L, Vertigan AE, Altman KW, Birring SS. Treatment of unexplained chronic cough: CHEST guideline and expert panel report. *Chest.* 2016; 149(1):27–44.

3. Irwin R, Boulet L, Cloutier M, et al. Managing cough as a defence mechanism and as a symptom: a consensus report for the American College of Chest Physicians. *Chest*. 1998;114(2):133S (147).

4. Macedo P, Zhang Q, Saito J, et al. Analysis of bronchial biopsies in chronic cough. *Respir Med*. 2017;127:40–44.

5. Birring S, Prudon B, Carr A, Singh S, Morgan M, Pavord I. Development of a symptom specific health status measure for patients with chronic cough: Leicester Cough Questionnaire. *Thorax*. 2003;58:339–343.

6. Vertigan AE, Bone SL, Gibson PG. Development and validation of the Newcastle Laryngeal Hypersensitivity Questionnaire. *Cough*. 2014;10(1):1.

7. Jacobson H, Johnson A, Grywalski C, Silbergleit A, Jacobson G, Benninger M. The Voice Handicap Index (VHI): development and validation. *Am J Speech Lang Pathol*. 1997;6:66–70.

8. Davenport P. Urge to cough: what can it teach us about cough. *Lung*. 2008;186(S1):107–111.

9. Leech J, Mazzone SB, Farrell MJ. Brain activity associated with placebo suppression of the urge-to-cough in humans. *Am J Resp Crit Care Med*. 2013;188(9):1069–1075.

10. Ando A, Smallwood D, McMahon M, Irving L, Mazzone SB, Farrell MJ. Neural correlates of cough hypersensitivity in humans: evidence for central sensitisation and dysfunctional inhibitory control. *Thorax*. 2016;71(4):323–329.

11. Hartley NA, Thibeault SL. Systemic hydration: relating science to clinical practice in vocal health. *J Voice*. 2014; 28(5):28.

12. Verdolini K, Titze I, Druker D. Changes in phonation threshold pressure with induced conditions of hydration. *J Voice*. 1990;4:142–151.

13. Chamberlain SAF, Garrod R, Clark L, et al. Physiotherapy, and speech and language therapy intervention for patients with refractory chronic cough: a multicentre randomised control trial. *Thorax*. 2016;72(2):129–136.

14. Vertigan A, Theodoros D, Gibson PG, Winkworth A. Efficacy of Speech pathology management for chronic cough: a randomised placebo controllled trial of treatment efficacy. *Thorax*. 2006;61(12):1065–1069.

15. Ryan NM, Vertigan AE, Bone S, Gibson PG. Cough reflex sensitivity improves with speech language pathology management of refractory chronic cough. *Cough*. 2010;6(1):1–8.

16. Gibson PG, Vertigan AE. Management of chronic refractory cough. *BMJ*. 2015;14(351).

17. Ryan N, Birring S, Gibson P. Gabapentin for refractory chronic cough: a randomised, double-blind, placebo-controlled trial. *Lancet*. 2012;380(9853):1583–1589.

18. Morice A, Menon M, Mulrennan S, et al. Opiate therapy in chronic cough. *Am J Resp Crit Care Med*. 2007;175(4): 312–315.

19. Jeyakumar A, Brickman TM, Haben M. Effectiveness of amitriptyline versus cough suppressants in the treatment of chronic cough resulting from postviral vagal neuropathy. *Laryngoscope*. 2006;116(12):2108–2112.

20. Chung KF. Advances in mechanisms and management of chronic cough: the Ninth London International Cough Symposium 2016. *Pulm Pharmacol Ther*. 2017;47:2–8.

21. Vakil N, van Zanten SV, Kahrilas P, Dent J, Jones R. The Montreal definition and classification of gastroesophageal reflux disease: a global evidence-based consensus. *Am J Gastroenterol*. 2006;101(8):1900–1920.

22. Kahrilas P, Smith J, Dicpinigaitis P. A causal relationship between cough and gastroesophageal reflux disease (GERD) has been established: a pro/con debate. *Lung*. 2014;192(1):39–46.

23. Kahrilas PJ, Altman KW, Chang AB, et al. Chronic cough due to gastroesophageal reflux in adults: CHEST guideline and expert panel report. *Chest*. 2016;150(6):1341–1360.

24. Chang A, Lasserson T, Kiljander T, Connor F, Gaffney J, Garske L. Systematic review and meta-analysis of randomised controlled trials of gastro-oesophageal reflux interventions for chronic cough associated with gastro-oesophageal reflux. *BMJ*. 2006;332(7532):11–17.

25. Chang AB, Lasserson TJ, Gaffney J, Connor FL, Garske LA. Gastro-oesophageal reflux treatment for prolonged non-specific cough in children and adults. *Cochrane Database Syst Rev*. 2006;18(4).

26. Kahrilas PJ, Howden CW, Hughes N, Molloy-Bland M. Response of chronic cough to acid-suppressive therapy in patients with gastroesophageal reflux disease. *Chest*. 2013;143(3):605–612.

27. Shaheen NJ, Crockett SD, Bright SD, et al. Randomised clinical trial: high-dose acid suppression for chronic cough—a double-blind, placebo-controlled study. *Aliment Pharmacol Ther*. 2011;33(2):225–234.

28. Boeckxstaens G, El-Serag HB, Smout AJ, Kahrilas PJ. Symptomatic reflux disease: the present, the past and the future. *Gut*. 2014;63(7):1185–1193.

29. Zalvan CH, Hu S, Greenberg B, Geliebter J. A comparison of alkaline water and Mediterranean diet vs proton pump inhibition for treatment of laryngopharyngeal reflux. *JAMA Otolaryngol Head Neck Surg*. 2017;143:1023–1029.

30. Smith JA, Decalmer S, Kelsall A, et al. Acoustic cough-reflux associations in chronic cough: potential triggers and mechanisms. *Gastroenterology*. 2010;139(3):754–762.

31. Song W-J, Chang Y-S, Morice A. Changing the paradigm for cough: does 'cough hypersensitivity' aid our understanding? *Asia Pac Allergy*. 2013;4(1):3–13.

32. Vertigan AE, Theodoros DG, Gibson PG, Winkworth AL. Voice and upper airway symptoms in people with chronic cough and paradoxical vocal fold movement. *J Voice*. 2007; 21(3):361–383.

33. Vertigan AE, Bone SL, Gibson PG. Laryngeal sensory dysfunction in laryngeal hypersensitivity syndrome. *Respirology*. 2013;18(6):948–956.

34. Haque R, Usmani O, Barnes P. Chronic idiopathic cough: a discrete clinical entity? *Chest*. 2005;127(5):1710–1713.

35. Morice A. The cough hypersensitivity syndrome: a novel paradigm for understanding cough. *Lung*. 2010;188 (suppl 1):S87–S90.

36. O'Neill J, McMahon S, Undem B. Chronic cough and pain: Janus faces in sensory neurobiology? *Pulm Pharma Therapeu.* 2010;26(5):476–485.

37. Niimi A, Chung KF. Airway inflammation and remodelling changes in patients with chronic cough: do they tell us about the cause of cough? *Pulm Pharmacol Ther.* 2004;17(6):441–446.

38. Abdullah H, Heaney LG, Cosby SL, McGarvey LP. Rhinovirus upregulates transient receptor potential channels in a human neuronal cell line: implications for respiratory virus-induced cough reflex sensitivity. *Thorax.* 2014; 69(1):46–54.

CHAPTER 43

Globus

Jacqueline Allen

INTRODUCTION

The sensation of a lump or foreign body or pressure or constriction in the throat is a common complaint in otolaryngology clinics the world over. Previously this was presumed to be a hysterical complaint until Malcolmson coined the term "globus pharyngeus" in 1968 after recognizing that most patients did not exhibit psychiatric disorders.[1] Recently better appreciation of organic causes of this sensation have emerged. It is still unclear why certain individuals experience the sensation more so than others, but it is likely multifactorial in nature. The difficulty is that infrequently it may represent a malignancy within the oro- or hypopharynx or the esophagus, and therefore must be investigated before reassurance can be given to the patient. Many investigations can be ordered and undertaken and it is a balance between ruling out serious pathology and over-investigating a benign complaint that requires largely lifestyle management.[2] With advances in current endoscopic equipment, this has become easier and credence should be given to patients complaining of globus sensation as significant improvements can be achieved now with both management regimens and eliminating serious pathologies.

DEFINITION

Globus pharyngeus is the reported subjective feeling of a lump or foreign body within the pharynx. It is a symptom.

CASE PRESENTATION

A 63-year-old woman presents with 3-month history of sensation of mass in throat and needing to clear the throat frequently. Associated symptoms are sensation of post-nasal drip and intermittent mild voice. No weight loss, odynophagia, otalgia, heartburn, or cough. Occasionally extra effort is required to swallow solid food and she reports intermittent belching and bitter taste in the pharynx. A non-smoker, Ms X also reports mouth-breathing during sleep.

Social: Non-smoker, minimal alcohol, mild hypercholesterolemia

Medications: Omeprazole 20 mg OD, simvastatin, cetirizine

Nil known allergies.

INITIAL ASSESSMENT

History

Red flag symptoms (otalgia, bleeding [hematemesis or oropharyngeal bleeding], pain, weight loss, significant voice change, marked dysphagia). Presence of these symptoms warrants urgent investigation, including full endoscopy (transnasal esophagoscopy [TNE]/gastroscopy), CT neck and chest and fluoroscopic swallow exam. Standard other history includes nature of complaint, triggers and moderators, previous and current therapies, plus social history (smoking/alcohol/stress) and medications.

Examination

Head and neck examination including thyroid gland (red flag findings: neck mass, trismus, nerve palsies, gross dysphonia)

Endoscopy

At a minimum a nasopharyngoscopy should be performed however this Author would suggest unsedated in-office TNE if available. This allows immediate rule-out of pharyngoesophageal carcinoma, assessment of upper esophageal sphincter (UES) compliance, evaluation of esophageal mucosa for reflux damage, and detection of hiatal hernia. Biopsies may be obtained if there is irritation, mass, or possible Barrett's metaplasia.

Scenario 1

Office head and neck examination is normal. Flexible transnasal esophagoscopy demonstrates a 2.5 cm mass in the left vallecula abutting the epiglottis and occupying the piriform inlet. Mass is smooth, well mucosalized, yellow in color (Figure 43–1). The rest of the piriform fossae, larynx, and pharynx is normal.

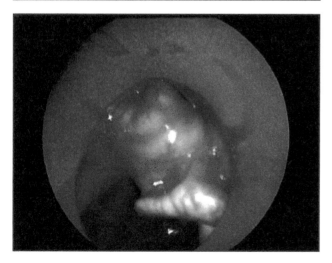

Figure 43–1. Endoscopic photomicrograph of vallecula cyst on tongue base.

Diagnosis

Vallecula cyst

Investigations

Nil

Management

Pharyngoscopy and de-roofing of vallecula cyst with gold laser.

Scenario 2

Office head and neck examination is normal. Flexible TNE is performed. Pharynx normal. Mild laryngeal edema with vocal fold pseudosulcus. Moderately tight pass of upper esophageal sphincter. Distal esophagus demonstrates grade A esophagitis, hiatal hernia, and a Shatzki's ring is present. Stomach is normal except for a Hill's grade 2 flap valve (mild laxity) on retroflexed view. Biopsies taken if:

- the squamocolumnar junction (SCJ) is markedly irregular,
- there are endoscopic findings consistent with Barrett's epithelium,
- gastritis is present (for *Helicobacter pylori*),
- there are esophageal findings (or history) suggestive of eosinophilic esophagitis (eg, ringed esophagus, multiple microabscesses/ white maculae within the esophageal body),
- there is an identifiable mass, or
- at strictures.

Diagnosis

Multifactorial globus sensation—combination of reflux events (likely both acid and non-acid volume reflux), pharyngeal drying (mouth breathing, cetirizine), and esophageal hypo/dysmotility.

Investigations

Initially, nil.
If symptoms persist despite initial therapy—pH and impedance study ± high resolution manometry, and/ or videofluoroscopic swallow study (VFSS).

Management

- Hydration
- Reassurance (everything has been visualized, review video with patient)
- Neck massage and stretching
- If possible, stop cetirizine
- Reflux lifestyle modifications: eat early, stay upright after eating for 90 minutes, sleep head elevated, avoid refluxogenic foods (caffeine, alcohol)
- Lubrication: steam, gargles, nasal cares, lozenges, fluids, alginate
- Review in 4 to 6 weeks

AT REVIEW

If there is no symptomatic relief, then arrange additional investigations as appropriate:

1. VFSS and pH-impedance study: If VFSS shows poor motility, or impedance demonstrates proximal reflux events (acid or non-acid), consider prokinetic agents (domperidone, metoclopramide, or erythromycin [low dose]). If pH study is positive for acid reflux events, consider H2 antagonist or proton pump inhibitor (PPI) therapy (as a block of treatment, not indefinitely).
2. Can consider breath urease test for *H. pylori*, although this is unlikely if no gastritis was seen on endoscopy. Treatable with triple therapy.

If there is marked dysmotility present, consider blood workup for systemic disease (autoimmune disorders, rheumatic disorders, diabetes mellitus) and esophageal manometry. If suggestive of a specific disorder, then referral to rheumatology, gastroenterology or appropriate service.

Management 2

Where additional investigations suggest proximal or high volume reflux that is unresponsive to medical (antacids, blocking agents, prokinetics) and lifestyle therapies (elevating head of bed, not reclining or exercising within 90 minutes of eating, avoiding refluxogenic foodstuffs such as caffeine, alcohol, and tomatoes, stopping smoking and losing weight), consider referral for fundoplication (usually this requires a positive symptom

association on pH/impedance study, coupled with fluoroscopic and endoscopic evidence of escape reflux in an anesthetically fit patient).

A manometry study may provide diagnostic information suggestive of primary or secondary motility disorders. Specific disorders may be amendable to directed treatment, such as achalasia to balloon disruption or Heller's myotomy. If identified, motility disorders should be referred to the gastroenterology department for ongoing management. Trial of prokinetic medication can also be utilized such as domperidone 10mg TDS. Medication interactions must be considered as these medications interact with selective serotonin uptake inhibitors (SSRI's) such as escitalopram, and may have an effect on prolonging QT interval in those with pre-existing cardiac arrythmia.

Scenario 3

Level II lymph node identified in left neck. Nasopharyngoscopy demonstrates tongue base asymmetry with irregular surface contours in the left vallecula region (Figure 43–2). Mobile vocal folds bilaterally, edema of aryepiglottic fold on left side.

Immediately: perform immediate transnasal esophagoscopy (TNE) for staging and screening metachronous tumor; consider in-office biopsy (depending on bleeding risk) or schedule for urgent panendoscopy following imaging.

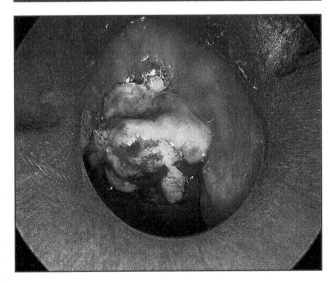

Figure 43–2. Endoscopic photomicrograph of malignant tumour of tongue base.

Diagnosis

Oropharyngeal malignancy (squamous cell carcinoma)

Management

- CT neck/chest, PET/CT fusion for staging
- Consider formal biopsy under anesthetic for tongue base mass. Request human papilloma virus evaluation (p16 vs polymerase chain reaction)
- Dental assessment and scanning dental radiograph
- Multidisciplinary team review (tumor board)
- Further treatment depending on diagnosis—chemoradiation vs surgery and postoperative radiation
- Pain management, nutrition assessment

DIFFERENTIAL DIAGNOSIS

There is a wide differential diagnosis in globus sensation. This may represent a true mass (sometimes a "lump in the throat feeling" is due to a lump in the throat!), whether that is benign (vallecula cyst, lymphoid hyperplasia, squamous papilloma, hamartoma, thyroid enlargement, fibroepithelial polyp, lingual thyroid, enlarged and pendulous uvula) or malignant (squamous cell carcinoma, lymphoma, salivary malignancy, rhabdomyosarcoma, melanoma). However, it may also be due to altered physiology and vagally-mediated feedback that acts as an "early warning system" to protect the airway and glottis.

Structural

- Benign
- Malignant
- Strictures—malignant, anastomotic, caustic, post-radiation

Functional

- Muscular: cricopharyngeal irritation (manometry usually demonstrates normal pressures at the UES but the sphincter may be irritated by a combination of factors,

especially dryness), neuromuscular disease (inclusion body myositis [IBM], myotonic dystrophy [MD], dermatomyositis, amyotrophic lateral sclerosis [ALS], Shy–Drager syndrome).
- Mucosal: dryness and exposure to chemicals/irritants (dust, industrial volatile substances, high air flows including talking/fans/air conditioning, refluxate, smoking)
- Neurogenic: following stroke (cerebrovascular accident) or above conditions (ALS, IBM, MD, dermatomyositis)
- Traumatic: injury, treatment-related (post-radiation), iatrogenic (post-surgical, such as anterior cervical decompression and fusion [ACDF], thyroid surgery)
- Inflammatory/infective: osteophytosis (friction trauma) (Figure 43–3), candida, neck abscess

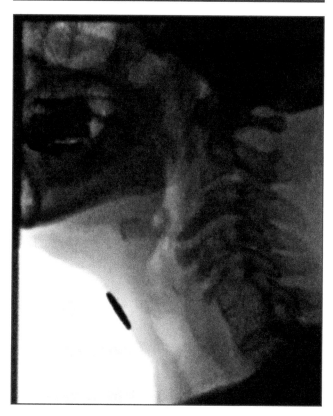

Figure 43–3. Lateral fluoroscopic view of pharynx demonstrating moderate osteophytosis of the spine at levels C3–5 impinging into pharyngeal lumen.

MANAGEMENT

Management is dependent on the diagnosis and must be tailored to the individual (Table 43–1). As illustrated by the varying scenarios above, it may range from reassurance and lifestyle advice through to surgical extirpation or oncologic therapy. In treating globus sensation it is important to rule out serious diagnoses before assigning the patient to a reassurance strategy. For this reason, I find it particularly useful to perform a full endoscopy (transnasal esophagoscopy) in the office at the time of presentation. This allows me to rule out an esophageal carcinoma or pharyngeal mass and thereby tailor medical therapy to the patient's symptom burden, bearing in mind that often establishing lack of a tumor or serious condition, and providing a clear explanation of how multiple factors may generate symptoms can be enough for patients to be satisfied and relieved of concern. In some cases, this is all the patient desires and further workup or intervention may be unwarranted.

In cases of tumor, early identification improves prognosis and possibility of curative treatment and avoids delayed diagnosis or misdiagnosis. Availability of intervention will vary from institution to institution; however, it is often multidisciplinary, involving otolaryngology, speech language pathology, gastroenterology, physiotherapy, general surgery, and respiratory services. Throughout the process, clear explanation of symptom generation and rationale for treatment is very useful in assisting the patient with symptom management and engendering compliance with strategies.

PITFALLS

The key is to avoid attributing globus sensation to nonorganic or psychological causes without completely ruling out mass lesions or neurologic disease. Globus sensation requires a full workup to enable reassurance and conservative multifocal treatment to be given, with each individual then receiving a tailored and targeted treatment plan.

Table 43–1. Possible Causes of Globus Sensation

Reported Cause	Hypothesized Mode of Action
Gastroesophageal or extra-esophageal reflux	1. Direct irritation of laryngopharynx from esophagopharyngeal escape
	2. Vagally mediated hyperfunction or hypersensitivity of esophagus
Psychological factors and stress	Increased anxiety and attention to the symptom complex
Heterotopic gastric mucosal patches in esophagus (CHGM)	Secretion of gastric hormones in the upper esophagus
Lingual tonsil hypertrophy	Direct contact with posterior pharyngeal wall or epiglottic tip
Osteophytosis	Friction related discomfort with swallowing or head movements
Rarely tumors or growths in the laryngopharynx	Squamous cell carcinoma of the laryngopharynx, hamartomata, salivary neoplasms, rare conditions
Esophageal motility disorders	Non-specific motility problems or specific manometric diagnoses, eg, ineffective esophageal motility
Upper esophageal sphincter dysfunction	Hypertensive upper esophageal sphincter—pathological vs compensatory response
Salivary dysfunction	Hyposalivation and xeropharyngia
Thyroid disease or nodules	Deeply located or anteriorly located thyroid nodules >3 cm diameter
Pharyngeal inflammation—Post-nasal drip, pharyngitis,	Chronic irritation or inflammation of the pharyngolaryngeal mucosa from infection, post-nasal drainage

DISCUSSION

Because globus sensation is a symptom and there is no diagnostic test for its presence or indeed even to quantify the degree of symptomatology, and because there seem to be a number of factors that contribute to presence, sustenance, or aggravation of the symptom, it is very difficult to compare treatment effectiveness or even to advocate for a particular treatment over others.[2] Inherent in the discussion of possible treatments is the complete evaluation of the complaint. To ensure diagnosis of treatable conditions, a complete evaluation is necessary. For expediency, in-office endoscopy of the pharyngolarynx and esophagus performed at initial consultation is hugely helpful, enabling reassurance regarding malignant growths, identification of mass lesions, evaluation of reflux damage, biopsy of mucosa, and assessment of the nasal airways and glottis.[3] This immediately allows a targeted treatment approach to be devised and can direct further investigations if required at the outset. If everything is normal and there are no "red flag" symptoms in the history, this enables the clinician to utilize a conservative approach of reassurance and pharyngolaryngeal hygiene. Because the natural history of globus sensation is not fully understood, we need to avoid misattribution of improvement to administered treatments. Published studies suggest 50 to 60% improvement in symptoms over 5 to 7 years without specific treatments.[4,5] Conversely, half of patients have persistent symptoms but learn to live with the symptoms much like patients with tinnitus. In a study following 74 globus sufferers for over 7 years, although half had persistent symptoms, none of these patients developed upper aerodigestive tract malignancy.[5]

WHAT IS THE CAUSE?

Current literature on globus spans associations with allergy and positive skin prick testing, psychological disorders and depression, cervical osteophytosis, xerostomia or hyposalivation, thyroid disease, esophageal motility disorders, gastroesophageal reflux disease, extra-esophageal reflux, and gastric heterotopic mucosa (gastric inlet patches).[1,6–13] Treatments suggested encompass the whole range too, with options from high dose proton pump therapy, prokinetics including traditional rikkunshito (Japanese traditional medicine), hydration techniques, to amitriptyline and gabapentin, or mood enhancers such as paroxetine.[2,11,13] Interestingly, other strategies for addressing the complaint have included education, endoscopy to demonstrate normal findings to patients, hypnotherapy and speech language therapy for reframing sensory feedback.[2,3,13,14] Akin to other neurologic-based symptom complexes, these approaches look to empower patients regarding their symptoms and action workable approaches to self-management. They have been highly successful in select groups where problematic organic disease has been ruled out.[13,14]

Possibly this is the key—that there is no one pathologic entity that causes globus, but many different contributors in differing amounts.

PSYCHOLOGICAL ASPECTS

One of the key aspects of research, though, is that the symptom is not merely hysterical or psychologic. While there may be some contribution from heightened perceptions or association with particular personality types, it appears that there is an organic component to symptom generation in most patients.[6] Nonetheless a psychological component is also present and medications that modulate mood and neural functions have shown some success in alleviating globus sensation.[15–18] Low dose amitriptyline was more efficacious in reducing reported symptoms over 1 to 6 months compared with daily dose of pantoprazole in 34 patients with functional esophageal disorders.[15] A randomized trial of 148 subjects reporting globus sensation compared treatment with either PPI, amitriptyline, or paroxetine and demonstrated physiological reduction in UES pressure using either paroxetine or amitriptyline but not PPI. Symptomatic improvement was greatest in the paroxetine group (72% vs 46% vs 14% for paroxetine, amitriptyline, and lansoprazole, respectively) with additional improvements in sleep quality and emotional well-being.[17] Gabapentin has also been used to treat refractory globus sensation that did not respond to initial high dose proton pump inhibitor therapy.[18] Fifty-seven percent (8/14) of patients non-responsive to PPI reported improvement on gabapentin.[18] Further cognitive-behavioral interventions demonstrating success in management of globus sensation include hypnotherapy, electroconvulsive therapy, education, reframing, and mood enhancers, such as selective serotonin reuptake inhibitors (SSRIs).[16,18,19] Kiebles reported success using hypnotically assisted relaxation (HAR) in 10 patients unresponsive to previous anti-secretory medication.[14] Manometry in these subjects demonstrated normal resting UES pressures, and 9/10 (90%) subjects reported relief of symptoms following a seven-session protocol.[14] Speech therapy has also demonstrated success in treatment of globus symptoms where other pathology has been excluded.[19,20] Some of the value may be in demonstrating alternative behaviors and providing education and reassurance.[20]

REFLUX AND UPPER ESOPHAGEAL SPHINCTER ASPECTS

It has been hypothesized that globus symptoms are due to reflux disease; however, typical reflux symptoms are uncommon in these patients. Only 37% of patients presenting with globus sensation reported heartburn in a study of 160 patients; however, 80% of the same group responded (symptomatic improvement) to acid suppression therapy of some type.[21] Hill et al studied 26 patients with globus sensation performing 24-hr pH study, manometry, esophagogastroduodenoscopy, and esophageal biopsies.[6] They also performed psychological profiles in these patients and a control group. Results of pH-metry were positive in 30% of those with globus vs 5% of controls ($p <0.05$) but no other factors differed between groups, including the psychological profiles.[6] Sinn et al studied 64 patients with globus and divided them into two groups—those with clinical diagnosis of GERD and those without.[22] All patients were given two weeks of rabeprazole treatment. Those with GERD symptoms and globus did not differ in response rate to PPI compared with those with globus alone; however, the globus symptom score was higher in those where GERD symptoms were also present.[22] Zelenik et al compared pH studies in patients with globus complaints using both a pH<4 level and pH<5.[23] At the lower pH level, 24% of studies were positive for acid reflux. Including pH<5 as abnormal added a further 8.7%, providing a combined total of a third of globus patients demonstrating abnormal acid exposure times.[23] Although there does appear to be a group of patients with globus who achieve symptom improvement on acid suppression therapy, it is not a universal response. This suggests that reflux is not the only player in generation of the globus symptom and that there are cofactors involved. Corso et al provide explanation for this variance.[24] Their study evaluated manometry, pH metry, and symptoms. The rate of globus sensation in those with hypertensive UES on manometry was 28%

(28/101) compared with only 3% (17/650) in those with normal UES pressures.[24] There was no concordance with pH-measured gastroesophageal reflux in this study for either group.[24] Kwiatek and colleagues demonstrated a hyperdynamic UES in patients with globus compared with those with GERD alone or asymptomatic controls.[25] Much larger pressure fluctuations were seen in measured UES pressures in those with globus during respiration (37 mm Hg vs <10 mm Hg).[25] Therefore, it may be that globus sensation is generated from the upper esophageal sphincter in response to irritation which may include refluxate, but may also include other stimuli such as dryness, turbulent airflow, heat, cold, position, stress, inhaled or ingested irritants, and viral attacks.[12] In this regard then, globus would be a "neurogenic symptom," which would make much more sense in the overall picture of globus presentation when one considers its waxing and waning nature and the association with stressful events. These findings are also important in considering treatment recommendations and duration of therapy given the side effect profile of proton pump inhibitors in particular. If there is not a clear associated symptom or quantitative evidence to support GERD, it may be prudent to limit empiric trials of PPI to short duration in order to prevent medication-induced acid rebound or malabsorption issues. Furthermore, referring patients for surgical anti-reflux procedures must be undertaken with caution as positive results of fundoplication or other lower esophageal sphincter enhancing surgeries for extra-esophageal symptoms are much lower than for those of typical GERD symptoms.[26–28]

OTHER GASTROINTESTINAL ASPECTS

Other gastrointestinal disorders have been linked to globus generation. Motility disorders of the esophagus span a wide range but have been associated with increased complaint of globus.[29–31] Esophageal motility is abnormal in 47 to 67% of those presenting with globus sensation evaluated by VFSS and manometry.[29–32] In 119 patients complaining of globus sensation and failing empiric PPI therapy, manometry demonstrated abnormal esophageal motility in 48% with ineffective esophageal motility the most common manometric diagnosis.[32] Poor bolus clearance was also noted to be more common in those with globus complaints in a VFSS study of 72 patients versus 33 control subjects.[33] A study of 21 patients with globus sensation reported 67% incidence of esophageal motility disorder, 24%

incidence of abnormal pH metry, and 25% incidence of psychiatric diagnosis using DSM criteria.[30] Identification of abnormal motility by fluoroscopic study or manometry (which is the gold standard in diagnosis) provides impetus for offering prokinetic treatment such as domperidone. Treatment with prokinetic medications offers benefit and relief of globus sensation as well as dyspeptic symptoms if present. *H. pylori* gastritis is a common finding in the general population. It was identified in 60% (75/123) of a cohort of patients presenting with globus sensation for which no other cause was identified.[34] Treatment of *H. pylori* resulted in improvement of symptoms in 50% of eradicated cases.[34] Gastric inlet patches are areas of heterotopic gastric mucosa found in the proximal esophagus. They contain parietal cells capable of acid production, and an association of cervical heterotopic gastric mucosa (CHGM) and globus sensation has been identified (Figure 43–4).[35,36] Lancaster reported four cases of CHGM associated with globus symptoms in which treatment with acid suppression resulted in relief of symptoms.[35] Treatment of the tissue by argon plasma coagulation also seems to improve symptoms regardless of underlying gastroesophageal reflux.[37,38] Von Rahden proposed a classification of CHGM based on association of symptoms, findings, and dysplasia or malignant transformation.[39] Type I HGM patients are asymptomatic, but type II HGM is associated with extra-esophageal symptoms. Types III and IV were associated with anatomic abnormalities (strictures) and development of a neoplasm, respectively.[39]

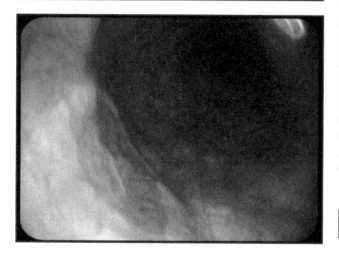

Figure 43–4. Endoscopic photomicrograph of heterotopic gastric mucosa in the proximal esophagus.

PHYSICAL ASPECTS

Physical or anatomic variants may result in the sensation of lump. Thyroid nodules that are larger (>3 cm) or sit anterior to the trachea have been associated with significant globus perception.[40] Excision of nodules in some instances may provide relief, although surgery has not been proposed as a primary treatment for globus as yet.[40] Burns and Timon interviewed 200 patients undergoing thyroid surgery preoperatively and postoperatively for prevalence of globus sensation.[41] Prior to treatment, 58/200 (29%) reported globus, while following thyroid surgery 80% of patients reported resolution of the symptom.[41]

Osteophytosis, particularly anterior marginal osteophytes located at C5 and C6 have also shown some association with reported globus sensation (see Figure 43–3).[8,42] Typically identified on lateral projections of videofluoroscopic swallowing studies, osteophytes are rarely large enough to warrant surgery where this is a significant risk to the pharyngeal plexus that can result in dysphagia. Anti-inflammatory medication may be considered to manage friction-driven discomfort.

NEOPLASTIC ASPECTS

Although this is by far the least common cause of globus sensation, it is the most crucial to rule out or identify early. For this reason, complete workup should be undertaken before reassurance is given. Both benign and malignant tumors of the pharyngolarynx and esophagus may give rise to a feeling of lump in the throat as, of course, that is what they are. Benign hamartomata, post-cricoid lymphangioma, vallecula cysts, inflammatory pseudotumor, and smooth muscle tumors have been found and squamous cell carcinoma of the oropharynx, supraglottis, or hypopharynx or rare tumors such as melanoma, salivary tumors, or lymphoma are documented.[43-45] Management of such lesions will be specific to the tumor itself, with appropriate imaging for staging, histological diagnosis, and patient status determining the final therapeutic paradigm.

SUMMARY

Globus sensation is a symptom that may be generated by a variety of stimuli and respond to several different interventions. It is rarely associated with sinister pathology; however, this must be ruled out initially, allowing subsequent treatment to focus on appropriate aspects of care for the individual concerned. Early flexible pharyngoesophagoscopy is helpful in ruling out serious illness and may be combined with additional investigations ranging from fluoroscopic swallowing studies, pH metry, and manometry to CT scan in some cases. A combination of inputs may be more effective in managing the condition than monotherapy, including education and behavioral therapies, pharmacotherapy, and in targeted cases only, surgery.

REFERENCES

1. Malcomson KG. Globus hystericus vel pharynges (a reconnaissance of proximal vagal modalities). *J Laryngol Otol*. 1968; 82:219–230.

2. Lee B, Kim G. Globus pharyngeus: a review of its etiology, diagnosis and treatment. *World J Gastroenterol*. 2012; 18:2462–2471.

3. Cheng CC, Fang TJ, Lee TJ, et al. Role of flexible transnasal esophagoscopy and patient education in the management of globus pharyngeus. *J Formos Med Assoc*. 2012; 111:171–175.

4. Timon C, O'Dwyer T, Cagney D, Walsh M. Globus pharyngeus: long-term follow-up and prognostic factors. *Ann Otol Rhinol Laryngol*. 1991;100:351–354.

5. Rowley H, O'Dwyer TP, Jones AS, Tion CI. The natural history of globus pharyngeus. *Laryngoscope*. 1995;105: 1118–1121.

6. Hill J, Stuart RC, Fung HK, Ng EK, Cheung FM, Chung CS, van Hasselt CA. Gastroesophageal reflux, motility disorders, and psychological profiles in the etiology of globus pharyngis. *Laryngoscope*. 1997;107:1373–1377.

7. Jaruchinda P, Saengsapawiriya A, Chakkaphak S, Somngeon S, Petsrikun K. The study of allergic skin test in patients with globus pharyngeus: a preliminary report. *J Med Assoc Thai*. 2009;92:531–536.

8. Chen CL, Tsai CC, Chou AS, Chiou JH. Utility of ambulatory pH monitoring and videofluoroscopy for the evaluation of patients with globus pharyngeus. *Dysphagia*. 2007;22:16–19.

9. Kirch S, Gegg R, Johns MM, Rubin AD. Globus pharyngeus: effectiveness of treatment with proton pump inhibitors and gabapentin. *Ann Otol Rhinol Laryngol*. 2013; 122:492–495.

10. Lancaster JL, Gosh S, Sethi R, Tripathi S. Can heterotopic gastric mucosa present as globus pharyngeus? *J Laryngol Otol*. 2006;120:575–578.

11. Nakano S, Iwasaki H, Kondo E, et al. Efficacy of proton pump inhibitor in combination with rikkunshito in patients complaining of globus pharyngeus. *J Med Invest*. 2016;227–229.

12. Baek CH, Chung MK, Choi JY, So YK, Son YI, Jeong HS. Role of salivary function in patients with globus pharyngeus. *Head Neck*. 2010;32:244–252.

13. Riehl ME, Keefer L. Hypnotherapy for esophageal disorders. *Am J Clin Hypn*. 2015;58:22–33.

14. Kiebles JL, Kwiatek MA, Pandolfino JE, Kahrilas PJ, Keefer L. Do patients with globus sensation respond to hypnotically assisted relaxation therapy? A case series report. *Dis Esophagus*. 2010;23:545–553.

15. You LQ, Liu J, Jia L, Jiang SM, Wang GQ. Effect of low-dose amitriptyline on globus pharyngeus and its side effects. *World J Gastroenterol*. 2013; 19:7455–7460.

16. Cybulska EM. Globus hystericus—a somatic symptom of depression? The role of electroconvulsive therapy and antidepressants. *Psychosom Med*. 1997;59:67–69.

17. Chen DY, Jia L, Gu X, Jiang SM, Xie HL, Xu J. Comparison of paroxetine and amitriptyline in the treatment of refractory globus pharyngeus. *Dig Liver Dis*. 2016;48:1012–1017.

18. Kirch S, Gegg R, Johns MM, Rubin AD. Globus pharyngeus: effectiveness of treatment with proton pump inhibitors and gabapentin. *Ann Otol Rhinol Laryngol*. 2013:122: 492–495.

19. Millichap F, Lee M, Pring T. A lump in the throat: should speech language therapists treat globus pharyngeus? *Disabil Rehabil*. 2005;27:187–190.

20. Khalil HS, Bridger MW, Hilton-Pierce M, Vincent J. The use of speech therapy in the treatment of globus pharyngeus patients. A randomised controlled trial. *Rev Laryngol Otol Rhinol (Bord)*. 2003;124:187–190.

21. Park JH, Lee DH, Kim JY, et al. Gastroesophageal reflux disease with laryngopharyngeal manifestation in Korea. *Hepatogastroenterol*. 2012;59:2527–2529.

22. Sinn DH, Kim JH, Kim S, Son HJ, Kim JJ, Rhee JC, Rhee PL. Response rate and predictors of response in a short-term empirical trial of high-dose rabeprazole in patients with globus. *Aliment Pharmacol Ther*. 2008;27:1275–1281.

23. Zelenik K, Matousek P, Urban O, Schwarz P, Stárek I, Komínek P. Globus pharyngeus and extraesophageal reflux: simultaneous pH <4.0 and pH <5.0 analysis. *Laryngoscope*. 2010;120:2160–2164.

24. Corso MJ, Pursnani KG, Mohiuddin MA, et al. Globus sensation is associated with hypertensive upper esophageal sphincter but not with gastroesophageal reflux. *Dig Dis Sci*. 1998; 43:1513–1517.

25. Kwiatek MA, Mirza F, Kahrilas PJ, Pandolfino JE. Hyperdynamic upper esophageal sphincter pressure: a manometric observation in patients reporting globus sensation. *Am J Gastroenterol*. 2009; 104:289–298.

26. Oelschlager BK, Eubanks TR, Oleynikov D, Pope C, Pellegrini CA. Symptomatic and physiologic outcomes after operative treatment for extraesophageal reflux. *Surg Endosc*. 2002;16:1032–1036.

27. Catania RA, Kavic SM, Roth JS, et al. Laparoscopic Nissen fundoplication effectively relieves symptoms in

patients with laryngopharyngeal reflux. *J Gastrointest Surg.* 2007;11:1579–1587.

28. Yan C, Liang WT, Wang ZG, Hu ZW, Wu JM, Zhang C, Chen MP. Comparison of Stretta procedure and Toupet fundoplication for gastroesophageal reflux disease-related extra-esophageal symptoms. *World J Gastroenterol.* 2015;21:12882–12887.

29. Manabe N, Tsutsui H, Kusunoki H, Hata J, Haruma K. Pathophysiology and treatment of patients with globus sensation—from the viewpoint of esophageal motility dysfunction. *J Smooth Muscle Res.* 2014;50:66–70.

30. Färkkilä MA, Ertama L, Katila H, Kuusi K, Paavolainen M, Varis K. Globus pharyngis, commonly associated with esophageal motility disorders. *Am J Gastroenterol.* 1994;89:502–508.

31. Moser G, Vacariu-Granser GV, Schneider C, et al. High incidence of esophageal motor disorders in consecutive patients with globus sensation. *Gastroenterology.* 1991;101:1512–1521.

32. Tsutsui H, Manabe N, Uno M, et al. Esophageal motor dysfunction plays a key role in GERD with globus sensation—analysis of factors promoting resistance to PPI therapy. *Scand J Gastroenterol.* 2012;47:893–899.

33. Adachi J, Ohmae Y, Karaho T, et al. Relationship between globus sensation and esophageal clearance. *Acta Otolaryngol.* 2010;130:138–144.

34. Kasap E, Ayhan S, Yüceyar H. Does Helicobacter pylori treatment improve the symptoms of globus hystericus? *Turk J Gastroenterol.* 2012;23:681–685.

35. Lancaster JL, Gosh S, Sethi R, Tripathi S. Can heterotopic gastric mucosa present as globus sensation? *J Laryngol Otol.* 2006;120:575–578.

36. Alaani A, Jassar P, Warfield AT, Gouldesbrough DR, Smith I. Heterotopic gastric mucosa in the cervical oesophagus (inlet patch) and globus pharyngeus: an under-recognised association. *J Laryngol Otol.* 2007:121:885–888.

37. Meining A, Bajboug M, Preeg M, et al. Argon plasma ablation of gastric inlet patches in the cervical esophagus may alleviate globus sensation: a pilot trial. *Endoscopy.* 2006;38:566–570.

38. Frieling T, Kuhlbusch-Zicklam R, Weingardt C, Heise J, Kreysel C, Blank M, Muller D. Clinical impact of esophageal function tests and argon plasm coagulation in heterotopic gastric mucosa of the esophagus and extraesophageal reflux symptoms—a prospective study. *Z Gastroenterol.* 2015;53:101–107.

39. Von Rahden BH, Stein HJ, Becker K, Liebermann-Meffert D, Siewert RJ. Heterotopic gastric mucosa of the esophagus: literature review and proposal of a clinicopathological classification. *Am J Gastroenterol.* 2004;99:543–551.

40. Nam IC, Choi H, Kim ES, Mo EY, Park YH, Sun DI. Characteristics of thyroid nodules causing globus symptoms. *Eur Arch Otorhinolaryngol.* 2015;272:1181–1188.

41. Burns P, Timon C. Thyroid pathology and the globus symptom: are they related? A two-year prospective trial. *J Laryngol Otol.* 2007;121:242–245.

42. Caylaki F, Yavuz H, Erkan AN, Ozer C, Ozluoglu LN. Evaluation of patients with globus pharyngeus with barium swallow pharyngoesophagography. *Laryngoscope.* 2006;116:37–39.

43. Graefe H, Stellmacher F, Sotlar K, Wollenberg B, Gehrking E. Inflammatory pseudotumour of the hypopharynx: clinical diagnosis, immunohistochemical findings and treatment of this rare disease. *In Vivo.* 2008;22:817–820.

44. Husamaldin Z, Aung W, McFerran DJ. Smooth muscle tumour of the pharynx: a rare tumour presenting with globus pharyngeus symptoms. *J Laryngol Otol.* 2004;118:885–887.

45. Smith NM, Stafford FW. Post cricoid lymphangioma. *J Laryngol Otol.* 1991;105:220–221.

CHAPTER 44

Anterior Glottoplasty for Voice Feminization

Marc Remacle and Anna Pamela C. Dela Cruz

CASE DESCRIPTION

The patient is a 34-year-old male-to-female transgender who presented following several sessions of speech therapy for transgender dysphonia. Her voice sounded female at rest but voicing was effortful and was associated with vocal fatigue and instability, especially in the evenings. She was then offered a surgical option for voice feminization. An anterior glottoplasty was performed successfully, providing an effortless feminine voice with a mean frequency improved from 91 Hz to 198 Hz. Patient followed up regularly and had sustained F0, and satisfactory results based on the self-evaluation questionnaire (Transgender patient Voice Questionnaire–Male to Female [TVQ-MtF]) improved from 62 to 7. However, a few months later, the patient opted for another procedure to attain a higher pitch. A laser-assisted voice adjustment (LAVA) procedure was then performed 8 months later, providing an additional gain of 50 Hz in fundamental frequency. The voice of the patient after the two procedures was clearly identified as female by experts and naïve listeners.

DISCUSSION POINTS

1. Describe the fundamental principles for pitch elevation.
2. Discuss the surgical options for voice feminization in patients undergoing male-to-female gender transition.

One of the most common challenges that male-to-female transgender individuals relate to is having a masculine-sounding voice. Male-to-female transgenders usually undergo several procedures to align their physical appearance with their gender and congruence between voice and gender being a critical part of successful gender transition. For this reason, they are prompted to seek methods to improve perceptual femininity of their voice. Several approaches for voice feminization have been used and are described in literature, including hormonal therapy, conservative management with speech therapy, and surgery.

Transgender patient patients are usually on hormonal therapy during transition. In male-to-female transgender patients, hormone therapy is able to accomplish secondary female characteristics such as breast development, female pattern of fat distribution, and elimination of male pattern hair growth. In female-to-male transgender patients, testosterone therapy has helped in achieving physical changes to become more masculine and in deepening the voice. However, hormonal therapy with anti-androgens and estrogen has minimal effect on the properties of voice of male-to-female transgender patients.[1,2] Consequently, they retain a masculine voice and are advised to seek other options such as speech therapy or surgery.

Speech therapy has been used widely as a non-invasive approach for voice feminization. The goal of therapy is to increase the fundamental frequency (F0) whose perceptual correlate is pitch, to approximate that of females.[3] Male-to-female transgender patients with a higher mean F0 were perceived as more feminine by speech language therapists and naïve listeners.[4-6] Studies on speech therapy, however, show that it is time intensive, requiring several sessions, and results may vary between individuals.[3] Also, the male voice may reemerge during non-verbal vocalisations like yawning, coughing, and laughing.[7]

For more consistent and long-term results, surgery is one of the options offered for voice feminization. The fundamental speech frequency (F0) can be surgically altered and is determined by tension, mass, and length of the vocal folds and these are the principles upon which surgical approaches for pitch elevation are based. Raising the pitch may be done by either increase in vocal fold tension, alteration of the vocal fold mass, or density or vocal fold shortening.[7]

CASE RESOLUTION

Initial Evaluation

Physical Examination and Complementary Tests

The problem of having a masculine voice among male-to-female transgender patients following speech therapy is one of the reasons for referral to a laryngeal surgeon. Most patients usually have undergone several sessions of speech therapy when they seek surgical intervention. In a long-term study on the maintenance of fundamental frequency with speech therapy done by Dacakis, out of the 10 male-to-female transgender patients included, only 2 were able to maintain the gains in F0 achieved during therapy.[3] A study done by Gelfer and Tice also evaluated the speaking fundamental frequency of male-to-female transgender patients immediately after 8 weeks of speech therapy and 15 months after the termination of therapy, and results showed that not all gains in F0 were maintained in the long-term.[8] Surgery, on the other hand, offers patients a more consistent feminine voice with more favorable long-term outcomes.

This patient came into our clinic for a surgical opinion on voice feminization after having several speech therapy sessions. Upon consultation, initial assessment was done by transnasal videoendoscopy and stroboscopy. This allows visualization of the vocal folds and identification of any laryngeal pathologies. In our patient, the vocal folds were normal, with symmetric and periodic mucosal waves, and there were no detectable lesions.

Following the examination of the vocal folds, voice assessment was done through a multifaceted approach and included acoustic analysis, self-report measures, and auditory perceptual assessment.

Objective Evaluation

The acoustical measurement that is usually evaluated for outcome assessment is the mean fundamental frequency. Other acoustical measures that may also be assessed include intonation, frequency shift, formant frequency, maximum phonation time, and phonation quotient. Among the acoustic parameters, fundamental frequency or pitch is reported to be the most distinguishing characteristic between male and female voices.[9,10] In a study by Spencer, speakers using a fundamental frequency below 160 Hz were perceived as male, while those using higher fundamental frequencies were perceived as female.[11]

Subjective Evaluation

Another way of evaluating success of intervention is through self-report measures of vocal functioning by the patient. The individual's self-perception of voice and its impact on everyday life is considered an important component in assessment.[12] Examples of these measures include the Voice Handicap Index (VHI), Voice Related Quality of Life (V-RQOL) scale, Transgender Self-evaluation of Voice Questionnaire (TSEQ), and the TVQ.[12,13]

Perceptual Evaluation

Perceptual assessment is also regarded as a valuable measure in determining the success of treatment. The patient was asked to make a voice recording by reading aloud the "Rainbow Passage" using her usual speaking voice at a comfortable pitch and intensity, preoperatively and postoperatively. This was evaluated by a group of speech-language pathologists and blinded listeners, according to their perception of the recorded voice, whether it was feminine or masculine.

Patient Preferences and Expectations

Although the patient already had a female-sounding voice with speech therapy, she was dissatisfied because of the effort she had to make to produce a feminine voice. She also readily experienced vocal fatigue and voice instability especially in the evening. Among patients who have been speaking at an artificially elevated pitch for several years, many of them may produce voice with a degree of strain.[14] Also, even though speech therapy is a non-invasive way of raising the pitch, results are often inconsistent and voice is not natural sounding. Patient was informed of the surgical options for voice feminization. After discussing the benefits and possible complications of doing surgery for voice feminization, patient agreed to undergo anterior glottoplasty based on Wendler's technique.[15–17]

Surgical Treatment

Indications

Surgical alteration of vocal pitch is a good option for the patient considering her concerns after speech therapy. In her case, elevation of the pitch by creation of an anterior web, also known as Wendler's glottoplasty, was proposed. Anterior glottoplasty via a transoral approach was first described by Wendler in 1990.[15] In this technique, the endolarynx is exposed by suspension laryngoscopy. De-epithelialization of the anterior part of the vocal folds is done and then firmly sutured to obtain a V-shaped anterior commissure. The resulting shortened vocal folds and reduced vibrating mass, in principle, raise the pitch. Using this approach, Gross reported his results in endoscopic vocal fold shortening. In his study, among the 10 male-to-female transgender patient patients who underwent this surgical technique, there was a general increase in mean spontaneous frequency of 9.2 semitones (mean F0 preop of 116.8 Hz and mean F0 postop of 201.0 Hz). He demonstrated that there was also a decrease in range for the lower frequencies such that even in uncontrolled situations, no deep voice is possible.[7]

Contraindications

There are no absolute contraindications for this patient to undergo anterior glottoplasty. Patient also has no known comorbidities that may preclude her to undergo general anesthesia.

Expected Results

Remacle et al presented a case series of 15 male-to-female transgender patients who underwent anterior glottoplasty based on Wendler's technique but using CO_2 laser for de-epithelialization of the anterior part of

the vocal folds instead of cold instruments. The mean follow-up period was 7.2 months postoperatively; their results showed an increase in median fundamental frequency (F0) from 150 Hz to 194 Hz.[16] In a follow-up study by Mastronikolis et al, there was a significant increase in mean fundamental frequency (F0) from 135.8 Hz to 206.3 Hz in 31 male-to-female transgender patients who underwent anterior glottoplasty. The mean follow-up period was 9.2 months. They also noted that there was a higher mean F0 postoperatively for patients younger than 40 years old. It was also described that patients were advised speech therapy after healing and obtaining the anterior web.[17]

Risk-Benefit Analysis

The procedure of creating an anterior web endoscopically was explained well to the patient. This technique has been demonstrated to significantly elevate the pitch among male-to-female transgender patients. In a meta-analysis done by Song and Jiang on pitch elevation among male-to-female transgender patients, it was shown that the largest increase in fundamental frequency was seen with endoscopic shortening techniques, with a gain of 78.98 Hz in mean fundamental frequency. This was followed by cricothyroid approximation, with a mean difference of 44.97 Hz and then followed by laser reduction technique with a mean difference of 36.89 Hz.[18] The endoscopic shortening approach has the advantages of avoiding an external incision with better long-term results for pitch elevation.

The possible risks such as suture dehiscence and incomplete reduction of the vocal fold length which may result from inadequate elevation of pitch were also explained to the patient.[17]

ALTERNATIVE SURGICAL APPROACHES FOR VOICE FEMINIZATION

Surgical Approaches for Increasing Vocal Fold Tension

Cricothyroid Approximation

There are other surgical approaches for voice feminization, the most popular of which is cricothyroid approximation. Also known as the type IV thyroplasty, this technique was first described by Isshiki.[19,20] In this procedure, simulating the contraction of the cricothyroid muscles is done by approximating the cricoid and thyroid cartilage together using sutures, which increases tension in the vocal folds, thereby raising the pitch. This technique was later modified by Lee and Sataloff, respectively.[21,22]

This approach often has good early results; however, there is an observed pitch decline within 6 to 18 months.[7] Yang et al reported their study on 20 patients undergoing primary cricothyroid approximation with a mean follow-up of 22 months. There was increase in mean fundamental frequency on sustained vowels from 145 Hz to 202 Hz after surgery, and on reading tasks from 134 Hz to 185 Hz postoperatively. However, they also noted that in some of their patients, there is a gradual decline in the postoperative pitch.[14] Van Borsel et al also investigated the effectiveness of cricothyroid approximation in voice feminization in 9 male-to-female transgender patient patients from a perceptual perspective. Results of their study showed that it can effectively raise the pitch in male-to-female transgender patients but is not sufficient to create a voice that is perceived as totally female.[6]

Anterior Commissure Advancement

This technique was developed by LeJeune et al to increase the tension of the vocal folds. Tightening of the thyroarytenoid ligament was done in six patients by advancement of the anterior commissure of the glottis via a limited thyrotomy.[23] Tucker later modified this technique by placing a tantalum splint. Included in his study were nine patients with various conditions presenting with lax vocal folds, and two of them were male-to-female transgender patients who underwent the procedure to address the low-pitched voice.[24]

Surgical Approaches for Altering the Vocal Fold Mass

Laser-Assisted Vocal Adjustment

This technique was described by Orloff et al in which vaporization using CO_2 laser is performed 1 to 2 mm lateral to the free edge of the vocal fold extending along the superior surface of the vocal fold from the vocal process to as far anterior as possible. This results in a decrease in mass and increase in stiffness resulting from the scarring process of vocal fold tissue and accounts for the rise in vocal pitch. The results of their study with 31 patients showed an increase in mean

fundamental frequency of 26 Hz, with a mean preoperative F0 of 142 Hz and a mean postoperative F0 of 168 Hz.[25]

Laser Reduction Glottoplasty

Koçak et al presented their approach for voice feminization via a modified laser-assisted voice adjustment technique known as laser reduction glottoplasty. They reported their results in six patients who had unsatisfactory outcomes with cricothyroid approximation. In this technique, the vocal fold cover, ligament, and medial fibers of the vocalis muscle are ablated longitudinally using CO_2 laser while preserving the medial vibrating cover. Results of their study showed a mean elevation in fundamental frequency of 45.17 ± 8.47 Hz (from a mean F0 of 158.33 ± 12.14 Hz preoperatively to a mean F0 of 203.50 ± 13.34 Hz after surgery), with a follow-up of up to 12 months postoperatively.[26]

Surgical Approaches for Vocal Fold Shortening

Vocal Fold Shortening via an External Approach

Donald described a surgical procedure to shorten the vibrating length of the vocal fold via an external approach. The anterior commissure is approached via a laryngofissure and is divided at the midline. The anterior third of each true vocal fold is then de-epithelialized by sharp dissection and then approximated with three sutures. In his study of three patients, he reported improvement in vocal pitch and satisfactory results in terms of vocal quality in all subjects.[27] Acoustical measurements and results of self-evaluation or perceptual evaluation were not described in the study.

Endoscopic Vocal Fold Shortening

Wendler first described the technique on vocal fold shortening via an endoscopic approach.[15] As previously discussed, anterior glottoplasty for voice feminization among male-to-female transgender patients was later used and reported in studies by Gross, Remacle, and Mastronikolis.[7,16,17] Kim also reported his results on vocal fold shortening and retrodisplacement of the anterior commissure in 362 patients, with 313 male-to-female transgender patients included among them. The procedure is also done by creating an anterior web, but includes de-epithelialization and suturing of the subglottis aside from the anterior third of the vocal folds. His results showed an increase in mean F0 of 73.6 Hz among male-to-female transgender patients following voice rehabilitation.[28] A study by Casado et al also demonstrated a significant increase in mean fundamental frequency from 136.03 Hz preoperatively to 229.4 Hz postoperatively in 18 male-to-female transgender patient patients after Wendler's glottoplasty. Their technique involved creation of an anterior web and additionally performing vaporization of the upper surface of the vocal folds from the vocal process to the anterior commissure.[29]

The endoscopic technique of shortening the vocal folds is gaining wide acceptance due to avoidance of an external incision and better long-term results and is now the more commonly used method for effectively raising the vocal pitch among male-to-female transgender patients.

TECHNIQUES AND RESULTS

Anesthesia and Perioperative Care

The procedure was performed under general anesthesia with jet ventilation. This is preferred over laser-compatible tubes to provide an unimpeded surgical access to the larynx. A constant communication between the surgeon and the anesthesiologist is important when doing a transoral laser microsurgery with jet ventilation. The inspired fraction of oxygen (FiO_2) is usually adjusted to a value below 0.4 when the laser is in use to avoid combustion.

Instrumentation and Procedural Technique

The endolarynx was exposed through a rigid suspension laryngoscope. An operating microscope was brought into position with the micromanipulator and CO_2 laser machine connected to it. The anterior part of the vocal folds was de-epithelialized using the CO_2 laser (settings: 10 watts intensity, continuous wave, repeat mode with a delay of 0.1 seconds, and a 2-mm-wide circular beam), with caution not to injure the vocal ligament. The corresponding tissue of the vocal folds was firmly sutured to obtain a V-shaped anterior commissure. Four 3-0 resorbable threads, two for each vocal fold, were used. One thread was passed through the vocal ligament at the junction between the anterior and the middle third. The second was passed more anteriorly to the first. The same

procedure was performed on the contralateral fold. The anterior thread was ligated together with one knot inferior to the glottic plane and the other knot superior to the glottic plane. The same procedure was performed for the more posterior two threads. Laparoscopic forceps was used to hold the needle in place and a knot pusher to secure the suture. Fibrin glue was then applied to strengthen the suture.[16,17]

The patient was advised absolute voice rest for 2 weeks to limit tension forces and prevent the dehiscence of suture points. Patient was treated with antibiotics (amoxicillin + clavulanic acid: 1 g three times daily) for 1 week, proton pump inhibitors for 6 weeks, and inhaled steroids twice daily for 1 week.[16,17]

Results and Procedure-Related Complications

First postoperative follow-up was done at 3 weeks, which showed good approximation of the anterior one-third of the true vocal folds on endoscopic examination (Figure 44–1). Patient was allowed low intensity voice use after 2 weeks of absolute voice rest. She was also advised speech therapy. Follow-up visits were then scheduled around every 3 weeks until the postoperative result was achieved. After anterior glottoplasty, the patient had an increase in mean fundamental frequency of 100 Hz.

Self-evaluation by the patient showed that she was satisfied with the outcome of surgery, using the TVQ-MtF. Perceptual assessment by speech-language pathologists and naïve listeners also revealed that she was mostly identified as female.

Eight months postoperatively, the patient expressed that she wanted another procedure to further elevate the pitch. After discussion of possible options, a LAVA was proposed to the patient. Postoperative results after LAVA in our patient demonstrated an additional gain of 50 Hz in mean fundamental frequency. Perceptual evaluation of the patient's voice recording by speech-language pathologists and blinded listeners also showed that she was identified as female. Patient was advised to continue speech therapy postoperatively.

Although there was a significant increase in mean fundamental frequency, patient later on was dissatisfied that a further increase in pitch cannot be reached. This is the psychological problem sometimes with these patients. They identify and liken themselves to a female model, wishing to reproduce a high-pitched female voice. Counseling is thus important to confirm that these patients have realistic expectations.

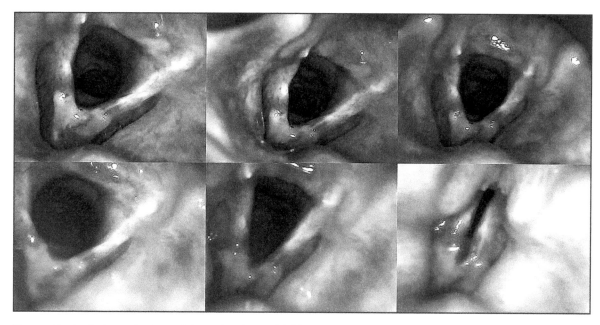

Figure 44–1. Endoscopic view of the patient's vocal folds at 3 weeks after anterior glottoplasty.

Some studies also pointed out that there are other factors aside from pitch that distinguish between male and female voices. Resonance, formant patterns, intonation, breathiness also influence the perception of a person's voice as male or female.[5,10,30]

LONG-TERM MANAGEMENT

Outcome Assessment and Referral

Outpatient follow-up with videolaryngoscopy and stroboscopy with measurement of the mean fundamental frequency should be routinely performed. This is done to check whether the patient is able to maintain the increase in F0. Postoperative speech therapy is also recommended for optimal long-term results. Several studies have suggested post-surgical voice therapy to be a part of the management of patients undergoing voice feminization.[16,17,28,29] In a study by Casado et al, patients who underwent Wendler's glottoplasty were advised postoperative speech therapy. Ten out of the 18 patients consented and received 24 sessions of post-surgical voice therapy. Results showed that those who received voice therapy post-surgery had a higher

mean F0 of 243.2 Hz compared with those who did not, with a mean F0 of 212.0 Hz.[29]

REFERENCES

1. Edgerton MT. The surgical treatment of male transgender patients. *Clin Plastic Surg.* 1974;1:285–323.
2. Gooren L. Hormone treatment of the adult transgender patient patient. *Horm Res.* 2005;64(suppl. 2):31–36.
3. Dacakis G. Long-term maintenance of fundamental frequency increases in male-to-female transgender patients. *J Voice.* 2000;14(4):549–556.
4. McNeill EJM, Wilson JA, Clark S, Deakin J. Perception of voice in the transgender client. *J Voice.* 2008;22:727–733.
5. Gelfer MP and Schofield KJ. Comparison of acoustic and perceptual measures of voice in male-to-female transgender patients perceived as female versus those perceived as male. *J Voice.* 2000;14(1):22–33.
6. Van Borsel, J., Van Eynde, E., De Cuypere, G., Bonte, K. Feminine after cricothyroid approximation? *J Voice.* 2008; 22:379–384.
7. Gross M. Pitch-raising surgery in male-to-female transgender patients. *J Voice.* 1999;13:246–250.
8. Gelfer MP and Tice RM. Perceptual and acoustic outcomes of voice therapy for male-to-female transgender individuals immediately after therapy and 15 months later. *Journal of Voice.* 2013;27(3):335–347.

9. Gelfer MP, Mikos VA. The relative contributions of speaking fundamental frequency and formant frequencies to gender identification based on isolated vowels. *J Voice.* 2005;19:544–554.

10. Wolfe VI, Ratusnik DL, Smith FH, Northrop G. Intonation and fundamental frequency in male-to-female transgender patients. *J Speech Hearing Disord.* 1990;55:43–50.

11. Spencer LE. Speech characteristics of male-to-female transgender patients: a perceptual and acoustic study. *Folia Phoniatr.* 1988;40:31–42.

12. Dacakis G, Davies S, Oates JM, Douglas JM, Johnston JR. Development and preliminary evaluation of the Transgender patient Voice Questionnaire for male-to-female transgender patients. *Journal of Voice.* 2013;27(3): 312–320.

13. Dacakis G, Oates J, Douglas J. Beyond voice: perceptions of gender in male-tofemale transgender patients. *Curr Opin Otolaryngol Head Neck Surg.* 2012;20:165–170.

14. Yang CY, Palmer AD, Murray KD, Meltzer TR, Cohen JI. Cricothyroid approximation to elevate vocal pitch in male-to-female transgender patients: results of surgery. *Ann Otol Rhinol Laryngol.* 2002;111(6):477–485.

15. Wendler J. Vocal pitch elevation after transexualism male to female. In: *Proceedings of the Union of the European Phoniatricians.* Salsomaggiore, Italy; 1990.

16. Remacle M, Matar N, Morsomme D, Verduyckt I, Lawson G. Glottoplasty for male-to-female transgender patientism: voice results. *J Voice.* 2011;25:120–123.

17. Mastronikolis N, Remacle M, Biagini M, Kiagiadaki D, Lawson G. Wendler glottoplasty: an effective pitch raising surgery in male-to-female transgender patients. *J Voice.* 2013;4:516–522.

18. Song TE, Jiang N. Transgender phonosurgery: a systematic review and meta-analysis. *Otolaryngol Head Neck Surg.* doi: 10.1177/0194599817697050

19. Isshiki N, Morita H, Okamura H, Hiramoto M. Thyroplasty as a new phonosurgical technique. *Acta Otolaryngol.* 1974;78:451–45.

20. Isshiki N, Taira T, Tanabe M. Surgical alteration of vocal pitch. *J Otolaryngol.* 1983;12:135–154.

21. Lee SY, Liao TT, Hsieh T. Extralaryngeal approach in functional phonosurgery. In: *Proceedings of the 20th Congress of the IALP.* Tokyo, Japan; 1986:482–483.

22. Sataloff RT. *Professional Voice: The Science and Art of Clinical Care.* 2nd ed. San Diego, CA: Singular Publishing Group; 1997:630–631.

23. LeJeune FE, Guice CE, Samuels PM. Early experiences with vocal ligament tightening. *Ann Otol Rhinol Laryngol.* 1983;92(5 pt. 1):475–477.

24. Tucker HM. Anterior commissure laryngoplasty for adjustment of vocal fold tension. *Ann Otol Rhinol Laryngol.* 1985;94:547–549.

25. Orloff LA, Mann AP, Damrose JF, Goldman SN. Laser-assisted voice adjustment (LAVA) in transgender patients. *Laryngoscope.* 2006;116:655–660.

26. Kocak I, Akpınar ME, Cakır ZA, Dogan M, Bengisu S, Celikoyar MM. Laser reduction glottoplasty for managing androphonia after failed cricothyroid approximation surgery. *J Voice.* 2010;24:758–764.

27. Donald PJ. Voice change surgery in the transgender patient. *Head Neck Surg.* 1982;4:433–437.

28. Kim HT. A new conceptual approach for voice feminization: 12 years of experience. *Laryngoscope.* 2017;127:1102–1108. doi:10.1002/lary.26127

29. Casado JC, Parra MJR, Adrian JA. Voice feminization in male-to-female transgendered clients after Wendler's glottoplasty with vs. without voice therapy support. *Eur Arch Otorhinolaryngol.* 2016. doi: 10.1007/s00405-016-4420-8.

30. Oates J, Dacakis G. Voice change in transgender patients. *Venereology.* 1997;10:178.

CHAPTER 45

The Larynx in Systemic Inflammation

Angela Zhu, Jason Rudman, and David E. Rosow

Systemic inflammatory conditions consist of allergic, autoimmune, metabolic, and traumatic dysfunction of multiple anatomic locations and organ systems. Many patients with systemic conditions may complain of laryngeal symptoms, either as the initial manifestation of a disease or as a secondary symptom. The larynx is a complex organ involving the interplay of fine neuromuscular control, vascular supply, and critical bony and cartilaginous structures, and it is therefore vulnerable to conditions affecting any of these systems, often relatively early in the disease process. The subglottic region lies in a watershed area between two microvascular beds, which further contributes to its susceptibility. It is not surprising then that the vocal folds and cricoarytenoid joints are commonly affected areas in laryngeal disease. In the adult population, laryngitis is often due to chronic, noninfectious causes. These conditions can cause inflammation, dryness, or friability and scarring of the laryngeal mucosa, which can in turn cause symptoms of dyspnea, dysphagia, hoarseness, globus sensation, or coughing. Symptoms may wax and wane over time, or may progress to the point of aphonia, frank aspiration, or airway compromise. Because each different systemic disease can manifest with such a wide range of symptoms, understanding how to differentiate them is essential for pinpointing the correct diagnosis. With improvements in conservative endoscopic laryngeal procedures giving patients a wider array of surgical options for treatment, learning how to recognize and manage laryngeal manifestations of systemic inflammation is therefore of great interest to practicing otolaryngologists. This chapter discusses case presentations of the several systemic conditions

and their laryngeal manifestations: Wegener's granulomatosis (granulomatosis with polyangiitis [GPA]), relapsing polychondritis, sarcoidosis, amyloidosis, immunoglobulin (Ig)G4-related disease, pemphigus vulgaris, and bullous pemphigoid.

CASE 1

A 29-year-old woman presents with progressive exertional dyspnea, stridor, as well as a saddle nose deformity and episodic epistaxis. Anterior rhinoscopy shows nasal septal crusting and intranasal synechiae. Laryngoscopy shows a beefy red subglottic larynx with moderate to severe stenosis (Figure 45–1), with inflammation on biopsy. No involvement of the trachea is seen on tracheoscopy; pemphigoid is ruled out. Cytoplasmic antineutrophil cytoplasmic antibodies (c-ANCA) is positive. Diagnosis: GPA.

Patient Assessment

Presenting Symptoms

Dyspnea on exertion is the most common symptom. Stridor, cough, wheezing, dysphonia, dysphagia, and a change in voice are also possible.

Patient Demographics

Male > female (1.5:1) although in subglottic disease female > male, age 35–55, Northern European > black

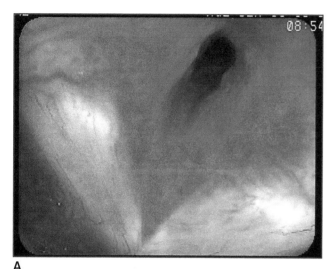

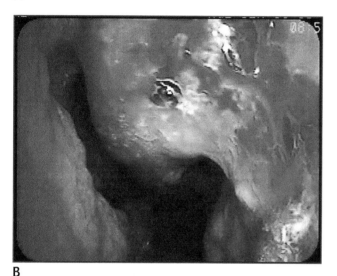

Figure 45–1. (A) Larynx of patient with GPA demonstrating significant infraglottic and subglottic narrowing, beefy red stenosis. (B) Nasal cavity of same patient demonstrates severe friability, inflammation, and crusting.

Medical History

Recurrent epistaxis, saddle-nose deformity

Social History

None

Review of Symptoms

Chest infections, arthralgia, blocked nose.

Physical Exam Findings

Dyspnea, stridor. Nasal crusting, sinusitis, nasal septal perforation, epistaxis, saddle-nose deformity, and serous otitis media may be present.

Imaging/Endoscopy

Fiberoptic endoscopy for larynx visualization. Appears reddish, friable, circumferential narrowing.[1,2]

Other Tests to Confirm/Rule Out Diagnosis

- c-ANCA is positive more frequently than perinuclear (p)-ANCA; however, in one study only 57% of patients with stenosis had a positive ANCA test. In another study, 20% of patients with subglottic stenosis have negative ANCA.[3] Patients may become ANCA positive later in their disease course. Serial ANCA titers are not necessary for monitoring laryngeal disease because they do not correlate with subglottic stenosis progression.
- CT scan: Can reveal laryngotracheal stenosis.
- Pulmonary function testing: Abnormal in 60% of patients.[2] Inspiratory and expiratory curve flattening[3] is correlated with necessity of surgical intervention.[2]
- Biopsies: Biopsy can reveal caseating necrosis and granuloma formation, including giant cells and a necrotic center surrounded by lymphocytes. Small vessel vasculitis is observed. However, biopsies are not always positive, especially in GPA patients with subglottic stenosis. Biopsies and other tests used to manage systemic GPA treatment should not be used as grounds for assessing patient status for laryngeal procedures.

Rule Out Pemphigoid

Immunofluorescence can reveal characteristic staining pattern and loosening of the dermal-epidermal junction. Laryngoscopic exam reveals fibrinous base with a halo of erythema. Blebs are usually absent because the mucosal surface is sloughed upon swallowing.

Discussion

Wegener's granulomatosis, also known as GPA, is an ANCA-associated small vessel vasculitis (inflammation of small blood vessels): capillaries, venules, small arteries, and arterioles. GPA also causes necrotizing granulomatous inflammation of various tissues, leading to organ damage. Classically, it affects the upper and lower respiratory tracts, lungs, and kidneys. Ninety percent of GPA patients report some otolaryngologic findings.[4] Although involvement of the larynx only is rare in GPA, subglottic stenosis is a potentially life-threatening condition and the most common complication of tracheobronchial GPA, reported to occur in 16 to 23% of cases.[1,5–7] It can lead to dyspnea, stridor, cough, hemoptysis, and sputum production, and narrowing of the upper airway at the level of the cricoid cartilage or upper tracheal rings. Prompt diagnosis and treatment of GPA is critical, as the mortality rate of untreated GPA is 90% in 2 years, due to either renal or respiratory failure. Treating the airway symptoms in GPA poses a challenge, however, because airway disease does not respond to monotherapy with either surgery or immunosuppressive treatment for the systemic component of the disease. Treatment is therefore tailored specifically to the patient's airway symptoms and usually consists of a combination of endoscopic surgery with adjuvant immunosuppression.

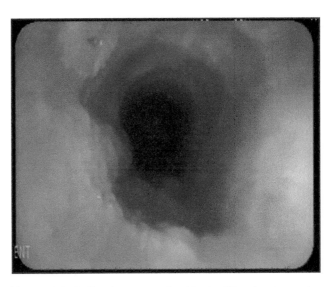

Figure 45–2. Tracheoscopy of patient with relapsing polychondritis revealing diffuse mucosal inflammation with weakened cartilaginous framework.

CASE 2

A 31-year-old woman presents with progressive exertional dyspnea, voice changes, and intermittent external ear pain. Physical examination reveals mildly erythematous, deformed auricles. Flexible laryngoscopy reveals infraglottic edema and circumferential subglottic stenosis, with a hypoplastic appearance to the laryngeal framework (Figure 45–2). Diagnosis: relapsing polychondritis.

Patient Assessment

Presenting Symptoms

Fever, malaise, fatigue, episodic pain and tenderness in auricles, worsening shortness of breath, anterior neck discomfort, stridor, dysphonia.

Patient Demographics

Male = female, although airway involvement is reported to be more common in females,[8] age 40 to 60, Caucasian. Linked to human leukocyte antigen DR4.

Medical History

One-third of patients have coexisting autoimmune disease.

Social History

Done

Physical Exam Findings

Dyspnea, wheezing, inspiratory stridor, dysphonia, nonproductive cough, obstructive respiratory failure

Imaging/Endoscopy

- CXR: possible findings include tracheal narrowing, opacities from infection or atelectasis due to obstruction, calcification of laryngeal or tracheal cartilage.
- CT: high resolution CT focusing on the larynx and trachea is useful in assessing tracheal wall thickening, luminal narrowing, and cartilage calcification.[9,10] Glottic, subglottic, laryngeal, or tracheobronchial stenosis may be observed. However, CT is limited in that it cannot distinguish between inflammation or fibrosis as causes of narrowing. Calcified deposits in tracheal cartilages can be seen in chronic relapsing polychondritis.

Table 45–1. Summary of Systemic Diseases of the Larynx

	Presenting Symptoms	Exam Findings	Key Lab Findings	Imaging Findings	Histology	Treatment
Wegener's Granulomatosis (Granulomatosis with Polyangiitis)	Dyspnea, stridor, cough, hemoptysis, wheezes, crackles. Nasal crusting, sinus pain, nasal obstruction, purulent nasal discharge.	Smooth diffuse swelling, crusting, erythema of laryngeal tissues. "Cobblestoning" nasal mucosa, nodules, or ulcerated inflammatory masses. Subglottis stenosis.	Positive c-ANCA (anti-proteinase 3)	CT or MRI: diffuse circumferential tracheal thickening.	Central mass of epithelioid and giant cells, surrounded by lymphocytes and inflammatory cells. Central necrosis or caseation.	Immunosuppressive therapy: Glucocorticoids combined with either rituximab or cyclophosphamide (2 mg/kg daily for 12 months) (Polychronopoulos, Nouraei), then maintenance with methotrexate or azathioprine. However, upper airway stenosis is not usually improved by immunosuppression. 1. Reduce surgical manipulation during flares (Gluth). 2. Endoscopic dilation is first line treatment. Laser or cold-knife lysis can be useful. Stenting is controversial. 3. Adjuvant options: Intralesional glucocorticoid injection or topical mitomycin C (Hoffmann, Roediger) 4. Tracheostomy as a last resort or during acute obstructive airway inflammation (Alaani, Langford, Gluth) 5. Laryngotracheal reconstruction with costal cartilage graft (LTR)– recommended when systemic disease is controlled
Relapsing Polychondritis	Fever, malaise, fatigue, pain and tenderness in the area of cartilage involved	Pain above thyroid gland, dyspnea, wheezing, inspiratory stridor, dysphonia, nonproductive cough, obstructive respiratory failure	Elevated CRP, ESR	CT or MRI: laryngobronchial wall thickening, narrow lumen, and cartilage calcification	Inflammatory cell infiltration of cartilage, breakdown of cartilage matrix	1. Immunosuppression with prednisone or dapsone. Second line agents are azathioprine, cyclophosphamide, or methotrexate for systemic disease. 2. Nebulized racemic ephedrine (Gaffney) 3. Nasal continuous positive airway pressure (CPAP) or bilevel positive airway pressure (BiPAP) are temporary solutions in patients with diffuse respiratory disease (Ishikawa). 4. Surgical resection of inflammatory masses when systemic disease is in remission 5. Expanding metal or silicon stents, but comes with a risk of stent migration, inflammation, and airway collapse proximal and distal to the stent (Eng, Dunne) 6. External tracheal fixation to vascular adventitia of aorta with pericardium, dura, or Gore–Tex implant (Eng). 7. Neodymium yttrium aluminum garnet (Nd:YAG) laser ablation (Sacco) 8. Tracheotomy in refractory disease. However, will not be effective for distal or diffuse airway stenosis and can induce inflammation and iatrogenic fibrosis.

Disease	Symptoms	Exam findings	Labs	Imaging	Histology	Treatment
Sarcoidosis	Dysphonia, dyspnea, dysphagia, dry cough, enlarged lymph nodes, stridor, throat pain.	Edema, erythema, nodules, ulcerations, and masses	Increased gamma-globulin, serum calcium, liver transaminases, ESR, and ACE	CT or CXR: bilateral hilar adenopathy, reticular opacities	Noncaseating granulomas	1. Corticosteroids 2. Methotrexate 3. Intralesional glucocorticoids 4. Laser reduction with or without mitomycin C (James 2004)
Amyloidosis	Hemoptysis, dysphonia, odynophagia, breathlessness, hoarseness, stridor, airway obstruction	Smooth, yellow or pink-gray mass, intact epithelium. Swollen subglottic region, significant luminal narrowing	–	–	Polarized apple–green birefringence with Congo Red staining, eosinophilic deposits	1. Laser-based surgical resection (Kourelis) or conventional surgery. 2. Intralesional corticosteroid injection
IgG4–RD	Dysphonia, dysphagia, odynophagia, globus sensation, throat pain	Non-malignant hyperplasia and/or fibrosis of the larynx; diffuse or focal enlargement, masses, and nodules	IgG4:IgG ratio of 2:1; IgG4 serum levels >135 mg/dL	–	IgG4 + cell infiltration, storiform fibrosis, obliterative phlebitis	1. High-dose corticosteroids
Pemphigus Vulgaris	Progressive hoarseness, stridor, or dyspnea	Ulceration with gray membranes, fragile, painful blisters, scarring, laryngeal edema, stenosis	Increased desmoglien-3 antibodies	–	Reticular inter-keratinocyte staining on skin biopsy	1. Corticosteroids 2. Dapsone 3. Immunosuppressants (azathioprine, cyclophosphamide, rituximab) 4. Tetracycline
Bullous Pemphigoid	Hemoptysis, sore throat, or hoarseness, dyspnea	Ulceration, scarring, supraglottic narrowing; white fibrinous base surrounded by erythema	Increased auto-antibodies to BP180 and BP230	–	Linear deposits of IgG at the basement membrane or dermal-epidermal junction	1. Corticosteroids 2. Dapsone 3. Immunosuppressants (azathioprine, cyclophosphamide, rituximab)

- MRI: shows hyperintensity of soft tissue inflammation on T2-weighted images. Gadolinium-enhanced regions are seen on T1-weighted images.
- Spirometry: inspiratory and expiratory flow volume loops can detect abnormalities in the airway, such as extrathoracic/intrathoracic obstruction or dynamic laryngeal collapse due to weakened cartilage support. Spirometry can also be used to quantify the degree of obstruction.

Other Tests to Confirm/Rule Out Diagnosis

- Biopsy: pathology of cartilage tissue shows inflammatory cell infiltration (polymorphonuclear leukocytes, lymphocytes, plasma cells, or eosinophils) and breakdown of the cartilage matrix (loss of mucopolysaccharides)
- Laboratory findings: nonspecific, but can be used to rule out other diagnoses. Markers of inflammation include increased erythrocyte sedimentation rate (ESR) and increased C-reactive protein (CRP), and absence of their elevation can be used to rule out relapsing polychondritis (RPC). Anemia is usually seen on complete blood count with differential.

Rule Out Granulomatosis with Polyangiitis

GPA and RPC share many features and can manifest similarly in the larynx. RPC can coexist with vasculitides like GPA and connective tissue diseases in up to one third of patients.[12] However, some distinguishing features in each disease can distinguish the two, such as cavitary pulmonary nodules in GPA and, when present, dynamic tracheobronchial collapse or aortic aneurysms in RPC. Bronchoscopy in GPA can show diffuse vessel erythema and edema of the tracheobronchial mucosa.

Discussion

Relapsing polychondritis is a rare disease of inflamed cartilaginous structures rich in glycosaminoglycans.[11] RPC affects laryngeal, tracheal, and bronchial cartilages in over 50% of RPC patients,[12] with 25% of patients having laryngotracheal strictures. Although the etiology is unknown, 25 to 35% of patients have a history of autoimmune disease.[13,14] The disease is frequently episodic in nature, and chronic inflammation may result in tracheobronchomalacia or laryngomalacia, predisposing the weakened cartilage to collapse during inspiration. Among patients with RPC, laryngotracheal involvement causes one third of deaths.[8] Involvement of the laryngeal, tracheal, and bronchial cartilages can compromise airway patency either via internal (poorly draining respiratory secretions) or external (compression) lesions. Mechanisms of respiratory compromise may be due to central airway fibrosis via laryngotracheal cartilage destruction or peripheral airway inflammation and narrowing.[15] Symptomatically, laryngeal chondritis can present as pain above the thyroid gland, dysphonia/aphonia, or hoarseness. The disease can lead to laryngotracheal stenosis or sialometaplasia of the larynx, which can be misdiagnosed as a carcinoma.[16] Other than biopsy, there is no confirmatory test for RPC, and diagnosis is made based on the appropriate clinical picture.[17] Due to the rarity of the disease, treatment has not been standardized but generally consists of long-term immunosuppression (see Table 45–1).

CASE 3

A 50-year-old African American woman was referred for evaluation of hoarseness and dyspnea. Complaints of "noisy breathing" for the past year, initially diagnosed as asthma, progressively worsened until she cannot tolerate walking more than one block. Exam shows a hoarse, raspy voice with inspiratory stridor. Flexible laryngoscopy revealed profound, beefy edema and stenosis of the supraglottis, with a laryngeal aperture of only about 3 to 4 mm (Figure 45–3). Suspicious pulmonary nodules were identified on imaging; biopsy confirmed sarcoidosis. The patient underwent an awake tracheostomy to secure the airway.

Patient Assessment

Presenting Symptoms

Fever, adenopathy

Patient Demographics

Female > male. 20 to 50 years old. African American > Caucasian

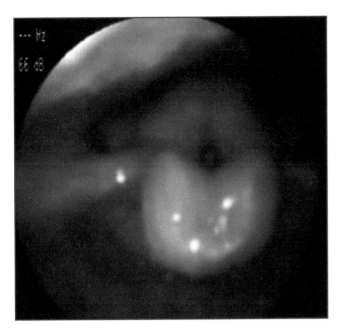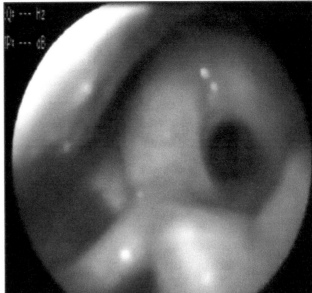

Figure 45–3. Sarcoidosis affecting supraglottic larynx with swelling and malformation of epiglottis (*left*) and circumferential supraglottic stenosis (*right*).

Physical Exam Findings

Dysphonia, dyspnea, dysphagia, dry cough, enlarged lymph nodes, stridor, throat pain. Hoarseness is usually not present, as the true vocal folds are spared.

Associated Comorbidities

Obstructive sleep apnea[18]

Imaging/Endoscopy

- Laryngoscopy: the appearance of the epiglottis is described as "turban-like" and nodular due to swelling of the epiglottis rim.[19] Edema, erythema, nodules, ulcerations, and masses may also be visible.
- Chest CT: epiglottis enlargement, vocal cord thickening, subglottic stenosis
- Chest x-ray: bilateral hilar adenopathy, reticular opacities

Other Tests to Confirm/Rule Out Diagnosis

- Biopsy: epithelioid non-caseating granulomas with asteroid bodies and Schaumann bodies, lymphocytic infiltration

- Laboratory tests: increased gamma-globulin, increased serum calcium, elevated liver transaminases, increased ESR, and increased angiotensin-converting enzyme[17]
- Pulmonary function test (PFT): measures the severity of airway involvement. PFTs may reveal a restrictive lung disease pattern, but normal PFTs do not exclude pulmonary involvement.
- CD4:CD8 ratio is typically 4:1 or greater.
- Arterial blood gas may reveal hypoxemia and hypocapnia.

Discussion

Sarcoidosis is a rare disease of non-caseating granulomas of different organs. Otolaryngologic involvement in sarcoidosis is rare, with only 3 to 5% of patients manifesting disease in the head and neck.[20] Laryngeal presentation is even more rare, at less than 1%.[21–23] The supraglottic region of the larynx, including the vallecula, aryepiglottic folds, and epiglottis, is the area most commonly affected due to the rich lymphatic supply.[23] The subglottis is less commonly affected and true vocal fold involvement is rare because these areas have fewer lymphatic channels.[19] Hoarseness is not a common symptom because the vocal folds are typically spared.[24] The granulomas are not painful but will present with airway obstruction or laryngeal nerve impingement if large enough.[25] Vocal fold paralysis and hoarseness can result from mediastinal adenopathy severe enough to involve the recurrent laryngeal nerves.[26] The mechanisms responsible for severe airway obstruction are via extrinsic compression by large lymph nodes or intrinsic stenosis by mucosal edema/scarring. The course of sarcoidosis is slow, with periods of disease relapse and remittance. Often, sarcoidosis involving the larynx is initially misdiagnosed as asthma, a much more common etiology for the presenting symptoms. Severe cases of sarcoidosis in the larynx can grossly resemble GPA/Wegener's on laryngoscopy. Sarcoidosis is treated with systemic steroids and immunomodulators such as methotrexate. Locally, endoscopic CO_2 laser reduction or inhaled/intralesional glucocorticoids can reduce supraglottic disease.[27]

PROTEIN DEPOSITION DISEASES

Case 4

A 31-year-old woman was referred for hoarseness. Videostroboscopy revealed pronounced erythema and bulging of the left supraglottis with heaped-up yel-

lowish tissue extending onto the superior surface of the left vocal fold (Figure 45–4). The tissue interfered with the mucosal wave. Biopsy was consistent with amyloidosis.

Patient Assessment

Presenting Symptoms

For disease limited to the larynx: hoarseness. For disseminated disease: nephrotic range proteinuria, restrictive cardiomyopathy, fatigue, unintentional weight loss.

Patient Demographics

Male > female (7:3), median age at diagnosis is 64 years

Physical Exam Findings

Hemoptysis, dysphonia, odynophagia, breathlessness, hoarseness, stridor, airway obstruction.

Imaging/Endoscopy

Laryngoscopy: smooth, yellow, or pink-gray mass. The epithelium is usually intact. The subglottic region may be swollen. Nodules or polypoid lesions causing significant luminal narrowing.

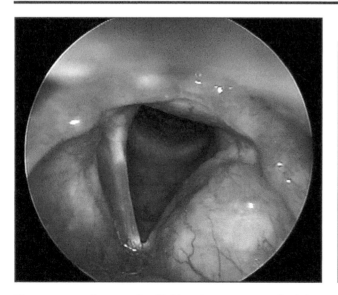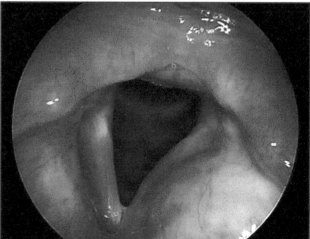

Figure 45–4. Preoperative (*left*) and postoperative (*right*) laryngoscopic view of patient with isolated laryngeal amyloidosis.

Other Tests to Confirm/Rule Out Diagnosis

- Biopsy: the diagnosis of amyloidosis is confirmed by tissue biopsy. Histological stain visualized by polarized light microscopy with Congo red dye reveals apple-green birefringence. Cellular eosinophilic material on non-polarized light microscopy. Metachromatic on crystal violet or methyl violet stain. Electron microscopy reveals fibrillary deposits.
- Bone marrow aspiration can reveal plasma cells if multiple myeloma is the cause.

Rule Out Other Causes of Amyloidosis

Etiology of amyloid deposition will influence patient management. If the patient has amyloid light-chain (AL) amyloidosis, chemotherapy to treat the underlying plasma cell dyscrasia is necessary. Protein fragments can be distinguished by mass spectrometry–based protein analysis.

Discussion

Amyloidosis is caused by extracellular deposition of insoluble protein subunits in various organs, including the larynx. Amyloidosis is comorbid with autoimmune disease 7% of the time[28] or it can be idiopathic. Amyloidosis is a generic term and constitutes several subclasses, including AL (immunoglobulin light chain) caused by plasma cell dyscrasias and AA (fragments of acute phase reactant serum amyloid A) caused by chronic inflammation, although most localized amyloidosis is caused by the AL (primary) type.[29] Primary amyloidosis deposits in the head and neck in 19% of cases[30] and the larynx is the most commonly involved site[31–33] in the head and neck with the following order of involvement: ventricular fold, aryepiglottic fold, and subglottis.[34] Overall, laryngeal deposits constitute 0.2% of all benign laryngeal tumors.[35,36] However, amyloidosis in the larynx is almost always symptomatic and may cause respiratory mortality. In a study at the Mayo Clinic of 413 patients with localized immunoglobulin light chain amyloidosis, 98% of patients with laryngeal deposits reported symptoms and were likely to have two or more recurrences compared with amyloidosis in other organs.[28] Deposition of proteins is typically subepithelial. The true and false vocal folds are commonly involved, presenting as dysphonia.[33,37] Unlike treatment in inflammatory diseases, steroids or radiation is not helpful in treatment.[32] Conservative endoscopic surgical excision of lesions and close follow-up for recurrence and repeat excision are recommended.[38,39] If the cause is AL amyloidosis, chemotherapy such as melphalan should be initiated in cases of systemic disease. Although recurrence of localized amyloidosis lesions in the larynx is common, long-term prognosis is favorable.[38,40]

CASE 5

A 65-year-old man is referred for hoarseness and globus sensation for 5 months. Laryngoscopic exam revealed fullness and erythema of the entire left vestibular fold, partially obscuring visualization of the left vocal fold (Figure 45–5). After surgical excision, pathology revealed plasma cell granuloma with scattered IgG4-positive cells throughout. Diagnosis: IgG4 disease.

Patient Assessment

Presenting Symptoms

Dysphonia, dysphagia, odynophagia, globus sensation, throat pain

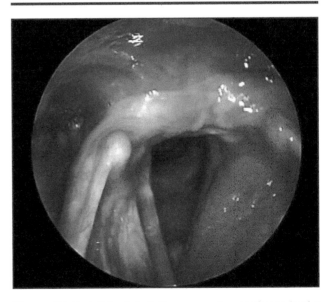

Figure 45–5. IgG4-related disease causing erythema in the larynx.

Patient Demographics

Male > female (2.8–3.5:1) overall, although male:female ratio is 1:1 in head and neck disease,[41] fourth decade and older

Physical Exam Findings

Stridor, hoarseness, ulceration or fibrosis of the larynx

Imaging/Endoscopy

Laryngoscopy: non-malignant hyperplasia and/or fibrosis of the larynx; diffuse or focal enlargement, masses, and nodules

Other Tests to Confirm/Rule Out Diagnosis

- Biopsy: histologic diagnosis of IgG4:IgG ratio of >2:1. Infiltration of lymphocytes and plasmacytes (IgG4 positive), swirling "storiform" fibrosis, obliterative phlebitis, increased eosinophils
- Laboratory tests: elevated serum IgG4 in 60–70% cases (>135 mg/dL), although other diseases may present with elevated IgG4 (Sjogren syndrome, mixed connective tissue disease) or tissue infiltration of IgG4-positive cells (ANCA-associated vasculitis, Epstein–Barr virus lymphadenopathy, mastoiditis).[42]

Rule Out Malignant Head and Neck Cancer and Amyloidosis

Malignant head and neck cancer, if advanced, may present with destruction of underlying laryngeal cartilage and bone. Because IgG4-related disease (RD) is postulated to have an autoimmune etiology, both mass lesions may appear metabolically active on PET-CT or other imaging modalities. Biopsy of the affected site may distinguish malignancy from amyloidosis or IgG4-RD, although inflammatory infiltrate and the presence of IgG4 cells may be present in malignancy, autoimmune diseases, and IgG4-RD. Western blot analysis of immunoglobulin heavy chain fragments is recommended.[42]

Discussion

IgG4-RD is a recently recognized group of chronic inflammatory disorders with similar pathologic and clin-

ical characteristics. They can present as pseudotumors, also known as inflammatory myofibroblastic tumors (IMTs). The head and neck region is the second-most commonly involved site in IgG4-RD, after the pancreas.[41] Most commonly, IgG4-RD presents as a space-occupying mass in the head and neck that results in fibrosis and responds to corticosteroid treatment. IgG4 disease can present similarly to amyloidosis, as both diseases manifest as protein deposits in various organs and cause fibrosis and obliterative phlebitis. IgG4-RDs may also appear as malignant tumors of the head and neck. However, IgG4-RD mass lesions will not involve destruction of underlying bone, unlike malignant cancers.[42] IgG4 disease is treated with high dose corticosteroids and immunosuppressants, and surgical resection is generally not recommended.[41,43]

BLISTERING CUTANEOUS DISEASES

Case 6

A 45-year-old man presents with 6 weeks of progressive hoarseness, hemoptysis, and dysphagia, along with oral pain. In the last few weeks he has developed skin lesions of the face and hands that slough off with gentle rubbing. Laryngoscopy shows supraglottic erythema with supraglottic ulcerations along the laryngeal aspect of the epiglottis. Laryngeal biopsy with direct immunofluorescence shows intercellular IgG. Laryngoscopic examination is shown in Figure 45–6. Diagnosis: pemphigus vulgaris.

Patient Assessment

Presenting Symptoms

Progressive hoarseness, stridor, or dyspnea

Patient Demographics

Mean age 40 to 50 years. Possible correlation with UV radiation and pesticides. More common in Ashkenazi Jews and Mediterranean populations.[44]

Medical History

May coexist with other autoimmune diseases

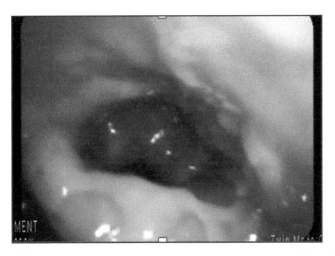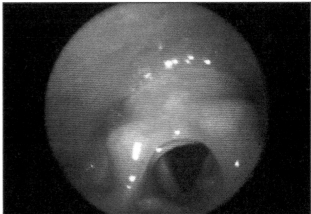

Figure 45–6. Pemphigus vulgaris causing ulceration (*left*) with resulting mild stenosis (*right*) of the larynx.

Social History

None pertinent

Family Hx

May have family history of autoimmune disease

Physical Exam Findings

Affects oral mucosa first in 70% of cases, usually with ulceration with gray membranes. May involve pharynx, larynx, esophagus, nasal cavity. On the skin, fragile, painful blisters may be present. It is very rare to have larynx as the only site of disease,[44] although prevalence of laryngeal involvement overall has been reported to be as high as 85%.[45]

Laryngoscopy

Ulceration, unruptured blisters, scarring, laryngeal edema, or—in later stages—stenosis may be present in the supraglottis or glottis.

Imaging

None typically required

Other Tests to Confirm/Rule Out Diagnosis

- Biopsy: intra-epithelial acantholytic lesions with direct immunofluorescence showing a reticular, intracellular fluorescence pattern from IgG deposits in keratinocytes.
- Laboratory findings: indirect immunofluorescence measures amount of circulating anti-desmosome (desmoglein 3) antibodies.[46] Titers may correlate with disease progression or response to treatment.

Discussion

Pemphigus vulgaris (PV), the most common of the pemphigus diseases, is a rare autoimmune disease affecting mucous membranes and skin. Pemphigus is typically considered a type II hypersensitivity reaction with antibodies formed against desmosomes, leading to separation of layers within the epidermis or stratified epithelial layers. It is very rarely isolated to the larynx and is typically first identified in oral mucosa, nasal mucosa, or skin. However, laryngeal complaints are more common when nasal symptoms are also present and typically consist of hoarseness, progressive stridor, or dyspnea.[47]

Laryngoscopy may reveal supraglottic ulcerations with a tan or gray base, as the blisters that are typically seen on skin are sloughed off by swallowing or coughing. A later finding of disease may be supraglottic narrowing and scarring. Diagnosis requires tissue biopsy which typically reveals intra-epithelial acantholysis.[24]

Treatment is typically with immunosuppressant systemic medications, with high dose corticosteroids remaining the treatment of choice in the acute phase.

In more serious cases, corticosteroids may be combined with other immunosuppressants (cyclosporine, cyclophosphamide, azathioprine, rituximab).[48] Other therapeutic options for pemphigus include plasmapheresis, tetracyclines, and dapsone. Surgical intervention is limited to biopsy or endoscopic dilation when necessary.

CASE 7

An 87-year-old woman presents with tense skin blisters of the lower torso skin and scant hemoptysis. Oral exam shows a large de-roofed blister of the soft palate. Laryngoscopy shows bullae and ulcerations of the laryngeal aspect of the epiglottis (Figure 45–7). Biopsy of the oropharyngeal lesion showed subepidermal bullae with fibrin and eosinophils between the interface of the basement membrane and epidermis.[49] Serum testing is positive for BP180. Diagnosis: bullous pemphigoid.

Patient Assessment

Presenting Symptoms

Patients tend to present with pruritic tense skin blisters associated with oral or laryngopharyngeal symptoms of hemoptysis, sore throat, or hoarseness. May have symptoms of dyspnea from mucosal scarring and laryngeal stenosis if chronic.

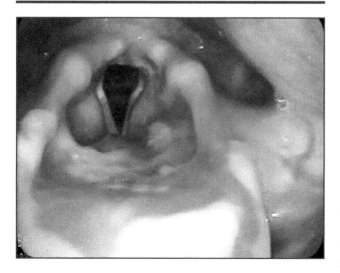

Figure 45–7. Blistering laryngeal lesions consistent with bullous pemphigoid.

Patient Demographics

Older individuals, fourth decade and older

Medical History

May have a history of autoimmune disease or prior skin bullae

Physical Exam Findings

Tense blisters 1 to 3 cm on skin of flexural surfaces and trunk, sometimes involving upper aerodigestive tract mucosa (1/3 of cases). Associated with pruritis, sore throat, voice changes, inspiratory stridor, hemoptysis, or laryngeal edema.

Laryngoscopy

Ulceration or scarring of mucosa of upper aerodigestive tract leading to supraglottic narrowing; white fibrinous base surrounded by erythema.[50]

Imaging

None

Other Tests to Confirm/Rule Out Diagnosis

- Biopsy: mast cell degranulation, edema, eosinophil-rich subepithelial blisters with leukocytic infiltrate, with continuous linear deposits of IgG or C3 in the basement membrane.
- Laboratory findings: auto-antibodies to BP180 and BP230, associated with hemidesmosomes.[46] These are not present in patients with other blistering diseases.[51]

Differential Diagnosis

Mucous membrane pemphigoid (MMP), also known as cicatricial pemphigoid (CP), epidermolysis bullosa acquisita (EBA).[52]

Discussion

Bullous pemphigoid is a subepithelial autoimmune blistering disease with auto-antibodies against epidermal basement membrane proteins. It rarely affects the larynx, but laryngoscopy may show large tense blisters of the supraglottis, or more commonly ruptured blisters or ulcers with the blister surface sloughed off. In the chronic phase, if untreated, there can be laryngeal stenosis from chronic scarring. Bullous pemphigoid tends to have a chronic course with exacerbations and partial or full remissions. Treatment consists of systemic glucocorticoids, dapsone, and/or other immunosuppressive medications.[51] Critical airway narrowing may warrant surgical intervention.

REFERENCES

1. Alaani A, Hogg RP, Drake Lee AB. Wegener's granulomatosis and subglottic stenosis: management of the airway. *J Laryngol Otol.* 2004;118(10):786–790.
2. Langford CA, Sneller MC, Hallahan CW, et al. Clinical features and therapeutic management of subglottic stenosis in patients with Wegener's granulomatosis. *Arthritis Rheum.* 1996;39(10):1754–1760.
3. Polychronopoulos VS, Prakash UB, Golbin JM, Edell ES, Specks U. Airway involvement in Wegener's granulomatosis. *Rheum Dis Clin North Am.* 2007;33(4):755–775, vi.
4. Jennette JC, Falk RJ. Small-vessel vasculitis. *N Engl J Med.* 1997;337(21):1512–1523.
5. Gluth MB, Shinners PA, Kasperbauer JL. Subglottic stenosis associated with Wegener's granulomatosis. *Laryngoscope.* 2003;113(8):1304–1307.
6. Stappaerts I, Van Laer C, Deschepper K, Van de Heyning P, Vermeire P. Endoscopic management of severe subglottic stenosis in Wegener's granulomatosis. *Clin Rheumatol.* 2000;19(4):315–317.
7. Nouraei SA, Obholzer R, Ind PW, et al. Results of endoscopic surgery and intralesional steroid therapy for airway compromise due to tracheobronchial Wegener's granulomatosis. *Thorax.* 2008;63(1):49–52.
8. Puechal X, Terrier B, Mouthon L, Costedoat-Chalumeau N, Guillevin L, Le Jeunne C. Relapsing polychondritis. *Joint Bone Spine.* 2014;81(2):118–124.
9. Behar JV, Choi YW, Hartman TA, Allen NB, McAdams HP. Relapsing polychondritis affecting the lower respiratory tract. *AJR Am J Roentgenol.* 2002;178(1):173–177.
10. Lin ZQ, Xu JR, Chen JJ, Hua XL, Zhang KB, Guan YJ. Pulmonary CT findings in relapsing polychondritis. *Acta Radiol.* 2010;51(5):522–526.
11. Trentham DE, Le CH. Relapsing polychondritis. *Ann Intern Med.* 1998;129(2):114–122.
12. Kent PD, Michet CJ, Jr., Luthra HS. Relapsing polychondritis. *Curr Opin Rheumatol.* 2004;16(1):56–61.
13. Heman-Ackah YD, Remley KB, Goding GS, Jr. A new role for magnetic resonance imaging in the diagnosis of laryngeal relapsing polychondritis. *Head Neck.* 1999;21(5):484–489.
14. Hansson AS, Holmdahl R. Cartilage-specific autoimmunity in animal models and clinical aspects in patients—focus on relapsing polychondritis. *Arthritis Res.* 2002;4(5):296–301.
15. Faix LE, Branstetter BFt. Uncommon CT findings in relapsing polychondritis. *AJNR Am J Neuroradiol.* 2005;26(8):2134–2136.
16. Wenig BM. Necrotizing sialometaplasia of the larynx. A report of two cases and a review of the literature. *Am J Clin Pathol.* 1995;103(5):609–613.
17. Loehrl TA, Smith TL. Inflammatory and granulomatous lesions of the larynx and pharynx. *Am J Med.* 2001;111 Suppl 8A:113S–117S.
18. Ahmed M, Sulaiman I, Rutherford R, Gilmartin JJ. First presentation of sarcoidosis with severe obstructive sleep apnoea and epiglottic involvement. *Sarcoidosis Vasc Diffuse Lung Dis.* 2013;30(2):146–148.
19. McLaughlin RB, Spiegel JR, Selber J, Gotsdiner DB, Sataloff RT. Laryngeal sarcoidosis presenting as an isolated submucosal vocal fold mass. *J Voice.* 1999;13(2):240–245.
20. Badhey AK, Kadakia S, Carrau RL, Iacob C, Khorsandi A. Sarcoidosis of the head and neck. *Head and neck pathology.* 2015;9(2):260–268.
21. Ellison DE, Canalis RF. Sarcoidosis of the head and neck. *Clin Dermatol.* 1986;4(4):136–142.
22. Plaschke CC, Owen HH, Rasmussen N. Clinically isolated laryngeal sarcoidosis. *Eur Arch Otorhinolaryngol.* 2011;268(4):575–580.
23. Polychronopoulos VS, Prakash UBS. Airway involvement in sarcoidosis. *Chest.* 2009;136(5):1371–1380.
24. Leahy K. Laryngeal and tracheal manifestations of systemic disease. In: P Flint, et al, eds, *Cummings Otolaryngology: Head and Neck Surgery.* 5th ed. Maryland Heights, MO: Mosby; 2010:889–893.
25. Coffey CS, Vallejo SL, Farrar EK, Judson MA, Halstead LA. Sarcoidosis presenting as bilateral vocal cord paralysis from bilateral compression of the recurrent laryngeal nerves from thoracic adenopathy. *J Voice.* 2009;23(5):631–634.
26. el-Kassimi FA, Ashour M, Vijayaraghavan R. Sarcoidosis presenting as recurrent left laryngeal nerve palsy. *Thorax.* 1990;45(7):565–566.
27. Sims HS, Thakkar KH. Airway involvement and obstruction from granulomas in African-American patients with sarcoidosis. *Respir Med.* 2007;101(11):2279–2283.
28. Kourelis TV, Kyle RA, Dingli D, et al. Presentation and outcomes of localized immunoglobulin light chain amyloidosis: the Mayo Clinic experience. *Mayo Clin Proc.* 2017;92(6):908–917.
29. Grindle CR, Curry JM, Cantor JP, Malloy KM, Pribitkin EA, Keane WM. Localized oropharyngeal amyloidosis. *Ear Nose Throat J.* 2011;90(5):220–222.
30. Penner CR, Muller S. Head and neck amyloidosis: a clinicopathologic study of 15 cases. *Oral Oncol.* 2006;42(4):421–429.
31. Alaani A, Warfield AT, Pracy JP. Management of laryngeal amyloidosis. *J Laryngol Otol.* 2004;118(4):279–283.
32. Mitrani M, Biller HF. Laryngeal amyloidosis. *Laryngoscope.* 1985;95(11):1346–1347.
33. Behranwala KA, Ali Asgar B, Borges A, Marfatia PT. Laser in treatment of laryngeal amyloidosis. *Indian J Otolaryngol Head Neck Surg.* 2004;56(1):46–48.

34. O'Reilly A, D'Souza A, Lust J, Price D. Localized tongue amyloidosis: a single institutional case series. *Otolaryngol Head Neck Surg*. 2013;149(2):240–244.

35. Thompson LD, Derringer GA, Wenig BM. Amyloidosis of the larynx: a clinicopathologic study of 11 cases. *Mod Pathol*. 2000;13(5):528–535.

36. Stevenson R, Witteles R, Damrose E, et al. More than a frog in the throat: a case series and review of localized laryngeal amyloidosis. *Arch Otolaryngol Head Neck Surg*. 2012;138(5):509–511.

37. Behnoud F, Baghbanian N. Isolated laryngeal amyloidosis. *Iran J Otorhinolaryngol*. 2013;25(70):49–52.

38. Pribitkin E, Friedman O, O'Hara B, et al. Amyloidosis of the upper aerodigestive tract. *Laryngoscope*. 2003;113(12):2095–2101.

39. Kennedy TL, Patel NM. Surgical management of localized amyloidosis. *Laryngoscope*. 2000;110(6):918–923.

40. Pietruszewska W, Wagrowska-Danilewicz M, Klatka J. Amyloidosis of the head and neck: a clinicopathological study of cases with long-term follow-up. *Arch Med Sci*. 2014;10(4):846–852.

41. Mulholland GB, Jeffery CC, Satija P, Cote DW. Immunoglobulin G4-related diseases in the head and neck: a systematic review. *J Otolaryngol Head Neck Surg*. 2015;44:24.

42. Takano K, Yamamoto M, Takahashi H, Himi T. Recent advances in knowledge regarding the head and neck manifestations of IgG4-related disease. *Auris Nasus Larynx*. 2017;44(1):7–17.

43. Shaib Y, Ton E, Goldschmeding R, Tekstra J. IgG4-related disease with atypical laryngeal presentation and Behcet/granulomatous polyangiitis mimicking features. *BMJ Case Rep*. 2013;2013.

44. Vasiliou A, Nikolopoulos TP, Manolopoulos L, Yiotakis J. Laryngeal pemphigus without skin manifestations and review of the literature. *Eur Arch Otorhinolaryngol*. 2007;264(5):509–512.

45. Fernandez S, Espana A, Navedo M, Barona L. Study of oral, ear, nose and throat involvement in pemphigus vulgaris by endoscopic examination. *Br J Dermatol*. 2012;167(5):1011–1016.

46. Tabuchi K, Nomura M, Murashita H, et al. Coexistence of pemphigus vulgaris and bullous pemphigoid in the upper aerodigestive tract. *Auris Nasus Larynx*. 2006;33(2):231–233.

47. Kavala M, Altintas S, Kocaturk E, et al. Ear, nose and throat involvement in patients with pemphigus vulgaris: correlation with severity, phenotype and disease activity. *J Eur Acad Dermatol Venereol*. 2011;25(11):1324–1327.

48. Gregoriou S, Koutsoukou XA, Panayotides I, et al. Pemphigus vulgaris of the epiglottis successfully treated with rituximab. *J Eur Acad Dermatol Venereol*. 2015;29(9):1845–1846.

49. Lee CM, Leadbetter HK, Fishman JM. A case of oropharyngeal bullous pemphigoid presenting with haemoptysis. *Case Rep Otolaryngol*. 2015;2015:631098.

50. Ohki M, Kikuchi S, Ohata A, Baba Y, Ishikawa J, Sugimoto H. Features of oral, pharyngeal, and laryngeal lesions in bullous pemphigoid. *Ear Nose Throat J*. 2016;95(10–11):E1–E5.

51. Yancey KB, Egan CA. Pemphigoid: clinical, histologic, immunopathologic, and therapeutic considerations. *JAMA*. 2000;284(3):350–356.

52. Higgins TS, Cohen JC, Sinacori JT. Laryngeal mucous membrane pemphigoid: a systematic review and pooled-data analysis. *Laryngoscope*. 2010;120(3):529–536.

CHAPTER 46

Pemphigus Vulgaris

Theodore Athanasiadis and Kimon Toumazos

INTRODUCTION

Laryngeal pemphigus is a rare and potentially fatal entity, with patients usually exhibiting lesions in other locations and organ systems. Managing these patients usually involves multidisciplinary care with involvement from immunologists, respiratory physicians, and otolaryngologists. Immunosuppression is the mainstay of treatment, with newer immunomodulating agents showing some promise. Historically, preserving the mucosal and skin surfaces has been advocated, while surgical treatment has been seen as a last resort in these patients.

DEFINITION

Pemphigus vulgaris (PV) is a form of pemphigus, a subgroup of the autoimmune bullous diseases (ABDs), which are characterized by a disruption in the host immune system resulting in blister formation affecting skin and or mucosa.

CASE PRESENTATION

We present a case of PV in a 53-year-old male with bullae affecting his skin and mucous membranes of the nose and paranasal sinuses extending down to his laryngeal and subglottic airway. PV had been diagnosed in him by his dermatologist and immunologist 12 months previously after a number of skin biopsies were taken. There was a history of previous extensive functional endoscopic sinus surgery under a rhinologist. Referral to a laryngologist was made due to increasing dyspnea, dysphonia, and dysphagia as well as odynophagia. The patient managed a national landscape gardening supply business and found it increasingly difficult to conduct his business due to these symptoms. He is a non-smoker who does not drink alcohol, with no other previous medical comorbidities.

Medications: Prednisolone 25 mg OD

Nil known allergies

Initial Assessment

History

Symptoms included breathing restriction, reduced exercise tolerance, voice change, dysphagia, hemoptysis. Inquiry regarding current treatment therapies and social history was undertaken.

Examination

Breathing characteristics, obvious skin lesions affecting head and neck, oral exam, nasal exam with nasendoscope, laryngoscopy. Examination looking for severity of dyspnea (stridor at rest may indicate need to expedite treatment) extent and spread of disease in terms of mucosal lesions. In-office transnasal esophagoscopy would be quite useful if available in order to evaluate the esophagus and stomach for possible mucosal lesions, as would in-office tracheoscopy in order to fully evaluate the trachea for lesions or scar tissue.

Scenario

A 53-year-old male has mild inspiratory stridor at rest and very strained rough voice. Body mass index is within normal limits. No cutaneous lesions on his face; however, multiple skin lesions affect his forearms. Oral cavity normal. Nasendoscopy revealed crusting throughout the nasal cavity and paranasal sinuses with dark brown blood-stained mucus and crusts dripping into the post-nasal space. Laryngeal exam revealed mucosal ulcerations affecting the supraglottis (mainly epiglottis), edematous vocal folds, subglottic crusting with some fresh blood, normal trachea below the sub-glottic region down to main stem bronchi. Significant scar tissue affects the arytenoids and false folds with severe airway restriction immediately superior to the glottis restricting airway to around 2 to 3 mm. (Video 1)

Diagnosis

Pemphigus vulgaris affects the upper airway with significant supraglottic stenosis likely to be related to healed ulceration—involvement of skin and nasal mucosa also, with relative sparing of the oral cavity.

Investigations

Biopsy of epiglottic ulcerations taken under local anesthetic. Immunofluorescence testing confirmed PV.

Previous:

- Autoimmune blood screen
- Skin biopsies analyzed with direct immunofluorescence
- CT neck, sinuses, chest

Management

Initial

- Close discussion with all treating parties—dermatologist, immunologist, rhinologist, primary care physician, patient and patient's family
- Observation initially

- Nose: topical saline flushes and intranasal corticosteroid
- Laryngeal lubrication with steam inhalation, gargles, sugar-free lozenges, regular sips of water
- Possible reflux treated with prophylactic alginate
- Topical steroid injections on two occasions (triamcinolone 40 mg/mL) to ulcerated regions under local anesthetic
- Oral prednisolone and methotrexate
- Decision made for 6 weekly laryngology reviews over 6 months, unless symptoms deteriorated further

Medium Term

- Two months into the above treatment he was also commenced on fortnightly rituximab infusions. There was significant resolution of all his cutaneous lesions over a period of 3 months. Crusting in the nose and paranasal sinuses as well as subglottis persisted; however, laryngeal mucosal lesions decreased and had completely subsided over 6 months.
- Supraglottic stenosis deteriorated further, leaving the patient restricted to his house due to dyspnea. He also had a number of urgent presentations to his local community hospital emergency department via ambulance with respiratory distress requiring nebulized adrenalin and oxygen. Patient was advised to seek medical attention earlier and was counseled regarding possible requirement for a tracheostomy.

Surgical Intervention

Given the degree of respiratory distress, a decision was made to proceed with upper airway surgery. The case was discussed with a number of prominent international airway surgeons, who mostly counseled in favor of further monitoring or tracheostomy. After extensive counseling of the patient and his family, he proceeded with microlaryngoscopy, CO_2 laser resection of supraglottic scar tissue, and injection of triamcinolone with the understanding that he may require a temporary tracheostomy. A Hunsaker–Mon jet device was used to provide subglottic jet ventilation, and the procedure

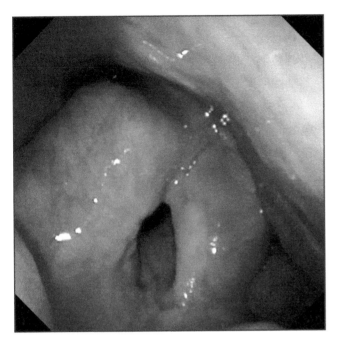

Figure 46–1. Pemphigus preoperative supraglottis.

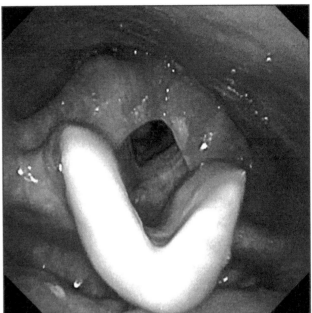

Figure 46–3. Pemphigus postoperative supraglottis.

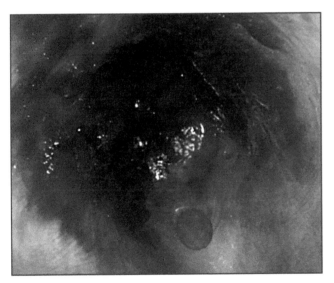

Figure 46–2. Pemphigus subglottis.

proceeded uneventfully (see Figures 46–1, 46–2, and 46–3). The patient was monitored in the intensive care unit for 5 days with marked supraglottic edema; however, he did not require intubation or tracheostomy insertion. After 2 further days on the ward he was dis-

charged home with an increased dose of prednisolone tapered down to baseline over 2 weeks.

Follow-up over the next 12 months revealed a delighted patient who could return to his premorbid physical activities, including water skiing, gardening, and overseas travel without any airway symptoms. On laryngoscopy he has maintained a significantly improved supraglottic airway with no supraglottic restriction. The subglottic crusting remains.

DISCUSSION

Pemphigus encompasses 78% of ABDs, while other subgroups of ABDs include bullous pemphigoid (BP), 12.5%; dermatitis herpetiformis, 6.5%; epidermolysis bullosa, 3%; and linear immunoglobulin A (IgA) bullous dermatosis.[1]

The two major forms of pemphigus are pemphigus vulgaris and pemphigus foliaceus (PF), accounting for approximately 84% and 16% of pemphigus, respectively.[2] Other, rarer subtypes of pemphigus include pemphigus erythematosus, pemphigus herpetiformis, endemic pemphigus foliaceus (*fogo salvagemin brazil*), IgA pemphigus, paraneoplastic pemphigus (PNP), and drug-induced pemphigus.[3]

EPIDEMIOLOGY

Pemphigus has an incidence of roughly 1 per 100,000 population per year with mean age at diagnosis of 49.7 years (although this can range from ages 10 to 92) and has a slight female predominance, with F:M ratio of 1.54:1.[4,5] Crude mortality rate for pemphigus is 0.033 per 100,000.[6]

PATHOPHYSIOLOGY

Pemphigus is characterized by circulating autoantibodies (IgG) to desmoglein (Dsg) molecules Dsg1, Dsg2, and Dsg3.[7] Dsg2 is contained in all tissues containing desmosomes, hence the various forms of pemphigus vary in their differing effects on Dsg1 and Dsg3.[7] Dsg 1 is found only in the epidermis and is expressed in the more superficial layers, while Dsg3 is found in stratified epithelia, including both epidermal and mucosal epithelium, and are expressed mostly in the deeper layers.[7] PV has two subforms, the mucosal form, which involves mostly Dsg3 antigens, and the mucocutaneous form, which involves both Dsg3 and Dsg1 antigens.

Disruption of Dsg's by autoantibodies leads to loss of cell-to-cell cohesion, causing the histological feature of acantholysis. The presence of acantholysis differentiates pemphigus from pemphigoid disease. IgG deposition on the epithelial cell surfaces are evident on direct immunofluorescence (DIF), and hence DIF is the gold standard for pemphigus diagnosis.[8]

CLINICAL MANIFESTATIONS

PV localized to the mucosae with no skin involvement, mucosal PV (18%), is differentiated from pemphigus vulgaris that also involves the skin, mucocutaneous PV (70%).[4] Both, however, most commonly begin with painful non-healing mucosal ulcerations, and common sites include oral (62–100%), pharyngeal (61–64.9%), laryngeal (40–59%), nasal (22–36.6%), conjunctiva, and vaginal.[4,9–11]

PV lesions compared with PF lesions have a more moist appearance, and this is due to the keratinocyte Dsg's targeted in PV which lie deeper in the epithelium.[12] PV easily ruptures, leaving sharp outlined erosions, and heal without scarring. Lesions are often described as itching or burning.[4] Itching as well as involvement of the

Table 46–1. Frequency of Ear, Nose, and Throat Symptoms in PV Patients

Symptoms	Frequency
Oral pain	75.6%
Odynophagia	58–70.7%
Sore throat	48–56%
Hoarseness	25–39%
Otalgia	26.8%
None	12.2%

pharyngeal or nasal mucosa, a positive Nikolsky sign, and severe skin involvement have greatest impact on PV patients' quality of life.[13]

Eighty percent of patients with laryngeal or nasal symptoms have evidence of pemphigus involvement on ENT evaluation.[14] Nasal symptoms seem to have non-specific manifestations such as epistaxis, crusting, or discharge.[10] The frequency of ENT symptoms are shown in Table 46–1.[10,11]

On ENT evaluation, laryngeal lesions occur on the epiglottis, supraglottis, piriform sinuses, ventricular folds, and vocal cords in decreasing frequency.[11]

Gross morphology of PV lesions include bullae, erosions, crustings, and, rarely, apthous-like ulcers.[15] PV lesions in the ear and nose are exclusively seen as erosions.[10] Oral, pharyngeal, and laryngeal lesions are predominantly erosions; however, bullae and ulcers are commonly seen.[10]

DIAGNOSIS/INVESTIGATIONS

Guidelines for the diagnosis of pemphigus developed by the European Dermatology Forum involve four criteria and have been summarized below[16]:

1. Clinical presentation (mentioned above)
2. Histopathology: 4 mm punch excision for a fresh (<24 h) small vesicle or 1/3 of the peripheral portion of a blister and 2/3 perilesional skin (in 4% formalin solution). Intra-epidermal suprabasal acantholysis is seen in PV and PNP, while acantholysis at the granular layer is seen in PF.

3. DIF: perilesional skin (up to 1 cm from fresh lesion) in cryotube or saline or Michel's fixative. IgG and/or C3 deposits at the surface of epidermal keratinocytes.
4. Serology: indirect immunofluorescence (IIF) to detect serum autoantibodies.

Gold standard investigation for diagnosis of pemphigus is DIF of perilesional skin.[8] Serological tests such as enzyme-linked immunosorbent assay (ELISA) of Dsg1/3 or IIF microscopy can be an alternative, with 86% and 89% sensitivity, respectively, compared with DIF.[8]

MANAGEMENT

Knudson et al neatly categorize treatment in mucous membrane involvement of pemphigus vulgaris treatment[17]:

- Mild, non-progressive oral disease can be treated with high potency topical corticosteroids 2–3 times daily.
  Dapsone therapy (125–150 mg daily) can be introduced early.
  Tetracycline (2 g/day) and nicotinamide (1500 mg/day) can be considered.
- Severe mucous membrane involvement or concurrent cutaneous involvement requires oral corticosteroids such as prednisone (0.5–1 mg/kg/day) plus adjuvant immunosuppressive therapy such as azathioprine (1.5–3 mg/kg/day), mycophenolate mofetil (2–2.5 g/day divided in two doses), cyclophosphamide (50–200 mg/day), cyclosporine (5 mg/kg/day), or methotrexate (10–17.5 mg/week). Control of disease can lead to tapering of adjuvant immunosuppression.
- Refractory cases may require intravenous Ig, plasmapheresis, and rituximab to be considered, with or without corticosteroids and an immunosuppressant.

The efficacy of rituximab in patients who were unresponsive to systemic steroids shows some promise.[18] Furthermore, a recent study suggests rituximab used as first-line treatment combined with short-term prednisone provides a better 24-month remission rate of 89% compared with 34% of patients receiving prednisone alone.[19]

PROGNOSIS

Duration to complete remission varies greatly in PV patients. In patients not on therapy the range is from 4 months to 10 years, while PV patients on therapy can enter remission anytime from 1.5 months to 3.5 years.[20] The majority of PV patients remain on long-term medications for 5 to 10 years.[20] Mortality in PV patients between 2001 to 2010 internationally has been reported as 5.2% (this includes deaths from all causes).[20] Mortality among PV patients is 2.4 times greater than for the general population, mainly due to infections such as pneumonia and septicemia.[21] This can be attributed to the immunosuppressive therapy offered to PV patients, predisposing them to opportunistic infections, as well as the impaired mucosal barrier by PV itself.[22] Cardiovascular disease and malignancy are also seen in significantly higher incidence in PV patients.[21,22]

SUMMARY

This rare case of pemphigus vulgaris affecting the upper airway illustrates the utility of multi-team and multi-modality treatment. Immunomodulating medication (rituximab) had a significant positive effect on the presence of mucocutaneous lesions and should be considered in those not responsive to more traditional therapies. Given the severity and ongoing progression of the airway symptoms in this case, observation was no longer ideal and surgical intervention was warranted. There is a significant risk of permanent mucosal injury with airway surgery in pemphigus vulgaris patients, and thus the possibility of a tracheostomy becoming a permanent fixture was raised. With good mucosal control of disease, however, in certain situations surgery should be considered and can be performed with good results.

REFERENCES

1. Sobhan M, Farshchian M, Tamimi M. Spectrum of autoimmune vesiculobullous diseases in Iran: a 13-year retrospective study. *Clin Cosmet Investig Dermatol.* 2016; 11(9):15–20. doi: 10.2147/CCID.S97214.
2. Heelan K, Mahar AL, Walsh S, Shear NH. Pemphigus and associated comorbidities: a cross-sectional study. *Clin Exp Dermatol.* 2015;40(6):593–599. doi: 10.1111/ced.12634

3. Vassileva S, Drenovska K, Manuelyan K. Autoimmune blistering dermatoses as systemic diseases. *Clin Dermatol*. 2014;32(3):364–375. doi: 10.1016/j.clindermatol.2013.11.003

4. Chams-Davatchi C, Valikhani M, Daneshpazhooh M, et al. Pemphigus: Analysis of 1209 cases. *Int J Dermatol*. 2005;44(6):470–476. doi: 10.1111/j.1365-4632.2004.02501.x

5. Baum S, Astman N, Berco E, Solomon M, Trau H, Barzilai A. Epidemiological data of 290 pemphigus vulgaris patients: a 29-year retrospective study. *Eur J Dermatol*. 2016;26(4):382–387. doi: 10.1684/ejd.2016.2792

6. Baibergenova AT, Weinstock MA, Shear NH. Mortality from acquired bullous diseases of skin in Canadian adults 2000–2007. *Int J Dermatol*. 2012;51(11):1325–1328. doi: 10.1111/j.1365-4632.2011.05227.x

7. Delva E, Tucker DK, Kowalczyk AP. The desmosome. *Cold Spring Harbor Perspect Biol*. 2009;1(2):a002543. doi: 10.1101/cshperspect.a002543

8. Giurdanella F, Diercks GF, Jonkman MF, Pas HH. Laboratory diagnosis of pemphigus: direct immunofluorescence remains the gold standard. *Br J Dermatol*. 2016;175(1):185–186. doi: 10.1111/bjd.14408

9. Su O, Onsun N, Meric Teker A, et al. Upper airway tract and upper gastrointestinal tract involvement in patients with pemphigus vulgaris. *Eur J Dermatol*. 2010;20(6):792–796. doi: 10.1684/ejd.2010.1121

10. Robati RM, Rahmati-Roodsari M, Dabir-Moghaddam P, et al. Mucosal manifestations of pemphigus vulgaris in ear, nose, and throat; before and after treatment. *J Am Acad Dermatol*. 2012;67(6):e249–e252. doi: 10.1016/j.jaad.2011.06.022

11. Mahmoud A, Miziara ID, Costa KC, Santi CG, Maruta CW, Aoki V. Laryngeal involvement in pemphigus vulgaris: a proposed classification. *J Laryngol Otol*. 2012;126(10):1041–1044. doi: 10.1017/S0022215112001375

12. Waschke J. The desmosome and pemphigus. *Histochem Cell Biol*. 2008;130(1):21–54. doi: 10.1007/s00418-008-0420-0

13. Ghodsi SZ. Quality of life and psychological status of patients with pemphigus vulgaris using Dermatology Life Quality Index and General Health Questionnaires. *J Dermatol*. 2012;39(2):141–144. doi: 10.1111/j.1346–8138.2011.01382.x

14. Hale EK, Bystryn JC. Laryngeal and nasal involvement in pemphigus vulgaris. *J Am Acad Dermatol*. 2001;44(4):609–611. doi: 10.1067/mjd.2001.112225

15. Kavala M, Altıntaş S, Kocatürk E, et al. Ear, nose and throat involvement in patients with pemphigus vulgaris: correlation with severity, phenotype and disease activity. *J Eur Acad Dermatol Venereol*. 2011;25(11):1324–1327. doi: 10.1111/j.1468-3083.2011.03981.x

16. Hertl M, Jedlickova H, Karpati S, et al. Pemphigus. S2 Guideline for diagnosis and treatment—guided by the European Dermatology Forum (EDF) in cooperation with the European Academy of Dermatology and Venereology (EADV). *J Eur Acad Dermatol Venereol*. 2015;29(3):405–414. doi: 10.1111/jdv.12772

17. Knudson RM, Knudson RM, Kalaaji AN, Bruce AJ. The management of mucous membrane pemphigoid and pemphigus. *Dermatol Ther*. 2010;23(3):268–280. doi: 10.1111/j.1529-8019.2010.01323.x

18. Sami N. Nasal, pharyngeal, and laryngeal pemphigus vulgaris successfully treated with rituximab. *Ear Nose Throat J*. 2017;96(4-5):E35–E38. https://www.ncbi.nlm.nih.gov/pubmed/28489243

19. Joly P, Maho-Vaillant M, Prost-Squarcioni C, et al. First-line rituximab combined with short-term prednisone versus prednisone alone for the treatment of pemphigus (Ritux 3): a prospective, multicentre, parallel-group, open-label randomised trial. *Lancet*. 2017. doi: 10.1016/s0140-6736(17)30070-3

20. Cholera M, Chainani-Wu N. Management of pemphigus vulgaris. *Adv Ther*. 2016;33(6):910–958. doi: 10.1007/s12325-016-0343-4

21. Kridin K, Sagi SZ, Bergman R. Mortality and cause of death in patients with pemphigus. *Acta Derm Venereol*. 2017;97(5):607–611. doi: 10.2340/00015555-2611

22. Leshem YA, Gdalevich M, Ziv M, David M, Hodak E, Mimouni D. Opportunistic infections in patients with pemphigus. *J Am Acad Dermatol*. 2014;71(2):284–292. doi: 10.1016/j.jaad.2014.03.020

CHAPTER 47

Relapsing Polychondritis and the Airway

Andrew J. Kinshuck and James H. Hull

INTRODUCTION

Relapsing polychondritis (RP) is a condition that causes inflammation of cartilaginous structures throughout the body. It is a rare, immune-mediated disease which is characterized by recurrent and progressive inflammation and destruction of cartilage. This condition most commonly involves the cartilaginous areas of the ears, nose, and airway but may also include non-cartilaginous structures within the eyes, the audiovestibular apparatus, skin, heart, and the nervous system. The incidence RP is reported to be between 2 to 3.5 per million population[1-3] and it has a variable course and prognosis. However, respiratory involvement is associated with more severe symptoms and a poorer prognosis. The management of RP should be approached in a multidisciplinary fashion with involvement of multiple medical specialties. High dose corticosteroids and immunosuppressants are most often used as front-line treatments, although there is currently no definitive trial indicating the optimal approach. Surgical intervention is sometimes required, especially for laryngotracheal involvement to maintain airway patency.

DEFINITION

Relapsing polychondritis is a progressive immune-mediated destructive inflammation of the cartilaginous structures. When RP involves the larynx and the tracheobronchial, it carries a significant mortality.

CASE PRESENTATION

A 39-year-old male non-smoker presented with increased shortness of breath. He had no symptoms of cough, hemoptysis, dysphagia, or weight loss. He initially had attended his local hospital and was reviewed by both ENT and respiratory specialists. He was found to have an obstructive picture on spirometry and had been started on continuous positive airway pressure (CPAP). His symptoms were initially worse at night and he was diagnosed as having sleep apnea. His body mass index (BMI) was high at 33 and this was thought to be a contributing factor. It was later noted that he had a saddle-nose deformity and thickening of both pinnas with no palpable cartilage. Following a delay, the clinical diagnosis of RP was made and he was started on systemic oral corticosteroids (prednisolone) and immunosuppressants (methotrexate).

Despite this treatment, his symptoms worsened and due to ongoing difficulties with his breathing, he was referred to a tertiary airway and respiratory center for further management.

Initial Assessment

History

A comprehensive history is required due to the multiple systems involved by RP. There is often a delay in diagnosis and patients will have had numerous investigations and treatments. The respiratory history should cover breathing difficulties including sleep apnea, exercise tolerance, cough, and hemoptysis. The ENT history should include changes in the shape of pinna, warmth, and discomfort of the ear (eg, when lying at night), hearing loss, nasal deformity, voice change, and breathing difficulties. A complete history should include questions regarding rheumatological problems, ie, early morning joint discomfort and ocular symptoms.

Examination

A multisystem examination is required due to RP involving cartilage throughout the body but also has associated dermatological, ophthalmological, and neurological signs. On examination of the ENT system: the pinna should be palpated for presence of cartilage and loss of structure. Hearing test may also be indicated. The nasal examination may reveal a saddle nose deformity and septal perforation. Any voice change or strain should be looked for and respiratory signs of increased work of breathing should be noted. Due to laryngotracheal involvement there can be an audible wheeze on auscultation or even stridor.

Nasendoscopy

Findings can include septal perforation and laryngeal stenosis. Nasendoscopy can also assess for signs of other differential diagnoses, including vasculitis or granulomatosis within the nasopharynx and larynx.

SCENARIO 1

ENT examination revealed a saddle nose deformity and bilateral thickened pinnas. The larynx appeared uninvolved, with mobile symmetrical vocal folds. Respiratory examination revealed a resting respiratory rate at 29 breaths per minute. On auscultation there was a reduced chest expansion and a loud expiratory wheeze throughout.

Diagnosis

Relapsing polychondritis with tracheal involvement

Investigations

Blood Tests

The first line of investigations included blood tests: full blood count, renal function, erythrocyte sedimentation rate (ESR), C-reactive protein (CRP), antinuclear antibodies (ANA), rheumatoid factor (RF), immuno-

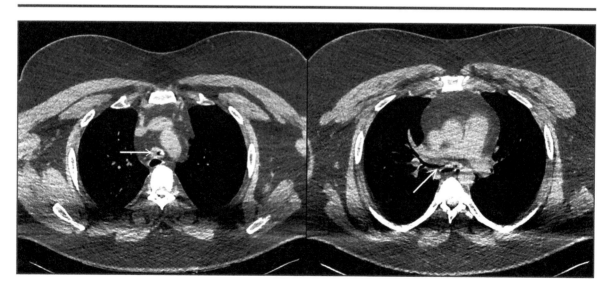

Figure 47–1. CT chest with arrows demonstrating diffuse thickening of the trachea and bronchial stenosis, respectively.

globulins (Ig), anti-neutrophil cytoplasmic antibodies (ANCA), myeloperoxidase (MPO), and proteinase 3 (PR3). The inflammatory markers were mildly elevated with autoantibody screen negative.

Cartilage Biopsy

A biopsy of the pinna cartilage was not arranged due to the lack of cartilage and other diagnostic criteria being met.

Imaging

A high-resolution CT neck and chest were arranged. The CT scan revealed diffuse thickening of the trachea and both main bronchi (Figure 47–1). There was severe narrowing of the proximal main bronchi.

Pulmonary Investigations

The oxygen saturations were 95% in room air. The peak expiratory flow rate (PEFR) was 145 L/min with a predicted PEFR of 550 L/min.

Pulmonary function tests included forced expiratory volume in 1 sec (FEV_1) of 27% predicted, forced vital capacity (FVC) of 67% predicted and FEV_1/FVC ratio of 31%. There was evidence of significant flow oscillation on the expiratory limb of the flow-volume loop (Figure 47–2).

Management

The patient was treated as severe progressive RP with pulmonary involvement. The case was discussed in a multidisciplinary setting and the options presented to the patient. The corticosteroids were increased and further immunosuppressants were offered to the patient. Due to the significant airway collapse and deterioration in his breathing, an urgent procedure was arranged for airway assessment under general anesthesia and insertion of a Montgomery® T-tube. This was planned as a staged procedure with a tracheostomy tube initially until the stoma healed. During the general anesthetic there were significant challenges for the anesthetic team and in ventilating the patient. The assessment identified significant collapse of the trachea and both bronchi. A cuffed tracheostomy tube was inserted while the tracheostomy tract healed and a T-tube was planned for insertion 6 weeks later. The patient returned for conversion to a Montgomery T-tube

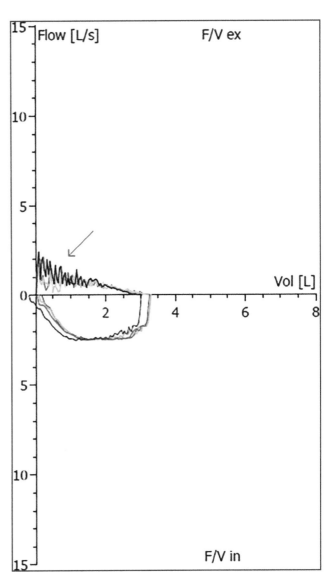

Figure 47–2. Flow-volume loop with the arrow demonstrating oscillation on expiratory limb. Bronchoscopy was performed under sedation and revealed collapsing of the airway on expiration. There were no discernible tracheal cartilage rings (Figure 47–3).

and the upper limb and lower limb were kept as long as possible to allow maximum stenting of the trachea.

Over the next 6 months the disease progressed despite increasing the steroids and resulted in further laryngeal involvement. This resulted in minimal support for the arytenoids, and the vocal cords appeared shortened, with a degree of stenosis at the level of the glottis. However, the airway remained stable with the

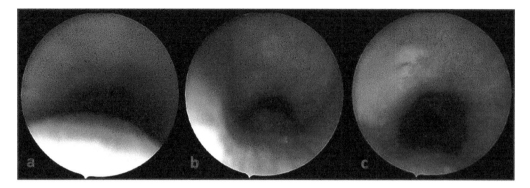

Figure 47–3. Bronchoscopy images (A) collapse of trachea (B) collapse on expiration (C) airway on inspiration.

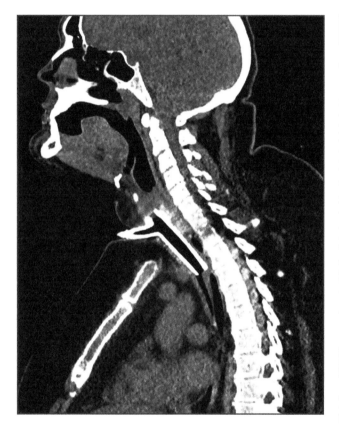

Figure 47–4. Sagittal CT scan demonstrating position of T-tube and evidence of laryngeal stenosis.

T-tube in situ and some vocalization was possible with the T-tube capped off. He managed at home with regular saline nebulizers and suction to maintain his airway and secretions. Figure 47–4 demonstrates the position of the T-tube in the airway.

DIFFERENTIAL DIAGNOSIS

The diagnosis of RP can be challenging and there are other local and systemic conditions that cause cartilage inflammation and destruction. Inflammation of the pinna can be caused by an infective process resulting in perichondritis. Nasal bridge collapse and saddle nose deformity can also be caused by vasculitis and granulomatosis conditions. Ocular involvement seen in RP can be similar to keratitis and scleritis, which is seen in other systemic conditions such as rheumatoid arthritis (eg, Reiters syndrome) and granulomatosis with polyangitis (Wegener's granulomatosis). Large airway collapse is also seen in tracheobronchomalacia and excessive dynamic airway collapse (EDAC). Tracheobronchomalacia is due to weakness in the cartilage of the airway causing collapse. EDAC is airway collapse and stenosis of more than 50% with intact cartilage.

DISCUSSION

RP is a rare condition which was first described in 1923 by Rudolf von Jaksch, a physician working in Prague, and was called polychondropathia.[4] Pearson et al in 1960 described two patients with the condition and named it relapsing polychondritis[5] due to its episodic nature.

RP normally presents in the fourth and fifth decades and occurs equally in both men and women. The incidence is reported as 2 to 3.5 per million population.[1–3] Although the etiology is unknown, an autoimmune process has been hypothesized. This is due to antibodies to type II cartilage being demonstrated in up to a third of patients.[6] The destruction of cartilage is caused by the release of proteolyitc enzymes (including matrix metalloproteinases [MMPs]) by inflammatory cells, chondrocytes, and other cell components.[7] The histological features of RP show the chondrocytes being vacuolated and necrotic before being replaced by fibrous tissue.[7]

Diagnosis of RP

RP can be a difficult diagnosis to be made due to its rarity and variety of presenting features and involved systems. Thus a delay in diagnosis is not unusual, and in a series of 36 patients it took an average of almost 3 years for a diagnosis of RP to be made following the onset of symptoms.[8]

The diagnosis can be made clinically with features of cartilage involvement. In 1976 McAdam et al[9] presented a diagnostic criteria for RP based on the clinical features. A certain diagnosis would be made if there were three of the following: (i) bilateral auricular chondritis, (ii) non-erosive sero-negative inflammatory polyarthritis (iii) nasal chondritis (iv) ocular inflammation (v) respiratory tract chondritis (vi), and audiovestibular dysfunction. Modified criteria were proposed by Damiani and Levine in 1979.[10] They reported a further 10 cases of the condition and suggested for diagnosis that patients have (i) at least three or more diagnostic criteria (histological confirmation not necessary), (ii) one or more of McAdam's signs with positive histological confirmation, or (iii) chondritis in two or more separate anatomical locations with response to steroids. Michet made further changes to the diagnostic criteria.[11] The change in criteria required the presence of proven inflammation of two or three areas, including the pinna, nasal, or laryngotracheal cartilage—or inflammation in one of these cartilage areas plus two other signs, including ocular inflammation, vestibular dysfunction, sero-negative inflammatory arthritis, and hearing loss.[11]

A cartilage biopsy can be helpful if positive but is not always necessary to make the diagnosis. Biopsy of the auricular (pinna) cartilage is undertaken due to auricular chondritis being seen in the majority of patients with RP[9] and is well tolerated under local anesthetic. However, the cartilage is gradually replaced by fibrous tissue and therefore is not always present on biopsy. Initial histological assessment demonstrates perichondral infiltration of lymphocytes and plasma cells.[7] Further inflammatory cells invade the cartilage as the disease progresses, and proteolyitc enzymes cause further destruction to the cartilage.[7]

The initial blood tests look for signs of inflammation and infection as well as an autoimmune screen for other differential diagnosis such as vasculitis and granulomatosis. Blood tests include: full blood count, renal function, ESR, CRP, ANA, RF, Ig, ANCA, MPO, and PR3. A raised ESR can be seen in RP and can be used as a guide for active disease.[5] In a 10-patient case series from Singapore of RP, the ESR was raised in 80% and CRP elevated in 50% of cases at presentation.[12] Antibodies directed against type 2 collagen are present during acute exacerbations of RP and their serum concentration correlates with disease severity.

Clinical Manifestations of RP

RP can affect multiple systems, including ENT, respiratory, cardiovascular, musculoskeletal, ocular, renal,

Table 47–1. Different RP Diagnostic Criteria

McAdam[9] (three of the following)	Damiani and Levine[10]	Michet[11]
(i) bilateral auricular chondritis	Three out of six McAdam's criteria	(i) Proven inflammation in two out of three cartilages: auricular, nasal and laryngotracheal
(ii) non-erosive sero-negative inflammatory	One out of six McAdam's criteria and histological confirmation	(ii) Proven inflammation in one of the above and two other signs from ocular inflammation, hearing loss, vestibular dysfunction, or seronegative inflammatory arthritis
(iii) nasal chondritis	Two out of six McAdam's criteria and response to corticosteroid	
(iv) ocular inflammation		
(v) respiratory tract chondritis		
(vi) audiovestibular dysfunction		

dermatological, and neurological. Skin lesions have been reported in up to half the patients with RP.[13] The skin manifestations reported include ulceration, purpura, and involvement.[13] Ocular involvement include a variety of manifestations such as edema, extraocular muscle palsy, episcleritis, scleritis, conjunctivitis, corneal infiltrate, peripheral ulcerative keratitis, corneal thinning, retinopathy, exudative retinal detachment, and optic neuritis.[14] Cardiovascular manifestations include aortic valve incompetence and mitral valve regurgitation. Renal involvement is rare but IgA nephropathy and nephritis have been documented.[15] Peripheral or central nervous systems can be involved, resulting in cranial nerve palsy.[16] There have been suggestions in the literature of associations with hematological malignancies. There are a few small series and case reports that have reported RP and concomitant myelodysplastic syndrome (MDS).[17–19] MDS is an acquired bone marrow neoplastic disorder. The reasons for this are unknown but most likely multifactorial due to immunosuppression and a sustained inflammatory process.

In a study by Hazra et al[20] in the UK, 61 confirmed RP cases were looked at in detail. They noted that the most frequent reported clinical feature was ear inflammation (70%), followed by arthritis (36%) (Table 47–2).

ENT Manifestations of RP

A combined review of 337 patients[3] found auricular/pinna chondritis to be the most frequent manifestation of RP, seen in 89% of patients. Other otological manifestations include tinnitus, vestibular dysfunction, and conductive and sensorineural hearing loss.[21]

Pinna or auricular chondritis is seen in the majority of RP patients during the course of their disease[22]

Table 47–2. Clinical Features of RP in a Cohort of 61 Patients in the UK[20]

Clinical Features	Reported
External ear inflammation	70%
Arthritis	36%
Nasal inflammation	26%
Eye inflammation	20%
Skin (vasculitis)	12%
Major airway disease	12%

and results in a misshapen pinna. The pinna can be thickened due to fibrosis and even ossify sometimes, resulting in a cauliflower or boxer's ear. Nasal cartilage involvement may start with inflammation of the nasal bridge of the nose. Further destruction of the cartilaginous septum results in nasal bridge collapse and saddle nose deformity. Larnygotracheal involvement is seen in 50% of patients with RP and is associated with a poor prognosis.[9] Laryngeal involvement causes collapse of the laryngeal cartilage, resulting in stenosis. This can present as dysphonia and result in aphonia, with patients requiring a tracheostomy for an adequate airway.

Respiratory Manifestations

Tracheobronchial involvement is the most severe manifestation of RP. It is uncommon at presentation but occurs in nearly half of patients during the course of the disease. Symptoms include dyspnea, cough, wheeze, stridor, and dysphonia. Pulmonary involvement is associated with poorer prognosis. In a small series of five patients with RP and airway involvement, two patients died despite airway stent insertion and ventilatory support.[23] Due to the steroid response, patients can be misdiagnosed with asthma or chronic obstructive pulmonary disease (COPD).[24] An important differential is also tracheobronchomalacia and excessive dynamic airway collapse (EDAC), which also cause large airway collapse. Tracheobronchomalacia is due to weakness in the cartilage of the airway causing collapse. It can be congenital and is associated with prematurity and associated with laryngeal clefts and tracheo-esophageal fistula. EDAC is defined as airway collapse and stenosis of more than 50%. However, the cartilage is intact and the stenosis is due to laxity of the posterior wall of the trachea. EDAC can be seen in COPD and asthma.[25]

CT imaging of the chest can aid the diagnosis demonstrating smooth and lateral tracheal wall thickening with sparing of the posterior wall highly suggestive of RP.[26] Other features on the CT scan include luminal narrowing and calcification of the tracheal rings. Expiratory phase scans can show the dynamic collapse of the airway. Magnetic resonance imaging (MRI) and positron emission tomography (PET) have also been used to assess airway and cartilaginous involvement.[27,28]

Bronchoscopy can also be used to exclude other differential diagnoses and demonstrate dynamic collapse of the airway. However, bronchoscopy should be performed with caution due to risks of respiratory obstruction and causing further respiratory distress.

Prognosis

Prognosis of RP is varied due to the unpredictable nature of the disease. In a Hungarian epidemiological study of 256 patients, there was a 10-year survival of approximately 80%.[2] However, other studies have found a much lower survival, with Michet et al describing a 55% survival at 10 years after diagnosis.[11] In a UK population base cohort study of 106 patients, the standardized mortality ratio was 2.16 (95% CI: 1.24, 3.51), $p < 0.01$.[28] Where there is cardiac, aorta, or laryngotracheal involvement, the condition can be fatal. RP can also be life threatening due to associated malignancy, vasculitis, and infection risk related to immunosuppressants.[20]

Management

The management of patients with RP is a multidisciplinary approach due to the number of different systems that can be affected. Treatments are available for managing disease control as well as symptom relief. The treatment of RP depends on the extent and the severity of the disease process. In mild cases, nonsteroidal anti-inflammatory drugs (NSAIDs) and oral corticosteroids are used to control symptoms. In more severe cases, high dose corticosteroids and different immunosuppressive medication have been used. Second-line medications include methotrexate, azathioprine, cyclophosphamide, cyclosporine, sulfasalazine, and monoclonal antibodies such as infliximab. There are only small series in the published literature on these different treatments, and the evidence is unclear about the optimum regime.[29-31]

A UK cohort study by Hazra et al[20] looked at the treatment of 117 patients with RP between 1990 and 2012. The most frequently used drugs after diagnosis were glucocorticoids (64%) and NSAIDs (45%) (Table 47–3). Biologic agents such as infliximab had not been introduced yet into routine clinical practice and were not used in this cohort.

Numerous surgical procedures may be required depending on the system involved—for example, surgery for aneurysms, aortic valve replacements, ocular complications, and laryngotracheal surgery to maintain an adequate airway. Tracheobronchial stenting, tracheostomy, and ventilatory support are all used for airway stenosis. Tracheostomy tubes are required if there is laryngeal stenosis but also provide some stenting to the distal trachea. Tracheostomy tubes can

also be fitted to ventilatory support and suctioning to keep an airway patent. The authors prefer the use of Montgomery T-tube (Boston Medical Products) for RP patients (Figures 47–5 and 47–6). T-tubes are made of a soft silicone material that can have a customized length to the upper and lower limbs. T-tubes are similar to tracheostomy tubes but have an upper limb which can stent the subglottis and a lower limb to stent the distal trachea. T-tubes have their own risks compared with tracheostomy tubes, as they do not have an

Table 47–3. Medications Used in the Treatment of RP in a UK Cohort[20]

Drug Class	1 Year Before Diagnosis (%)	Once Diagnosed (%)
NSAID	34	45
Glucocorticoids	39	64
Methotrexate	9	24
Azathioprine	2	13
Hydroxychloroquine	8	8
Dapsone	2	6
Colchicine	2	4
Sulfasalazine	2	0

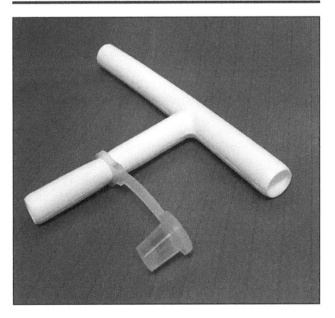

Figure 47–5. Montgomery® T-tube with cap.

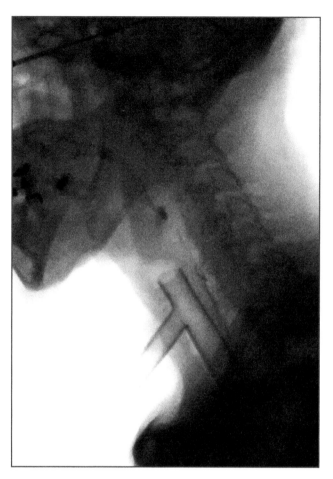

Figure 47–6. T-tube in situ demonstrated on lateral neck x-ray.

inner tube. Thus, the patient and medical staff need to be trained on how to care for them and keep them patent. Patients often prefer them to tracheostomy tubes as they do not require neck tapes, there is no flange, and patients can keep it capped off when talking. They normally require a general anesthetic to change them every 6 to 12 months.

There are published reports in the literature of tracheobronchial stents being used to keep the airway patent in RP. There are different indwelling airway stents used, including: silicone stents,[32] self-expandable metallic stents (SEMS),[33] and Y-shape stents. The authors occasionally use stents, in the short term, to open a stenosed airway segment and allow future placement of tracheostomy and T-tubes. However, stents have their own complications, including infection, granulation, erosion, migration, and bronchial tears.[34] Laryngotracheal reconstruction has also been reported for treating

laryngeal stenosis using a hyoid bone pedicled on sternohyoid muscle to expand the larynx.[35]

SUMMARY

RP is a rare condition that causes inflammation of cartilaginous structures throughout the body. It has a variable course and can affect many different symptoms. Corticosteroids are the first-line treatment option; however, individual management plans are required due to the variability of involved systems and disease severity. Pulmonary involvement is associated with a poor prognosis and mortality. Laryngotracheal involvement provides specific challenges that require a multidisciplinary approach. Surgical interventions including tracheostomy, T-tube, and stent insertion are necessary in severe cases to prevent airway collapse.

REFERENCES

1. Ludvigsson J, van Vollenhoven R. Prevalence and comorbidity of relapsing polychondritis. *Clin Epidemiol*. 2016; 8:361–362.
2. Horváth A, et al. A nationwide study of the epidemiology of relapsing polychondritis. *Clin Epidemiol*. 2016; 8:211–230.
3. Kent P, Michet C, Luthra H. Relapsing polychondritis. *Curr Opin Rheumatol*. 2004;16(1):56–61.
4. R J-W, Polychondropathia. *Wien Arch F Inn Med*. 1923; 6:93–100.
5. Pearson C, Kline H, Newcomer V. Relapsing polychondritis. *N Engl J Med*. 1960;263:51–58.
6. Foidart JM, et al. Antibodies to type II collagen in relapsing polychondritis. *N Engl J Med*. 1978;299(22):1203–1207.
7. Arnaud L, et al. Pathogenesis of relapsing polychondritis: a 2013 update. *Autoimmun Rev*. 2014;13(2):90–95.
8. Trentham D, Le C. Relapsing polychondritis. *Ann Intern Med*. 1998;129(2):114–122.
9. McAdam LP, et al. Relapsing polychondritis: prospective study of 23 patients and a review of the literature. *Medicine (Baltimore)*. 1976;55(3):193–215.
10. Damiani J, Levine H. Relapsing polychondritis—report of ten cases. *Laryngoscope*. 1979;89(6 pt 1):929–946.
11. Michet CJ, et al. Relapsing polychondritis. Survival and predictive role of early disease manifestations. *Ann Intern Med*. 1986;104(1):74–78.
12. Chuah T, Lui N. Relapsing polychondritis in Singapore: a case series and review of literature. *Singapore Med J*. 2017;58(4):201–205.

13. Francès C, et al. Dermatologic manifestations of relapsing polychondritis. A study of 200 cases at a single center. *Medicine (Baltimore).* 2001;80(3):173–179.

14. Yoo J, Chodosh J, Dana R. Relapsing polychondritis: systemic and ocular manifestations, differential diagnosis, management, and prognosis. *Semin Ophthalmol.* 2011;26 (4–5):261–269.

15. Chang-Miller A, et al. Renal involvement in relapsing polychondritis. *Medicine (Baltimore).* 1987;66(3):202–217.

16. Lin DF, et al. Clinical and prognostic characteristics of 158 cases of relapsing polychondritis in China and review of the literature. *Rheumatol Int.* 2016;36(7):1003–1009.

17. Myers B, Gould J, Dolan G. Relapsing polychondritis and myelodysplasia: a report of two cases and review of the current literature. *Clin Lab Haematol.* 2000;22(1):45–48.

18. Hebbar M, et al. Association of myelodysplastic syndrome and relapsing polychondritis: further evidence. *Leukemia.* 1995;9(4):731–733.

19. Heo SW, et al. A case of relapsing polychondritis associated with myelodysplastic syndrome with erythroid hypoplasia/aplasia. *Korean J Intern Med.* 2003;18(4):251–254.

20. Hazra N, et al. Incidence and mortality of relapsing polychondritis in the UK: a population-based cohort study. *Rheumatology (Oxford).* 2015;54(12):2181–2187.

21. Bachor E, et al. Otologic manifestations of relapsing polychondritis. Review of literature and report of nine cases. *Auris Nasus Larynx.* 2006;33(2):135–141.

22. Puéchal X, et al. Relapsing polychondritis. *Joint Bone Spine.* 2014;81(2):118–124.

23. Sarodia B, Dasgupta A, Mehta A. Management of airway manifestations of relapsing polychondritis: case reports and review of literature. *Chest.* 1999;116(6):1669–1675.

24. Gorard C, Kadri S. Critical airway involvement in relapsing polychondritis. *BMJ Case Rep.* 2014.

25. Buitrago DH, et al. Current concepts in severe adult tracheobronchomalacia: evaluation and treatment. *J Thorac Dis.* 2017;9(1):E57–E66.

26. Lee KS, et al. Relapsing polychondritis: prevalence of expiratory CT airway abnormalities. *Radiology.* 2006; 240(2):565–573.

27. Oddone M, et al. Relapsing polychondritis in childhood: a rare observation studied by CT and MRI. *Pediatr Radiol.* 1992;22(7):537–538.

28. Lei W, et al. (18)F-FDG PET-CT: a powerful tool for the diagnosis and treatment of relapsing polychondritis. *Br J Radiol.* 2016;89(1057):20150695.

29. Longo L, et al. Relapsing polychondritis: a clinical update. *Autoimmun Rev.* 2016;15(6):539–543.

30. Park J, Gowin K, Schumacher H. Steroid sparing effect of methotrexate in relapsing polychondritis. *J Rheumatol.* 1996;23(5):937–938.

31. Mathian A, et al. Relapsing polychondritis: A 2016 update on clinical features, diagnostic tools, treatment and biological drug use. *Best Pract Res Clin Rheumatol.* 2016;30(2):316–333.

32. Sacco O, et al. Severe endobronchial obstruction in a girl with relapsing polychondritis: treatment with Nd: YAG laser and endobronchial silicon stent. *Eur Respir J.* 1997;10(2):494–496.

33. Nobukiyo S, et al. A case of relapsing polychondritis involving placement of an expandable metallic stent. *Auris Nasus Larynx.* 2003;30(suppl):S141–S144.

34. Chapron J, et al. Bronchial rupture related to endobronchial stenting in relapsing polychondritis. *Eur Respir Rev.* 2012;21(126):367–369.

35. Xie C, et al. Laryngotracheal reconstruction for relapsing polychondritis: case report and review of the literature. *J Laryngol Otol.* 2013;127(9):932–935.

SECTION IV
DYSPHAGIA/SWALLOWING

CHAPTER 48

Impaired Laryngeal Response to Cough Reflex Testing

Maggie-Lee Huckabee, Phoebe Macrae, and Emma Wallace

Dysphagia is a common outcome of a number of acute and chronic conditions. Prevalence in stroke is estimated to be 78%,[1] in Parkinson's disease at 81%[2] and head and neck cancer at 50%,[3] to name a few. With malnutrition, dehydration, and pneumonia as consequences, the accurate diagnosis of swallowing impairment—and appropriate management—is necessary to reduce consequent patient morbidities and mortalities, as well as health care costs. Fundamental obstacles in the clinical assessment of swallowing arise from the paucity of observable clinical behaviors to suggest impairment and the impact of sensory impairment on these behaviors. Although thyroid movement can be palpated during swallowing, adequacy of movement as it impacts epiglottic deflection and upper esophageal sphincter (UES) opening cannot be judged. Patient reactions to pathophysiology, such as coughing, throat clearing, and struggling behavior, are unlikely to occur in the presence of peripheral or central sensory deficits. Thus, it becomes unclear on clinical assessment if the patient has no swallow impairment or if evidence of underlying impairment is masked by sensory inhibition (so-called silent aspiration).[4] In response, cough reflex testing is gaining traction in clinical swallowing assessment with the primary aim of detecting integrity of vagal nerve sensory fibers and consequent risk of silent aspiration.[5]

A patient with a small focal brainstem lesion exemplifies the complexity of clinical dysphagia diagnosis. With critical motor and sensory nuclei and their central and peripheral connections confined to a structural region less than one inch in diameter,[6] a small focal lesion can produce broadly differing presentations. As highlighted in the case report below, differential diagnosis when cough response is absent on initial clinical swallowing assessment requires instrumental assessment to clarify physiology and contribute to the diagnostic picture.

DEFINITIONS

Three key terms are particularly relevant to this case.

- Aspiration: entry of food or liquid into the airway below the level of the vocal cords
- Silent aspiration: aspiration without a cough or clearance response
- Cough reflex testing: stimulation of cough receptors via inhaled tussigenic agents. Used to provide information about integrity of laryngeal sensory processing for cough.

Specific to cough reflex testing, methodological variations exist in the literature, including tussive agents, methods of delivery, and test endpoint.

- The tussive agents can be categorized as acid vs non-acid. Commonly used acid agents include citric acid and tartaric acid, with the most commonly used non-acid tussive being capsaicin.[7]
- Methods of tussive agent delivery include single-dose, or dose response.[8] Single dose

methods are used to establish presence or absence of a cough response at a given concentration. Dose-response methods aim to determine thresholds by testing cough response at incremental concentrations.[7] The tussive agent may be delivered in a single breath inhalation, or tidal breathing over a fixed time.[8] Methods of citric acid cough reflex testing are summarized below (Figure 48–1).

- The cough reflex test endpoint also differs according to protocol.[8] Commonly used outcome measures are cough frequency, or the presence or absence of C2 and/or C5 response. C2 and C5 responses are defined as the concentration that elicits at least 2 or 5 coughs, respectively.[9]

In the case discussion below, the method of cough reflex testing is derived from a method previously described in clinical studies of cough sensitivity after stroke.[10] It utilizes a single dose of citric acid (0.6 mol/L) delivered over 15 s and requires a C2 response for two out of three trials.

CASE PRESENTATION

A 58-year-old male was admitted to the emergency department with reports of nausea, vomiting, lethargy, and vertigo. Mild left sided weakness of the upper extremity was detected on examination. Blood pressure on admission was elevated. CT scan was clear for acute lesion. On cranial nerve examination, the patient presented very slight dysphonia with weak vocal quality, and lateralizing features of mild left-sided impairment to cranial nerve (CN) XII. MRI was consequently completed which identified no clear lesion; however, small lesions—even those with clinical manifestations—may not be always seen on MRI. MR angiogram, however, revealed narrowing of right vertebral artery. He was provided a diagnosis of small medullary infarct based on clinical presentation. As per common stroke admission protocols, he was screened by nursing staff for swallowing impairment.[11] With presentation of mild dysphonia during speech, and with questionable wet dysphonia following oral intake, he was subsequently referred to speech-language pathology for formal swallowing assessment.

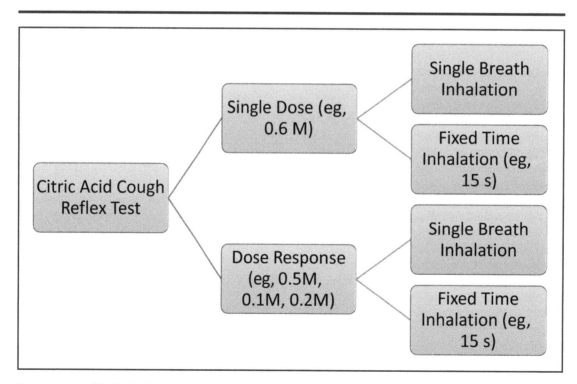

Figure 48–1. Methods of citric acid cough reflex testing.

Initial Assessment

The patient received formal swallowing assessment on the second day of admission, consisting of cognitive/communication screening, dysphagia specific history, and CN examination, cough reflex testing, and observation of oral intake. The patient was alert and engaged and able to answer questions, follow commands, and provide his own apparently reliable history. Clinical presentation on CN examination was without evidence of significant motor impairment for CN 5, 7, 9, and 10, with the exception of mild dysphonia during connected speech. This was imperceptible to most, although recognized by the patient and his partner; improvement was observed with increased phonatory effort. This was also true for lateralization and strength of tongue movement, which was mildly impaired on initial examination, suggesting potential involvement of CN XII. Sensory integrity was questioned by the patient's report of taste changes, raising concern primarily for CN VII sensory. He commented that meals since his stroke have been less flavorsome. Gag response was absent on direct assessment; relevance of this finding is not convincing given variability in this response in healthy individuals.[12] More notably, the patient presented no cough to inhalation of nebulized citric acid at 0.6 mol/L when presented via facemask at a restricted flow rate of 6.6 L/min.[13] Volitional cough was judged to be audibly strong but non-productive.

In the presence of marginal CN findings, despite the absence of cough on cough reflex testing, the decision was made to proceed with oral trials as a component of the clinical examination. Liquids were ingested with no apparent struggling behaviors for controlled sips. Rapid ingestion appeared to be executed efficiently. Mild wet dysphonia was observed on 3/6 trials, which was not spontaneously cleared but, when cued, was cleared sufficiently to baseline. No cough response was produced. The patient reported being nervous about ingesting solids and semi-solids and behaviorally was cautious. Oral bolus manipulation of solids was generally prompt and efficient, with only slight lateral lingual residual post intake. Occasionally, solid bolus intake resulted in multiple swallows to subjectively clear.

Given the etiology of brainstem stroke with its likelihood for producing significant dysphagia,[14] subtle signs of dysphagia on oral ingestion and evidence of suspected sensory deficits, particularly an absence of reflexive cough, instrumental assessment of swallowing was considered appropriate. The presence of sensory deficits in particular would render clinical assessment of swallowing unreliable for ruling out significant pharyngeal phase dysphagia and silent aspiration.

The two most frequently conducted imaging techniques for diagnosing swallowing impairment are videofluoroscopy and videoendoscopy. There are specific strengths and weaknesses to both and selection of the approach will depend on the general physical health and stability of the patient, the suspected pathophysiologic features inferred from clinical observation, and the very specific goals of the examination process.

A videoendoscopic swallowing study (VESS) has the benefits of direct visualization of the pharynx and larynx for assessment of superficial structural integrity. It is superior to videofluoroscopy for identifying specific laryngeal physiology, and may provide more direct evaluation of laryngeal sensitivity through touch or by observation of subtle responses that do not produce audible indicators. Critically, in acute settings, VESS can be executed at bedside, allowing glottal assessment in acutely unwell patients or those with medical needs that prohibit transfer to a radiology suite. This assessment, however, is less informative for understanding pharyngeal biomechanics, such as hyoid excursion, and the integration of oral and pharyngeal kinematics.

Conversely, videofluoroscopic swallowing study (VFSS) provides a more holistic representation of swallowing and bolus flow from the oral cavity into the esophagus. Dynamics and timing of pharyngeal motility are clear; however, laryngeal mechanics are not clearly visualized. Importantly, intrinsic pharyngeal structures and movement patterns are clearly observed. For pharyngeal dysphagia, this information may play a critical role in devising physiologically specific rehabilitation approaches. VFSS offers less flexibility—this is a key point when patients are unstable and/or unable to transfer off the ward, or radiology resources are in high demand. VFSS also imposes radiation exposure,[15] which although relatively small, should nonetheless be considered.

Although patients with brainstem infarct are known to have significant pharyngeal pathophysiology that typically requires concentrated rehabilitation, the presence of dysphonia, albeit mild, and concerns for laryngeal sensation justify VESS as an initial assessment. The following scenarios describe divergent differential diagnoses based on initial and then subsequent instrumental assessment, highlighting the potential strengths and weaknesses of cough reflex testing in dysphagia service delivery.

SCENARIO 1: IMPAIRED SENSATION AND IMPAIRED MOTOR FUNCTION: WALLENBERG'S SYNDROME (LATERAL MEDULLARY INFARCT)

Investigation

Endoscopic evaluation revealed asymmetric palatal elevation on phonation with apparent mild left sided weakness. In the pharyngeal region, there was no significant pooling of secretions. On visualization of the larynx, there was slight asymmetry in laryngeal adduction for phonation and cough, which is improved with effort and Valsalva maneuver. For liquid boluses, pre-swallow pooling was observed to the aryepiglottic regions with supraglottic penetration, presumably due to reduced glossopalatal approximation; upon volitional bolus transfer, there was a further delay in swallowing onset, with bolus inconsistently reaching pyriform sinuses and trace interarytenoid penetration with no cough or clearing response. With onset of swallowing, the initiation of arytenoid adduction was observed prior to "white-out" associated with pharyngeal closure on the endoscope. Post-swallowing, there was moderate, diffuse pharyngeal residue, somewhat more predominant in the pyriform sinuses and on heavier bolus textures. As seen on clinical examination, there were multiple swallows observed on textured boluses, which did not fully clear residual. Aspiration of liquids was observed immediately on visualization of the larynx; further aspiration occurred post-swallow from the pyriforms on one bolus. No cough response was elicited. Using the tip of the endoscope to touch the lateral pharyngeal walls, aryepiglottic folds, and ventricular folds, the patient denied perception of touch, although a partial laryngeal adductor response was observed.

Based on initial endoscopic assessment, pharyngeal residual and aspiration are clearly observed. The underlying biomechanics that allow for post-swallow aspiration of residual cannot be determined. Therefore, further evaluation of pharyngeal physiology with VFSS and high-resolution manometry (HRM) was recommended for rehabilitation planning.

In brief, VFSS revealed functional velopharyngeal closure and upper pharyngeal pressure to inhibit nasal redirection. Glossopalatal approximation was inconsistent, allowing for pre-swallow pooling with delayed swallowing on liquids and pre-swallow intermittent silent aspiration, as was observed on endoscopy. Ante-rior hyoid movement (consistent with intact trigeminal motor input) appeared substantial to facilitate adequate epiglottic deflection, but there also appeared to be specific resistance to bolus flow through the upper esophageal sphincter consistent with impairment of vagal nerve motor fibers. Although cricopharyngeal prominence was not observed, UES closure occurred prior to full transfer of the bolus into the esophagus with consequent pyriform > vallecular residual. This was aspirated intermittently post-swallow, again with no cough. To clarify if pharyngeal residual was entirely an issue of UES premature closure or if this was paired with poor pharyngeal pressure generation, HRM was completed. This assessment revealed pharyngeal pressure generation in the hypopharynx to be at the low end of normal range. UES nadir pressure and duration of UES opening were both outside the 95% confidence interval.[16]

Diagnosis

Significant pharyngeal phase dysphagia with delayed onset of swallowing, allowing for pre-swallow aspiration, paired with decreased duration of UES opening and consequent post-swallow aspiration of pyriform residual. No protective airway responses were observed. Consistent with Wallenberg lateral medullary stroke presentation.

Management

1. Remain nil by mouth (NBM) with nutritional support via nasogastric (NG) or percutaneous endoscopic gastrostomy (PEG) tube. Aspiration is persistent and produces no protective response, thus the safest course of action is to withhold oral trials until cough returns or physiology improves to the extent that aspiration is not present.
2. Oral trials of a cold, sour, or carbonated bolus may be therapeutically trialled with instructions for volitional cough after each trial to clear any airway invasion. This sensory stimulation may facilitate increased sensory response in the pharynx, although clear efficacy data for this approach are lacking.[17,18] This should be done within the constraints of therapeutic feeding and only following execution of

oral hygiene to decrease potential for oral bacterial aspiration, which is known to increase pneumonia risk.[19]

3. There are numerous options for therapeutic resolution of UES noncompliance or premature closure. In the acute phase when potential for spontaneous recovery is not yet determined, medical (injection of botulinum toxin into cricopharyngeus muscle) or surgical approaches (cricopharyngeal dilatation, cricopharyngeal myotomy) are not recommended. Behavioral rehabilitation approaches such as execution of Mendelsohn maneuver[20] with prophylactic floor of mouth muscle strengthening exercises[21] are considered more appropriate. Additionally, gaining increased conscious control over UES opening extent and duration using HRM as a biofeedback modality may prove beneficial. Recent research is advocating for the use of skill-based rehabilitation approaches for pharyngeal phase impairment,[22] which may apply to targeted aspects of pharyngeal swallowing such as modulation of the duration and extent of UES opening.

SCENARIO 2: IMPAIRED SENSATION AND NORMAL MOTOR FUNCTION—ACUTE COUGH SUPPRESSION VERSUS DEJERINE'S SYNDROME (MEDIAL MEDULLARY INFARCT)

Investigation

Initial instrumental assessment with VESS. Endoscopic evaluation revealed symmetric palatal elevation on phonation. Pre-swallow pooling to the pyriform sinuses was observed, although the patient was able to hold the bolus orally on command. This suggests an intact capacity for motor sufficiency in glossopalatal approximation, but with an apparent sensory deficit and resulting delay in swallowing onset. With onset of swallowing, the initiation of arytenoid adduction was observed prior to "white-out" associated with pharyngeal closure on the endoscope. Post-swallowing, there was diffuse mild coating throughout the pharynx, somewhat more predominant on heavier textures. As seen on clinical examination, there were multiple swallows observed on textured boluses, which fully cleared residual. No penetration or aspiration was observed on any texture. Using the tip of the endoscope to touch the lateral pharyngeal walls, aryepiglottic folds, and ventricular folds, the patient denied perception of touch, although a partial laryngeal adductor response was observed.

Diagnosis

The presence of isolated sensory impairment with no significant associated motor impairment suggests one of two potential etiologies. Post-acute cough suppression[23] may be seen in the presence of normal or subclinical motor impairment and represents a compensatory protective response to an acute neurological event. Disturbances in reticular formation often co-occur with post-acute cough suppression,[23] which may explain the patient's lethargy. An alternative etiology is Dejerine's syndrome, the clinical picture arising from a medial medullary stroke. Laryngeal sensory deficits and silent aspiration have been linked with Dejerine's syndrome, with 71% of patients with medial medullary infarction (MMI) showing signs of silent aspiration.[24] Vertigo, contralateral hemiparesis with sensory impairment, and ipsilateral tongue weakness may be additional signs of Dejerine's syndrome.[25]

Irrespective of etiology, pharyngeal coating, reduced pharyngeal sensation, and absent cough, with few indicators of motor pathway involvement, suggest primary deficits of sensation.

Management

1. Initiate oral trials as tolerated, restricted only by patients' comfort level and confidence.
2. No restriction of liquids.
3. Multiple volitional swallows per bolus on heavier textures to clear pharyngeal residue.
4. As a general precaution in the presence of reduced laryngeal sensitivity, the patient was advised to implement rigorous oral hygiene practice and maintain mobility after meals to decrease risk of chest infection in the event of intermittent, incidental aspiration. The patient was advised to produce a forceful cough if vocal quality appeared "wet" post-swallowing.
5. Speech and language pathology follow-up was suggested to evaluate for return of cough prior to discharge. Duration of inhibited cough due to acute cough suppression should resolve promptly.

Investigation

Initial instrumental assessment with VESS. Endoscopic evaluation revealed symmetric palatal elevation on phonation. The bolus remained in the oral cavity with glossopalatal approximation prior to swallowing, and no apparent delay in swallowing onset. With onset of swallowing, the initiation of arytenoid adduction was observed prior to "white-out" associated with pharyngeal closure on the endoscope. Post-swallowing, there was trace coating throughout the pharynx on textured boluses that was not clinically significant. Additional swallows fully cleared this coating. No supraglottic penetration or aspiration was observed on any texture. Using the tip of the endoscope to touch the lateral pharyngeal walls, aryepiglottic folds, and ventricular folds, the patient confirmed perception of touch, and a complete laryngeal adductor response was observed.

Diagnosis

Patient presents with intact pharyngolaryngeal sensation and normal swallowing physiology. Cough reflex test (CRT) did not accurately identify sensory deficits.

Management

1. No restriction of foods.
2. No restriction of liquids.
3. Discharge from speech-language pathology, no further follow-up required.

DIFFERENTIAL DIAGNOSIS

Structural Laryngeal Anatomy, Receptor Sites, Types of Receptors

The vagus nerve (CN X) innervates sensory receptors throughout the pharyngolaryngeal mucosa. Pharyngolaryngeal sensory receptors are multi-modal, meaning they respond to a range of stimuli including tactile, wa-ter and acid,[26] to elicit a hierarchy of airway protective responses.

The internal branch of the superior laryngeal nerve (ibSLN) innervates the mucosa of the laryngeal vestibule and pyriform recesses and plays an important role in eliciting the laryngeal cough reflex at a supraglottic level.[27,28] Interestingly, sensory fibers from the SLN can bypass the nucleus tractus solitarius (NTS) and travel directly to the nucleus ambiguus (NA) to modify motor output during swallowing,[29] allowing for rapid elicitation of the laryngeal cough reflex in the event of airway invasion. The inferior laryngeal nerve, the terminal branch of the recurrent laryngeal nerve, supplies sensory innervation to the lower part of the larynx, and may play a role in eliciting the cough reflex subglottically. The pharyngeal branch of the vagus nerve, together with branches of the glossopharyngeal nerve, form the pharyngeal plexus, and provide sensory innervation to the mucous membrane of the pharynx, the base of tongue, and upper surface of the epiglottis.

Sensory nuclei of the vagus and glossopharyngeal nerves lie in the NTS in the lateral medulla, thus, any lesion, albeit small, can impair sensation in the pharyngeal and laryngeal mucosa. Given the position of the NTS, it's likely that a lateral medullary lesion (Wallenberg's syndrome), may result in profound sensory loss to the pharynx and larynx, in addition to impaired motor function, carried by efferent nerves originating in the NA, as seen in scenario 1. A medial medullary lesion is likely to compromise the pyramidal tracts, medial lemniscus, and hypoglossal nerve nucleus,[25] resulting in limb and proprioceptive impairments and lingual weakness. However, given the crowded landscape of the medulla, lesions in the medial medulla may comprise interconnecting reticular fibers between NTS and NA and explaining, in part, a relatively high presentation of silent aspiration associated with this type of lesion.

Functional (Table 48–1)

Management Need for Careful Evaluation

Careful evaluation of patients presenting with absent cough reflex is necessary in order to inform appropriate management decisions. Of importance, clinical evaluation alone is inadequate for identifying pharyngo-

Table 48–1. Potential Clinical Scenarios Resulting from Absent CRT Response Following Small Focal Brainstem Infarct

Scenario 1	Scenario 2	Scenario 3
Wallenberg's syndrome (lateral medullary infarct)	Dejerine's syndrome (medial medullary infarct) vs. Global Suppression	CRT missed the mark
Neurogenic Motor ✗	Neurogenic Motor ✗/✓	Neurogenic Motor ✓
Asymmetry in soft palate Asymmetry in laryngeal adduction for phonation and cough Reduced gloss-palatal approximation (pre-swallow pooling) Reduced pressure in hypopharynx Duration of UES opening reduced	May present clinically significant motor impairments observed on instrumental assessment.	No clinically significant motor impairments observed on instrumental assessment.
Neurogenic Sensory ✗	Neurogenic Sensory ✗/✓	Neurogenic Sensory ✓
Delay in swallowing initiation Silent penetration and aspiration Absent perception of touch to lateral pharyngeal walls, aryepiglottic folds, and ventricular folds	Absent perception of touch to lateral pharyngeal walls, aryepiglottic folds and ventricular folds.	No clinically significant sensory impairments observed on instrumental assessment.

laryngeal sensorimotor impairments and informing treatment planning for this patient population.

The consequences of oropharyngeal and UES motor impairments, such as premature spillage and diffuse pharyngeal residual—as seen only on instrumental assessment—is concerning for patients with impaired sensation and absent cough reflex. Such patients are vulnerable to penetration and aspiration and require adequate airway protective mechanisms. An absent cough reflex, in the presence of impaired swallowing biomechanics, requires conservative management, particularly in the acute phase. Such patients are candidates for non-oral feeding, such as NG and PEG tubes, to maintain adequate nutrition and hydration while swallowing rehabilitation is under way.

Management of patients with impaired sensation and intact swallowing biomechanics will differ, as such patients pose less risk of persistent aspiration and penetration, thus are less reliant on their cough reflex. Management involving patient education (eg, oral hygiene practices) and minimizing risks in the event of incidental silent aspiration (eg, mobility post oral intake, volitional coughing if voice is "wet") is advised.

Of importance, differential diagnosis of the above patient group requires instrumental assessment to affirm the diagnostic picture and ensure appropriate

management. Few empirically determined treatments for pharyngolaryngeal sensory deficits exist in the dysphagia literature, which challenges management of patients with impaired pharyngolaryngeal sensation. However, some studies have shown promising evidence for rehabilitation of pharyngolaryngeal sensation in the neurodegenerative patient population.[30,31]

PITFALLS

Cough reflex testing has been used in respiratory medicine for more than 50 years but is relatively new in assessment of patients with dysphagia. Protocols of the "best" method of citric acid cough reflex testing in the dysphagic population continue to be developed. The current clinical method has advantages for patients with cognitive deficits who struggle to follow directions or patients who cannot form an adequate lip seal over a mouthpiece. In addition, the use of a suppressed cough method is more likely to represent a patient's true cough reflex, and avoid the influence of suggestion.

Limitations of the current method of cough reflex testing exist in the percentage of healthy individuals who do not respond to 0.6 M citric acid. Monroe, Manco,

Bennett, and Huckabee found that 21.9% of healthy individuals could suppress a cough response across a range of 0.1–2.6 mol/L citric acid.[32] Such individuals may—or may not—display additional airway protective mechanisms (eg, throat clear, voicing, swallowing, laryngeal adduction) when asked to suppress their cough. While this constitutes a failed response on CRT, it suggests intact or semi-intact laryngeal sensation and should be noted on testing. In addition, judgment of reflexive cough strength remains challenging. It's likely that individuals will attenuate their cough response when asked to suppress, giving the false impression of a weak cough response. For this reason, judgment of cough strength should be interpreted with caution for the suppressed cough protocol. While CRT adds valuable information to the clinical picture, it should not be the sole determinant of the integrity of pharyngolaryngeal sensation.

DISCUSSION

The clinical case above highlights the complexity of differential diagnosis for patients with medullary infarction who present with absent cough reflex on CRT. Depending on the size and location of the infarct, neurogenic sensory deficits can occur in the presence or absence of neurogenic motor deficits, as seen in scenarios 1 and 2, respectively. Such deficits are not apparent on clinical evaluation and require instrumental assessment to elucidate the diagnostic picture. The three possible scenarios and outcomes are discussed in detail below.

Impaired Sensory and Motor Function Following Medullary Infarct (Wallenberg's Syndrome)

Patients with pharyngolaryngeal sensory and motor deficits (scenario 1) are perhaps the most vulnerable patient group. Wallenberg's syndrome is the clinical picture resulting from a lateral medullary infarct. Dysphagia, resulting from diminished pharyngeal reflexes, facial sensory impairments, dysarthria, lingual palsy, and UES impairments are widely reported in patients with Wallenberg's syndrome.[33,34] While cough reflex testing is not reported in previous studies of patients with Wallenberg's syndrome, Kwon et al note that 31%

of patients present with silent aspiration, suggesting impaired pharyngolaryngeal sensation, in the presence of aforementioned oropharyngeal motor deficits.[24] Importantly, many of the signs of dysphagia associated with Wallenberg's syndrome are not apparent on clinical evaluation (ie, pharyngeal sensory deficits, silent aspiration, and UES impairment), highlighting the importance of instrumental assessment. The prevalence of dysphagia is grossly underrepresented in this patient population, as few studies use instrumental assessment to confirm the diagnostic picture, relying solely on clinical signs and patient reported symptoms.

Given the crowded landscape of the medulla, even small, focal lateral medullary infarcts may result in severe dysphagia.[35] Furthermore, vital swallowing nuclei, the NTS and the NA, are located in the lateral medulla and are likely to be involved in lateral medullary infarct. A negative MRI should not rule out Wallenberg's syndrome in the presence of clinical signs of dysphagia.

Studies have shown that long term prognosis of patients with Wallenberg's syndrome is good. However, presence of dysphagia and aspiration pneumonia are significantly more prevalent in patients with poorer prognoses.[36] Specifically, presence of dysphagia on initial assessment was independently associated with poorer outcomes at 1 year.[36] Given the presence of sensory and motor swallowing deficits, conservative management of Wallenberg's syndrome is initially required. Dysphagia is often severe enough to require non-oral feeding in the acute phase with spontaneous recovery and return to oral feeding expected within 1 to 2 months post stroke.[37,38]

Impaired Sensory and Intact Motor Function

Laryngeal sensory deficits may occur in the presence of subclinical motor deficits, as seen in scenario 2. Dejerine's syndrome is the clinical picture resulting from medial medullary infarct (MMI). It is a relatively uncommon stroke syndrome. Given the involvement of the lemniscus and pyramidal pathway and hypoglossal nerve nuclei with an MMI, absent cough and pharyngolaryngeal sensory or motor deficits are unexpected in this patient cohort. However, Kwon et al identified silent aspiration in 71% of patients with Dejerine's syndrome using instrumental assessment.[24] While the precise neurological deficits of this clinical presentation are unclear, lesions of the surrounding reticular formation that interconnects the NTS and NA may explain the presence of silent aspiration in Dejerine's syndrome,[24] rather than specific involvement of the NTS and NA.

Consideration of the intricate relationship between sensory and motor function must be given in scenario 2. Oropharyngolaryngeal sensory and motor function are not mutually exclusive, and sensory input directly influences motor output. While the patient presents with subclinical motor impairments, it's likely that a loss of sensation in the pharynx and larynx will have a direct influence on swallowing biomechanics. Reduced sensation in the pharyngolaryngeal area may result in pre-swallow pooling or delayed initiation of arytenoid adduction, particularly in the presence of additional stress, such as reduced attention or fatigue. Inability to detect bolus position may result in delay in initiation of protective airway reflexes and in reflexive swallow patterns, despite intact motor pathways. Additionally, sensory feedback systems are necessary for modulating motor output, thus subtle biomechanical changes are feasible in the presence of intact motor substrates.

As an alternative etiology to isolated laryngeal deficits, post stroke "brainstem shock" is described by Addington et al and may be apparent following medullary stroke.[23] Reticular or respiratory drive disturbances are often seen alongside absent cough reflex. While the neurological nature of such impairments can be challenging to determine, regardless of etiology, management of both conditions is somewhat similar. It's possible that patients with "brainstem shock" may also exhibit respiratory-swallowing timing difficulties due to deficits in respiratory drive that may not be apparent with Dejerine's syndrome.

CRT Predicted Sensory Deficits Inaccurately

Scenario 3 highlights the importance of differential diagnosis and careful evaluation in patients with absent cough reflex. Sensitivity and specificity of the citric acid CRT at 0.6 M is 71% and 60%, respectively.[13] While this is considerably better than other individual components of the clinical swallowing evaluation, it requires cautious interpretation and careful clinical reasoning. The CRT should be interpreted in conjunction with other findings from the clinical swallowing evaluation. The importance of affirming an absent cough response on instrumental assessment is important to avoid unnecessary conservative management in such patients.

REFERENCES

1. Daniels SK, Foundas AL. Lesion localization in acute stroke patients with risk of aspiration. *J Neuroimag*. 2009; 9(2):91.
2. Coates C, Bakheit AMO. The prevalence of verbal communication disability in patients with Parkinson's disease. *Disab Rehabil*. 1997;19(3):104–107. doi:10.3109/09638289709166834
3. García-Peris P, Parón L, Velasco C, et al. Long-term prevalence of oropharyngeal dysphagia in head and neck cancer patients: impact on quality of life. *Clin Nutr*. 2007; 26(6):710–717. doi:10.1016/j.clnu.2007.08.006
4. Ramsey D, Smithard D, Kalra L. Silent aspiration: what do we know? *Dysphagia*. 2005;20(3):218–225. doi:10.1007/s00455-005-0018-9
5. Holmes S. A service evaluation of cough reflex testing to guide dysphagia management in the postsurgical adult head and neck patient population. *Curr Opin Otolaryngol Head Neck Surg*. 2016;24(3):191–196. doi:10.1097/moo.0000000000000256
6. Koehler PR, Haughton VM, Daniels DL, Williams AL, Yetkin Z, Charles HC, Shutts D. MR measurement of normal and pathologic brainstem diameters. *AJNR Am J Neuroradiol*. 1985;6(3):425–427.
7. Morice AH, Kastelik JA, Thompson R. Cough challenge in the assessment of cough reflex. *British J Clin Pharmacol*. 2001;52(4):365–375.
8. Morice AH, Fontana GA, Belvisi MG, et al. ERS guidelines on the assessment of cough. *Euro Resp J*. 2007;29(6):1256.
9. Dicpinigaitis PV. Clinical cough III: measuring the cough response in the laboratory. *Handb Exp Pharmacol*. 2009; (187):297–310. doi:10.1007/978-3-540-79842-2_15
10. Miles A, Zeng IS, McLauchlan H, Huckabee ML. Cough reflex testing in dysphagia following stroke: a randomized controlled trial. *J Clin Med Res*. 2013;5(3):222–233. doi:http://dx.doi.org/10.4021/jocmr1340w
11. Swigert NB, Steele C, Riquelme LF. Dysphagia screening for patients with stroke: challenges in implementing a joint commission guideline. *The ASHA Leader*. 2007; 12(3):4–29. doi:10.1044/leader.FTR1.12032007.4
12. Bleach NR. The gag reflex and aspiration: a retrospective analysis of 120 patients assessed by videofluoroscopy. *Clin Otolaryngol Allied Sci*. 1993;18(4):303–307.
13. Miles A, Moore S, McFarlane M, Lee F, Allen J, Huckabee ML. Comparison of cough reflex test against instrumental assessment of aspiration. *Physiol Behav*. 2013; 118:25–31. doi:http://dx.doi.org/10.1016/j.physbeh.2013.05.004
14. Kruger E, Teasell R, Salter K, Foley N, Hellings C. The rehabilitation of patients recovering from brainstem strokes: case studies and clinical considerations. *Top Stroke Rehabil*. 2007;14(5):56–64. doi:10.1310/tsr1405-56.
15. Kim HM, Choi KH, Kim TW. Patients' radiation dose during videofluoroscopic swallowing studies according

to underlying characteristics. *Dysphagia*. 2013;28(2):153–158. doi:10.1007/s00455-012-9424-y

16. Jungheim M, Schubert C, Miller S, Ptok M. [Normative data of pharyngeal and upper esophageal sphincter high resolution manometry]. *Laryngorhinootologie*. 2015;94(9): 601–608. doi:10.1055/s-0034-1395532

17. Bulow M, Olsson R, Ekberg O. Videoradiographic analysis of how carbonated thin liquids and thickened liquids affect the physiology of swallowing in subjects with aspiration on thin liquids. *Acta Radiol*. 2003;44(4):366–372.

18. Logemann JA, Pauloski BR, Colangelo L, Lazarus C, Fujiu M, Kahrilas PJ. Effects of a sour bolus on oropharyngeal swallowing measures in patients with neurogenic dysphagia. *J Speech Hear Res*. 1995;38(3):556–563.

19. Langmore SE, Terpenning MS, Schork A, Chen Y, Murray JT, Lopatin D, Loesche WJ. Predictors of aspiration pneumonia: how important is dysphagia? *Dysphagia*. 1998;13(2):69–81. doi:10.1007/pl00009559

20. Kahrilas PJ, Logemann JA, Krugler C, Flanagan E. Volitional augmentation of upper esophageal sphincter opening during swallowing. *Am J Physiol*. 1991;260(3 pt 1): G450–456.

21. Shaker R, Kern M, Bardan E, et al. Augmentation of deglutitive upper esophageal sphincter opening in the elderly by exercise. *Am J Physiol*. 1997;272(6 pt 1):G1518–G1522.

22. Lamvik K, Jones R, Sauer S, Erfmann K, Huckabee ML. The capacity for volitional control of pharyngeal swallowing in healthy adults. *Physiol Behav*. 2015;152:257–263.

23. Addington WR, Stephens RE, Widdicombe J, Rekab K. Effect of stroke location on the laryngeal cough reflex and pneumonia risk. *Cough*. 2005;1:4. doi:10.1186/1745-9974-1-4

24. Kwon M, Lee JH, Kim JS. Dysphagia in unilateral medullary infarction: lateral vs medial lesions. *Neurology*. 2005;65(5):714–718. doi:10.1212/01.wnl.0000174441.39903.d8

25. Paliwal VK, Kalita J, Misra UK. Dysphagia in a patient with bilateral medial medullary infarcts. *Dysphagia*. 2009; 24(3):349–353. doi:10.1007/s00455-008-9194-8

26. Storey AT. A functional analysis of sensory units innervating epiglottis and larynx. *Exp Neurol*. 1968;20(3):366–383.

27. Widdicombe JG. Studies on afferent airway innervation. *Am Rev Resp Dis*. 1977;115(S):99–105. doi:10.1164/arrd.1977.115.S.99

28. Yamamoto Y, Hosono I, Atoji Y, Suzuki Y. Morphological study of the vagal afferent nerve endings in the laryngeal mucosa of the dog. *Ann Anat*. 1997;179(1):65–73. doi:10.1016/S0940-9602(97)80138-0

29. Miller AD, Bianchi AL, Bishop BP. *Neural Control of the Respiratory Muscles*. Boca Raton, FL: CRC Press; 1997.

30. Ebihara S, Ebihara T. Cough in the elderly: A novel strategy for preventing aspiration pneumonia. *Pulm Pharmacol Ther*. 2011;24(3):318–323. doi:10.1016/j.pupt.2010.10.003

31. Ebihara T, Takahashi H, Ebihara S, et al. Capsaicin troche for swallowing dysfunction in older people. *J Am Geriatr Soc*. 2005;53(5):824–828. doi:10.1111/j.1532-5415.2005.53261.x

32. Monroe MD, Manco K, Bennett R, Huckabee M-L. Citric acid cough reflex test: establishing normative data. *Speech, Lang Hear*. 2014;17(4):216–224. doi:10.1179/2050572814Y.0000000041

33. El Mekkaoui A, Irhoudane H, Ibrahimi A, El Yousfi M. Dysphagia caused by a lateral medullary infarction syndrome (Wallenberg's syndrome). *Pan Afr Med J*. 2012; 12:92.

34. Kameda W, Kawanami T, Kurita K, Daimon M, Kayama T, Hosoya T, Kato T. Lateral and medial medullary infarction: a comparative analysis of 214 patients. *Stroke*. 2004;35(3):694–699. doi:10.1161/01.str.0000117570.41153.35

35. Buchholz DW. Clinically probable brainstem stroke presenting primarily as dysphagia and nonvisualized by MRI. *Dysphagia*. 1993;8(3):235–238.

36. Kim TJ, Nam H, Hong J-H, et al. Dysphagia may be an independent marker of poor outcome in acute lateral medullary infarction. *J Clin Neurol*. 2015;11(4):349–357. doi:10.3988/jcn.2015.11.4.349

37. Aydogdu I, Ertekin C, Tarlaci S, Turman B, Kiylioglu N, Secil Y. Dysphagia in lateral medullary infarction (Wallenberg's syndrome): an acute disconnection syndrome in premotor neurons related to swallowing activity? *Stroke*. 2001;32(9):2081–2087.

38. Kim H, Chung CS, Lee KH, Robbins J. Aspiration subsequent to a pure medullary infarction: lesion sites, clinical variables, and outcome. *Arch Neurol*. 2000;57(4): 478–483.

CHAPTER 49

Voice and Swallowing Difficulties in Parkinsonian-type Multiple System Atrophy

Sebastian Doeltgen and Jane Bickford

INTRODUCTION

Multiple system atrophy (MSA) is a rare neurodegenerative disorder affecting areas of the spinal cord, brainstem, and cortex and is characterized by cell loss primarily affecting the autonomic and motor systems. The estimated global incidence is approximately 0.6/100,000 per annum, with a higher incidence of 3/100,000 per annum in those aged over 50 years.[1] The mean onset age is 50 to 70 years[2] and average life expectancy from onset of symptoms is approximately 7 years.[3]

There are different subtypes of MSA, commonly described as parkinsonian-type MSA (MSA-p) or cerebellar-type MSA (MSA-c), depending on whether parkinsonian or cerebellar symptoms predominate. Key symptoms of the MSA-c subtype include urinary dysfunction, cerebellar ataxia, and postural hypotension, whereas parkinsonian symptoms, such as tremor and difficulty initiating movements, are predominant in the MSA-p subtype. Often, these do not adequately respond to levodopa therapy. Corticospinal tract involvement may also be present, as well as imbalance, constipation, mild intellectual impairment, and neuropsychiatric symptoms, including depression, insomnia, hallucinations, and dementia,[4] especially as the disease progresses.

The neuropathological mechanisms underlying MSA are not yet fully understood, although environmental and dietary influences have been suggested.[5] Based on the key symptoms of MSA, which involve degeneration of striatonigral, olivopontocerebellar, and central autonomic networks, the underlying neuropathology is likely multifactorial and often overlapping.[6]

It is difficult to distinguish MSA from idiopathic Parkinson's disease (PD) at initial presentation, as symptoms are very similar. Key distinguishing features include autonomic failure (such as bladder dysfunction and orthostatic hypotension), poor response to levodopa, and akinetic parkinsonism or cerebellar ataxia.[7]

As with Parkinson's disease, MSA is often associated with significant impairment of communication, swallowing, and phonation. These typically occur much earlier, are associated with a shorter life expectancy,[8] and often decline more rapidly than in PD.[9] A small but growing body of evidence is now informing our understanding of the specific functional impairments resulting from MSA as they relate to communication, swallowing, and phonation. Cardinal features of MSA-p include progressive, hypokinetic dysarthria (which may have ataxic and/or spastic features),[10,11] oropharyngeal dysphagia, as well as neurogenic dysphonia, characterized by breathy (or hoarse) voice of low volume, reduced pitch, and shorter length of utterances.[12]

In this chapter, we present the journey of a 62-year-old man, in whom ultimately MSA-p was diagnosed, in the context of the biopsychosocial model.[13] We discuss the multidisciplinary contributions to the diagnostic and management planning processes and outline some of the psychosocial aspects relating to this case.

DEFINITION

MSA is a rare neurodegenerative disorder characterized by degeneration of cells in areas of the spinal cord, brainstem, and cortex, affecting primarily the autonomic and motor systems.

CASE PRESENTATION

A 62-year-old former high school teacher (R.K.) presents with recent history of unsteady gait, increasingly bradykinetic gross movements, and progressive deterioration in handwriting legibility. Recent medical history is sketchy as R.K. increasingly withdrew from friends and family since the passing of his wife 8 years ago. The only familial contact is his daughter, D.T., who does not accompany R.K. to the initial consultation. R.K. lives at his own home, where he recently had an (otherwise inconsequential) fall. He also had a bout of pneumonia and his daughter reports that she has trouble understanding his quiet and often unintelligible voice over the phone. R.K.'s general practitioner (GP) queried early stage PD and referred R.K. for differential diagnosis of possible PD with oropharyngeal/ laryngeal impairment to a multidisciplinary PD outpatient clinic at the local hospital.

INITIAL CONSULTATION

History

R.K. attends the multidisciplinary clinic by himself. During the initial laryngology assessment, he appears cognitively intact and is able to answer simple questions regarding his medical and personal history. He reports no history of smoking, no excessive alcohol consumption, and no major medical episodes. He mentions that he generally has lost interest in life since the passing of his wife. He recently went into early voluntary retirement as the workload at his school became unmanageable for him. R.K. is mobile but reports increasing difficulty walking due to unsteadiness and bouts of unexplained dizziness. He also mentions lack of appetite and that he may have lost some weight.

Examination

R.K. presents with a gradual deterioration in speech and mobility. He has a mild hoarseness characterized by a monopitch and monoloud voice. It is graded at 1 (mild dysphonia) on the GRBAS auditory-perceptual rating scale.[14] His speech is slow with imprecise consonant production and intermittent rushes of speech, both contributing to overall reduced intelligibility and consistent with hypokinetic dysarthria.

R.K. mentions significantly prolonged mealtimes, which he mainly attributes to slow chewing rather than any problems with his swallowing as he has not had any episodes of choking and reports eating a normal diet. No formal swallowing assessment is undertaken at this stage.

Management

The clinic's multidisciplinary team discusses the initial assessment findings that afternoon and agree on a probable diagnosis of early stage PD. His symptoms appear to be consistent with stage 3 PD.[15] The consulting neurologist prescribes R.K. with levodopa. In the week following the appointment, D.T., R.K.'s daughter, contacts the clinic with a request for clarification of her father's situation. She reports that she lives in a remote country town 350 kilometers from the clinic. She has young children and only gets to see her father once a month. She and her father only recently organized for D.T. to have power of attorney, as she had been concerned that her father's health was declining. The team make a time to videoconference with her and learn from D.T. about her father's recent admission to two occasions of urinary incontinence, which he was extremely embarrassed about. A wait-and-see approach is taken to evaluate the efficacy of levodopa and monitor progression of symptoms.

18 MONTHS FOLLOW-UP

Eighteen months after the initial consultation, R.K. is accompanied to the laryngology clinic by his daughter for a follow-up assessment. His motor symptoms continued to decline since the last consultation and he had another bout of pneumonia. Levodopa initially improved symptoms but both R.K. and his daughter feel that the improvements are only marginal. R.K. has had further falls, in particular in the last 3 months.

Examination

R.K. now presents with moderate rigidity of the head and neck with a resting tremor, predominantly in the right upper limb. His voice remains monotone and weak. R.K. speaks little, but when prompted he tends to use short phrases and his speech becomes progressively quieter over the consult. Intermittent horizontal nystagmus is evident. R.K. complains of worsening urinary incontinence and constipation and reports diminished appetite, impaired taste sensation, and difficulty swallowing pills. Duration of mealtimes continues to be an issue and he has had a weight loss of 5 kilograms since the initial consult. R.K.'s daughter also mentions that her father complains of insomnia and often appears fatigued.

Endoscopy

In-office, fiberoptic nasopharyngoscopy and videostroboscopy are completed jointly with the clinic's consulting speech pathologist.

Assessment of Larynx

Glottis: healthy appearance and mild atrophy of structures. Consistent with normal aging.

Glottic Competence. During quiet breathing

- Regular vocal fold edges

During phonation tasks (sustained /ee/ and /ah/ and conversational speech)

- Adequate vocal fold adduction, symmetrical closure, and no evidence of supraglottic activity (eg, anterior-posterior [AP] or lateral compression of the ventricular folds).
- Mild bilateral bowing of the vocal folds, reducing vocal fold closure and amplitude of mucosal wave.
- Vocal quality noted to be rough, breathy, and weak.

Voluntary cough

- Vocal folds adduct, but quality is weak.

R.K.'s presentation is consistent with mild atrophy of the vocal folds in line with normal aging. Further assessment is required to classify his dysphonia.

Swallowing Assessment

Due to history of recurrent pneumonia, swallowing function is evaluated using thin and moderately thick liquids (International Dysphagia Diet Standardisation Initiative[16] [IDDSI] levels 0 and 3) as well as a small (1 × 1 cm) piece of toast.

R.K. presents with oral phase dysphagia characterized by impaired oral bolus control and bolus formation, resulting in prolonged mastication, and poor and effortful bolus propulsion into the pharynx. Premature spillage of both liquid and solid boli is noted. No evidence of penetration or aspiration, although diffuse pharyngeal residue is noted. Laryngeal movement is decreased during palpation on all consistencies.

Multidisciplinary Consult

A joint consult with the speech pathologist and nutritionist is arranged on the same day after R.K.'s laryngology appointment.

Oromotor Skill Screening Revealed the Following

- Full dentition but poor oral hygiene (buildup of plaque and coated tongue).
- Loss of facial expression
- Periodic adventitious movements of the perioral musculature
- Reduced range of motion (ROM) of all articulators
- Reduced lip strength
- Reduced tongue strength
- Normal elicitation of gag reflex
- Irregular, imprecise, and slowed oral diadochokinetic rate
- Variable breakdown in articulatory precision in connected speech, characterized by sound omissions and distortions, repetitions of sounds and syllables, prolongations of sounds, periodic instances of phrases, and sentence repetition

Additional Swallowing Assessments Included

- Timed Water Swallow Test (TWST)[17]
- R.K. required nine swallows and 20 seconds to drink approximately 125 mL of the 150 mL of room-temperature water. This equates to a volume per swallow of 13.9 mL, an average time per swallow of 2.2 sec, and a swallowing capacity (volume/time) of 6.25 mL/s, which is below the average for his age group (see Video 1_drinking).
- Test of Masticating and Swallowing Solids (TOMASS):
  Similar to the TWST, the TOMASS revealed an increased number of masticatory cycles (70) and swallows (5) per cracker compared with the established age-controlled group means.[18]

Voice and Speech

Additional voice and speech assessments occur in a quiet consulting room and include auditory-perceptual assessment of vocal quality, maximum phonation time (MPT), acoustic assessment of fundamental frequency, and intensity and dysarthria assessment. An audio recording is made using a good quality digital recorder situated 30 centimeters from R.K.'s mouth. R.K. is asked to complete the voice tasks specified by the Consensus Auditory-Perceptual Evaluation of Voice (CAPE-V),[19] including a sustained /a/ at comfortable level, glissando productions of /a/, and connected speech.

- Auditory-perceptual voice assessment CAPE-V results:
  Overall severity-mild and consistent pattern. Mild roughness and breathiness. Nil strain. Normal resonance (see Video 2_hmm).

Mildly reduced pitch range and loudness. Monosoft, worsened over session (see Video 3_reading aloud).

- Maximum phonation time (MPT) 9 seconds (see Video 4_sustained ahhh)
- Acoustic assessment using PRAAT[20]
  Fundamental frequency (F0)
    Modal (habitual): 120 Hz (PD 123.57Hz ± 17.43 Hz), healthy subjects 116.8Hz ± 20.50 Hz)[21]
    Range: 115 to 150 Hz
    Speaking fundamental frequency (SF0): 123 Hz

  Perturbation: low jitter/high shimmer = breathy
- Acoustic assessment using a sound level meter
  Intensity (dB) (see Video 5_counting1-10)
    Counting 1 to 10: 45 to 50 dB
    Counting 1 to 10 louder: up to 60 dB
    Connected speech (reading): 58 to 60 dB

R.K. reported he perceived he was very loud when he tried to project his voice. His intelligibility improved with increased loudness.

Dysarthria Assessment

A full dysarthria assessment was completed using the Frenchay Dysarthria Assessment 2,[22] as presence and severity of dysarthria appear to be cardinal features of MSA-p. R.K. is asked to do a range of oromotor and speech tasks. He is also asked to read aloud.

- Reflexes: Mild dribbling
- Lips: Tremor with lip spread
- Palate: Nil of note
- Laryngeal: Monopitch and monoloud
- Tongue: Tremor and reduced range of motion for protrusion, elevation, lateral, and alternate movements (see Video 6_tongue elevation and Video 7_tongue lateral).
- Diadochokinetic rate (eg, ka-la): syllable rate: 14 repetitions (28 syllables) in 5 seconds or 5.6 syllables/second. This is within the normal range of 2.5 to 9 syllables/second[23] (see Video 8_ka-la).
- Prosody: Excess and equal stress, adequate rate and monotone (see Video 3_reading aloud)
- Intelligibility: Imprecise articulation and unable to maintain intelligibility over an utterance

Summary of Assessment

- Moderate mixed dysarthria with hypokinetic, spastic, and ataxic features significantly impacting communicative participation.
- Organic voice disorder: Type 5 (neurological, upper motor neuron with dysarthrophonia) as per the Diagnostic Classification for Voice Disorders[24]
- Moderate oral phase dysphagia as well as mild pharyngeal phase dysphagia

Management

At the multidisciplinary assessment team meeting that afternoon, the team discuss their concerns about R.K.'s deterioration and discuss ways to support R.K. to avoid hospital admission due to another bout of pneumonia or fall.

The following actions are recommended and discussed with D.T. over the phone after the meeting:

- R.K. to commence a short intensive of voice therapy targeting his vocal loudness[25] in order to facilitate his communicative participation and secondarily strengthen airway protection via increased vocal fold adduction.
- In light of R.K.'s declining health, recent history of several falls, pneumonia, and weight loss, the team further recommends that he move into a residential care facility (RCF) in the near future. R.K. and D.T. will be supported in this process by a social worker associated with the clinic.

Medication

The consulting neurologist reviews R.K.'s levodopa medication, amending the dose and introducing a monoamine oxidase type B (MAO-B) inhibitor in order to enhance the effects of levodopa.

Mealtime Management and Respiratory Safety

R.K. is placed on a pureed diet (IDDSI level 4) and mildly thickened fluids (IDDSI level 2) in an attempt to reduce mealtime duration by providing easier to chew foods. In addition, a strict oral hygiene protocol is to be implemented at the RCF to minimize the risk of recurrent aspiration pneumonia due to aspiration of bacteria-laden saliva and/or oral residue.

FOLLOW-UP ASSESSMENT 30 MONTHS LATER

R.K. attends the clinic for a follow-up appointment. His daughter D.T. attends with him. She reports that R.K. has become more apathetic and that he is now being fed by an attendant. He has had another bout of pneumonia and two episodes of choking on pureed food. She is also concerned about her father's memory and general well-being, stating that he is forgetting things, withdrawing from participation in activities, and is completely sedentary. It is also clear to the team that R.K.'s communication is difficult to follow and a source of frustration for him and his daughter. Mealtime duration continues to be a problem, as R.K. increasingly fatigues and does not manage to finish his meals. R.K. has lost a further 5 kg since the last appointment. The RCF team are also concerned about his obvious decline and that the levodopa medication is not working at all anymore.

Multidisciplinary Consult

A joint consult with the clinic's speech pathologist and dietitian is arranged that afternoon.

Oromotor Skill Screening

Compared with the last assessment, the clinical impression has worsened for all assessed items, in particular:

- Reduced ROM of all articulators
- Reduced lip strength, with anterior loss of saliva noted
- Reduced tongue strength, fasciculations noted
- Diadochokinetic rate (eg, ka-la): Syllable rate: 6 repetitions (12 syllables) in 5 seconds or 2.4 syllables/second. This is below the normal range of 2.5 to 9 syllables/second

Clinical Assessment of Swallowing Trials

The speech pathologist decides to trial mildly and moderately thick fluids as well as pureed vegetables and chicken. R.K. hesitantly trials the mildly thick fluid, stating that it will probably "go down the wrong tube." He produces a weak cough a few seconds after the first swallow. His voice sounds somewhat wet after the second and third mildly thick trials. He does not cough after the moderately thick trial. His underlying dysphonia makes it difficult to determine clinically if significant amounts of fluid and food are misdirected, although his history of recurrent pneumonia does suggest this may be the case. A VFSS is arranged for the following week to confirm the biomechanical characteristics and severity of the suspected pharyngeal phase dysphagia and trial potential postural compensatory strategies.

Voice and Communicative Participation Assessment

R.K. reports he tried the voice therapy recommended after his last visit. He says he had some short term improvement with his voice and speech but the effects did not last. He also found the therapy tiring. A further voice evaluation is completed.

- Auditory-perceptual voice assessment
  CAPE-V results:
  Overall severity: mild-moderate and consistent pattern.
  Mild-moderate roughness and breathiness.
  Mild strain.
  Normal resonance.

Moderately reduced pitch range and loudness. Mono-soft, worsened over session.

- Maximum phonation time (MPT): 6 seconds
- Acoustic assessment using PRAAT[20]
  Fundamental frequency (F0)
      Modal (habitual): 138 Hz (PD 123.57Hz ± 17.43, healthy subjects 116.8Hz ± 20.50 Hz)[21]
      Range: 110 to 140 Hz
      Speaking fundamental frequency (SF0) 142 Hz
      Perturbation: Low jitter/high shimmer = breathy
- Acoustic assessment using a sound level meter
  Intensity (dB)
      Counting 1 to 10: 35 to 40 dB
      Counting 1 to 10 louder: up to 50 dB
      Connected speech (reading): 40 to 52 dB

The Communicative Participation Item Bank,[26] a 10-question survey is given to R.K. to complete. He scores 10, and this is a low score, indicating he experiences a high degree of interference impacting his communicative participation.

Referral for Dietetics Assessment

R.K. is at significant risk of cachexia due to dysphagia, reduced oral intake, and recurrent chest infections. Indicators for monitoring by a dietitian include >5% weight loss from normal weight, body mass index (BMI) <18.5 kg/m^2, and reduced oral and/or fluid intake. R.K. is referred to the RCF's consulting dietitian for assessment and consideration of a high calorie, high protein diet.

Other Relevant Information

At the team meeting that afternoon, the following relevant information is shared between the team members who consulted with R.K. today:

- R.K.'s incontinence and constipation persist.
- His dysarthria continues to significantly affect his communication and participation at the RCF.
- Gains with voice therapy are not maintained.
- Insomnia and disturbed sleep patterns contribute to daytime fatigue which affects his participation in activities and further aggravates the issues around mealtime and swallowing.
- His ongoing weight loss is of significant concern.

Management

Communication

R.K. requires support to increase his communicative participation. It is important to liaise with both the RCF and his family about how they can support him. The following strategies are recommended for implementation at the RCF:

- Avoid communicating in loud or noisy environments.
- Communication partners should face R.K. directly when talking with him.
- Encourage R.K. to use shorter sentences or key words instead of long complex sentences.
- Where necessary, ask R.K. to repeat key words or rephrase.
- Spell out words and/or use topic cues (or combination of both).
- Encourage R.K. to ask communication partners if they have understood him by asking, "Did you get that?" or using gesture to indicate success, such as thumbs up or thumbs down.
- To reduce the demand for talking, communication partners can use the following question types to elicit what R.K. wants/needs:
  - Closed questions (eg, do you want A or B?)
  - Yes/no questions

- Consider using simple alphabet charts and speech apps if communication becomes really frustrating and/or fatiguing for R.K.

REVISED DIAGNOSIS

Based on rapid decline and non-PD cerebellar and autonomic nervous system symptoms, R.K. is given a revised diagnosis from PD to probable MSA-p. He is taken off the levodopa altogether; his other medications are reviewed.

OUTCOME OF VIDEOFLUOROSCOPIC SWALLOWING STUDY

VFSS 1 week later reveals significant impairment in the oral and pharyngeal stages of swallowing. R.K. presents with severe oral phase dysphagia characterized by poor oral control and anterior spillage especially of thin liquids. Preparation of a cohesive bolus is also impaired due to reduced jaw and tongue movement. Tongue tremor is evident prior to onset of swallow and repetitive tongue rocking is associated with multiple attempts to initiate a swallow and significantly increased oral transit time. Prior to onset of swallow, premature spillage is observed for all consistencies. A swallow response is initiated when bolus fills the valleculae space.

R.K. also presents with pharyngeal phase dysphagia, characterized by significantly reduced laryngeal anterior-superior excursion and consequently incomplete epiglottic deflection. Diffuse post-swallow residue is noted and there is aspiration of mildly and moderately thick liquids in two of three trials for each consistency.

During the investigation, the speech pathologist trialed the effortful swallow and chin tuck maneuvers. The effortful swallow somewhat reduced post-swallow residue and the chin tuck helped reduce premature spillage into the pharynx, but increased anterior spillage, especially with mildly thickened fluids.

Updated Management Plan

Based on the outcomes of the instrumental swallowing assessment, the speech pathologist recommends R.K. only consume moderately thickened fluids (IDDSI level 3) using a chin tuck position and effortful swal-

lowing, as possible. Due to the limited prospect of consistent implementation of these strategies during mealtimes, the multidisciplinary team discusses the situation with R.K.'s daughter via teleconference the following week. The possible benefits of a percutaneous endoscopic gastrostomy (PEG) are discussed with D.T., which include maintaining R.K.'s nutritional intake while bypassing the oropharyngeal intake route and his weight. R.K. will continue to be able to join mealtimes and with the help of an attendant consume small amounts of thickened fluids and pureed foods. D.T. is hesitant to accept this as a viable option as she perceives this step as a final phase in her father's disease management, which she finds difficult to accept. She agrees to consider the team's recommendation but prefers to see how her father copes with the newly recommended moderately thick diet. Another follow-up appointment is scheduled in 6 months time, or prior, if required.

In order to improve R.K.'s ability to communicate with others, the use of the communication strategies, including the use of simple questions, an alphabet chart, and speech apps are also reinforced.

FOLLOW–UP ASSESSMENT 36 MONTHS LATER

R.K. attends the scheduled follow-up appointment with his daughter and a care worker from the RCF. Apart from another bout of pneumonia, the RCF staff have become increasingly concerned about R.K.'s unsteady gait and postural hypotension, which has seen him faint on two occasions. As a consequence, the consulting GP at the RCF has recommended that R.K. self-propel in a wheelchair as possible. R.K.'s mixed dysarthria has worsened. His speech intelligibility is poor and he speaks very softly. The care worker reports snoring and bouts of gasping for breath (sleep apnea) at night. R.K. continues to struggle at mealtimes, even on the moderately thick diet and has experienced further weight loss. The care worker reports concerns regarding R.K.'s significantly reduced fluid intake and a recent bout of urinary tract infection. R.K. also presents with audible inspiratory stridor during the consultation.

Endoscopy

In-office, fiberoptic nasopharyngoscopy is completed.

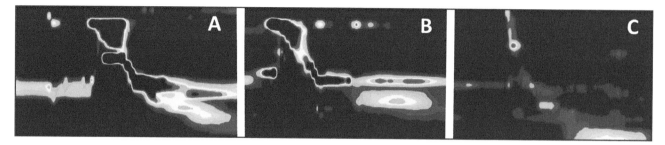

Figure 49–1. High-resolution manometric traces of a 5 mL thin liquid bolus of (**A**) a young control participant (25 y.o. male), (**B**) an older control participant (66 y.o. male), and (**C**) R.K. (62 y.o. male with MSA-p). Note the significantly reduced vigor of the pharyngeal contraction and hypotonic UES high pressure zone. Impedance-based pressure flow analysis revealed a significantly reduced transition of the bolus across the UES as well as a significantly increased bolus presence time in the hypopharynx.[27]

Assessment of Larynx

Glottis: mild-moderate atrophy of structures, consistent with disease progression.

Glottic Competence. During quite breathing

- Regular vocal fold edges and vocal folds resting in paramedian position. Mild-moderate laryngeal (inspiratory) stridor noted. This is consistent with weakness of the posterior cricoarytenoid muscles (abductors) and usually signals late stages of the disease.

During phonation tasks (sustained /i/ and /a/ and conversational speech)

- Inadequate vocal fold adduction, symmetrical closure, and no evidence of supraglottic activity (eg, AP or lateral compression of the ventricular folds). Vocal quality noted to be harsh, breathy, and grade 3 (severe dysphonia) on the GRBAS.[14]

Voluntary cough

- Vocal folds do not fully adduct during voluntary cough; cough is strained, breathy, and weak

Other Relevant Information—High-Resolution Pharyngeal Manometry

Since the last appointment, R.K. and his family were approached by a research team who conducted an investigation of oropharyngeal motility in neuro-degenerative diseases. As R.K. always had a passion for education and science, he and his daughter agreed to his participation in the one-off investigation. A brief report of findings was forwarded to the clinic and included the following (Figure 49–1).

CASE DEBRIEF

Two weeks after the 36 month consult, R.K. receives a PEG tube; however, he continues to join mealtimes in the RCF and with the assistance of a carer consumes small amounts of moderately thick fluids and liquidized solids (IDDSI level 3). Over the subsequent 3 years, R.K.'s condition deteriorates further and he transitions into a palliative care home, where he passes away approximately 6 years following the initial consult.

DISCUSSION

R.K.'s pathway to diagnosis of MSA-p is not atypical and highlights the importance of frequent reviews and a multidisciplinary approach. His initial presentation with parkinsonian-like symptoms resulted in the implementation of a number of medical and behavioral treatment options. Levodopa and the intensive vocal loudness training provided him short term relief. However, rapid progression of his symptoms and the presence of new symptoms (eg, urinary incontinence, constipation, vertigo, postural hypotension) gave his treating health practitioners additional information. The differential diagnosis of MSA-p came 30 months after he was diagnosed with Parkinson's disease. The health professionals used both comprehensive assessment tools and clinical evaluations to support their clinical reasoning.

Very few relevant clinical guidelines or pathways for MSA are accessible to health practitioners. The ones that are pertain to medical diagnosis and management[28,29] of PD.[30] However, a person-centered approach to disease management is widely accepted in health care.[31] In Australia, a patient-centered approach can face unique challenges. The vast geographical distances and reduced community supports or expertise can result in multidisciplinary teams having to provide extensive supports and education. The use of technology (eg, teleconferencing) has facilitated this need.

In R.K.'s care, the biopsychosocial model[13] and use of the International Classification of Functioning framework[32] assisted the multidisciplinary team to take a person-centered approach. This was evident with the team's concern and attempts to support R.K.'s psychosocial well-being. A significant environmental factor for R.K. was that his social supports and relationships were limited and his only next of kin, his daughter, lived remotely from R.K. Where possible, the team included R.K. and his daughter D.T. in management decisions. For example, case meetings with D.T. were arranged via video-conference and teleconference or a team member liaised directly with her when she was unable to attend R.K.'s appointments.

Members of the multidisciplinary team spent time educating and preparing R.K. and his daughter for R.K.'s likely deterioration. They also provided information and guidance to R.K.'s care workers at his RCF. The multidisciplinary team valued the support D.T. was willing to give R.K. and noted that D.T. had been granted power of attorney for R.K. The team was aware that D.T. was constrained by her own personal circumstances (eg, living in a distant geographic location, primary carer responsibilities for her own children).

In this chapter the focus has been on swallowing and communication assessment and support for R.K. The speech pathologist and otolaryngologist worked jointly with the other members of the multidisciplinary team throughout R.K.'s care. This ensured that all professions were aware of developments in R.K.'s medical diagnosis as well as that they were able to communicate with other team members their assessment findings and recommendations.

Speech, Voice, and Communication Summary

A range of screening tools and assessments were used to assess R.K.'s speech, voice, and communication skills over time. Like many people with MSA-p, R.K.'s skills in these domains in the early stages of the diseases appeared similar to early PD. The nasendoscopic evaluations at 18 and 36 months provided valuable information about his glottal efficiency and sufficiency. The early visualization of R.K.'s larynx revealed the absence of functional laryngeal deficits and mild atrophy consistent with normal aging. It also provided an important baseline for future assessment. The speech pathologist conducted a comprehensive case history and assessed R.K.'s speech intelligibility using a standardized dysarthria assessment at the 18-month visit. His voice was also assessed using a range of auditory-perceptual rating scales of pitch, loudness, and vocal quality. These measures were complemented by acoustic analysis of the fundamental frequency, speaking fundamental frequency, intensity, and perturbation of a range of R.K.'s speech samples (eg, sustained vowel, conversational speech, reading aloud). R.K.'s communicative participation was assessed by using a short standardized self-report questionnaire.

R.K.'s speech and voice patterns were similar to PD and characterized by mixed dysarthria with hypokinetic, spastic and ataxic features, and hypophonia. A possible distinguishing speech pattern for MSA-p sufferers is that they are more likely to experience spastic and ataxia dysarthria and are more likely to produce fewer syllable repetitions per second than PD patients who experience hypokinetic dysarthria. At the 18-month assessment R.K. was still able to produce a comparable syllable rate, but at the 30-month follow-up his syllable rate was below normal.

As the disease progressed, R.K. experienced laryngeal stridor. This is consistent with weakness of the posterior cricoarytenoid muscles (abductors) and usually signals late stages of the disease. It was noted at the 36-month follow-up. The decline in R.K.'s speech and voice skills also impacted his ability to communicate and participate in important social activities such as talking and interacting with others. Difficulties with expressing himself caused him frustration and appeared to impact his mental health.

A range of direct and indirect interventions were used to manage R.K.'s speech, voice, and communication issues. A short intensive of voice therapy targeting vocal loudness had short term benefits but unfortunately these benefits were not sustained. This outcome is inconsistent with a diagnosis of Parkinson's disease. There is increasing evidence that vocal loudness therapy can be used to treat dysarthrophonia resulting from Parkinson's disease.[25] Later, the speech pathologist recommended the use of alternative and augmentative communication aids to support R.K.'s communication.

The indirect intervention involved educating R.K., his daughter, and care workers. This education included strategies to increase R.K.'s communicative participation. The speech pathologist emphasized ways R.K. could modify his verbal messages and how communication partners could play active and important roles in supporting R.K. to communicate successfully. These strategies were reviewed and reinforced regularly. They were also provided in written form.

Swallowing Summary

R.K.'s swallowing function appeared unimpaired at the first consult, although there were some innocuous signs that a subclinical swallowing impairment might be present, including reported weight loss (likely resulting from reduced nutritional intake) and early signs of oral phase impairment (resulting in prolonged mealtimes). His swallowing function dramatically declined over the ensuing 18 months, which is in keeping with a more rapid decline in MSA compared with Parkinson's disease.[8] The impairment of oral phase movements, in particular of the tongue, is typical in parkinsonian-type disorders and often characterized by a back and forth rocking of the tongue when attempting to initiate a swallow. This leads to a significantly prolonged oral phase and often results in premature spillage of the bolus into the pharynx, increasing the risk of pre-swallow aspiration. Within 30 months, R.K.'s swallowing continued to decline significantly, being characterized by severe oral and pharyngeal phase impairment. As was evident from both the VFSS and high-resolution manometry reports, hyolaryngeal excursion, pharyngeal contractile vigor, and upper esophageal sphincter (UES) opening were significantly impaired, resulting in severely limited and inefficient bolus flow across the pharyngoesophageal segment. Paired with significant oral phase issues leading to poor oral bolus containment and premature spillage, R.K. is at great risk for ongoing pulmonary aspiration of liquids, foods, and saliva.

Although aspiration alone does not inevitably result in aspiration pneumonia,[33] R.K. presents with several factors that increase his overall risk, including a sedentary lifestyle and poor oral hygiene. The latter is a significant issue, especially as R.K. is reliant on the care of others to maintain good oral hygiene. It is a main concern of the consulting speech pathologist to educate the care staff at the RCF regarding the link between poor oral hygiene and aspiration pneumonia.

Placement of the PEG tube is perceived as a significant milestone by R.K.'s daughter and seen as a gesture of "giving up." It is important to highlight that placement of a PEG tube does not necessarily mark the end of all oral intake, but instead provides a means of maintaining sufficient nutritional and hydration intake without the pressure of having to consume adequate amounts per os. As such, earlier placement of a PEG tube is increasingly considered an option to bypass the oral intake route and maintain nutritional status and BMI in neurodegenerative conditions. A multidisciplinary approach is required to provide adequate education and counseling for patients and their families in this decision-making process.

CONCLUSION

We present the case of R.K. whose clinical presentation appeared consistent with Parkinson's disease and was initially characterized by bradykinesia, festinating gait, hypophonia, and micrographia. Over the course of the early stages of the disease, several parkinsonian-atypical symptoms were noted, including urinary incontinence, constipation, vertigo, and postural hypotension, as well as mixed hypokinetic dysarthria with spastic and ataxic features, producing fewer syllable repetitions per second than commonly seen in PD patients. In addition, R.K. did not respond to levodopa therapy. These key features help differentiate MSA from PD but are often not evident at first consult. Clinically, these key features are also often assessed by, or reported to, different health professions. R.K.'s pathway to a diagnosis of MSA-p thus highlights the benefits and necessity of a multidisciplinary approach to patient-centered care. All health professions involved provided important clinical information that jointly contributed to the final diagnosis. Both comprehensive assessment tools and thorough clinical evaluations supported their clinical reasoning. The comprehensive multidisciplinary collaboration also enabled the implementation of appropriate and timely support for R.K. and his daughter. From a review of the literature it is evident that formal care pathways for MSA, as are available for acute stroke care, are critically lacking. Such pathways would enable more widespread and formalized provision of multidisciplinary support for people with MSA and would allow patients and clinical stakeholders to advocate for optimal clinical care.

REFERENCES

1. Ubhi K, Low P, Masliah E. Multiple system atrophy: a clinical and neuropathological perspective. *Trends Neurosci.* 2011;34(11):581–590.
2. Jamora RD, Gupta A, Tan AK, Tan LC. Clinical characteristics of patients with multiple system atrophy in Singapore. *Ann Acad Med Singapore.* 2005;34(9):553–557.
3. Coon EA, Sletten DM, Suarez MD, et al. Clinical features and autonomic testing predict survival in multiple system atrophy. *Brain.* 2015;138(12):3623–3631.
4. Stefanova N, Buecke P, Duerr S, Wenning GK. Multiple system atrophy: an update. *Lancet Neurol.* 2009;8(12):1172–1178.
5. Vidal JS, Vidailhet M, Elbaz A, Derkinderen P, Tzourio C, Alpérovitch A. Risk factors of multiple system atrophy: a case-control study in French patients. *Mov Disord.* 2008;23(6):797–803.
6. Swan L, Dupont J. Multiple system atrophy. *Phys Ther.* 1999;79:488–494.
7. Ciolli l, Krismer F, Nicoletti F, Wenning, GK. An update on the cerebellar subtype of multiple system atrophy. *Cerebell Atax.* 2014;1(14):1–12.
8. Müller J, Wenning GK, Verny M, McKee A, Chaudhuri KR, Jellinger K, Litvan I. Progression of dysarthria and dysphagia in postmortem-confirmed parkinsonian disorders. *Arch Neurol.* 2001;58(2):259–264.
9. Fanciulli A, Wenning GK. Multiple-system atrophy. *New Engl J Med.* 2015;372(3):249–263.
10. Kluin KJ, Foster NL, Berent S, Gilman S. Perceptual analysis of speech disorders in progressive supranuclear palsy. *Neurol.* 1993;43:563–566.
11. Knopp DB, Barsottini OGP, Ferraz HB. Multiple system atrophy speech assessment: study of five cases. *Arquivos de Neuro-Psiquiatria.* 2002;60:619–623.
12. Penner H, Miller N, Walters M. *Motor speech disorders in three parkinsonian syndromes: a comparative study.* Paper presented at: the 16th International Congress of Phonetic Sciences (ICPhS); 2007.
13. Engel GL. The clinical application of the biopsychosocial model. *Am J Psychiatry.* 1980;137(5):535–544.
14. Hirano M. *Clinical Examination of Voice.* New York, NY: Springer; 1981.
15. Hoehn MM, Yahr MD. Parkinsonism: onset, progression, and mortality. *Neurology.* 1967;17:427–442.
16. International Dysphagia Diet Standardization Initiative. Retrived November 2, 2017, from http://iddsi.org/
17. Hughes TAT, Wiles, CM. Clinical measurement of swallowing in health and in neurogenic dysphagia. *Quart J Med.* 1996;89:109–116.
18. Huckabee ML, McIntosh T, Fuller L, et al. The Test of Masticating and Swallowing Solids (TOMASS): reliability, validity and international normative data. *Int J Lang Commun Disord.* 2017; doi: 10.1111/1460–6984.12332. [Epub ahead of print]
19. American Speech-Language-Hearing Association, T. (2006). *Consensus Auditory-Perceptual Evaluation of Voice (CAPE-V).* ASHA SID 3-Voice and Voice Disorders. Retrieved 18 Sept. 2017, from http://www.asha.org/
20. Boersma P, Weenink D. Praat: Doing phonetics by computer (Version 6.0.32). Retrieved from http://www.praat.org/ 2017.
21. Huh YE, Park J, Suh MK, Lee SE, Kim J, Jeong Y, Kim HT, Cho JW. Differences in early speech patterns between Parkinson variant of multiple system atrophy and Parkinson's disease. *Brain Lang.* 2015;147:14–20.
22. Enderby PM, Palmer R. *Frenchay Dysarthria Assessment 2 Edition.* 2008. Austin, TX: Pro-Ed.
23. Pierce JE, Cotton S, Perry A. Alternating and sequential motion rates in older adults. *Int J Lang Commun Disord.* 2013;48(3):257–264.
24. Baker J, Ben-Tovim D I, Butcher A R, Esterman A, McLaughlin K. Development of a modified diagnostic classification system for voice disorders with inter-rater reliability study. *Logopedic Phoniatric Vocology.* 2007;32(3):99–112.
25. Yorkston KM, Hakel M, Beukelman DR, Fager S. Evidence for effectiveness of treatment of loudness, rate, or prosody in dysarthria: a systematic review. 2007. *Database of Abstracts of Reviews of Effects (DARE): Quality-Assessed Reviews.*
26. Baylor C R, Yorkston K, Eadie T L, Kim J, Chung H, Amtmann D. The Communicative Participation Item Bank (CPIB): item bank calibration and development of a disorder-generic short form. *J Speech Lang Hear Res.* 2013;56(4):1190–1208.
27. Cock C, Omari T. Diagnosis of swallowing disorders: how we interpret pharyngeal manometry. *Curr Gastroenterol Rep.* 2017;19:11. doi: 10.1007/s11894-017-0552-2
28. Gilman S, Wenning GK, Low PA, et al. Second consensus statement on the diagnosis of multiple system atrophy. *Neurol.* 2008;71(9):670–676.
29. Perez-Lloret S, Flabeau O, Fernagut PO, et al. Current concepts in the treatment of multiple system atrophy. *Mov Dis Clin Prac.* 2015;2:6–16.
30. National Institute for Health and Care Excellence. (2017). Parkinson's disease pathway (pp. 1–6). Retrieved October 23, 2017, from http://www.nice.org.uk/
31. Hughes JC, Bamford C, May C. Types of centredness in health care: themes and concepts. *Med Health Care Phil.* 2008;11:455–463.
32. World Health Organization. *International Classification of Functioning, Disability and Health—Short Version.* Geneva, Switzerland: WHO; 2001.
33. Langmore SE, Terpenning MS, Schork A, Chen Y, Murray JT, Lopatin D, Loesche WJ. Predictors of aspiration pneumonia: how important is dysphagia? *Dysphagia.* 1998;13(2):69–81.

CHAPTER 50

Lower Cranial Nerve Palsy

Maggie Kuhn

INTRODUCTION

The lower cranial nerves maintain the critical functions of the laryngopharynx: breathing passage, lower airway protection, and phonation. These functions require intact motor supply and sensory feedback provided by cranial nerves. Cranial nerve impairment can occur in isolation or combination. The impact on voice and swallowing is variable and depends on severity of deficits, cognition, motivation, comorbidities and other neurological injuries.[1] In cranial nerve injury, all stages of swallowing can be affected by deficits, including poor oral containment, decreased pharyngeal propulsion, reduced laryngeal closure, and cricopharyngeal (CP) dysfunction.[2]

DEFINITION

The lower cranial nerves include the vagus nerve (X) as well as the glossopharyngeal nerve (IX), accessory nerve (XI), and hypoglossal nerve (XII). Cranial nerve (CN) impairment results when focal or systemic diseases affect these nerves centrally (brainstem), proximally (skull base), or peripherally (neck).

ANATOMY

The vagus nerve's motor fibers originate from the nucleus ambiguus of the medulla and cross the premedullary cistern to leave the skull base through the jugular foramen. The nodose ganglion via nucleus tractus solitaris receives sensory input. The internal branch of the superior laryngeal nerve (SLN) carries sensory information from the larynx above the vocal folds. The external branch innervates the cricothyroid muscle. Along with cranial nerves IX and X, the vagus nerve contributes to the pharyngeal plexus. The vagus nerve descends in the carotid sheath through the parapharyngeal space. On the right side, the recurrent laryngeal nerve (RLN) arises at the cervicothoracic junction and passes posteriorly around the right subclavian artery. On the left side, the RLN arises at the level of the aortic arch posterior to the ligamentum arteriosum. The RLN supplies the intrinsic muscles of the larynx and sensory innervation to the larynx below the vocal folds.[3,4]

Laryngeal impairment may result from high (brainstem, skull base, proximal CNX) or low (SLN, RLN, pharyngeal plexus) nerve injuries. Nearly all patients with CNX impairment experience dysphonia and up to 40% of patients with unilateral vocal fold immobility (UVFI) have swallowing impairment, including aspiration, pharyngeal discoordination, CP muscle dysfunction or velopharyngeal insufficiency. Variable motor and sensory connections between the RLN and SLN have been described and may explain the spectrum of presentations and compensations in UVFI.[5] In up to 15% of cases of UVFI, the etiology is a high CNX injury.[6] Deficits in such cases, from combined SLN and RLN impairment, are more severe.[7]

CASE PRESENTATION

A 46-year-old man with a left vagal schwannoma was referred for evaluation of hoarseness and dysphagia 1 week following surgical excision.

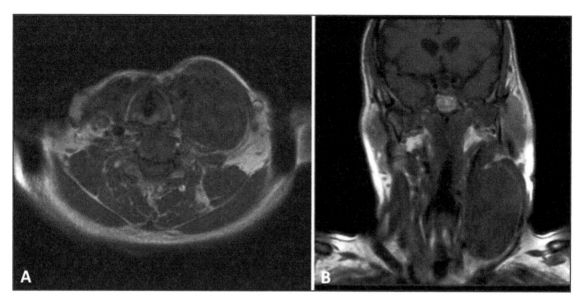

Figure 50–1. Axial (**A**) and coronal (**B**) views of T1-weighted MRI neck demonstrating a 3 × 5 cm left vagal schwannoma. It appears as a vertically oriented, homogeneous mass posterior to the carotid bifurcation.

Definition

Schwannomas arise from cranial, peripheral, and autonomic nerve sheath cells. They comprise 5% of all benign soft tissue tumors.[8] While the head and neck is an unusual location for schwannomas, in this region most are extracranial and non-vestibular, arising from the sympathetic chain or CN X.[9] They frequently present as asymptomatic neck masses confirmed with characteristic radiographic findings (Figure 50–1).[10] Hoarseness is a presenting symptom in up to 20% of patients.[11] Definitive treatment for vagal schwannomas is surgical resection with attempted nerve preservation.[11–13] However, there is up to 85% incidence of vocal fold immobility after vagal schwannoma resection.[14]

INITIAL ASSESSMENT

History

Initial evaluation includes a comprehensive description of symptoms, most importantly dysphonia and dysphagia. Vocal quality, endurance, fluctuation, and pain should be elicited. Patient-reported symptom instruments (Voice Handicap Index 10 [VHI-10] or Voice-Related Quality of Life [VRQOL]) are useful. Charac-

teristics of swallowing should be discussed, including quality of dysphagia (solids, liquids, pills, multiple), onset, and sequelae (weight loss, malnutrition, pneumonia). The Eating Assessment Tool (EAT-10) is useful for gauging patients' swallowing symptoms. Cough strength, frequency of throat clearing, and breathing quality should be solicited.

A thorough history should include pertinent medical and surgical comorbidities. Of particular importance are cardiovascular, neurologic, respiratory, oncologic, and traumatic histories. Any surgery involving the head, neck, spine, or chest should be completely discussed. Prior and present exposure to toxic substances (tobacco, alcohol) is relevant.

Examination

Physical examination in suspected CN injury begins with a general assessment including voice quality, speech intelligibility, secretion management, and ease of breathing. A volitional cough should be prompted and assessed for quality and productiveness. Involuntary cough with palpation of a lateral neck mass indicates vagal schwannoma.[15] The face and neck should be carefully inspected for evidence of prior trauma or surgery as well as for the anticipated healing of known, recent surgical wounds. The mouth is evaluated for trismus, dentition, oral hygiene, saliva production, and mucosal health.

Careful attention must be paid to CN function. In many disease states, multiple cranial nerves may be affected, increasing morbidity and prolonging rehabilitation.[4]

Comprehensive evaluation includes tests of olfaction (CN I), visual acuity (CN II), ocular motion (CN III/IV/VI), facial sensation and masticatory muscle function (CN V), facial movement (CN VII), palate elevation (CN IX/X), shoulder function (CN XI), and tongue function (CN XII).

Endoscopy

Endoscopic visualization of the laryngopharynx is critical and may include both halogen flexible indirect laryngoscopy as well as videostroboscopy for fine evaluation of vocal fold function. During endoscopy, vocal fold mobility and positioning are assessed as well as compensatory findings. Pharyngeal strength and symmetry are noted. Sensation and presence of the laryngeal adductor reflex are examined. Secretion status can be assessed by the presence of pooling, penetration, or regurgitation. Videostroboscopy provides additional information about vocal fold structure, glottic closure, and vocal fold height symmetry.

Swallowing Evaluation

A more careful assessment of swallowing is performed when clinically warranted. A non-instrumental evaluation is the clinical swallow evaluation and is typically performed by a speech-language pathologist who assesses for swallowing safety through examination, questioning, and swallowing trials. Instrumental evaluations include flexible endoscopic evaluation of swallowing (FEES) and videofluoroscopic swallow study (VFSS). These tests depict deglutitive anatomy and function simultaneously. In possible CN palsy, they're valuable to assess timing, pharyngeal coordination, airway closure, laryngopharyngeal sensation, and pharyngoesophageal segment function.

SCENARIO 1

The patient's operative report describes schwannoma enucleation and vagal nerve preservation. The patient reports a raspy voice and vocal fatigue as well as occasional choking with liquids since the surgery. His VHI-10 is 32 and EAT-10 is 13. Perceptually, his voice is breathy and his cough is weakened. His tongue and uvula are midline.

Diagnosis

Incomplete CN X palsy following nerve-sparing vagal schwannoma resection

Investigations

Stroboscopy: For a chief complaint of dysphonia following vagal schwannoma, videostroboscopy is performed. The left vocal fold is immobile and lateralized, resulting in a glottic gap. The ipsilateral aryepiglottic fold is deviated toward midline. There is increased false vocal cord and anterior-posterior compression.[16] Pooled secretions may be seen in the ipsilateral hypopharynx (Figure 50–2B).

Computed Tomography

Though not required when the cause of vocal fold immobility is fairly certain, CT is the preferred imaging modality to investigate vagal nerve palsy. Thin slices through the larynx demonstrate dilation of ipsilateral pyriform sinus, thickening and medial positioning of the aryepiglottic fold, dilation of laryngeal ventricle, atrophy of the posterior cricoarytenoid muscle, and fatty replacement of the thyroarytenoid muscle.[17] Furthermore, inferior pharyngeal constrictor atrophy and ballooning of pharyngeal walls may be observed.[18] See Figure 50–3.

Management

The patient is recommended left type I thyroplasty and arytenoid adduction. Without significant swallowing complaints or findings, symptoms are managed with counseling and behavioral therapy including positioning (chin tuck, head turn), maneuvers (surpraglottic swallow), and texture modification.

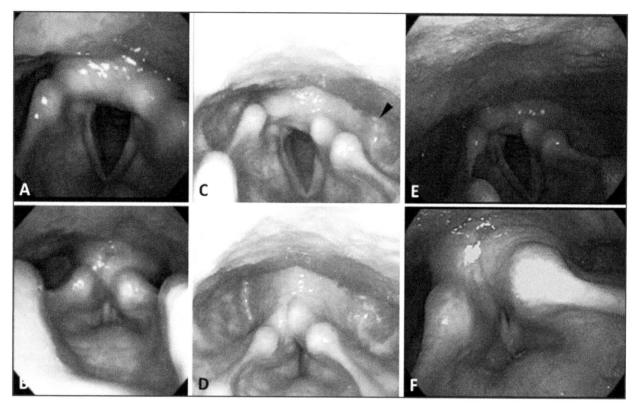

Figure 50–2. Videostroboscopic images from a patient with a left vagal schwannoma. Prior to left vagal schwannoma resection (A and B), the larynx appears normal. Following left vagal schwannoma resection (C and D), the left vocal fold is immobile and lateralized, the left arytenoid is medially displaced, glottis closure is incomplete, and the left pyriform contains scant pooled secretions. After medialization thyroplasty with arytenoid adduction (E and F), glottis closure is improved, arytenoid is repositioned, and hypopharynx contains no secretions.

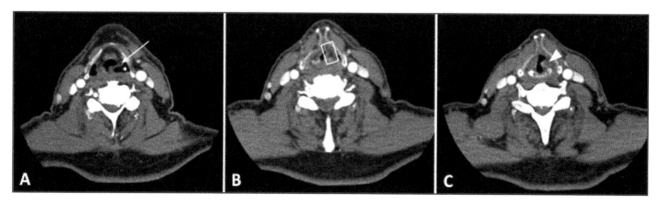

Figure 50–3. Axial views of a contrast-enhanced neck CT in a patient with left CN X palsy. (A) The left pyriform sinus is dilated (*asterisk*) and the left aryepiglottic fold is displaced (*white arrow*). (B) The left ventricle is enlarged (box). (C) The left arytenoid is anteriorly displaced (*arrowhead*).

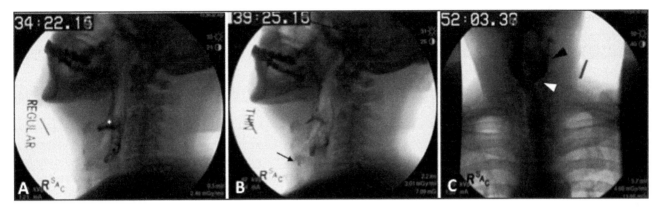

Figure 50–4. Videofluoroscopic swallow study following CN X sacrifice. (**A**) Lateral view demonstrates vallecular (*white asterisk*) and hypopharyngeal (*black asterisk*) residue. (**B**) Lateral view with silent aspiration (*black arrow*) after the swallow. (**C**) Anterior-posterior view showing left pharyngeal dilation (*black arrowhead*) and left impaired pharyngoesophageal segment opening (*white arrowhead*).

The patient's operative report describes intended CN X preservation but concern for malignant transformation prompted vagus nerve sacrifice. He reports a breathy voice with very weak cough. He becomes exhausted with speaking and his voice has a wet quality. VHI-10 is 34. He chokes with both solids and liquids. He has not had a fever since surgery but has lost 2 to 3 lbs. His EAT-10 is 36. On exam his tongue is midline but his palate deviates slightly to the right.

Diagnosis

High left vagal nerve injury with resultant combined motor and sensory laryngopharyngeal impairment following nerve sacrificing vagal schwannoma resection

Investigations

Stroboscopy: Endoscopic evaluation is performed confirming immobile left vocal fold positioned as described above. FEES at the same time demonstrates impaired hyolaryngeal excursion, deep laryngeal penetration, and residue in both valleculae and hypopharynx. Sensory testing shows impaired left hemilaryngeal sensation. Videofluoroscopic evaluation of swallowing is

warranted. During the study, dilation of left pyriform sinus, bolus diversion to paralyzed side, and unilateral cricopharyngeus muscle dysfunction are observed.[19] Additionally, pharyngeal residue and silent aspiration on thin liquids are noted (Figure 50–4). Attempted maneuvers (supraglottic swallow, Mendelson maneuver) and positioning (chin tuck) improve but do not eliminate aspiration and pharyngeal residue.

Management

The patient is recommended type I thyroplasty and arytenoid adduction with CP myotomy and possible hypopharyngeal pharyngoplasty. Additionally, he is counseled regarding his swallowing impairment and taught to maintain good oral hygiene. Behavioral therapy includes swallowing exercises (super supraglottic swallow, Masako), positioning, and prophylactic strategies (post-swallow throat clear).

Myriad conditions may cause lower cranial nerve palsy resulting in laryngeal impairment leading to dysphonia and dysphagia. Possible causes and their diagnostic clues are listed in Table 50–1.

Table 50–1. Possible Causes of High Vagal Lesions

Cause	Diagnostic Clues
Schwannoma	• Neck mass • CT/MRI
Cerebellar pontine tumor	• Other CN palsies (VII, VIII) • Audiogram • MRI
Cerebrovascular accident (Wallenberg's syndrome)	• Ipsilateral CN deficits • Contralateral trunk/extremity sensory deficits • Ataxia • CT/MRI
Trauma (skull base)	• History (mechanism) • Associated facial fractures • CSF leak • CT
Paraganglioma	• Neck mass • CT/MRI
Cerebral aneurysm, AVM	• History (headache, tinnitus) • CT/MRI • Angiography
Lymphoma	• History (constitutional symptoms) • Lymphadenopathy • CBC
Metastatic disease	• History • PETCT
Meningioma	• History • CT/MRI
Carotid artery aneurysm	• Neck mass/bruit • CTA/MRA
Chiari malformation, type 1	• History (headache, nausea, tinnitus) • CT/MRI
Multiple sclerosis	• History • CSF • MEP • MRI
Infection (eg, Lyme disease)	• History (exposure) • CBC, Ab • CSF

PITFALLS

Controversy surrounds the management of benign cervical and skull base lesions. Surgical extirpation carries potentially devastating functional consequences for lesions intimately related to the lower cranial nerves, which at times present little immediate or potential harm to patients. However, for such lesions, including vagal schwannoma, conservative approaches may not be advantageous as generally benign soft tissue tumors may undergo malignant transformation, and surgery may become riskier as a tumor expands.[20]

In evaluating such patients, it should be remembered that dysphonia and dysphagia are symptoms rather than diagnoses. Appropriate assessment of hoarseness and swallowing dysfunction and ultimately their effective treatment requires multidisciplinary evaluation and care. In the complex motor and sensory deficits resulting from cranial nerve palsy, management should be guided by the multidimensional appraisal of overall patient condition and symptoms as well as objective evaluation of dysfunction.

DISCUSSION

A variety of conditions cause lower CN palsy, and often deficits occur iatrogenically in the treatment of malignant or locally advanced benign tumors. Although surgical resection is the mainstay of treatment for such lesions, the impact on laryngopharyngeal function (when CN X is at risk) ought to be carefully considered. We rely on retrospective series and heterogeneous reviews to inform the prognosis and rehabilitative techniques in such patients.

Prognosis Lower Cranial Nerve Palsy

Voice and swallowing prognoses vary among reported case series and reviews. In the worst case, surgery at the skull base, adjacent to the lower cranial nerves, has historically been reported to cause aspiration in up to 75% of patients.[21] This is likely explained by the cumulative effect of multiple lower cranial neuropathies.

Recent reports suggest a more optimistic outcome. In Fang's 2011 series of 17 patients who had high-vagal injuries (of various cause), 12 were initially feeding tube dependent. All of these patients had sudden onset of CN X dysfunction (iatrogenic or cerebrovascular accident). Four patients improved with time and swallowing therapy, allowing for feeding tube removal. All but one of the remaining feeding tubes were removed following laryngoplasty with or without arytenoid adduction.[6]

A systematic review of 35 cases of surgically managed vagal schwannomas found that 26.4% had no postoperative complications. Hoarseness was reported by 22.6% even though UVFI was found confirmed in 35.8%. Of those, 47.4% experienced full or partial recovery.[11] With his group, Califano reported their experience with vagal schwannoma resection requiring CN X nerve sacrifice. They found that less than half of patients (40%) reported dysphagia, and when VFSS results were available, abnormalities were limited to aspiration by one patient and pharyngeal residue in two patients. No patients required feeding tube placement. In their cohort, all patients ultimately achieved Functional Oral Intake Scale (FOIS) 7 (normal diet) with swallow therapy with or without type I thyroplasty (performed in 70% of patients).[12]

With these outcomes in mind, concern for swallowing deficit should not prohibit early vagal schwannoma resection, as long as patients receive appropriate rehabilitation for swallow dysfunction and glottic incompetence.

Additional Assessment of Lower Cranial Nerve Palsy

Evolving technologies may assist in the accurate assessment and reliable prevention of debilitating lower CN palsy.

Electromyography

Increasingly used to predict long-term function in RLN injury, electromyography (EMG) may play a role in preserving motor nerve function during schwannoma resection. In their series of extracranial schwannomas, Ijichi and colleagues used EMG stimulation for nerve mapping during surgical schwannoma excision. They observed favorable results, with only 2 patients reporting dysphonia after vagal schwannoma resection. Both were reported to have improved within 1 year. Of the 15 patients managed with this nerve preservation technique, no tumor recurrence was reported.[22]

Manometry

Manometric evaluation of swallowing has evolved over the past several decades, and it is increasingly being applied outside of the esophagus—to the pharynx and upper esophageal sphincter (UES). Manometry can quantify pharyngeal deglutitive forces and detect failure of UES relaxation and the relative coordination of pharyngeal contraction and UES relaxation.[23] In a 1995 report on the use of solid-state manometry in UVFI, patterns of motility corresponded to site of lesion: UES dysfunction was observed with central lesions, whereas pharyngeal dysfunction was observed with peripheral lesion.[24]

Application of contemporary manometry technology, high-resolution manometry (HRM), reveals similar findings in patients with peripheral UVFI. UES residual pressure was abnormal in only a minority (one third) of patients, but all demonstrated abnormal pharyngeal pressures. This included both abnormally elevated and reduced pressure. HRM results were compared with VFSS findings. Thirty-two percent of patients aspirated on VFSS and were more likely to have low pharyngeal pressures compared with non-aspirators.[25]

Rehabilitation Techniques in Lower Cranial Nerve

Interventions for CN X palsy target dysphonia and related glottic insufficiency as well as dysphagia due to laryngopharyngeal motor and sensory deficits. The latter cannot be easily corrected, and impaired swallowing is likely to cause greater detriment to patient quality of life relative to short-term hoarseness. In mild or suspected temporary cases of swallowing impairment, specific maneuvers (head turn to affected side, supraglottic swallow, double swallow) and behaviors (alternating solids and liquids, carbonated beverage swallows, small bolus size) can be employed.[21] In other cases, procedural interventions (described below) may be more effective. Of course, interpretation of results and technique efficacy are often limited by missing standardized or objective assessment metrics.

Medialization Thyroplasty and Arytenoid Adduction

Type I thyroplasty converts previously lost subglottic air pressure into acoustic power. Furthermore, improving glottic closing pressure helps maintain pharyngeal pressures thought to assist bolus transport during deglutition.[26] However, despite improved glottic closing pressure, it is not completely normalized, which might explain why dysphagia and aspiration may persist following thyroplasty.[7,27]

A report from 1997 by Flint described 84 patients with UVFI, 10 of whom had combined SLN and RLN dysfunction. All patients reported dysphonia and 61% reported dysphagia, which was more common in the combined SLN/RLN dysfunction patient. Thyroplasty improved swallowing in all patients, resulting in feeding tube removal in all but 2 patients.[7]

In Pou's series of 35 patients with high vagal lesions, medialization with or without arytenoid adduction offered significant benefit. Aspiration was improved by 94%. Over three-quarters of patients with tracheostomies were decannulated. In 90% of patients, voice symptoms were subjectively improved.[4]

In the lateral skull base population, early thyroplasty yields acceptable voice and swallowing outcomes and avoids need for tracheostomy.[28]

In his series, Bielamowicz reported that arytenoid adduction alone for high vagal lesion improved voice in 76% of patients. Sixty-six percent required a feeding tube for an additional year and one-quarter went on to require thyroplasty.[1]

Reinnervation

Restoring laryngopharyngeal muscle tone or sensation through CN reinnervation has been an area of active clinical and research interest. The use of ansa cervicalis to RLN anastomosis has most commonly been evaluated.[29] Its utility for RLN palsy is debated. For high CN X lesions, direct vagal to RLN anastomosis has been proposed. Two cases were reported in a 2015 publication. A 49-year-old asymptomatic man with 3 cm vagal schwannoma who underwent vagus to RLN anastomosis at time of resection and CN X sacrifice reportedly recovered quite well. Specifically, maximum phonation time, glottis configuration, and VHI-10 normalized by 18 months.[30] This may represent a rehabilitation strategy moving forward in appropriate patients.

Cricopharyngeal Myotomy

To address CP dysfunction, myotomy has been added to glottic incompetence procedures. In his series of combined early thyroplasty type I and inferior constrictor/CP myotomy for postop skull base surgery patients, Montgomery describes subjective good outcomes, particularly when the medialization and CP myotomy are performed simultaneously rather than sequentially.[31]

The combined procedure was further supported by Woodson. In her series of 13 patients with combined laryngeal and pharyngeal paralysis, arytenoid adduction and CP myotomy were very effective in improving dysphonia and dysphagia. Of note, results were poorer in patients with central as opposed to peripheral nerve lesions.[32]

Pharyngoplasty

Another adjunct to thyroplasty and/or arytenoid adduction to address swallowing impairment is hypopharyngeal pharyngoplasty. This procedure, described by Woo in 2003, aims to both reduce excess pharyngeal dilation and improve pharyngeal tone or tautness.[19]

SUMMARY

Lower CN palsy, specifically involving the vagus nerve, yields a spectrum of voice and swallowing complaints. In general, with more central lesions or multiply affected CNs, greater clinical deficits are observed. In the setting of iatrogenic injury, many patients recover well without invasive intervention. Patients reporting dysphonia or dysphagia from suspected high vagal lesion should be objectively assessed for anatomic and functional deficits. When appropriate, these can be addressed in order to restore glottic competence and improve laryngopharyngeal motor and sensory deficits. We might improve our capacity to assess these patients and predict outcomes with application of new technologies, including HRM and EMG. For more systematic assessment of outcomes related to interventions, prospective record keeping and use of measurable functional outcomes is critical.

REFERENCES

1. Bielamowicz S, Gupta A, Sekhar LN. Early arytenoid adduction for vagal paralysis after skull base surgery. *Laryngoscope.* 2000;110(3 pt 1):346–351.
2. Perie S, Coiffier L, Laccourreye L, Hazebroucq V, Chaussade S, St Guily JL. Swallowing disorders in paralysis of the lower cranial nerves: a functional analysis. *Ann Otol Rhinol Laryngol.* 1999;108(6):606–611.

3. Myssiorek D. Recurrent laryngeal nerve paralysis: anatomy and etiology. *Otolaryngol Clin North Am.* 2004;37(1): 25–44, v.

4. Pou AM, Carrau RL, Eibling DE, Murry T. Laryngeal framework surgery for the management of aspiration in high vagal lesions. *Am J Otolaryngol.* 1998;19(1):1–7.

5. Sanders I, Li Y, Biller H. Axons enter the human posterior cricoarytenoid muscle from the superior direction. *Arch Otolaryngol Head Neck Surg.* 1995;121(7):754–757; discussion 758.

6. Fang TJ, Tam YY, Courey MS, Li HY, Chiang HC. Unilateral high vagal paralysis: relationship of the severity of swallowing disturbance and types of injuries. *Laryngoscope.* 2011;121(2):245–249.

7. Flint PW, Purcell LL, Cummings CW. Pathophysiology and indications for medialization thyroplasty in patients with dysphagia and aspiration. *Otolaryngol Head Neck Surg.* 1997;116(3):349–354.

8. Biswas D, Marnane CN, Mal R, Baldwin D. Extracranial head and neck schwannomas—a 10-year review. *Auris Nasus Larynx.* 2007;34(3):353–359.

9. Liu HL, Yu SY, Li GK, Wei WI. Extracranial head and neck schwannomas: a study of the nerve of origin. *Eur Arch Otorhinolaryngol.* 2011;268(9):1343–1347.

10. Kang GC, Soo KC, Lim DT. Extracranial non-vestibular head and neck schwannomas: a ten-year experience. *Ann Acad Med Singapore.* 2007;36(4):233–238.

11. Cavallaro G, Pattaro G, Iorio O, Avallone M, Silecchia G. A literature review on surgery for cervical vagal schwannomas. *World J Surg Oncol.* 2015;13:130.

12. Patel MA, Eytan DF, Bishop J, Califano JA. Favorable swallowing outcomes following vagus nerve sacrifice for vagal schwannoma resection. *Otolaryngol Head Neck Surg.* 2017;156(2):329–333.

13. Battoo AJ, Sheikh ZA, Thankappan K, Hicks W, Jr., Iyer S, Kuriakose MA. Nerve-sparing subcapsular resection of head and neck schwannomas: technique evaluation and literature review. *J Laryngol Otol.* 2013;127(7):685–690.

14. St Pierre S, Theriault R, Leclerc JE. Schwannomas of the vagus nerve in the head and neck. *J Otolaryngol.* 1985; 14(3):167–170.

15. Lahoti BK, Kaushal M, Garge S, Aggarwal G. Extra vestibular schwannoma: a two year experience. *Indian J Otolaryngol Head Neck Surg.* 2011;63(4):305–309.

16. Woodson GE. Configuration of the glottis in laryngeal paralysis. I: clinical study. *Laryngoscope.* 1993;103(11 pt 1): 1227–1234.

17. Chin SC, Edelstein S, Chen CY, Som PM. Using CT to localize side and level of vocal cord paralysis. *AJR Am J Roentgenol.* 2003;180(4):1165–1170.

18. Vachha B, Cunnane MB, Mallur P, Moonis G. Losing your voice: etiologies and imaging features of vocal fold paralysis. *J Clin Imaging Sci.* 2013;3:15.

19. Mok P, Woo P, Schaefer-Mojica J. Hypopharyngeal pharyngoplasty in the management of pharyngeal paralysis: a new procedure. *Ann Otol Rhinol Laryngol.* 2003;112(10): 844–852.

20. Ogawa T, Kato T, Ikeda A, et al. Case of malignant transformation of vagus nerve schwannoma to angiosarcoma. *Head Neck.* 2014;36(2):E17–E20.

21. Jennings KS, Siroky D, Jackson CG. Swallowing problems after excision of tumors of the skull base: diagnosis and management in 12 patients. *Dysphagia.* 1992;7(1): 40–44.

22. Ijichi K, Kawakita D, Maseki S, Beppu S, Takano G, Murakami S. Functional nerve preservation in extracranial head and neck schwannoma surgery. *JAMA Otolaryngol Head Neck Surg.* 2016;142(5):479–483.

23. Hila A, Castell JA, Castell DO. Pharyngeal and upper esophageal sphincter manometry in the evaluation of dysphagia. *J Clin Gastroenterol.* 2001;33(5):355–361.

24. Wilson JA, Pryde A, White A, Maher L, Maran AG. Swallowing performance in patients with vocal fold motion impairment. *Dysphagia.* 1995;10(3):149–154.

25. Pinna BR, Herbella FAM, de Biase N, Vaiano TCG, Patti MG. High-resolution manometry evaluation of pressures at the pharyngo-upper esophageal area in patients with oropharyngeal dysphagia due to vagal paralysis. *Dysphagia.* 2017.

26. Shin T, Umezaki T, Maeyama T, Morikawa I. Glottic closure during swallowing in the recurrent laryngeal nerve-paralyzed cat. *Otolaryngol Head Neck Surg.* 1989; 100(3):187–194.

27. Iwanaga Y, Maeyama T, Umezaki T, Shin T. Intracordal injection increases glottic closing force in recurrent laryngeal nerve paralysis. *Otolaryngol Head Neck Surg.* 1992; 107(3):451–456.

28. Netterville JL, Jackson CG, Civantos F. Thyroplasty in the functional rehabilitation of neurotologic skull base surgery patients. *Am J Otol.* 1993;14(5):460–464.

29. Paniello RC, Edgar JD, Kallogjeri D, Piccirillo JF. Medialization versus reinnervation for unilateral vocal fold paralysis: a multicenter randomized clinical trial. *Laryngoscope.* 2011;121(10):2172–2179.

30. Ward GM, Sauder C, Olson GT, Nuara MJ. Longitudinal voice outcomes following laryngeal reinnervation via vagus-to-recurrent laryngeal nerve anastomosis after vagal nerve sacrifice: a case series. *Ann Otol Rhinol Laryngol.* 2015;124(2):153–157.

31. Montgomery WW, Hillman RE, Varvares MA. Combined thyroplasty type I and inferior constrictor myotomy. *Ann Otol Rhinol Laryngol.* 1994;103(11):858–862.

32. Woodson G. Cricopharyngeal myotomy and arytenoid adduction in the management of combined laryngeal and pharyngeal paralysis. *Otolaryngol Head Neck Surg.* 1997;116(3):339–343.

CHAPTER 51

Vagal Injury Following Ruptured Carotid Pseudoaneurysm

Anna Miles and Jacqueline Allen

Cranial nerve damage can occur for a variety of reasons—blunt or penetrating trauma, surgery, inflammation, infection, and tumor being most common. It may be isolated to a single cranial nerve or involve more than one nerve, particularly those that are co-located. Injury may be partial or total and either transient or permanent. Given the crucial role that cranial nerves play in respiration, deglutition, communication, and control homeostasis, injury may have broad and serious repercussions and require significant input to reach satisfactory functional outcomes.

In the head and neck region there is little redundant tissue. Vital neurovascular structures are separated by only tens of millimeters at most. Therefore a seemingly small injury may result in significant damage to neurovascular structures and may have greater impact and more severe consequences than a similar sized injury elsewhere in the body. A high index of suspicion is needed regarding potential disruption to neurovascular bundles in the neck and face. Thorough examination and investigation assists in identifying injury and may avoid unexpected deterioration or worsening of injury.

DEFINITION

Cranial nerve injury is damage from any cause that results in dysfunction or non-function of the affected cranial nerve. Symptom manifestations depend on which cranial nerve(s) is(are) involved.

CASE PRESENTATION

A 58-year-old Polynesian man presents with a 2-month history of toothache and neck mass.

Social: Living on an isolated Pacific Island, conservation ranger, non-smoker

Medical history: Type II diabetes for 4 years, hypertension

Initial Assessment (Days 1–3)

History

Two-month history of enlarging left neck mass. Flown from the Pacific Island to a large, tertiary hospital in a neighboring developed country for further investigation and management.

Examination

On admission large left neck mass noted, tender to palpation, cranial nerve (CN) XII palsy present with dysphagia, dysarthria, and limitation of neck movement.

Endoscopy

Laryngeal displacement and skewing due to left parapharyngeal swelling with effacement of left pyriform fossa and displacement of the glottis to the right causing airway compromise. Mobile vocal folds and complete glottal closure. No ulcerated mass lesion within pharynx. A nasogastric tube was inserted due to aspiration risk.

Non-Contrast Neck CT (due to renal impairment)

Large mass filling left neck, 8.5 × 13 cm with multiple enlarged left supraclavicular lymph nodes, and significant displacement of larynx with mild airway narrowing.

Underwent an open biopsy of left cervical lymphadenopathy, pharyngoscopy, and biopsy of left tongue base, and open tracheostomy procedure (size 8 cuffed Portex tube placed, cuff deflated).

Head and Neck Multidisciplinary Team Discussion

Radiology suggestive of large necrotic metastatic squamous cell carcinoma. No distant metastatic disease noted. Biopsy results unknown as yet. Current plan to offer palliative radiotherapy pending biopsy result.

Day 6

Biopsy results reported as non-diagnostic.

Repeat Open Biopsies

Team plan recommended repeat open biopsies with frozen section.

In operating room, an open approach to left neck mass was undertaken. Sternocleidomastoid was retracted laterally and a large amount of organized hematoma identified which also appeared necrotic. Beneath the hematoma a large smooth mass was visualized—not expansile or pulsatile. As clots were suctioned, profound bleeding erupted and pseudoaneurysm of left internal carotid artery diagnosed. Severe active bleeding required pressure control and cavity packing. Urgent vascular consult was requested leading to salvage by use of covered endoluminal stents (Viabahn 7 mm and atrium 8 mm stents in a stepdown fashion) before the neck wound was closed.

Post-Surgical Contrast Computed Tomography Angiogram (CTA)

Confirmed left common carotid pseudoaneurysm likely at the carotid bifurcation. No signs of metastatic disease.

Diagnosis—Left Common Carotid Artery Pseudoaneurysm

Day 2 Post-Surgery Endoscopy

Severe pharyngeal/laryngeal edema with the laryngeal vestibule unable to be visualized due to edema and significant secretions throughout the pharynx. Silent aspiration of secretions noted (New Zealand Secretion Scale[1] [NZSS] 7)[1] (Figures 51–1 and 51–2, Table 51–1). Pharynx immobile, poor tongue motion. Palsy of CN X, XI, XII.

Postoperative Management (Weeks 2–3)

Multiple wound washouts and further evacuation of hematoma required. Intravenous cefazolin and metronidazole plus dexamethasone administered. Nasogastric tube feeding continued. Tracheostomy management.

Postoperative Management (Months 1–3)

Definitive carotid surgery performed with carotid artery interposition patch graft with procured vein from limb. Stable surgical site with healing and completion of 4-week antibiotic course. Pulmonary function stable. Decision made to decannulate tracheostomy despite laryngeal dysfunction.

Laryngeal Evaluation

Mobile right vocal fold (reduced adduction) with immobile, lateralized left vocal fold. Supraglottic edema and reduced pharyngeal sensation to endoscope contact. Incomplete glottal closure. Asthenic, breathy voicing, bovine cough, and poor secretion clearance.

Swallow Evaluation

Functional endoscopic evaluation of swallowing (FEES) by ward speech-language therapist and otorhinolaryngologist were completed. Despite some response observed to touching of vocal folds (laryngeal adductor reflex) with endoscope, there was continued silent aspiration of secretions (NZSS 7; Penetration-Aspiration Scale[2] [PAS] 8), with secretions pooling in left vallecula, left pyriform fossa, and across the apices of both pyriforms as well as filling the post-cricoid region. Pharyngeal squeeze absent. No regurgitation of secretions through pharyngoesophageal segment. Very poor bolus

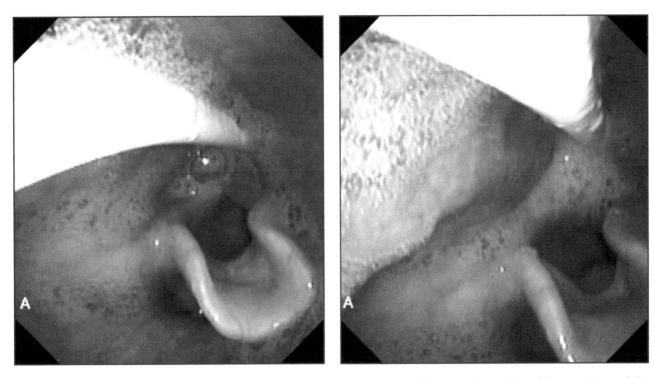

Figures 51–1 and 51–2. Flexible nasendoscopy views at week 1 post-rupture demonstrating a skewed larynx, edema of the interarytenoid region and gross foamy secretions filling the pharynx. There is aspiration of secretions and marked residue throughout the pharynx.

Table 51–1. Swallowing Outcome Measures

New Zealand Secretion Scale (NZSS) (Miles et al, 2018)[1]	New Zealand Secretion Scale (Miles et al., 2017)		
	Category	**Symptom**	**Score**
	Location	Nil significant pooled secretions in pyriform fossae or laryngeal vestibule	0
		Secretions in pyriform fossae (above 20%)	1
		Secretions in laryngeal vestibule (beyond healthy lubrication of mucosa)	2
	Amount in pyriform fossae	Nil significant pooled secretions in pyriform fossae (0–20%)	0
		Secretions in pyriform fossae, not yet full (20–80%)	1
		Secretions filling (80–100%) or overspilling pyriform fossae / inter-arytenoid space	2
	Response (*do not score if no significant pooling of secretions*)	*Normal airway responses in the pharynx or laryngeal vestibule may include spontaneous coughing, throat clearing, and/or swallowing*	
		Secretions in pyriform fossae or laryngeal vestibule effectively cleared	0
		Ineffective attempts to clear or no response to secretions in pyriform fossae	1
		Ineffective attempts to clear secretions from laryngeal vestibule	2
		No response to secretions in laryngeal vestibule	3
	TOTAL (maximum 7)		

(*continues*)

Table 51–1. (*continued*)

Penetration-Aspiration Scale (Rosenbek et al, 1996)[2]	1. Material does not enter the airway.
	2. Material enters the airway, remains above the vocal folds and is ejected from the airway.
	3. Material enters the airway, remains above the vocal folds, and is not ejected from the airway.
	4. Material enters the airway, contacts the vocal folds, and is ejected from the airway.
	5. Material enters the airway, contacts the vocal folds, and is not ejected from the airway.
	6. Material enters the airway, passes below the vocal folds, and is ejected into the larynx or out of the airway.
	7. Material enters the airway, passes below the vocal folds, and is not ejected from the trachea, despite effort.
	8. Material enters the airway, passes below the vocal folds, and no effort is made to eject.

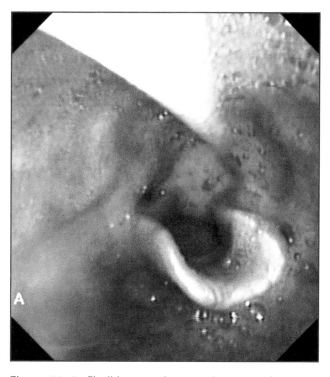

Figure 51–3. Flexible nasendoscopy view at week 1 post-rupture demonstrating blue discolouration of secretions due to swallowed food dye with aspiration of secretions and copious pharyngeal residue.

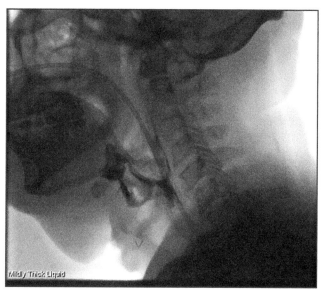

Figure 51–4. Lateral videofluoroscopic view one week following rupture demonstrating nasogastric tube in situ, grossly patulous piriform sinuses with valleculae and piriform residue.

transit. No clearance response to aspirated material (PAS 8) (Figure 51–3).

Conclusion

Moderate-severe oropharyngeal dysphagia characterized by pharyngeal weakness and reduced airway protection. Marked pharyngeal residue accumulates and spills from pyriform sinuses over the interarytenoid bar and aryepiglottic ligament into the laryngeal vestibule. Clearing swallows to reduce residue were only partially effective. Prompted cough to clear and repetitive swallow encouraged.

Videofluoroscopic Study of Swallowing

Severe-profound pharyngeal stage dysphagia characterized by minimal pharyngeal constriction and no pharyngoesophageal segment opening (Figure 51–4). Absent airway response to penetration/aspiration (PAS 8).

Nasogastric feeding converted to percutaneous endoscopic gastrostomy (PEG) and minimal oral intake with strict mouth care. Swallow rehabilitation program developed to allow return to home and family. Patient is primary breadwinner and keen to return to work. Swallowing rehabilitation program was to be supported with weekly email/video-chat review with speech-language therapist in Islands.

In view of the profound pharyngeal impairments, a combination of saliva frequency swallowing, effortful swallows, Masako swallows, and Chin Tuck Against Resistance (CTAR) was recommended (Table 51–2).

Table 51–2. Swallowing Rehabilitation Program

Task		Instruction
Task 1.	STOP spitting your saliva into tissues and START swallowing!	
Task 2.	**Saliva swallows** Purpose: To make you swallow your saliva more often and to stop saliva collecting in your mouth and throat.	Goal: In order to return to swallowing, you need to start swallowing. Exercise: 1. Sit comfortably and turn you head to the side. 2. Swallow every 30 seconds for 5 minutes
Task 3.	**Masako Maneuver** Purpose: The base of tongue plays an important role in pushing the food or liquid down the throat during a swallow. If the base of tongue and the back wall of the throat don't push against each other hard enough, food/drink can be left behind after the swallow.	Goal: To strengthen the back wall of the throat Exercise: Place your tongue between your front teeth and swallow your saliva. Complete the exercise 15 times (*extend number of times as you get stronger*)
Task 4.	**Effortful swallowing** Purpose: To continue to build up strength in the muscles in your throat that are important for swallowing—mainly the back wall of the throat. Also, this exercise is useful in helping you to swallow more difficult foods as it encourages you to get all the muscles working as much as they can, helping the food/drink to travel through your throat quickly and easily, leaving no residue behind.	Goal: To strengthen the back wall of the throat Exercise: Relax your muscles in your throat and then do a "hard swallow," exaggerating the muscle movements as best you can. If it helps, turn you head to the side. Repeat 15 times (*extend number of times as you get stronger*)
Task 5.	**Chin Tuck Against Resistance Exercise** Purpose: The neck muscles play an important role in closing the airway and opening the food pipe during a swallow. Without strong neck muscles, food and fluids goes into the airway or sticks around in the throat after a swallow.	Goal: To strengthen the throat muscles Exercise 1—HOLD: 1. Sit in a chair with the ball under your chin 2. Lower your chin to press the ball 3. Hold for 30 seconds (*extend this up to 60 seconds as you get stronger*) 4. Repeat the above 3 times with 1 minute breaks in between Exercise 2—REPETITIONS: 1. Keep the ball under your chin 2. Lower and raise your chin to press the ball 30 times (*extend this up to 60 times as you get stronger*) 3. Keep your shoulders relaxed

MANAGEMENT

- PEG feeding for nutritional needs
- Swallowing rehabilitation program—three times a week with therapist/three times a day exercises in home
- Review in 3 months

12-Month Review

Reviewed for first time at our Swallow Center. The speech-language therapist on the Island had been unable to contact the patient on his phone or email address during the 9-month period. Exercises had not been completed and 10 kg weight loss had occurred due to difficulties accessing PEG feeds at home.

FEES: no change in swallowing function. The oral cavity showed carious dentition and increasing gingivitis. Tongue mobility present and tongue dorsum was dry. Secretions continued to pool in the pharynx with continuing left vocal fold immobility and absent pharyngeal constriction on the left during pharyngeal squeeze activity.

MANAGEMENT

- Swallowing rehabilitation program—three times a week speech-language therapy support/three times a day exercise completion emphasized
- PEG feeds arranged and procured
- Review in 3 months at Swallow Center

15-Month Review

Swallowing rehabilitation program had been successfully implemented, with regular contact between patient and speech-language therapist.

FEES: minimal pooling of secretions in the pyriform apices (NZSS 2) and spontaneously swallowing his saliva. True vocal folds demonstrated asymmetry with a completely immobile left vocal fold and a fully mobile right vocal fold. Bilateral glottic edema with left vocal fold demonstrating pseudosulcus, slumping, and poor tension. The arytenoid is also hooded over the posterior aspect of the left true vocal fold. Glottal closure is incomplete, with a persistent 1 to 2 mm glottal gap which significantly impacts drinking liquids. Premature spill and direct penetration and aspiration of thin liquids is seen. Immediate cough response is seen (PAS 6) and ability to clear aspirated volume.

Compensatory left head turn and chin tuck resolved aspiration of puree and solid but there remained penetration and PAS 4 response to thin liquid contact with true vocal folds. No regurgitation was seen and improvement in pharyngeal strength was noted particularly on the right side; however, the left remained fairly atonic. Laryngeal sensation also improved with epiglottic touch triggering cough and laryngeal adductor reflex.

MANAGEMENT

- Recommended left vocal fold injection laryngoplasty.
- Microlaryngoscopy and left vocal fold injection laryngoplasty with calcium

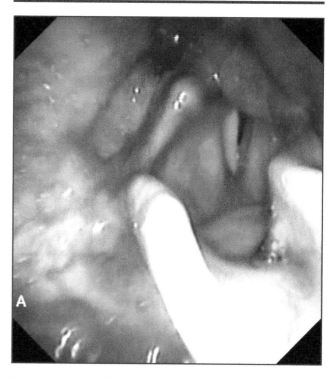

Figure 51–5. Flexible nasendoscopy view at 15 months post-rupture demonstrating reduced interarytenoid edema and laryngeal vestibule clear of most secretions and residue. Left vocal fold is paramedian and immobile. Posterior glottic gap still present but providing a respiratory function.

hydroxyapatite implant performed under general anesthetic. No complications.

- Purpose: improve airway protection during swallowing, increase cough efficiency and voice quality.
- FEES post-laryngoplasty: Right vocal fold mobile with left anterior vocal fold medialized. Anterior glottal contact achieved with improved voicing and cough. Posterior glottic gap still present but providing a respiratory function (Figure 51–5). Marked supraglottic compensation with both anterior and lateral squeeze (type II and type III closure pattern). Rough voice quality, however; patient feels voicing is easier and less tiring. Reduced secretions present in pharynx and swallow efficiency improved.

MANAGEMENT

- Increase to normal diet/normal fluids with a head turn to the left
- Removal of PEG
- Reduction of rehabilitation exercises

At 2 years post-injury patient remains on full oral diet with functional voicing and returned to full-time work as conservation ranger (Table 51–3).

DISCUSSION

While malignancy is common, and often late presenting when patients live in rural or remote areas with poor access to health care resources, there must be a high index of suspicion for other causes of neck mass in underdeveloped regions. Tropical infectious diseases are more common in island settings, and tuberculosis rates are significant in the Pacific Islands in general with around 24,000 new cases per year in the Western Pacific region.[3] Carotid pseudoaneurysm is a rare presentation of neck mass but has been described in the setting of infection including mycotic infections, direct injury to the neck, post-surgical injury, post-treatment tissue damage and spontaneously.[4–11] Trauma to the neck may result in significant injury to neurovascular structures, with lack of awareness of the nature of a mass increasing the risk of complications and iatrogenic injury.

Carotid pseudoaneursym may occur anywhere along the course of the carotid artery. Depending on location of the mass (skull base vs carotid bifurcation) symptoms and signs may include dysphagia, dysphonia, tongue weakness or atrophy, Horner's syndrome, conductive hearing loss, and autonomic dysfunction.[6,10,12,13] At times the mass may be expansile or pulsatile, but often this is not the case, particularly if partial or complete thrombosis has occurred. Any patient with high (proximal) vagal nerve disruption, whether

Table 51–3. Trajectory of Swallowing, Voice, and Cough Impairments Over Time

Impairment		On Hospital Discharge	After 4 Months of Swallowing Rehabilitation	After Left Vocal Fold Laryngoplasty
Voice	Perceptual Voice Profile	Severe breathy dysphonia with moderate strain.	Severe breathy dysphonia with moderate strain.	Mild-moderate breathy dysphonia.
		Wet voice quality.	Wet voice quality.	No wet quality.
	VHI	25 (severely elevated)	17 (mildly elevated)	7 (normal)
Oral intake	EAT-10	40 (severely elevated)	25 (moderately elevated)	12 (mildly elevated)
	FOIS	Nil-by-mouth	Minced/moist diet/normal fluids	Normal diet/fluids
Cough	Perceptual cough strength	Unable to cough, wet upper airways	Weak, wet bovine cough with inspiratory stridor	Adequate cough
	Reflexive cough	No response to aspiration saliva or oral trials	Ineffective response aspiration of oral intake	No aspiration observed
Nutritional status	Weight	53 kg	63 kg	67 kg

caused by infection, surgical trauma, other treatment (e.g., radiotherapy and/or inflammation), is likely to suffer from significant impairments in swallowing, cough, and voice abilities.[14] Depending on the cause of neural injury, various levels of recovery may be expected. Division of a cranial nerve is associated with long-term dysfunction, and level of recovery depends on whether neurorrhaphy is undertaken and age at injury. Injury whereby the neural elements remain intact within the neurolemma results in a greater range of recovery and, as in this case, may achieve good functional outcomes over time.[4,12] Diagnosis of vascular origin is best made by either angiography or computed tomography angiography (less invasive).[11,15] Open biopsy is not recommended and, as demonstrated by this case, can lead to catastrophic bleeding. In some cases bleeding may be the presenting symptom, often as epistaxis[6,16] but may also be pharyngeal. Carotid blowout is seen in patients with tumor progression or radiation-induced tissue degeneration[6,9] and can be a terminal event unless emergent management is undertaken. Control of bleeding may be achieved surgically, as in this case, with a stent or homograft to address the aneurysmal segment.[5,8,12,13,16,17] More recently endovascular control with stents, coils, or balloon occlusion has been successfully reported.[6,7,8,17]

In this case the patient presented with cranial nerve X and XII impairment and signs of skull base involvement consistent with other reported presentations of carotid pseudoaneurysm. CT scanning identified the mass responsible in the neck and extending to the skull base with direct pressure effects. Nasopharyngeal cancer is highly prevalent in Polynesian people and this was presumed to be the cause, although lack of definitive histopathological diagnosis from the initial biopsy should have alerted the team to a possible alternative diagnosis. The erroneous belief that necrotic tissue was due to malignancy resulted in the traumatic rupture of the pseudoaneurysm during the second surgical procedure. Once the cause of neck mass had been correctly identified, however, definitive treatment could be provided. This stabilized the neck and prevented further injury. Replacement of the covered stent with a homograft was required so that all diseased arterial tissue could be removed, preventing a relapse in the future. Long-term impairment was a result of the combination of pressure effects from the pseudoaneursym and post-surgical injury.

The response to therapy is important here. As the vascular structures were repaired and the neural pathways remained intact peripherally, gradual improvement was achieved. This was significantly enhanced by a graded program of rehabilitation, supported by speech language therapy and dietetic input. As demonstrated by the lack of response in the 6 to 12 month window, when no meaningful rehabilitative input was given, compared with the dramatic improvement at 12 to 18 months once a swallow rehabilitation program was instituted alongside glottal closure techniques, it is clear that providing ongoing and long-term support and guidance to patients recovering from cranial nerve trauma will achieve the best outcomes.

The end result of a return to a complete oral diet and ability to return to the workforce indicate substantial compensation and recovery of function.

SWALLOWING REHABILITATION PROGRAMS

There have been a number of studies exploring the effect of exercises on swallowing physiology after neurological diseases (stroke, Parkinson's disease) as well as after head and neck cancer and its treatments. Although duration and dosage remain poorly established, many rehabilitation studies show physiological change after a 6-week program. There is little evidence to guide rehabilitation of cranial nerve deficits or peripheral nerve damage as seen in a case such as this; however, it is reasonable to expect that similar functional improvement could be garnered from targeted exercises, compensatory maneuvers and strength programs. Recent literature supports purpose-specific rehabilitation rather than just strength, with biofeedback enabling participants to "see" their target and to aim to hit it rather than under- or overshooting. This control-based learning helps with complex motor tasks.[18] The exercise regimen recommended here is supported by literature demonstrating improvements in pharyngeal swallow parameters as follows.

Pharyngeal Constriction Impairments

Adequate retraction of the base of tongue toward the pharyngeal wall and overall pharyngeal constriction are critical for efficient transit of the bolus through the pharynx. The effortful swallow can be used as both a compensatory and a rehabilitative strategy by asking the patient to perform a hard effortful swallow.[19,20] Effortful swallow technique has been shown to improve base of tongue retraction, increase pharyngeal pressures, and lead to improved clearance of residue in patients after stroke.[20–23]

The Masako maneuver is an exercise designed to improve tongue retraction to the posterior pharyngeal wall. It is performed by placing the tongue tip between the front teeth and swallowing saliva.[20,24] In patients after stroke, the Masako maneuver has been shown to improve tongue pressures and improve movement of the posterior pharyngeal wall.[24–26] In patients with dysphagia following tongue-base resection, simultaneous videofluoroscopy-manometry Masako swallows showed increased pharyngeal contact to the base of the tongue and increase in hyolaryngeal pressures in comparison to non-maneuver swallows.[26]

Impaired Pharyngoesophageal Segment Opening

Antero-superior movement of the hyolaryngeal complex and opening of the pharyngoesophageal segment is critical for airway protection and transfer of the bolus into the esophagus. Exercises shown to improve hyolaryngeal excursion and pharyngoesophageal segment opening include Shaker head lift, Mendelsohn maneuver, and the more recent CTAR.

The Shaker head lift exercise program is completed while lying down with a regime of three times a day for 6 weeks and comprises both isometric (1 minute of sustained lifting of the head, looking toward toes) and isokinetic exercises (30 consecutive head-raise repetitions).[27] Improvements in hyolaryngeal excursion, width, and duration of pharyngoesophageal segment (PES) opening, and reduction in aspiration have been shown in both healthy adults and patients after stroke.[28–31]

CTAR is a more recent indirect rehabilitative technique for hyolaryngeal excursion and PES opening[32,33] and involves the same isometric and isokinetic exercises as the Shaker head lift program, but in this technique the patient places a ball under the chin and tucks the chin to press the ball.

> ## VOCAL FOLD AUGMENTATION IN DYSPHAGIA MANAGEMENT

Unilateral vocal fold paralysis is common and will inevitably lead to dysphonia[34] and in some cases aspiration (40%) due to incomplete glottal closure.[35] Injection medialization or laryngoplasty reduces this glottal gap

and such techniques have been shown to reduce aspiration and improve quality of life.[36–38] Early intervention (within first 6 months post-injury) also seems to reduce the need for possible framework surgery such as external thyroplasty in future.[39] Spontaneous recovery is dependent on mechanism of injury. Puccinelli et al report only a 10% spontaneous recovery rate in those with unilateral vocal fold paralysis (UVFP) following cardiothoracic procedures.[40] Fang et al report 17 patients with high vagal injury, 11 of whom had sudden onset traumatic injury and 6 with progressive compressive injury due to skull base tumors.[41] Those with sudden onset injuries demonstrated greater feeding tube dependence than those with slower onset swallow dysfunction, and recommendation for early laryngoplasty is made, particularly in the abrupt-onset group.[41] Both injection laryngoplasty and external thyroplasty have demonstrated benefit in management of swallow impairment. Hendricker et al report Gore-Tex thyroplasty in 57 patients with dysphagia and glottal incompetence.[42] Twenty of 57 (35%) were PEG dependent and 11/20 (55%) were able to discontinue PEG tube use following thyroplasty.[42]

Closure of the glottal gap does appear to improve symptomatic dysphagia as reported by Cates et al.[43] Self-reported dysphagia scores using the Eating Assessment Tool 10 showed significant improvement post-medialization of the affected vocal fold.[43] Graboyes and colleagues studied UVFP following thoracic surgery, demonstrating marked improvement from a nil-per-os (NPO) diet to oral intake in 94% of subjects who underwent injection laryngoplasty.[44] Ruddy et al reported improved voluntary cough parameters following medialization of immobile vocal folds, resulting in improved clearance of airway secretions and retained bolus in symptomatic patients.[38]

An alternative approach was used by Thakar et al. Type IV thyroplasty (cricothyroid approximation) was undertaken in five patients with combined superior and recurrent laryngeal nerve injuries.[45] All cases demonstrated improved vocal outcomes and safe swallowing by 6 weeks post-surgery. They felt that this approach repositioned the vocal folds in the same vertical plane and restored tension in the paralyzed fold achieving greater glottal competence.[45]

It is important to realize that, as in this case, swallow dysfunction is multifactorial. Particularly when multiple cranial nerve palsies are present, treatment for glottal incompetence may not resolve all swallow dysfunction. Nayak et al studied 67 patients who underwent glottal closure procedures (14 thyroplasties, 53 injection laryngoplasties) and reported a 24% rate of persistent aspiration.[36] Both intradeglutitive and post-deglutitive aspiration occurred and was related to pharyngeal dysfunction, presence of residue, and impaired hyolaryngeal elevation.[36] This reminds us that multiple strategies are needed to comprehensively manage traumatic neurogenic swallow dysfunction.

SUMMARY

Mycotic carotid artery aneurysm is an uncommon cause of neck mass; however, it may occur in young patients and may present with neurogenic dysfunction. Imaging prior to biopsy is recommended to avoid additional surgical trauma as demonstrated in this case. Swallow impairment due to multiple cranial nerve palsies requires a multifactorial approach. In this case, after a 4-month exercise program and a laryngoplasty, safe swallowing was achieved, allowing removal of feeding tube, return to a normal diet with improved voice quality, and a return to work.

REFERENCES

1. Miles A, Hunting A, McFarlane M, Caddy D, Scott S. Predictive value of the New Zealand Secretion Scale (NZSS) for pneumonia. *Dysphagia*. 2018;33(1):115–122 .
2. Rosenbek JC, Robbins JA, Roecker EB, Coyle JL, Wood JL. A penetration-aspiration scale. *Dysphagia*. 1996;11:93–98.
3. Viney K, Hoy D, Roth A, Kelly P, Harley D, Sleigh A. The epidemiology of tuberculosis in the Pacific. 2000 to 2013. *Western Pac Surveill Response J*. 205;19:59–67.
4. Majeed A, Ribeiro NP, Ali A, Hijazi M, Farook H. A rare presentation of spontaneous internal carotid artery dissection with Horner's syndrome, VIIth, Xth, XIIth nerve palsies. *Oxf Med Case Reports*. 2016;omw078:eCollection 2016 Oct.
5. Yousuf KM, Khan FG. Pseudoaneurysm of head and neck vessels has been frequently observed in road side bomb blast victims. *Surgeon*. 2016;14:142–146.
6. Dong F, Li Q, Wu J, Zhang M, Zhang F, Li B, Jin K, Min J, Liang W, Chao M. Carotid blowout syndrome after nasopharyngeal carcinoma radiotherapy: successful treatment by internal carotid artery occlusion after stent implantation failure. *Springerplus*. 2016. doi: 10.1186/s40064-016-3209-7. eCollection 2016.
7. Law Y, Chan YC, Cheng SW. Endovascular repair of giant traumatic pseudo-aneurysm of the common carotid artery. *World J Emerg Med*. 2015;6:229–232.
8. Pulli R, Dorigo W, Alessi Innocenti A, Pratesi G, Fargion A, Pratesi C. A 20-year experience with surgical management of true and false internal carotid artehry aneurysms. *Eur J Vasc Endovasc Surg*. 2013;45:1–6.
9. Girishkumar HT, Sivakumar M, Andaz S, Santosh V, Solomon R, Brown M. Pseudoaneurysm of the carotid bifurcation secondary to radiation. *J Cardiovasc Surg (Torino)*. 1999;40:877–878.
10. Oba M, Niizuma H, Kodama N, Endo M, Suzuki J. [Villaret's syndrome due to extra-cranial internal carotid aneurysm: a case report.] *No Shinkei Geka*. 1983;11:751–754.
11. Ooi GC, Irwin MG, Lam LK, Cheng SW. An unusual complication of emergency tracheal intubation. *Anaethesia*. 1997;52:154–158.
12. Hacein-Bey L, Blazum JM, Jackson RF. Carotid artery pseudoaneurysm after orthognathic surgery causing lower cranial nerve palsies: endovascular repair. *J Oral Maxillofac Surg*. 2013;71:1948–1955.
13. Fernandes CM, Robbs JV, Price AR. Septic erosion of the internal carotid artery. A case report. *J Laryngol Otol*. 1980;94:225–229.
14. Giraldez-Rodriguez LA, Johns M 3rd. Glottal insufficiency with aspiration risk in dysphagia. *Otolaryngol Clin North Am*. 2013; 46:1113–1121.
15. Desimpelaere J, Seynaeve P, Kockx M, Appel B, Gyselinck J, Mortelmans L. Mycotic pseudo-aneurysm of the extracranial carotid artery. *J Belge Radiol*. 1997;80: 170–171.
16. Bazina A, Mismas A, Hucika Z, Pavlisa G, Poljakovic Z. Endovascular treatment of internal carotid artery pseudo-aneurysm presenting with epistaxis. A case report. *Interv Neuroradiol*. 2014;20:743–745.
17. Miyachi S, Ishiguchi T, Taniguchi K, Miyazaki M, Maeda K. Endovascular stenting for pseudoaneurysms of the cervical carotid artery. *Interv Neuroradiol*. 1997;30 (suppl 2):129–132.
18. Huckabee M, McRae P. Rethinking rehab: skill-based training for swallowing impairment. *SIG 13 Perspect Swall Swall Dis (Dysphagia)*. 2014;23:46–53.
19. Groher M, Crary M. *Dysphagia: Clinical Management in Adults and Children*. 2nd ed. Maryland Heights, MO: Elsevier; 2016.
20. Johnson DN, Herring HJ, Daniels SK. *Curr Phys Med Rehabil Rep*. 2014;2:207. https://doi.org/10.1007/s40141-014-0059-9
21. Lever TE, Cox KT, Holbert D, Shahrier M, Hough M, Kelley-Salamon K. The effect of an effortful swallow on the normal adult esophagus. *Dysphagia*. 2007;22:312–325.
22. Nekl CG, Lintzenich CR, Leng X, Lever T, Butler SG. Effects of effortful swallow on esophageal function in healthy adults. *Neurogastroenterol Motil*. 2012;24:252–256.
23. Hind JA, Nicosia MA, Roecker EB, Carnes ML, Robbins J. Comparison of effortful and non-effortful swallows in healthy middle-aged and older adults. *Arch Phys Med Rehabil*. 2001;82:1661–1665.
24. Fujiu-Kurachi M. Developing the tongue holding maneuver. *Perspect Swallow Swallow Dis (Dysphagia) ASHA*. 2002;11:9–11.

25. Fujiu M, Logemann JA. Effect of a tongue-holding maneuver on posterior pharyngeal wall movement during deglutition. *Am J Speech-Lang Pathol.* 1996;5:23–30.

26. Lazarus C, Logemann JA, Song CW, Rademaker AW, Kahrilas PJ. Effects of voluntary manoeuvres on tongue base function for swallowing. *Foli Phoniatr Logop.* 2002; 54:171–176.

27. Easterling C, Grande B, Kern M, Sears K, Shaker R. Attaining and maintaining isometric and isokinetic goals of the Shaker exercise. *Dysphagia.* 2005;20:133–138.

28. Shaker R, Kern M, Bardan E, Taylor A, Stewart ET, Hoffmann RG, et al. Augmentation of deglutitive upper esophageal sphincter opening in the elderly by exercise. *Am J Physiol.* 1997;272(6 pt 1):G1518–G1522.

29. Shaker R, Easterling C, Kern M, et al. Rehabilitation of swallowing by exercise in tube-fed patients with pharyngeal dysphagia secondary to abnormal UES opening. *Gastroenterology.* 2002;122(5):1314–1321.

30. Don Kim K, Lee HJ, Lee MH, Ryu HJ. Effects of neck exercises on swallowing function of patients with stroke. *J Phys Ther Sci.* 2015;27(4):1005–1008.

31. Park T, Kim Y. Effects of tongue pressing effortful swallow in older healthy individuals. *Arch Gerontol Geriatr.* 2016;66:127–133.

32. Mishra A, Rajappa A, Tipton E, Malandraki GA. The recline exercise: comparisons with the head lift exercise in healthy adults. *Dysphagia.* 2015;30:730–737.

33. Kraaijenga SA, van der Molen L, Stuiver MM, Teertstra HJ, Hilgers FJ, van den Brekel MW. Effects of strengthening exercises on swallowing musculature and function in senior healthy subjects: a prospective effectiveness and feasibility study. *Dysphagia.* 2015;30:392–403.

34. Misono S, Merati A. Evidence-based practice: evaluation and management of unilateral vocal fold paralysis. *Otolaryngol Clin North Am.* 2012;45(5):1083–1108.

35. Toutounchi SJ, Eydi M, Golzari SE, Ghaffari MR, Parvizian N. Vocal cord paralysis and its etiologies: a prospective study. *J Cardiovasc Thorac Res.* 2015;6(1):47–50.

36. Nayak VK, Bhattacharyya N, Kotz T, Shapiro J. Patterns of swallowing failure following medialization in unilateral vocal fold immobility. *Laryngoscope.* 2002;112:1840–1844.

37. Andrade Filho P, Carrau R, Buckmire R. Safety and cost-effectiveness of intra-office flexible videolaryngoscopy with transoral vocal fold injection in dysphagic patients. *Am J Otolaryngol Head Neck Med Surg.* 2006;27:319–322.

38. Ruddy BH, Pitts TE, Lehman J, Spector B, Lewis V, Sapienza CM. Improved voluntary cough immediately following office-based vocal fold medialization injections. *Laryngoscope.* 2014;124:1645–1647.

39. Alghonaim Y, Roskies M, Kost K, Young J. Evaluating the timing of injection laryngoplasty for vocal fold paralysis in an attempt to avoid future type 1 thyroplasty. *J Otolaryngol Head Neck Surg.* 2013;42:24.

40. Puccinelli C, Modzeski MC, Orbelo D, Ekbom DC. Symptomatic unilateral vocal fold paralysis following cardiothoracic surgery. *Am J Otolaryngol.* 2018;39(2):175–179. doi: 10.1016/j.amjoto.2017.11.011

41. Fang TJ, Tam YY, Courey MS, Li HY, Chiang HC. Unilateral high vagal paralysis: relationship of the severity of swallowing disturbance and types of injuries. *Laryngoscope.* 2011;121:245–249.

42. Hendricker RM, deSilva BW, Forrest LA. Gore-Tex medialization laryngoplasty for treatment of dysphagia. *Otolaryngol Head Neck Surg.* 2010;142:536–539.

43. Cates DJ, Venkatesan NN, Strong B, Kuhn MA, Belafsky PC. Effect of vocal fold medialization on dysphagia in patients with unilateral vocal fold immobility. *Otolaryngol Head Neck Surg.* 2016;155:454–457.

44. Graboyes EM, Bradley JP, Meyers BF, Nussenbaum B. Efficacy and safety of acute injection laryngoplasty for vocal cord paralysis following thoracic surgery. *Laryngoscope.* 2011;121:2406–2410.

45. Thakar A, Sikka K, Verma R, Preetam C. Cricothyroid approximation for voice and swallowing rehabilitation of high vagal paralysis secondary to skull base neoplasms. *Eur Arch Otorhinolaryngol.* 2011;268:1611–1616.

CHAPTER 52

Dysphagia Following Head and Neck Cancer

Wendy Liu, Peter Loizou, and Faruque Riffat

STRUCTURAL PHARYNGEAL PROBLEMS, WITH A PRESENTATION ON POST CHEMORADIOTHERAPY STRICTURING OF HYPOPHARYNX AND ESOPHAGUS, AND A DIAGNOSIS OF MECHANICAL OBSTRUCTION

INTRODUCTION

Dysphagia, the sensation of hesitation or delay in the passage of food during swallowing, is a common and debilitating symptom. It can be subclassified by either location (oropharyngeal or esophageal) or by the circumstances in which it occurs (functional vs obstructive) (see "Differential Diagnosis" section). It is of particular relevance in head and neck cancer (HNC) and its treatment imposes significant immediate and long-term physical, emotional, and psychosocial burdens on both patients and carers. The complaint of dysphagia, especially if new-onset or progressive, is a red flag symptom and should always be taken seriously, as it may represent a neoplasm of the upper aerodigestive tract (UADT). A thorough medical history including focused closed questioning regarding onset, duration, presence of choking, and whether dysphagia is to liquids or solids should be ascertained. Further directed questions should comprise other red flag symptoms, which could also be associated with HNC, such as odynophagia, dysphonia, referred otalgia, and weight loss. This should then be followed up by a full head and neck examination including a flexible fiberoptic nasolaryngoscopy. Additional investigations such as esophagogastroduodenoscopy (± biopsy), barium swallow, and esophageal manometry can be undertaken to rule out other serious pathologies if the head/neck examination is unremarkable and the history is consistent with pathology more distal. Given its multifactorial etiology, successful management necessitates thorough clinical and instrumental assessment, multidisciplinary collaboration, targeted therapeutic interventions, and vigilant follow-up.

DEFINITION

Dysphagia, derived from the Greek words *dys* (with difficulty) and *phagein* (to eat), is the impairment of swallowing and represents an abnormality in the transit of solids or liquids from the oral cavity through the esophagus to the stomach.[1]

CASE PRESENTATION

History of Presenting Complaint

A 62-year-old man presents with a 5-week history of a left neck lump. He has also had the sensation of fullness in the throat and symptomatic difficulties with his swallowing over the last 2 weeks. However, there was no associated weight loss or hoarseness of voice. His diagnosis is T3N2aM0 supraglottic squamous cell carcinoma and he is commenced on primary modality chemoradiotherapy (CRT) (intensity-modulated radiotherapy [IMRT]) with curative intent.

Previous Medical History

Recent diagnosis of squamous cell carcinoma (SCC) of supraglottis.

Left-sided hearing impairment secondary to childhood measles infection.

Tonsillectomy.

Medications: Nil regular, undergoing chemoradiotherapy

Allergies: Nil known drug allergies

Family history: The patient's brother had bowel cancer and his father, who was a lifelong smoker, died of lung cancer.

Social history: The patient is a clerical worker who lives with his wife and three sons, ages 23, 25, and 27. He has never smoked but does drink socially.

Initial Assessment

History

Red flag symptoms (globus, dysphagia, odynophagia, weight loss, referred otalgia, and B symptoms [night sweats, anorexia, lethargy]). Presence of these symptoms warrants urgent investigation including flexible fiberoptic nasolaryngoscopy (FNE), CT or MRI of the head, neck, and chest as well as fluoroscopic swallow examinations. Standard other history including nature of the complaint, time course, aggravating or relieving factors, previous and current medical or surgical therapies, plus social history (smoking/alcohol/illicit drug use) and medications. Due to recent increased numbers of human papillomavirus (HPV)—related oropharyngeal cancers, clinicians should also include a sexual history in targeted patients.

On Examination

When performing an examination of the head and neck, it is important to include inspection of the oral cavity (including floor of mouth, lateral tongue, retromolar trigone, and buccal mucosa), salivary glands, and thyroid, as well as palpation of the cervical lymph node basins.

Red flag findings (head or neck masses, trismus, nerve palsies, gross dysphonia) are recorded.

Endoscopy

Nasendoscopy should include assessment of the nasal mucosa, posterior nasal space, hypopharynx, larynx, and post-cricoid area. Clinicians should inspect for salivary pooling in the valleculae and pyriform fossae, which could indicate submucosal pathology or pharyngeal weakness. Biopsies should be obtained if there is inflammation or mass.

SCENARIO 1

Six weeks after beginning treatment he presents with oral intake decrease, lethargy, and dehydration. He also reports associated weight loss, dysphonia, odynophagia, and nausea. He is unable to swallow solid food but can swallow pureed food and liquids with some difficulty. His voice at the time was noted to be perceptually mildly to moderately dysphonic.

On inspection, there was localized erythema and desquamation consistent with acute radiation. There was no associated skin necrosis or ulceration. Examination of the oral cavity revealed poor oral hygiene and dental caries of the upper and lower molars. Neck inspection revealed a prominent mass along the left upper neck involving levels II and III. Palpation of this area was consistent with a firm mass measuring approximately 5 to 6 cm at its greatest diameter.

On flexible fiberoptic nasolaryngoscopy, a left sided exophytic irregular mass was noted arising from the left pyriform fossa and abutting the epiglottis consistent with the primary tumor. The glottic area was free of tumor and both vocal cords were mobile and symmetrical.

Diagnosis

Chemotherapy induced nausea and vomiting, high grade mucositis

Investigations

Nil

Management

- Intravenous fluid therapy
- Pain management—xylocaine lozenge or viscous
- Proton pump inhibitor
- Dexamethasone 6 mg daily
- Multidisciplinary team review—consider CRT dosage reduction
- Speech pathology assessment and dietician input for trial of a modified diet and optimization of nutrition
- If ongoing coughing or dysphagia—videofluoroscopic swallow study (VFSS)

SCENARIO 2

Six months post IMRT for a supraglottic SCC, the patient initially tolerated minced textured diet and thickened fluids, later presents to hospital with voice changes, respiratory distress, and worsening aspiration.

Head and neck examination shows skin and mucosal changes consistent with localized radiation therapy sequelae.

Flexible nasolaryngoscopy reveals significant unilateral impaired vocal cord movement. Modified barium swallow showed an upper pharyngeal stricture and significant aspiration of all fluid and food consistencies.

Diagnosis

Post IMRT recurrent laryngeal nerve palsy plus upper pharyngeal stricture and radiation induced fibrosis

Investigations

- CT scan head and neck and chest—rule out recurrence or second primary causing cranial nerve palsy
- Modified barium swallow—to assess severity of aspiration
- Rigid esophagoscopy

Management

- Nil by mouth + intravenous fluid hydration
- Gastroenterology consult for PEG insertion
- Serial pharyngeal dilation
- Multidisciplinary team review—voice and swallow rehabilitation exercises

SCENARIO 3

Two years post IMRT for supraglottic SCC, the patient presents with worsening dysphagia to solids, decreased oral intake, and lethargy. He also reports associated weight loss and hoarse voice.

Head and neck examination on the left was consistent with chronic tissue fibrosis secondary to previous localized radiation therapy. Inspection on the right side revealed a fixed mass along the right upper neck involving levels III and IV. Palpation of this area was consistent with a firm immobile mass measuring approximately 3 cm at its greatest diameter.

Flexible nasolaryngoscopy revealed a midline exophytic irregular mass which involved both arytenoids and the suprahyoid epiglottis; the left cord was also immobile.

Diagnosis

Recurrence of supraglottic SCC

Management

- CT neck/chest, PET/CT fusion for staging
- Panendoscopy and formal biopsy (recurrence vs. second primary). Request HPV evaluation (p16 vs. polymerase chain reaction)
- Multidisciplinary team review—discussion regarding salvage surgery
- Pain management
- Nutritional assessment
- Gastroenterology consult for prophylactic percutaneous endoscopic gastrostomy (PEG) insertion
- See Figures 52–1 and 52–2.

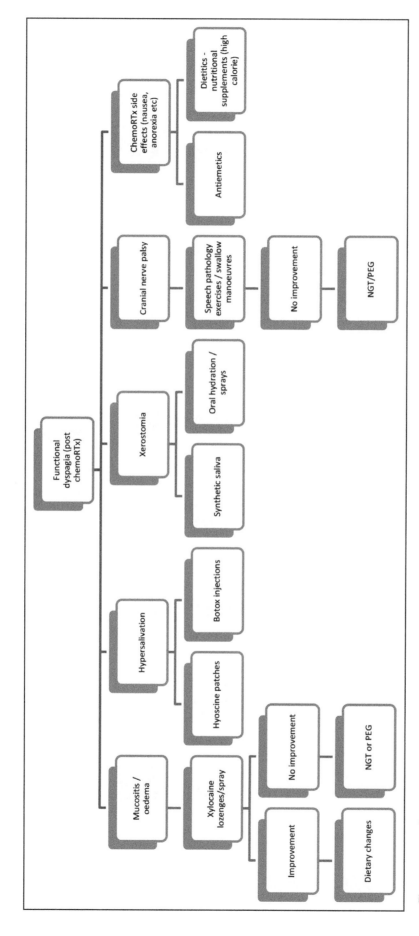

Figure 52–1. Functional dysphagia management.

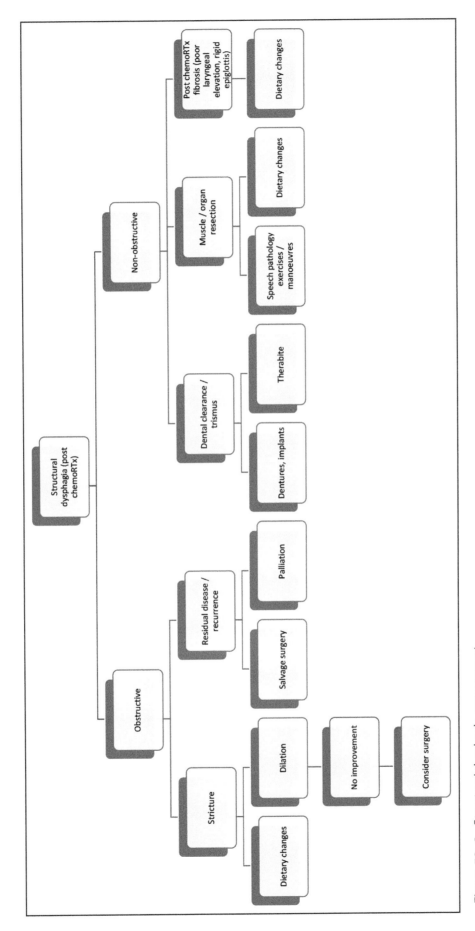

Figure 52–2. Structural dysphagia management.

DIFFERENTIAL DIAGNOSIS

In HNC patients, dysphagia usually presents as an obstruction of the UADT, the majority being intrinsic, such as oropharyngeal and hypopharyngeal tumors, but in some instances could be extrinsic, from a parapharyngeal or thyroid mass. In less common scenarios a mass may affect the cranial nerves or invade the skull base, from where they exit via their respective foraminae presenting as neurological dysphagia.

Dysphagia can be the only or just one of the presenting symptoms during initial consultation. Following the history and examination, further assessment by speech pathologists and input by dieticians can enable nutritional optimization. The swallow needs to be deemed safe if oral intake is to continue, with possible alteration of food consistency or thickening of fluids if necessary.

Structural

- Intrinsic

  - Benign—cleft lip and palate, pharyngeal or esophageal webs and diverticulae (Zenker's diverticulum)
  - Malignant—neoplasms
  - Strictures—malignant, anastomotic, caustic, post-radiation
  - Iatrogenic—surgical resection ± reconstruction, radiation fibrosis

- Extrinsic

  - Compression, encasement, or invasion—lung cancer, mediastinal lymphadenopathy, vascular abnormalities that compress the esophagus, cervical osteophytes, thyromegaly

Functional

- Oral—neurological disorders or stroke, loss of teeth, oral incompetence
- Mucosal—mucositis
- Muscular—neuromuscular disease (eg, myasthenia gravis, achalasia, multiple sclerosis, motor neuron disease), connective tissue diseases (polymyositis, muscular dystrophy)
- Neurogenic—cerebral infarction or intracranial hemorrhage (cerebrovascular accident), Parkinson's disease, delayed cranial nerve paresis, dementia, or the above conditions
- Psychiatric—psychogenic dysphagia
- Iatrogenic—medications

MANAGEMENT

Dysphagia is common after an oncological intervention and should be anticipated. Early detection and appropriate treatment tailored to the individual patient is needed to prevent or minimize serious secondary complications.[2] As demonstrated by the clinical scenarios above, management may vary from non-surgical lifestyle changes and reassurance to surgical dilatation or prophylactic PEG placement. It is useful to assess swallowing using subjective and objective (clinical and instrumental) measures to characterize the location, nature, and severity of the deficit. A more detailed assessment can be carried out by an otolaryngologist and speech pathologist in an inpatient or outpatient setting by a functional endoscopic evaluation of swallow (FEES) using different consistencies of fluid or food with or without the use of blue dye to assess for pooling and laryngeal penetration or aspiration. A videofluoroscopic swallowing exam (VFSE) or modified barium swallow (MBS) can also play a role in dynamic visualization of the mechanical aspects within each phase of swallowing, but this requires a radiographer and exposes the patient to x-ray radiation. A study by Szczesniak et al showed that the diagnostic sensitivity and specificity of videofluoroscopy in detecting strictures was 0.76 and 0.58, respectively, advising that when assessing causes of dysphagia in HNC patients, VFSE alone is inadequate to rule out strictures.[3] The psychosocial impairment of dysphagia can also be assessed using more validated subjective tools such as patient questionnaires, the most notable being the MD Anderson Dysphagia Inventory (MDADI).

Dysphagia at initial presentation requires appropriate assessment and investigation for the treating team to better predict the necessity of alternative methods for enteral nutrition such as a nasogastric tube (NGT) or a PEG/radiologically inserted percutaneous gastrostomy (RIG). An alternative method of enteral feeding may be required before treatment is commenced in order to nutritionally optimize a starving cachectic patient or in cases where treatment will compound the severity of the dysphagia.

Dysphagia is a potentially dose-limiting toxicity of HNC radiotherapy and has a complex multifactorial pathogenesis with acute inflammation, edema, xerostomia, and fibrosis contributing to neurological and muscular injury.[4] Local and systemic sequelae of chemotherapy (eg, mucositis, nausea, vomiting, fatigue) add to the swallowing impairment associated with other modalities of treatment.

Management of dysphagia post-CRT varies among institutions; however, given the multitude of contributory factors, it should always have a multidisciplinary approach involving a number of medical specialties and allied health professionals, including otolaryngology, oncology, gastroenterology, general surgery, speech language pathology, and dietetics. This enables the team to prepare the patient psychologically and understand the possible challenges that will be faced during and after treatment, thus educating patients and their support network and allowing for optimal motivation and rehabilitation planning. In HNC, it is important that patients and their families have a clear understanding that swallowing commonly does not recover to a baseline level, prior to oncological intervention.

In HNC we need to consider the functional deficit the patient would be left with from treatment and assess baseline dysphagia, pre-empt side effects of treatment, and involve speech pathology and dieticians early on to provide supportive care and rehabilitation.

PITFALLS

The key is to ensure that mass lesions, iatrogenic injury, or neurological disorders are ruled out as causes. Dysphagia post-CRT requires a full workup to enable prompt targeted therapies with aims to improve the patient's swallow and prevent serious associated complications.

In HNC patients, it is important that life-threatening causes such as residual disease, recurrence, or second primary are ruled out before attributing symptoms to short- or long-term side effects of previous surgical or CRT treatment. In patients with red flag symptoms deemed high risk for malignancy, additional investigations such as nasolaryngoscopy, modified barium swallow, and CT should be considered.

DISCUSSION

HNC is the sixth most common malignancy worldwide and almost two-thirds of patients present with locally advanced disease requiring aggressive multimodality treatment for cure.[5] While previously associated with tobacco and alcohol use, the epidemiology of the disease has changed in recent decades with an increased incidence of high-risk HPV-associated disease, predominantly HPV type 16. These patients are generally younger at the time of diagnosis, with a favorable prognosis for long-term survival.[6] Function-sparing treatment is of increased importance for this population; however, dysphagia remains a significant and common adverse effect of CRT.[7]

The occurrence of metachronous second primary malignancies is not unusual in HNC survivors and is a major cause of patient mortality. There are four key factors that determine a patient's risk of developing a second malignancy, these are (1) age at the time of radiation treatment, (2) genetic risk factors, (3) site of radiation, and (4) dose and volume of tissue being irradiated.[8] There is strong epidemiologic evidence that age at the time of radiotherapy is one the most important factors when determining a patient's likelihood of developing a secondary malignancy. The Life Span Study group, which followed atomic bomb survivors, estimated that relative risk decreased by about 17% per decade increase in age at exposure.[9] With HPV HNC being diagnosed in younger patient populations, there is a theoretical increased risk due to the carcinogenic properties of radiotherapy. A cohort study of 166 patients by Choe et al found that survival was significantly reduced in patients who had received previous concurrent CRT compared with patients who were CRT naïve, with a 2-year overall survival rate of 10.8% versus 28.4% ($p = 0.0043$).[10]

Over the past decade, with improved equipment and surgical techniques, transoral robotic surgery (TORS) has emerged as a minimally invasive alternative to more conventional non-surgical organ preservation techniques (eg, CRT). TORS has gained favor in the otolaryngology community due to documented advantages such as optimal 3D visualization of the surgical field, improved ergonomics and manual dexterity, and surgical precision. These factors are crucial in maintaining the structural integrity of the laryngopharynx for functional preservation and improving intra- and postoperative outcomes. Additionally, studies have shown that in appropriately selected patients, TORS has the potential to de-escalate radiotherapy to postoperative doses, or to avoid adjuvant chemotherapy (34–45%) or radiotherapy (9–27%) altogether.[11]

What Is the Cause?

Causes of dysphagia range from abnormalities in structure (structural dysphagia) or function (propulsive or motor dysphagia) of the cartilaginous, bony, muscle, or neural anatomy involved in the normal swallow. Oropharyngeal (transfer) dysphagia occurs due to disorders of the oropharyngeal area, typically from neurologic or myogenic abnormalities as well as tumors. Esopha-geal dysphagia occurs from disorders of the esophagus and is most commonly due to mechanical obstruction or altered esophageal motility.[12]

In HNC patients, surgical resection results in site-specific patterns of dysphagia and aspiration. The degree of impairment is dependent on baseline function, tumor size, and location; it increases with the extent of resection. Swallowing is a complicated mechanism requiring coordinated movement of various structures (Table 52–1); even expert reconstructive efforts cannot completely replicate original structure and function. Dental clearance and mandibular surgery affect mastication and interfere with suprahyoid muscle action. Tongue and tongue base resection results in com-

Table 52–1. Physiology of Swallowing—Swallowing Phases

Liquids	Solids
Oral Preparatory	Oral
Liquid is held in the anterior part of the floor of the mouth or on the dorsum of the tongue against the hard palate	Solids maneuvered by tongue onto the occlusal surfaces of the lower teeth for mastication.
Palatoglossal sphincter (uvula and tongue base) contracted to prevent passage of liquids into oropharynx	Food particles further softened by salivation until the bolus is adequate consistency for swallowing
Oral propulsive	Palatoglossal sphincter relaxed (open) permitting communication between the oral cavity and pharynx
Tongue base descends and contact with uvula is lost (opening of the palatoglossal sphincter)	Tongue, soft palate, and jaw move in a cyclical manner (food processing)
Gravity and sequential anterior to posterior contraction of the tongue against the palate propels the liquid into the oropharynx	Propulsion of a prepared food bolus by the tongue into the oropharynx can be interposed with food processing cycles
	Processed food often finds passage through the fauces to accumulate in the oropharynx and valleculae prior to the pharyngeal phase of swallowing
Pharyngeal	
Two crucial biological features, passage of food and liquid into the upper esophagus and airway protection	
Soft palate elevation, lingual thrust, laryngeal elevation and descent, pharyngeal muscle constriction and UES relaxation propel and draw (with negative pressure) the bolus into the upper esophagus along the path of least resistance	
Airway protection is afforded by closure of the true and false vocal cords, arytenoid flexion, and epiglottic retroversion	
Esophageal	
Gravity and ANS-mediated peristalsis deliver the bolus from the UES through the LES into the stomach	

ANS: autonomic nervous system.
UES: upper esophageal sphincter.
LES: lower esophageal sphincter.

promised lingual mobility, strength, and palatoglossal sphincter competency. Hard and soft palate resection predisposes to nasal regurgitation. Partial or total laryngectomy impacts on pharyngeal muscle coordination.[13]

Concurrent chemoradiotherapy is the recommended treatment for oropharyngeal carcinoma, with recent meta-analyses demonstrating significant survival benefits over radiotherapy alone. Timing and severity of radiotherapy-related dysphagia vary and are dependent on the intensity of the acute reactions, intrinsic radiosensitivity, and method of radiotherapy (fields, fractions, and dose). In the acute stages, edema and mucositis alter the normal contours of the swallowing apparatus, obliterating normal fossae and channels, impairing sensation, and inhibiting oral intake during treatment.[13] Long-term, fibrosis may develop affecting skin, connective tissue, and muscle and leading to stricture development and impaired range of motion of the hyolaryngeal complex, pharyngeal constrictors, and tongue base.[4] Concurrent CRT is associated with symptomatic stricture development in over 20% of patients and associated increase in PEG use.[14]

More than one causal mechanism may be present in HNC patients with dysphagia, e.g., adjuvant CRT may cause mucositis, esophageal stenosis, and reduced oral intake, compounding functional deficits with the patient's swallow attributable to the tumor itself and operative treatments.

Psychological Issues

It is well documented that HNC is arguably the most psychologically traumatic cancer to experience, with patients facing unique physical and emotional challenges. Not only are they affected by a potentially life-threatening diagnosis, but treatments often result in significant, highly visible disfigurement and impairment, disrupting day to day functions such as speech and swallowing.

Impairments in communication, emotional expression, and socially interactive activities such as mealtimes result in social isolation and distress.[15,16] Quality of life (QoL) is a multi-dimensional construct reflective of an individual's subjective assessment of the impact an illness or treatment has on his or her physical, psychological and social function, and general well-being.[17] It is inadequately addressed by traditional measures of treatment efficacy (eg, disease-free survival, overall survival, and tumor response rates).[18] A cohort study using standard psychiatric tests identified mood dis-

orders such as depression, anxiety, social phobia, and avoidance as clinically significant psychosocial issues both at baseline and after completion of treatment.[19]

In a systematic review by Parkar et al, several factors have been identified that may predict worse QoL outcomes, including the presence of a feeding tube, comorbidities, tracheostomy, disease location, and staging. Other studies observed an immediate decrease in QoL from diagnosis to 3 months after the start of therapy, returning toward baseline by 12 months in a majority of patients.[20] However, the evidence is still lacking to conclusively demonstrate a consistent positive relationship between functional outcomes, symptom burden, and a patient's QoL.[21]

Standardized questionnaires provide additional insight into the physical and psychosocial burdens of dysphagia, and a recent systematic review identified 17 clinician and patient-related scales such as the MDADI and Xerostomia Questionnaire. Although inconsistencies in design, volume, and heterogeneous reporting standards have prevented authors from combining data for clinical benefit, knowledge ascertained from such assessment tools may guide appropriate investigations, referral to other members of the multidisciplinary team, and interventions (eg, psychotherapy and antidepressant prophylaxis).[22]

It is important for clinicians to recognize that adherence to swallowing rehabilitation programs outlined by dieticians and speech pathologists requires long-term dedication and motivation from the patient. Studies failing to find benefit from exercise programs have noted patient compliance, participant withdrawal, and timing of interventions to be major factors hindering their results.[23] When considering nonsurgical management of dysphagia, patients and families should be advised that improvement can be protracted, if it occurs at all. To reducing the compounding factors of psychological issues leading to non-compliance with allied health led interventions, patients should undergo timely mental health assessment and commence psychotherapy or antidepressant prophylaxis if appropriate.

Nonsurgical Management

Education, dietary alterations, swallowing exercises, adaptive maneuvers, and orofacial prosthetics are the cornerstones of swallowing rehabilitation, and recent strategies focus on early intervention to overcome acute symptoms and sequelae of prolonged swallowing apparatus disuse. Preoperative assessment of a patient's dentition, including an orthopantomogram, is required to assist in the placement of orthodontics if dental clearance occurs. Langendijk et al[24] advocated the use of the "total dysphagia risk score" (TDRS), a summation of risk factors including T-classification, neck irradiation, weight loss, primary tumor site, and treatment modality as a predictive measure for swallowing dysfunction after curative radiotherapy for HNC. Subsequent studies have indicated its potential use in identifying patients appropriate for prophylactic PEG placement.[25]

Patients require tailored pre- and post-treatment written and verbal information regarding interventions and their impact, as well as the prognosis for their swallowing ability.[26] Dietary alterations, nutritional counseling, and oral nutritional supplementation to permit maintenance of an oral diet are protective against therapy-associated weight loss, interruption of radiotherapy, and continuation of oral intake following treatment.[27] Close monitoring is necessary to ensure that nutritional status is not compromised as HNC patients are more likely to experience nutrition deficiencies during all phases of illness compared with other cancer patients.[28] Preliminary evidence suggests that thickened liquids may prevent aspiration[29]; non-adherence to prescribed dietary modifications is associated with poor patient understanding and carries a significantly increased risk of aspiration pneumonia and death.[30] Enteral feeding via nasogastric or PEG tube is required when oral intake is insufficient, particularly in elderly patients (>60 years) with locally advanced disease, where chances of requiring enteral feeding exceed four times that of younger adults.[31]

Exercise-based swallowing preservation protocols have emerged as non-invasive, cost-effective interventions, improving functional swallowing outcomes and reducing gastrostomy tube feeding dependence and duration of hospital admission, particularly when commenced in the pre-treatment setting.[32] While there is a lack of consensus on key issues such as optimal frequency, intensity, and content of swallowing therapies, it is evident that prolonged disuse of structures critical to normal swallowing results in increased rates of dysphagia.[33] A prospective cohort study by Virani et al of 50 patients undergoing radiotherapy or CRT demonstrated significant benefits of targeted exercise regimens over water and saliva swallowing therapy in reducing PEG dependence and oral intake difficulties.[34] Similar findings were concluded in earlier randomized control trials, which demonstrated the superiority of active swallowing exercises in optimizing swallowing ability, salivation, and mouth opening and preventing muscle deterioration.[35] Martin-Harris et al proposed

a visual feedback guided mid-expiratory phase swallowing protocol with preliminary results demonstrating significant improvements in optimal phase patterning, laryngeal vestibular closure, tongue base retraction, pharyngeal residue, and penetration-aspiration scale scores.[36] Finally, adjunct measures such as transcutaneous neuromuscular electrical stimulation (NMES) initially showed promise in its ability to preserve swallowing function during CRT.[37] However, a more recent randomized control trial conducted by Langmore et al concluded that NMES did not add any additional benefit to traditional dysphagia therapy in postradiotherapy HNC patients. Surprisingly, the authors did note that all 170 patients reported significant improvements in both diet and quality of life, and further prospective evaluation is warranted.[38]

Surgical Management

Surgery is reserved for HNC patients with structural or functional derangements of swallowing that cannot be remedied by rehabilitation alone. Historically, PEG tubes have been placed therapeutically or reactively; however, prophylactic PEG placement has been in practice for many years. It remains a controversial topic with conflicting data, and most recommendations support its use primarily in high-risk patients with significant pre-treatment weight loss or comorbidities that may be aggravated by intense multimodality therapy, dysphagia, aspiration, or malnutrition.[39] Some authors have reported reduced aspiration and stricture rates, nutrition-related emergency department visits and hospitalizations, and costs compared with reactive PEG placement and higher proportions of chemotherapy cycles completed without associated PEG dependency.[40] However, not all studies have reached similar conclusions; Pohar et al found no benefits in treatment breaks, weight loss, or overall disease survival. Rather, it concluded prophylactic PEG insertion to be associated with higher rates of PEG dependence and strictures.[41] Currently, there is insufficient evidence to determine the optimal route of enteral feeding, and prophylactic PEG (or nasogastric) placement has not been conclusively demonstrated to offer significant advantages in nutritional outcomes, interruptions of treatment, and overall patient survival.[42]

Secretion management difficulties, strongly associated with dysphagia and known contributors to poor healing of malignancy and treatment-related fistulae, can be treated with aggressive wound care, pharmacologic inhibition, radiation, or surgery.[43] Botulinum toxin (BoNT) has emerged as a well-tolerated and effective treatment to reduce saliva flow. In a 2014 cohort study of 25 HNC patients, Steffen et al reported reduced salivary flow in all six fistula patients and improvements in functional hypersalivation in 11 patients. Advantages include ease of injection, minimal systemic medication interactions, duration of action, and shortened hospital stay, with an increasingly prominent role in elderly or palliative patients. Despite limitations of BoNT therapy, including the need for repeated administration after approximately 10 weeks and insufficient clinical effect in some patients, it offers HNC patients a new low-risk option for improved surgical recovery.[44]

Strictures develop in at least 7% of HNC patients within 3 years of treatment; while swallowing exercise showed some improvement, severe cases necessitated gastrostomy dependence following CRT.[4] In more recent years, management has shifted from open myotomy to endoscopic balloon dilation and carbon dioxide laser resection approaches. Advantages include reduced anesthesia time, length of stay, morbidity (pharyngocutaneous fistula, recurrent laryngeal nerve injury, hematoma, seroma, and infection), and mortality.[45] In a retrospective cohort study of 63 patients with pharyngoesophageal strictures, Agarwalla et al described an average of 3.3 dilations over a median of 4 weeks to achieve initial patency; however, recurrence occurred in 33% of patients, and 43% of patients harbored strictures refractory to dilation.[46] In another, larger single institution series, endoscopic dilation led to gastrostomy tube removal in 78% and 88% of patients at 1 and 2 years, respectively, following an average of 2.4 dilations.[47] For high-grade radiotherapy-related esophageal strictures, Francis et al reviewed 24 patients to report 42% returning to an oral diet and/or having their gastrostomy tube removed following a median of 9 dilations.[48] The importance of expedient stricture diagnosis and management had been emphasized, with a 2.4-fold increase in the odds of dilation failing to restore sufficient oral nutrition to permit gastrostomy tube removal if performed greater than 6 months after CRT. Perforation is the most frequent complication of balloon dilation and occurs in 1.8 to 4% of cases.[47] Carbon dioxide laser is a more recent advance in the endoscopic management of cricopharyngeal strictures. Dawe et al reported non-significant improvement in MBS impairment profile scores pre- and post-laser cricopharyngeal myotomy,[49] while Silver et al noted radiographic stricture improvements in all patients ($n = 10$) and complete resolution in 9.[50] Further prospective data with lengthier follow-up are required. Flexible transnasal esophagoscopy is an emerging technique of diagnostic and therapeutic value for esophageal stenosis. Advantageous in patients with trismus and cervical rigidity, and unfit for general anesthesia, it provides direct observation of secretions and swallowing anatomy, and can be undertaken in the office setting or operating room.

In a small retrospective series, Peng et al demonstrated significant improvements in mean functional outcome swallowing scale scores (4.4 to 2.7) and tolerance of oral diet in 75% of previously completely gastrostomy tube–dependent patients.[14] Lastly, Jamal et al explored the contributory role of epiglottic dysfunction in bolus obstruction and dysphagia after radiotherapy or CRT. Following transoral partial epiglottidectomy, six of seven patients reported improvements in swallowing, with these preliminary results suggesting a role for this technique in select HNC patients, particularly those with intact tongue base contraction and poor retroflexion of the epiglottis causing bolus obstruction at the level of the vallecula.[51]

SUMMARY

Dysphagia post-chemoradiotherapy in the HNC patient population poses unique challenges. The key to optimizing patient physical and psychosocial well-being and therapeutic outcomes is early identification of individuals at risk of dysphagia and initiation of preventative management strategies in the pre-treatment setting. Fiberoptic endoscopic evaluation of swallowing (FEES) and/or videofluoroscopy (MBS/VFSS) is considered to be the gold standard in dysphagia assessment and should be used in combination with questionnaires on quality of life and functional health status.[52] Repetition of outcome measures should be performed to monitor worsening side effects of oncological treatment, to detect spontaneous recovery, and to measure the effects of conservative or surgical interventions.[53] Treatment should be multidisciplinary in approach and tailored to the location and nature of an individual patient's swallowing deficit.

REFERENCES

1. Lembo A, Cremonini F. Chapter 35. Dysphagia. In: Henderson MC, Tierney LM, Jr., Smetana GW, eds, *The Patient History: An Evidence-Based Approach to Differential Diagnosis*. New York, NY: McGraw-Hill; 2012.
2. Jensen K, Bonde Jensen A, Grau C. The relationship between observer-based toxicity scoring and patient assessed

symptom severity after treatment for head and neck cancer. A correlative cross sectional study of the DAHANCA toxicity scoring system and the EORTC quality of life questionnaires. *Radiother Oncol.* 2006;78(3):298–305.

3. Szczesniak M, Maclean J, O'Hare J, et al. Videofluoroscopic swallow examination does not accurately detect cricopharyngeal radiation strictures. *Otolaryngol Head Neck Surg.* 2016;155(3):462–465.

4. Hutcheson K, Lewin J, Barringer D, et al. Late dysphagia after radiotherapy-based treatment of head and neck cancer. *Cancer.* 2012;118(23):5793–5799.

5. World Health Organization. Head and neck cancers. In: Stewart BW, Wild CP, editors. *World Cancer Report 2014* (ePUB). Lyon, France: World Health Organization Press; 2014:422–435.

6. Gillison ML, Koch WM, Capone RB, et al. Evidence for a causal association between human papillomavirus and a subset of head and neck cancers. *J Natl Cancer Inst.* 2000;92:709–720.

7. Trotti A, Pajak TF, Gwede CK, et al. TAME: development of a new method for summarising adverse events of cancer treatment by the Radiation Therapy Oncology Group. *Lancet Oncol.* 2007;8(7):613–624.

8. Ng J, Shuryak I. Minimizing second cancer risk following radiotherapy: current perspectives. *Cancer Management and Research.* 2014:1.

9. Preston DL, Ron E, Tokuoka S, et al. Solid cancer incidence in atomic bomb survivors: 1958–1998. *Radiat Res.* 2007;168:1–64.

10. Choe K, Haraf D, Solanki A, et al. Prior chemoradiotherapy adversely impacts outcomes of recurrent and second primary head and neck cancer treated with concurrent chemotherapy and reirradiation. *Cancer.* 2011;117(20): 4671–4678.

11. Sinclair CF, McColloch NL, Carroll WR, Rosenthal EL, Desmond RA, Magnuson JS. Patient-perceived and objective functional outcomes following transoral robotic surgery for early oropharyngeal carcinoma. *Arch Otolaryngol Head Neck Surg.* 2011;137(11):1112–1116.

12. Spieker M. Evaluating dysphagia. *Am Fam Physician.* 2000; 61:3639–3648

13. Russi EG, Corvo R, Merlotti A, et al. Swallowing dysfunction in head and neck cancer patients treated by radiotherapy: review and recommendations of the supportive task group of the Italian Association of Radiation Oncology. *Cancer Treat Rev.* 2012; 38:1033–1049.

14. Peng KA, Feinstein AJ, Salinas JB, Chhetri DK. Utility of the transnasal esophagoscope in the management of chemoradiation-induced esophageal stenosis. *Ann Otol Rhinol Laryngol.* 2015; 124:221–226.

15. Hammerlid E, Taft C. Health-related quality of life in long-term head and neck cancer survivors: a comparison with general population norms. *Br J Cancer.* 2001;84(2):149–156.

16 Archer J, Hutchison I, Korszun A. Mood and malignancy: head and neck cancer and depression. *J Oral Pathol Med.* 2008;37(5):255–270.

17. Murphy B, Ridner S, Wells N, Dietrich M. Quality of life research in head and neck cancer: a review of the current state of the science. *Crit Rev Oncol/Hematol.* 2007;62(3): 251–267.

18. Chen AY, Frankowski R, Bishop-Leone J, Geopfert H. The development and validation of a dysphagia-specific quality-of-life questionnaire for patients with head and neck cancer: the M. D. Anderson Dysphagia Inventory. *Arch Otolaryngol Head Neck Surg.* 2001;127:870–876.

19. Kohda R, Otsubo T, Kuwakado Y, et al. Prospective studies on mental status and quality of life in patients with head and neck cancer treated by radiation. *Psycho-Oncology.* 2005;14(4):331–336.

20. Hammerlid E, Silander E, Hrnestam L, Sullivan M. Health-related quality of life three years after diagnosis of head and neck cancer?A longitudinal study. *Head Neck.* 2001;23(2):113–125.

21. Parkar S, Shah M. A relationship between quality-of-life and head and neck cancer: a systemic review. *South Asian J Cancer.* 2015;4(4):179.

22. Smith J, Shuman A, Riba M. Psychosocial issues in patients with head and neck cancer: an updated review with a focus on clinical interventions. *Curr Psychiat Rep.* 2017;19(9).

23. Mortensen HR, Jensen K, Aksglaede K, et al. Prophylactic swallowing exercises in head and neck cancer radiotherapy. *Dysphagia.* 2015; 30:304–314.

24. Langendijk J, Doornaert P, Rietveld D, Verdonck-de Leeuw I, René Leemans C, Slotman B. A predictive model for swallowing dysfunction after curative radiotherapy in head and neck cancer. *Radiother Oncol.* 2009;90(2): 189–195.

25. Rütten H, Pop L, Janssens G, et al. Long-term outcome and morbidity after treatment with accelerated radiotherapy and weekly cisplatin for locally advanced head-and-neck cancer: results of a multidisciplinary late morbidity clinic. *Int J Radiat Oncol Biol Phys.* 2011;81(4):923–929.

26. Brockbank S, Miller N, Owen S, Patterson J. Pretreatment information on dysphagia: exploring the views of head and neck cancer patients. *J Pain Sympt Manage.* 2015;49(1): 89–97.

27. Bossola M. Nutritional interventions in head and neck cancer patients undergoing chemoradiotherapy: a narrative review. *Nutrients.* 2015;7(1):265–276.

28. Locher J, Bonner J, Carrol W. Prophylactic percutaneous endoscopic gastrostomy tube placement in treatment of head and neck cancer. *J Parenter Enter Nutr.* 2011; 35(3):365–374

29. Cichero J, Steele C, Duivestein J, et al. The need for international terminology and definitions for texture-modified foods and thickened liquids used in dysphagia management: foundations of a global initiative. *Curr Phys Med Rehab Rep.* 2013;1(4):280–291.

30. Low J, Wyles C, Wilkinson T, Sainsbury R. The effect of compliance on clinical outcomes for patients with dysphagia on videofluoroscopy. *Dysphagia.* 2001;16(2):123–127.

31. Sachdev S, Refaat T, Bacchus ID, et al. Age most significant predictor of requiring enteral feeding in head-and-neck cancer patients. *Radiat Oncol.* 2015;10:93–100.

32. Carroll W, Locher J, Canon C, Bohannon I, McColloch N, Magnuson J. Pretreatment swallowing exercises improve swallow function after chemoradiation. *Laryngoscope.* 2008; 118(1):39–43.

33. Schindler A, Denaro N, Russi E, et al. Dysphagia in head and neck cancer patients treated with radiotherapy and systemic therapies: literature review and consensus. *Crit Rev Oncol Haematol.* 2015;96:372–384.

34. Virani A, Kunduk M, Fink DS, McWhorter AJ. Effects of 2 different swallowing exercise regimens during organ-preservation therapies for head and neck cancers on swallowing function. *Head Neck.* 2015;37:162–170.

35. Kraaijenga S, Van der Molen L, Van den Brekel M, Hilgers F. Current assessment and treatment strategies of dysphagia in head and neck cancer patients: a systematic review of the 2012/13 literature. *Curr Opin Support Palliat Care.* 2014.

36. Martin-Harris B, McFarland D, Hill EG, et al. Respiratory-swallow training in patients with head and neck cancer. *Arch Phys Med Rehabil.* 2015; 96:885–893.

37. Bhatt A, Goodwin N, Cash E, et al. Impact of transcutaneous neuromuscular electrical stimulation on dysphagia in patients with head and neck cancer treated with definitive chemoradiation. *Head Neck.* 2015;37(7):1051–1056.

38. Langmore S, McCulloch T, Krisciunas G, et al. Efficacy of electrical stimulation and exercise for dysphagia in patients with head and neck cancer: a randomized clinical trial. *Head Neck.* 2015;38(S1):E1221–E1231.

39. National Comprehensive Cancer Network (NCCN). Principles of nutrition: management and supportive care (NUTR-A). In: *Clinical Practice Guidelines in Oncology: Head and Neck Cancers Version 2.* 2014.

40. Lewis SL, Brody R, Touger-Decker R, et al. Feeding tube use in patients with head and neck cancer. *Head Neck.* 2014; 36:1789–1795.

41. Pohar S, Demarcantonio M, Whiting P, et al. Percutaneous endoscopic gastrostomy tube dependence following chemoradiation in head and neck cancer patients. *Laryngoscope.* 2015;125:1366–1371.

42. Shaw SM, Flowers H, O'Sullivan B, et al. The effect of prophylactic percutaneous endoscopic gastrostomy (PEG) tube placement on swallowing and swallow-related outcomes in patients undergoing radiotherapy for head and neck cancer: a systematic review. *Dysphagia.* 2015;30: 152–175.

43. Bomeli S, Desai S, Johnson J, Walvekar R. Management of salivary flow in head and neck cancer patients—a systematic review. *Oral Oncol.* 2008;44(11):1000–1008.

44. Steffen A, Hasselbacher K, Heinrichs S, Wollenberg B. Botulinum toxin for salivary disorders in the treatment of head and neck cancer. *Anticancer Res.* 2014;34:6627–6632.

45. Bergeron J, Chhetri D. Indications and outcomes of endoscopic CO_2 laser cricopharyngeal myotomy. *Laryngoscope.* 2013;124(4):950–954.

46. Agarwalla A, Small AJ, Mendelson AH, et al. Risk of recurrent or refractory strictures and outcome of endoscopic dilation for radiation-induced esophageal strictures. *Surg Endosc.* 2015;29:1903–1912.

47. Chapuy CI, Annino DJ, Tishler RB, et al. Success of endoscopic pharyngoesophageal dilation after head and neck cancer treatment. *Laryngoscope.* 2013;123:3066–3073.

48. Francis DO, Hall E, Dang JH, et al. Outcomes of serial dilation for high-grade radiation-related esophageal strictures in head and neck cancer patients. *Laryngoscope.* 2015;1 25:856–862.

49. Dawe N, Patterson J, Hamilton D, Hartley C. Targeted use of endoscopic CO_2 laser cricopharyngeal myotomy for improving swallowing function following head and neck cancer treatment. *J Laryngol Otol.* 2014;128(12):1105–1110.

50. Silver N, Gal TJ. Endoscopic CO_2 laser management of chemoradiationrelated cricopharyngeal stenosis. *Ann Otol Rhinol Laryngol.* 2014;123:252–256.

51. Jamal N, Erman A, Chhetri DK. Transoral partial epiglottidectomy to treat dysphagia in posttreatment head and neck cancer patients: a preliminary report. *Laryngoscope.* 2014;124:665–671.

52 Speyer R, Baijens L, Heijnen M, Zwijnenberg I. Effects of therapy in oropharyngeal dysphagia by speech and language therapists: a systematic review. *Dysphagia.* 2010; 25(1):40–65.

53. Heijnen B, Speyer R, Kertscher B, et al. Dysphagia, speech, voice, and trismus following radiotherapy and/or chemotherapy in patients with head and neck carcinoma: review of the literature. *BioMed Research International.* 2016; 2016:1–24.

CHAPTER 53

Neurologically Impaired Pharynx

Lacey Adkins, Melda Kunduk, and Andrew J. McWhorter

INTRODUCTION

Concomitant chemotherapy and radiation therapy has been shown to have equivalent locoregional control rates compared with surgical interventions for select upper aerodigestive tract diseases.[1] With radiation treatment, the area treated usually consists of the primary tumor and its surrounding lymphatic drainage area. In head and neck cancer, this means that the structures involved with the swallowing mechanism are typically exposed to high doses of radiation, oftentimes resulting in dysphagia. The addition of chemotherapy not only improves locoregional control but also increases early and late complications. Early toxicities, such as mucositis, cause odynophagia and swallowing aversion and contribute to patients discontinuing oral food intake and subsequent weight loss, which is the most common reason for enteral and parental feeding during the acute phase of treatment. However, it is the later fibrosis-related functional and anatomical changes as well as decreased sensation that often cause more long-term dysphagia.[2–3]

Radiation therapy with or without chemotherapy in the head and neck cancer population is a known risk factor for development of swallowing problems and increases the risk of aspiration. Swallow dysfunction may present on a continuum from mild to severe and may result in altered diet, decline in nutritional intake, reduced quality of life, aspiration pneumonia, and overall morbidity. Concurrently, reduced oral nutritional intake may lead to malnutrition, disruption to cancer treatment, increased health care costs, and decline in prognosis. This life-threatening potential and patient health and safety impact make swallow disorders and malnutrition a significant concern in this population's treatment outcomes.

Current available research has sought to identify specific causes and examine swallowing-related outcomes in an effort to improve immediate and long-term swallowing function and quality of life. The swallow mechanism is influenced by the presence, function, and sensation of the organs of swallowing. Swallowing organs at risk include the superior pharyngeal constrictor muscles, middle pharyngeal constrictor muscles, inferior pharyngeal constrictor muscles, including the cricopharyngeal muscle component, esophageal inlet, cervical esophagus, base of tongue, supraglottic larynx, and glottic larynx. Patients also report changes to the perception of taste or loss of taste sensation, which often further intensifies the weight loss and malnutrition problems.

CASE PRESENTATION

A 61-year-old with history of T2N2bM0 squamous cell carcinoma of the base of tongue is now status post-concurrent chemotherapy and radiation completed 6 months ago. His treatment course was complicated by severe nausea and hyperemesis when eating per oral (PO) and he required percutaneous endoscopic gastrostomy (PEG) placement due to weight loss. His hyperemesis eventually subsided, and he is currently eating a soft diet with PEG feeds for supplemental nutrition. He is avoiding solids and meats because he feels too dry and they get stuck in his mouth. If this happens, he has to use a liquid wash to clear the food. He does note right sided odynophagia, worse when he wakes up in the morning, which improves throughout the day. He had lost 6 kg (15 lbs) in the 2 months following treatment but has recently begun to gain weight again. No fevers, chills, otalgia, hemoptysis, voice changes, or shortness of breath.

Social and medical history: former smoker with a two-pack-a-year smoking history, no alcohol. Hypertension

Medications: Lisinopril

Allergies: None

Initial Assessment

History

For a standard history, ask about the onset, location, duration, and character of the swallowing problems, including whether they are with solids, liquids, or both. Determine if there are any aggravating or relieving factors, as well as the timing and severity. Has there been any diet change or resulting weight loss due to the dysphagia? Also, look for any symptoms that are concerning for cancer recurrence, such as hemoptysis, otalgia, odynophagia, or voice changes. If these are present, this may indicate the need for further imaging or biopsy.

Examination

Complete head and neck exam, making sure to carefully examine and palpate the oral cavity and oropharynx for any evidence of recurrence. Given his persistent swallow complaints, also perform a flexible fiberoptic laryngoscopy to further evaluate the pharynx, hypopharynx, and larynx. Again, look for any lesions concerning for recurrence. Assess for any pooling of secretions and attempt to palpate with the tip of the endoscope to assess sensation. Given the radiation history, look for any long-term radiation effects such as chondronecrosis or fibrosis of the epiglottis, laryngeal or hypopharyngeal stenosis, or mobility abnormalities.

SCENARIO 1

Head and neck exam is normal with expected post-radiation fibrosis changes palpated within the neck.

Endoscopy reveals pooling of secretions within the vallecula, pyriform fossae, and posterior and lateral pharyngeal walls. During examination, secretions are seen pooling within the pyriform fossae with penetration into the laryngeal introitus, which is cleared with cued swallowing. Intermittent transient aspiration was also observed. Palpation of aryepiglottic folds and arytenoids occurred without any resulting cough reflex. Bilateral vocal folds mobile.

Diagnosis

Post-treatment swallowing dysfunction

Investigations

Initially, further evaluation of swallow function is needed, both to determine cause as well as assess safety and efficiency of the swallowing mechanism for a PO diet. This could be evaluated both by a functional endoscopic evaluation of swallowing (FEES) or a modified barium swallow (MBS). If it appears primarily to be due to motor incompetence, pharyngeal manometry may also be used for further evaluation.

Management

- Reassurance—continued cancer surveillance with no evidence of disease
- Speech and language pathology referral for swallowing function assessment and therapy
- Diet modifications as needed to address inefficient swallow
- Oral hygiene
- Hydration
- Diet modifications as needed, including enteral nutrition if persistent aspiration
- Follow-up in 4 to 6 weeks

SCENARIO 2

Head and neck exam is positive for post-radiation neck changes only. On endoscopy there is pharyngeal stenosis narrowing the transition between oropharynx and hypopharynx. There is significant radiation effect with thickening of the epiglottis and partial loss of the vallecula. No masses or lesions concerning for recurrence are noted; bilateral vocal folds mobile.

Diagnosis

Pharyngeal stenosis with swallow dysfunction

Investigations

Again, a FEES or MBS may be used to further evaluate the swallowing mechanism as well as further elucidate the role that the pharyngeal stenosis is playing in the swallow deficits. If the stenosis is a new finding, and particularly if it appears to be a source of the complaints of dysphagia, direct laryngoscopy and biopsy may be indicated.

Management

- Direct laryngoscopy with biopsy. If no recurrence noted, consider a pharyngoplasty to help relieve the area of stenosis.
- Balloon dilatation may be possible depending on the configuration of the stenotic segment.
- Speech and language pathology referral for swallowing function assessment and therapy
- Oral hygiene
- Hydration
- Diet modifications as needed, including enteral nutrition if persistent aspiration or inefficient swallow
- Follow-up in 4 to 6 weeks

DIFFERENTIAL DIAGNOSIS

Dysphagia in the setting of prior chemoradiation for an oropharyngeal cancer has multiple possible sources, as evidenced by prior studies. It may be an anatomical abnormality, such as stenosis or fibrosis altering the pharynx or hypopharynx. Another possibility is motor incompetence due to a delayed and uncoordinated pharyngeal swallow with pharyngeal contraction occurring later within the swallowing process relative to upper esophageal sphincter (UES) opening. There may also be reduced cricopharyngeal opening or fibrosis of the pharyngeal muscles with reduced pharyngeal constrictor function. Tongue base retraction to the posterior pharyngeal wall has also been shown to be reduced in patients treated with radiation as well as laryngeal elevation and closure. This predisposes to significant residue and pooling, increasing the risk of aspiration. Finally, some patients may also exhibit reduced pharyngeal sensation with/without motor deficits after chemoradiation.[2–3]

MANAGEMENT

Management is dependent upon the etiology. As demonstrated in the examples above, areas of stenosis may be treated surgically, whether it is a pharyngoplasty or dilation of pharyngeal or hypopharyngeal stenosis, dilation and botulinum injection into the cricopharyngeus muscle, or cricopharyngeal myotomy for cricopharyngeal dysfunction. However, if it appears to be motor or sensory incompetence, referral to a speech-language pathologist for swallowing therapy is a key aspect of management.

PITFALLS

Especially when the patient has a previous history of head and neck cancer, it is important to carefully assess for any evidence of recurrence before referring the patient to speech-language pathology. If there is any concern, whether in the history or exam, further imaging and/or endoscopy with biopsy should be performed before attributing complaints of dysphagia solely to motor or sensory incompetence.

DISCUSSION

While this particular case concentrates on swallow dysfunction that has developed well after treatment, there are many factors before and during treatment that may affect long-term swallowing that should be mentioned. During treatment, radiation to the neck, a high dose (defined as over 65 Gy), and use of three-dimensional conformal radiotherapy have been associated with a larger risk of critical weight loss.[4] In terms of long-term effects, studies have suggested that intensity-modulated radiation therapy as well as tumor positive for human papillomavirus result in less dysphagia and a decrease in feeding tube dependence.[5–7]

Research on prophylactic behavioral swallowing treatment protocols delivered either before or during the course of radiation demonstrated benefits for swallowing function.[8,9] Pre-radiation swallow therapy has been proven to be beneficial, particularly with such movements as epiglottis inversion and the position of the tongue base nearer the posterior pharyngeal wall during swallowing.[8] Similarly, in a study comparing therapy throughout the course of treatment and resulting muscle changes as seen on magnetic resonance imaging (MRI), the genioglossus, mylohyoid, and hyoglossus showed less deterioration in regard to the changes in their length and thickness compared with no treatment. The T2 relaxation time was also significantly reduced, suggestive of a reduction in muscle edema and fat infiltration.[9] Research comparing patients who have had prophylactic gastrostomy versus those who had reactive nasogastric tube placement suggests less severe swallow complaints, using both self-assessment with the MD Anderson Dysphagia Inventory and endpoints such as prolonged feeding tube use and admission for aspiration pneumonia.[10–11]

There are multiple ways to evaluate swallowing efficiency. At the basic level a bedside swallow is first employed; however, this has limitations, as visualization of the mechanics of oropharyngeal swallowing is not possible. Since there is no direct visualization, indicators frequently used include a wet dysphonic voice after swallowing or a cough. However, this test has been shown to be neither specific nor sensitive for detecting aspiration.[12] For visualization, both an MBS and FEES provide more information and are more accurate to determine the events before, during, and after the swallow that lead to penetration, residue, and aspiration resulting in compromised efficiency and safety of oral intake of food. Even though both imaging techniques allow determination of aspiration, each method has different strengths and weaknesses in the assessment of swallowing function.

An MBS allows real-time visualization of bolus transportation by watching a patient swallow barium contrast in liquid, paste, mixed, and solid consistencies under fluoroscopy. This can be seen both in the anteroposterior direction as well as the lateral direction, so that pooling, penetration, aspiration, and duration of transit can be evaluated, including any changes made by compensatory strategies. Unlike a FEES, it allows a more thorough evaluation of the oral phase of swallowing. Objective measurements are taken of both timing and displacement. Bolus transit time as well as the

time to movements such as hyoid displacement and UES opening are calculated. Motion and function of the hyoid and UES can only be determined by using MBS. Spatial measurements often include maximum hyoid displacement, maximum UES opening, and pharyngeal constriction ratio. The pharyngeal constriction ratio is a measure of pharyngeal area visible in lateral radiograph when bolus held in the oral cavity is divided by the pharyngeal area at the point of maximal pharyngeal contraction during swallow. This measurement is a validated surrogate measure for pharyngeal strength and again only available from MBS.[13] When pharyngeal contraction is impaired, the lower pharyngeal pressures can result in pooling/residue within the hypopharynx and increase the potential for aspiration after swallowing. MBS is an excellent tool for demonstrating physiological events before, during, and after the swallow to investigate the safety and efficiency of the swallowing mechanism. Figure 53–1 is an example of the post-chemoradiation MBS for the base of tongue patient. There is pooling of bolus within the vallecula and along the pharyngeal walls. As bolus passes distally, blunting of the epiglottis is evidenced while good UES opening is also seen. Limitations of MBS include exposure to radiation, 2D imaging of a 3D structure where superimposition of some structures occurs, use of barium as opposed to use of real food, limited time to evaluate, and lack of information regarding the management of saliva/secretions.

A FEES allows direct visualization of the pharynx during swallowing. In this way, any deficits in the movement of the palate, base of tongue, pharynx, or larynx can be identified while also identifying any pooling, penetration, or aspiration. By adding a sensory testing component, described below, the degree of sensation can be evaluated directly as well, whereas MBS only allows determination of sensation by response to deep penetration and the aspirated material.

When performing a FEES, there are several things to evaluate before proceeding to the actual swallowing component. With direct endoscopic evaluation, look for any abnormalities in tongue and soft palate motion, anatomical abnormalities, pharyngeal constriction, velopharyngeal closure, and laryngeal elevation. Also assess the status of secretions (their pooling, site, and amount as well as the patient response to them) and for any signs of aspiration. Often, the changes after treatment can be quite severe, as seen in Figure 53–2, which shows a patient with base of tongue cancer both before and after treatment. There is epiglottic thickening and edema with loss of vallecula form and fibrosis with copious pooling of secretions. Mobility of structures can

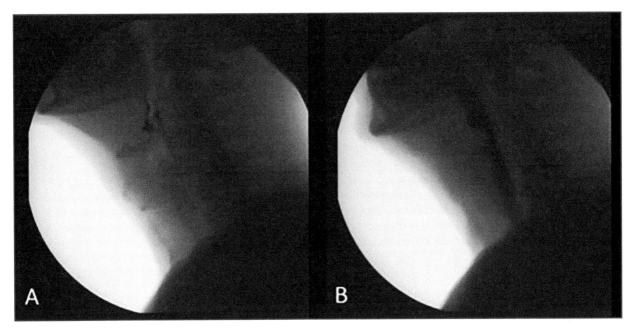

Figure 53–1. Modified barium swallow in a patient after chemoradiation. Barium residue is exhibited within the vallecula and along the pharyngeal walls (A) with the blunting of the epiglottis visible as the bolus passes (B).

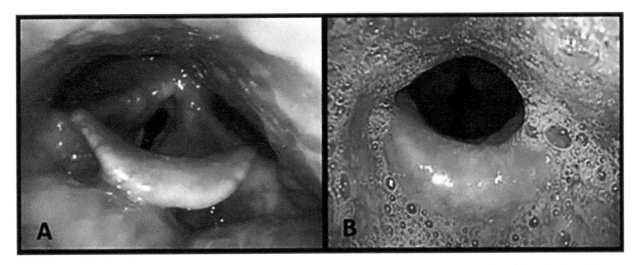

Figure 53–2. Flexible laryngoscopy view of a patient with base of tongue cancer both before (A) and after (B) chemoradiation. The patient has developed epiglottic thickening and edema with loss of vallecula and fibrosis with copious secretions pooling within the vallecula and along the pharyngeal walls.

be evaluated through having the subject perform a variety of phonatory tasks and dry swallows. Specifically, pharyngeal constriction and therefore its strength can be evaluated by having the patient say "eee" with a glide from lower pitch to higher pitch and watching for medial contraction of the lateral pharyngeal walls with narrowing of the pyriform sinuses and hypopharynx.[14–15] Also, accumulation of oropharyngeal secretions particularly within the laryngeal vestibule has been shown to be predictive of aspiration.[16] FEES allows the determination of presence and absence of secretions, their location, and the patient's reactions to them, whereas this information is not available from MBS.[17,18]

Once the initial examination is complete, then proceed with the swallowing test—typically this is performed using varying consistencies of food such as thin (water thin consistency), nectar thick, pudding, and solid consistency. Once the bolus enters the oral cavity, assess for premature oral leakage and base of tongue to posterior pharyngeal wall contact. Following the swallow, look for any signs of penetration, aspiration, or pooling. If there is evidence of penetration or aspiration, the effectiveness of cough can be evaluated. Information regarding penetration/aspiration during the swallow is usually not available due to "white out," which occurs as the endoscope contacts pharyngeal structures during hyolaryngeal movement. This information is available with MBS.

Sensory testing can be quantitatively evaluated during a flexible endoscopic evaluation of swallowing with sensory testing (FEESST) prior to any bolus preparation by blowing pulses of air onto laryngeal mucosa through the port of a flexible endoscope. This should stimulate the laryngeal adductor reflex, with the afferent limb being the internal branch of the superior laryngeal nerve and the efferent limb being the recurrent laryngeal nerve, causing brief bilateral contraction of the thyroarytenoid muscle. Should sensation be lacking, normal laryngopharyngeal reflexes will not be adequately initiated, resulting in increased risk of penetration and aspiration. The lowest pressure pulse of air that can elicit the reflex is defined as the threshold, with normal sensation reported as 4.0 mmHg and below. Moderately impaired sensation is between 4.0 and 6.0 mmHg, and more than 6.0 mmHg is defined as severely impaired.[19,20] If FEESST is not available, during FEES, gentle touching on the tip of epiglottis/aryepiglottic folds with the endoscope and asking/observing the patient's response may provide an indication regarding sensation. A triggered laryngeal adductor response is expected; however, this approach is not standardized and the results should be interpreted cautiously as it is a coarse method of testing of sensation.

More recently, pharyngeal manometry has been used to evaluate pharyngeal pressure, UES resting pressure and relaxation, and pharyngeal–UES coordination. It allows objective measurement of coordination and quantitative pressures. In a normal circumstance, the UES has a high pressure at rest due to cricopharyngeus muscle contraction. Upon swallowing initiation, the UES ceases tonic contractions and is forced open by bolus hydrostatic pressure combined with peristal-

tic constrictor contractions. A peristaltic wave is seen starting in the proximal sensors. On closing, the UES lumen will achieve sub-atmospheric pressure and then return to baseline pressure as the cricopharyngeus muscle activates.[21] Recently, high-resolution solid-state impedance manometry catheters have allowed the pressure structure to be evaluated without the use of radiology by giving a visual depiction of the pressure-flow characteristics during deglutition.[22]

If motor and sensory incompetence coexist, some form of aspiration or penetration is usually demonstrated. However, if pharyngeal contraction is intact, regardless of the sensory competence, the risk of aspiration with puree is low. However, if pharyngeal contraction is intact but there is severely impaired sensation, patients are more likely to aspirate thin liquids. With moderately impaired sensation, there is a higher prevalence of aspiration only among those with absent pharyngeal function.[23–24]

Once the nature of swallow dysfunction is known, whether sensory incompetence, motor incompetence, or both, and no other anatomical abnormalities are seen requiring surgical intervention (such as a concerning mass or stricture), referral to a speech-language pathologist is appropriate. Swallowing therapy may involve exercises to help improve strength and movement of the posterior pharyngeal wall or increase laryngeal or hyoid excursion and airway protection and decrease residue. Postural changes (such as chin tuck or head rotation) that reduce pharyngeal dimensions and redirect bolus movement can be utilized. Finally, maneuvers such as supraglottic swallow or the Mendelsohn maneuver may be implemented to change the timing or strength of particular movements of swallowing.

SUMMARY

The long-term effects of chemoradiation treatment of the head and neck on swallowing typically results in motor and/or sensory deficits. At-risk structures include the superior pharyngeal constrictor muscles, middle pharyngeal constrictor muscles, inferior pharyngeal constrictor muscles, cricopharyngeal muscle, esophageal inlet, cervical esophagus, base of tongue, supraglottic larynx, and glottic larynx. The most common motor abnormalities noted are delayed/incoordinated pharyngeal swallow and reduced pharyngeal constriction, cricopharyngeal opening, tongue base retraction, and laryngeal elevation. The exact etiology of swallow deficits can be determined with further imaging and evaluation, whether by MBS, FEES, or pharyngeal manometry. It is important to rule out any gross anatomical abnormalities requiring surgical intervention as well. However, if none are seen, the help of a speech-language pathologist is invaluable in attempting to improve immediate and long-term dysphagic symptoms.

REFERENCES

1. Argiris A. Update on chemoradiotherapy for head and neck cancer. *Curr Opin Oncol.* 2002;14(3):323–329.
2. Starmer HM, Tippett D, Webster K, et al. Swallowing outcomes in patients with oropharyngeal cancer undergoing organ-preservation treatment. *Head Neck.* 2014; 36(10):1392–1397.
3. Lazarus CL, Logemann JA, Pauloski BR, et al. Swallowing disorders in head and neck cancer patients treated with radiotherapy and adjuvant chemotherapy. *Laryngoscope.* 1996;106(9 pt 1):1157–1166.
4. Langius JA, Twisk J, Kampman M, et al. Prediction model to predict critical weight loss in patients with head and neck cancer during (chemo)radiotherapy. *Oral Oncol.* 2016;52:91–96.
5. Naik M, Ward MC, Bledsoe TJ, et al. It is not just IMRT: human papillomavirus related oropharynx squamous cell carcinoma is associated with better swallowing outcomes after definitive chemoradiotherapy. *Oral Oncol.* 2015;51(8):800–804.
6. Roe JW, Carding PN, Dwivedi RC, et al. Swallowing outcomes following intensity modulated radiation therapy (IMRT) for head & neck cancer—a systematic review. *Oral Oncol.* 2010;46(10):727–733.
7. Schwartz DL, Hutcheson K, Barringer D, et al. Candidate dosimetric predictors of long-term swallowing dysfunction after oropharyngeal intensity-modulated radiotherapy. *Int J Radiat Oncol Biol Phys.* 2010;78(5):1356–1365.
8. Carroll WR, Locher JL, Canon CL, Bohannon IA, McColloch NL, Magnuson JS. Pretreatment swallowing exercises improve swallow function after chemoradiation. *Laryngoscope.* Jan 2008;118(1):39–43.
9. Carnaby-Mann G, Crary MA, Schmalfuss I, Amdur R. "Pharyngocise": randomized controlled trial of preventative exercises to maintain muscle structure and swallowing function during head-and-neck chemoradiotherapy. *Int J Radiat Oncol Biol Phys.* 2012;83(1):210–219.
10. Goff D, Coward S, Fitzgerald A, Paleri V, Moor JW, Patterson JM. Swallowing outcomes for patients with oropharyngeal squamous cell carcinoma treated with primary (chemo)radiation therapy receiving either prophylactic gastrostomy or reactive nasogastric tube: a prospective cohort study. *Clin Otolaryngol.* 2017;42(6):1135–1140.
11. Ward MC, Bhateja P, Nwizu T, et al. Impact of feeding tube choice on severe late dysphagia after definitive chemoradiotherapy for human papillomavirus-negative head and neck cancer. *Head Neck.* 2016;38(suppl 1):E1054–E1060.
12. Splaingard ML, Hutchins B, Sulton LD, Chaudhuri G. Aspiration in rehabilitation patients: videofluoroscopy vs bedside clinical assessment. *Arch Phys Med Rehabil.* 1988;69(8):637–640.
13. Leonard R, Rees CJ, Belafsky P, Allen J. Fluoroscopic surrogate for pharyngeal strength: the pharyngeal constriction ratio (PCR). *Dysphagia.* 2011;26(1):13–17.
14. Fuller SC, Leonard R, Aminpour S, Belafsky PC. Validation of the pharyngeal squeeze maneuver. *Otolaryngol Head Neck Surg.* 2009;140(3):391–394.
15. Bastian RW. The videoendoscopic swallowing study: an alternative and partner to the videofluoroscopic swallowing study. *Dysphagia.* 1993;8(4):359–367.
16. Murray J, Langmore SE, Ginsberg S, Dostie A. The significance of accumulated oropharyngeal secretions and swallowing frequency in predicting aspiration. *Dysphagia.* 1996;11(2):99–103.
17. Bastian RW. Videoendoscopic evaluation of patients with dysphagia: an adjunct to the modified barium swallow. *Otolaryngol Head Neck Surg.* 1991;104(3):339–350.
18. Wu CH, Hsiao TY, Chen JC, Chang YC, Lee SY. Evaluation of swallowing safety with fiberoptic endoscope: comparison with videofluoroscopic technique. *Laryngoscope.* 1997;107(3):396–401.
19. Aviv JE, Martin JH, Sacco RL, et al. Supraglottic and pharyngeal sensory abnormalities in stroke patients with dysphagia. *Ann Otol Rhinol Laryngol.* 1996;105(2):92–97.
20. Aviv JE. Prospective, randomized outcome study of endoscopy versus modified barium swallow in patients with dysphagia. *Laryngoscope.* 2000;110(4):563–574.
21. Postma GN, Butler SG, Belafsky PC, Halum SL. Normal pharyngeal and upper esophageal sphincter manometry. *Ear Nose Throat J.* 2004;83(12):809.
22. Cock C, Omari T. Diagnosis of swallowing disorders: how we interpret pharyngeal manometry. *Curr Gastroenterol Rep.* 2017;19(3):11.
23. Setzen M, Cohen MA, Perlman PW, et al. The association between laryngopharyngeal sensory deficits, pharyngeal motor function, and the prevalence of aspiration with thin liquids. *Otolaryngol Head Neck Surg.* 2003; 128(1):99–102.
24. Aviv JE, Spitzer J, Cohen M, Ma G, Belafsky P, Close LG. Laryngeal adductor reflex and pharyngeal squeeze as predictors of laryngeal penetration and aspiration. *Laryngoscope.* 2002;112(2):338–341.

CHAPTER 54

Cricopharyngeal Dysfunction

Ashli O'Rourke

INTRODUCTION

Understanding pharyngoesophageal dysphagia is important as swallowing involves bolus transfer from the lips to the stomach and at any point in the swallowing continuum dysfunction can occur. While we may tend to think of dysphagia in stages (eg, oral preparatory, oral, pharyngeal, and esophageal), the swallowing mechanism is interrelated in timing, and dysfunction in one area can affect the other. Therefore, dysphagia clinicians need to understand, evaluate, and treat the swallowing mechanism as a whole.

An important cause of pharyngoesophageal dysphagia is cricopharyngeal (CP) muscle dysfunction. CP dysfunction is the failure of the upper esophageal sphincter (UES) to cease tonic contraction ("relax") and open during swallowing. CP pathology can be associated with a wide variety of disease states but oftentimes the etiology is unknown.

CASE PRESENTATION 1

A 68-year-old female presents with a 7-year history of worsening dysphagia. She primarily reports solid food and pill dysphagia. Her symptoms are alleviated by liquid swallows. She occasionally regurgitates undigested food during or immediately after a meal and often feels she must swallow multiple times on each bolus. She denies weight loss, dysphonia, odynophagia, or pulmonary symptoms. She has a history of heartburn that is adequately controlled on once daily proton pump inhibitor therapy.

Past medical history: Gastroesophageal reflux disease (GERD), essential hypertension

Past surgical history: None

Medications: Omeprazole 20 mg daily, lisinopril 10 mg

Allergies: None

Social: Denies tobacco or alcohol use

Initial Assessment

History

She does not exhibit any danger signs indicating malignancy. Weight loss, history of pneumonia or hemoptysis would be concerning. However, given her solid food dysphagia, further evaluation is warranted.

Examination

Reveals an overweight female in no acute distress. Her voice is within normal limits for age and gender. Head and neck examination is unremarkable and neurologic examination is normal.

Investigations

- Flexible endoscopic evaluation of swallowing (FEES) is completed. (Video 1). This reveals minimal to no pharyngeal residue immediately after her pharyngeal swallow,

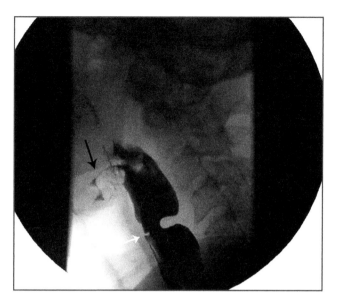

Figure 54–1. Esophagram image of CP bar with concomitant small anterior cervical web (*white arrow*). Note penetration during the swallow (*black arrow*).

but brisk regurgitation of swallowed solid food material from the esophagus into the pharynx (rising tide sign). No penetration or aspiration is noted. Pharyngeal contractility and sensation appear grossly intact.

- Esophagram is completed (Figure 54–1), which shows obstructive CP hypertrophy with a concomitant hypopharyngeal anterior web.

Diagnosis

Upper esophageal web and obstructive CP hypertrophy in the setting of symptomatically well-controlled reflux.

Management

 Endoscopic laser assisted CP myotomy (Video 2) is completed with resolution of symptoms.

CASE PRESENTATION 2

A 54-year-old male presents for evaluation of dysphagia 8 weeks following a brainstem cerebrovascular accident (CVA). He had a gastrostomy tube placed 1 week following his CVA and is not taking any nutrition by mouth due to aspiration-related pneumonia. He reports slurred speech.

Past medical history: Hypertension, hypercholesterolemia, poorly controlled diabetes type II, obesity

Past surgical history: Knee replacement surgery

Medications: Simvastatin, metformin, insulin, clopidogrel, aspirin

Allergies: Penicillin

Social: Former one pack per day smoker for 25 years, quit approximately 10 years ago. No alcohol consumption.

MRI of the brain revealed a left lateral medullary infarct.

Physical Examination

Examination revealed left facial nerve palsy with ptosis of left eye and nystagmus. Palatal myotonic movements noted. He was dysphonic and dysarthric and gait was ataxic.

Interventions

- Videofluoroscopic swallowing study (VFSS) was completed which showed adequate oral phase but decreased pharyngeal contractility. There was inadequate opening of pharyngoesophageal segment with penetration during the swallow with all liquid consistencies and silent aspiration with thin liquids after the swallow. Residue was most prevalent in the post-cricoid region.
- High-resolution manometry (HRM) revealed normal UES basal tone but inadequate opening duration and elevated relaxation pressures of the UES. He had normal distal esophageal motility.

Diagnosis

Cricopharyngeal hypertonicity due to lateral medullary (Wallenberg's) syndrome.

This syndrome is characterized by a pattern of symptoms such as vertigo, nystagmus, ataxia, palatal myoclonus, loss of pain and temperature sensation in the contralateral body and ipsilateral face, and ipsilateral Horner's syndrome (myosis, ptosis, and anhydrosis). Due to effects on the nucleus ambiguus, cranial nerve IX and X dysfunction are common, resulting in vocal fold paralysis and oftentimes severe dysphagia.[1] Since cricopharyngeal function is mediated by glossopharyngeal and vagal nerve branches,[2] CP dysfunction may be contributory to dysphagia in Wallenberg's syndrome.

Management

Endoscopic botulinum toxin A injection to CP muscle is completed with 30 units in 10 unit aliquots at three separate injection sites (Figure 54–2). For CP injections, a more concentrated solution than used with vocal fold injections is often desirable (eg, 100 units per mL).

Complete relaxation of the UES is achieved via a complex interaction of intrabolus pressure, hyolaryngeal mechanics, and neural inhibition. Failure of relaxation increases the risk of post-swallow pharyngeal residue and subsequent penetration or aspiration. CP botulinum toxin injections were first introduced in the literature by Schneider et al in 1994.[3] Investigations have shown improvement in swallow dysfunction following botulinum toxin injections in patients with neurologic CP dysfunction (ie, from vagal neuropathy or Wallenberg syndrome), particularly when some pharyngeal contractility is preserved.[4-6]

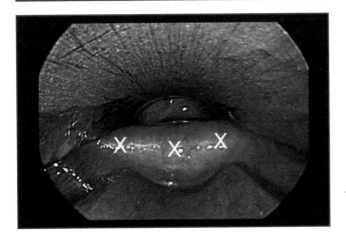

Figure 54–2. Endoscopic surgical view of the CP muscle. Injections are completed in three locations (*white X*).

Follow-Up

Patient had improvement in his symptoms following botulinum toxin injection but continued to have pharyngeal dysphagia issues. He participated in swallowing therapy and over the next 6 months improved to the point of tolerating a mechanical soft diet with thin liquids. No further botulinum toxin injections were completed. Prior investigations have shown that a single botulinum toxin injection in stroke patients may have longer lasting effects than could be expected from botulinum effects alone.[4]

CASE PRESENTATION 3

A 73-year-old female presents with a 7-year history of feeling that "all foods stick in my throat." Symptoms are not acutely worsening and onset was gradual. She reports difficulty with both solids and liquids, frequently coughing during meals. She has modified her diet to thicker liquids and softer solids that she chews well. She has lost 50 pounds over the last 6 years, mainly due to avoidance of certain consistencies. Denies voice changes, recent pneumonia, or odynophagia.

Prior to referral she underwent an esophagogastroduodenoscopy with bougie dilation to 42 French. This did not help her symptoms. The report indicated a tight UES and normal esophageal mucosa. No hiatal hernia.

Past medical history: Rheumatoid arthritis, coronary artery disease, hypothyroidism

Past surgical history: Coronary artery bypass graft, cholecystectomy

Medications: Atorvastatin, dicyclomine, lansoprazole, metoprolol, synthroid

Allergies: Sulfa drugs

Social: Quit smoking 22 years ago after 30-pack-year history, no alcohol use.

Interventions

- Esophagram was completed which revealed severe failure of relaxation of the CP muscle (Figure 54–3) and reduced primary esophageal peristalsis with tertiary

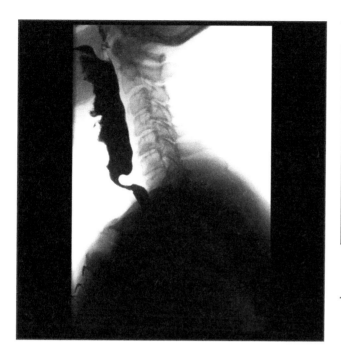

Figure 54–3. Esophagram image showing severe obstruction of the PES by a prominent CP muscle.

contractions. There were spondylitic degenerative changes of the cervical spine.
- HRM and pH testing were attempted but unable to pass the catheters into the esophagus and patient was intolerant of the examinations.

Diagnosis

Cricopharyngeal dysfunction, possible esophageal dysmotility

Management

- Endoscopic laser assisted cricopharyngeal myotomy was attempted but surgeon was unable to position scope to adequately view the cricopharyngeus, possibly due to osteophytic changes of the cervical spine.
- Converted to transcervical cricopharyngeal myotomy. Patient did well immediately postoperatively and was discharged home on postoperative day 3 tolerating soft diet.

Table 54–1. Ineffective Esophageal Motility Strategies

1. Eat small, frequent meals.
2. Eat in the upright position to allow gravity to help empty the esophagus.
3. Avoid lying down at least 2 hours after eating meals.
4. Avoid strenuous activity or exercise after eating.
5. If possible, try to swallow only once on each bite, allowing time (about 10–15 seconds) for the food to travel down the esophagus before taking another bite.
6. Be very careful swallowing pills. Take pills one at a time and with plenty of liquid. Consider liquid preparations of troublesome or large pills.

Follow-Up and Further Management

- Patient presented to clinic 3 weeks postoperatively. Swallowing function was much improved but she had new complaints of increased reflux symptoms, particularly complaining of acidic regurgitation into her throat upon lying down at night.
- HRM was completed which revealed ineffective esophageal motility (IEM).
- Patient was given IEM strategies (Table 54–1) to follow and started on liquid sodium alginate after each meal and at night before bed. After these failed to significantly relieve her symptoms, she was prescribed bethanechol 1 hour before meals.
- Since she was not a good surgical candidate for lower esophageal sphincter (LES) surgery due to her IEM, she was fitted for a Reza Band® (Somna Therapeutics, Germantown, WI) for use at night. The Reza Band is a device worn around the neck that applies external pressure to the cricoid cartilage. This improves pharyngoesophageal closure, thereby mechanically decreasing esophagopharyngeal reflux. She had good resolution of reflux symptoms and minimal dysphagia on this management.

CASE PRESENTATION 4

A 58-year-old male presents with a 5-year history of slowly progressive solid food dysphagia. He is avoiding meats, breads, and coarse solids. He reports a

10-pound weight loss over the last year that he attributes to diet modifications. He denies voice change, hemoptysis, hematemesis, otalgia, or odynophagia.

Past medical history: Hypertension, hyperlipidemia, lumbar spine degeneration

Past surgical history: Lumbar spine surgery

Medications: Atenolol, atorvastatin, gabapentin, occasional narcotic use for back pain

Allergies: Penicillin

Social: Current one pack per day smoker for past 40 years, moderate alcohol consumption

Physical Examination

Head and neck examination is unremarkable and there is no cervical lymphadenopathy.

Investigations

- Solid food dysphagia and weight loss are concerning symptoms in a patient with a history of tobacco and alcohol use. Evaluation for causes of dysphagia and assessment for possible upper aerodigestive tract malignancy are recommended.
- Flexible laryngoscopy was indicated after patient's gag prevented adequate assessment with mirror examination. No mucosal masses or lesions were noted. Normal vocal fold mobility. Pharyngeal contractility and sensation appeared grossly normal. Minimal residue and no aspiration or penetration noted when swallowing liquids or solids during laryngoscopy.
- Transnasal esophagoscopy was completed to evaluate for possible esophageal causes of solid food dysphagia, including malignancy. This revealed mild restriction at the UES but normal esophageal mucosa without stricture, masses, or lesions. No gastritis.
- Patient had an esophagram that revealed a CP bar with narrowing of the pharyngoesophageal lumen (Figure 54–4).
- HRM with impedance testing revealed normal basal UES tone with poor relaxation

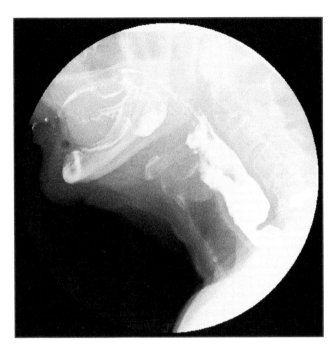

Figure 54–4. Esophagram image showing a narrow cricopharyngeal bar. Note anterior cervical osteophytes (*white arrow*) at the level of the bar, contributing to obstruction in this region.

opening duration and elevated relaxation pressures. There was fragmented esophageal peristalsis with 40% bolus transit (abnormal). Normal LES basal and relaxation pressures.
- pH-impedance testing was normal.

Diagnosis

Cricopharyngeal dysfunction in the setting of esophageal dysmotility

Management

Endoscopic botulinum toxin A injection to cricopharyngeus muscle is completed, 30 units in 10 unit aliquots at three separate injection sites.

Reevaluation

Patient presented to office 5 days following his procedure, complaining of significantly worsened dysphagia.

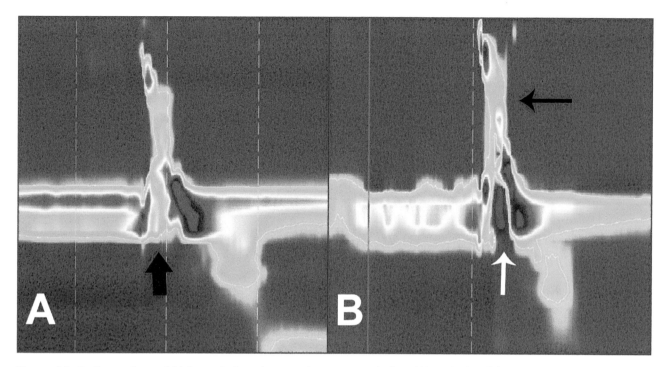

Figure 54–5. Comparison of high-resolution pharyngeal manometry before (**A**) and after (**B**) swallowing therapy without surgical intervention. There is decreased opening of the UES with increased intrabolus pressure (*wide black arrow*) that is improved following therapy (*white arrow*). Note also increased pharyngeal contractility (*thin black arrow*).

Voice was normal and laryngoscopy revealed normal vocal fold mobility. VFSS with concurrent HRM was completed. HRM revealed significantly decreased UES basal tone and decreased contractility of inferior pharyngeal constrictors (Figure 54–5). On videofluoroscopy, the cricopharyngeus was flaccid and obstructive (Video 56–3).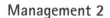

Management 2

- Reassessment was that the patient's etiology of CP dysfunction had been due to fibrosis or hypertrophy versus hypertonicity of the sphincter. Botulinum toxin in this patient, undertaken due to concern for esophageal dysmotility, actually worsened his symptoms. This was due to the creation of a flaccid obstruction of the CP muscle as well as diffusion of botulinum toxin to the inferior constrictors.
- The patient was treated with a modified diet and pyridostigmine 60 mg three times daily

with return to baseline swallowing function in less than a week. Pyridostigmine is a reversible acetylcholinesterase inhibitor used predominantly in the treatment of myasthenia gravis. Young and Halstead published a case series showing good efficacy of pyridostigmine in the improvement of severe adverse effects following laryngeal botulinum toxin injections.[7]

- Endoscopic laser assisted CP myotomy was completed approximately 6 weeks later with complete resolution of dysphagia.

DISCUSSION

Diagnosis

The diagnosis of cricopharyngeal dysfunction begins with a detailed history. Typically videofluoroscopy, via either a VFSS or esophagram, is completed that reveals failure of CP relaxation or a "CP bar." Other signs of

CP dysfunction may include appearance of shorter opening duration of the pharyngoesophageal segment (PES), post-cricoid residue, immediate retrograde flow from the PES (esophagopharyngeal reflux) or aspiration following the swallow.

Aside from videofluoroscopy, the preoperative workup for cricopharyngeal intervention is controversial. At the center of this controversy is whether CP myotomy may result in worsening esophagopharyngeal reflux. While a couple of studies have shown no increase in postoperative acidic reflux events following CP myotomy,[8,9] newer investigations with impedance technology and a focus on dysmotility issues are sparse. Migliore et al revealed several patients in their case series who required anti-reflux surgery following CP myotomy and recommended pharyngoesophageal manometry as a preoperative assessment.[10] Many otolaryngologists, chastened by their own adverse experiences or scattered case reports,[11] continue to question the role of preoperative pH-impedance and HRM evaluation. This controversy likely continues to exist because CP dysfunction represents a heterogeneous group of patients with different symptoms and etiologies.

A FEES examination or VFSS should be completed to assess the pharyngeal swallow in relation to UES function. If FEES is normal, a barium esophagram is obtained. If the patient has a VFSS with esophageal follow-through, then a formal esophagram may not be needed. The purpose of FEES or VFSS is to assess oropharyngeal swallowing in relation to PES function. Decreased pharyngeal contractility or impaired hyolaryngeal mechanics may affect proper PES functioning. In these cases, swallowing exercises or compensatory strategies may result in improved UES function without direct CP intervention.

While a barium esophagram showing symptomatic CP obstruction may suffice as a minimum, it is my opinion that a thorough investigation of the dysphagic patient is required for consistent and predictable outcomes. In patients at high risk for reflux or dysmotility, a thorough preoperative assessment allows for improved preoperative counseling with patients. In my practice, patients with suspected CP dysfunction routinely undergo HRM and pH-impedance testing prior to surgical intervention. This allows objective assessment of UES function and esophageal motility. Abnormal reflux can be addressed preoperatively and patient can be counseled regarding possible postoperative issues.

Transnasal esophagoscopy (TNE) may be completed in the office, but in my experience it is difficult to fully appreciate the function of the cricopharyngeus during unsedated examination. A full esophagoscopy is warranted in these patients, however, and is completed at the time of surgical intervention. If surgery is deferred, then TNE is completed for adequate evaluation.

HRM may be useful in differentiating spasm from a more static failure of relaxation. However, the limitation of both esophagram and HRM are that they cannot distinguish between failure of UES relaxation due to neurogenic causes or insufficient opening due to mechanical issues (eg, fibrosis).[12] Although electromyography (EMG) may help differentiate the two and guide the clinician to more specific treatment,[12] this is invasive and technically challenging, therefore not widely practiced.

Etiology

Cricopharyngeal dysfunction is a common cause of dysphagia encountered by otolaryngologists, although the frequency in dysphagic patients overall is fairly low. The incidence of cricopharyngeal bar seen on videofluoroscopy ranges from 6% to 15% in the literature, with incidence in patients over 60 years of age being higher at approximately 30%.[13,14]

There are several mechanisms that may lead to UES dysfunction, including spasm, failure of reduction in tonic contraction, fibrosis, and/or decreased hyolaryngeal superior-anterior movement. A thorough history is most likely to assist the clinician in identifying the correct cause of dysfunction; for example, fibrosis is most likely in a patient with history of head and neck radiation and a stroke patient may have decreased hyolaryngeal elevation and pharyngeal drive. Cricopharyngeal dysfunction can be due to many different disease states, some of which are rare and others that are more common (Table 54–2).[15] Categorization by dysfunction (ie, hypertrophy versus spasm) is likely the most clinically useful.

CP Dysfunction and GERD

The CP muscle is contracted at rest to prevent retrograde flow of gastroesophageal contents into the pharynx. It has been shown that UES tone increases with distal acid perfusion[16] and therefore cricopharyngeal hypertrophy may actually be a compensatory mechanism in the setting of esophageal dysmotility or reflux disease. There are few investigations that examine this phenomenon, but Chavez et al reported that nearly 1/3 of patients with impaired LES relaxation were

Table 54–2. Causes of UES Dysfunction

Neurologic
Stroke
Parkinson's disease
Vagal neuropathy
Idiopathic spasm
Amyotrophic Lateral Sclerosis
Esophageal dysmotility

Inflammatory
Myopathic
Polymyositis
Dermatomyositis
Inclusion body myositis
Gastroesophageal reflux
Caustic ingestion
Age related
Idiopathic
Iatrogenic
Recurrent laryngeal nerve injury
Instrumental damage (eg, gastroscopy injury)
Radiation fibrosis
Post-cricopharyngeal myotomy (intentional)

found to have UES abnormalities, the most common being hypertensive UES basal tone.[17] They also found that patients with impaired LES function were more likely to have UES dysfunction compared with normal controls.[17] Furthermore, in an interesting study by Wauters et al, the investigators found that UES mean relaxation and intrabolus pressure were significantly reduced after balloon dilation of the LES in achalasia patients.[18] Two other groups reported similar improvement in UES parameters following endoscopic LES myotomy.[19,20]

While not conclusive, these studies point to the possibility of compensatory CP hypertonicity and/or hypertrophy in esophageal body or LES dysfunction. Although most needle electromyography parameters have been shown to be normal in GERD patients,[21] prolonged foreburst duration was significantly correlated with reflux severity and may indicate irritation of the muscle caused by GERD.[22]

Treatment

The treatment of CP dysfunction depends on the cause and the severity of symptoms. Non-surgical options include swallowing therapy to improve pharyngeal contractility and bolus propulsion, compensatory maneuvers (eg, Mendelsohn maneuver, effortful swallow, head turn) designed to enhance CP opening, or diet modifications with avoidance of troublesome consistencies. Surgical options include cricopharyngeal botulinum toxin injections, dilation, and transcervical or endoscopic myotomy.

Botulinum Toxin Injection

Botulinum toxin injection is typically completed in the operating room, but authors have shown feasibility and efficacy with office based EMG guided injections.[7,12] Efficacy rates, typically evaluated by patient reported outcome measures, range from 43% to 100%.[23]

Adverse effects may include worsening dysphagia or rarely vocal fold immobility causing either dysphonia or airway constriction. These complications are typically due to too superficial of an injection (not intramuscular) leading to diffusion to inferior constrictors or too anterior of an injection leading to diffusion to the posterior cricoarytenoid muscles. To decrease adverse effects, unilateral injections are recommended with percutaneous EMG guided procedures and use of more concentrated, lower volume injections with operative laryngoscopic guided injections. It may be prudent to avoid dilation immediately following botulinum injection to decrease unwanted diffusion. Botulinum toxin type A is most commonly used and volumes range from 10 to 100 units in the literature.[7,24,25] An initial dose of 30 units botulinum A for bilateral injection (operative laryngoscopy) seems reasonable.

Dilation

Dilation of the cricopharyngeus may be accomplished by bougie or balloon procedure. While an overall safe technique, it often requires sedation or general anesthesia. In addition, reports reveal relatively short-term results with need for repeat dilation being common.[23]

Myotomy

Cricopharyngeal myotomy is completed by either an open transcutaneous or endoscopic laser assisted approach, with the latter gaining more popularity in recent years. In a comparison of success rates based on invasiveness of procedures, Kocdor et al found that myotomy (the most invasive) had a statistically higher success rate over botulinum toxin and balloon dilation procedures.[26] In addition, when comparing open with endoscopic myotomy procedures, logistic regression analysis revealed higher success rate with endoscopic procedures.[26] However, Ashman et al found in their systematic review that, due to the decreased incidence of adverse effects, the less invasive techniques of injection or dilation may be more appropriate for sicker or more elderly patients.[23]

SUMMARY

CP dysfunction is a heterogeneous disorder with multiple etiologies. There are several different possible interventions for CP dysfunction. The surgeon must consider the most likely cause of CP dysfunction along with patient related factors to choose the most appropriate intervention to alleviate dysphagic symptoms.

REFERENCES

1. Martino R, Terrault N, Ezerzer F, Mikulis D, Diamant NE. Dysphagia in a patient with lateral medullary syndrome: insight into the central control of swallowing. *Gastroenterology.* 2001;121(2):420–426.
2. Sasaki CT, Kim YH, Sims HS, Czibulka A. Motor innervation of the human cricopharyngeus muscle. *Ann Otol Rhinol Laryngol.* 1999;108(12):1132–1139.
3. Schenider I, Thumfart WF, Potoschig C, et al. Treatment of dysfunction of the cricopharyngeal muscle with botulinum A toxin: introduction of a new, noninvasive method. *Ann Otol Rhinol Laryngol* 1994;103:31–35.
4. Terré R, Panadés A, Mearin F. Botulinum toxin treatment for oropharyngeal dysphagia in patients with stroke. *Neurogastroenterol Motil.* 2013 Nov;25(11):e896–e702.
5. Woisard-Bassols V, Alshehri S, Simonetta-Moreau M. The effects of botulinum toxin injections into the cricopharyngeus muscle of patients with cricopharyngeus dysfunction associated with pharyngo-laryngeal weakness. *Eur Arch Otorhinolaryngol.* 2013;270(3):805–815.
6. Kim MS, Kim GW, Rho YS, Kwon KH, Chung EJ. Office-based electromyography-guided botulinum toxin injection to the cricopharyngeus muscle: optimal patient selection and technique. *Ann Otol Rhinol Laryngol.* 2017; 126(5):349–356.
7. Young DL, Halstead LA. Pyridostigmine for reversal of severe sequelae from botulinum toxin injection. *J Voice.* 2014;28(6):830–834.
8. Henderson RD, Hanna WM, Henderson RF, et al. Myotomy for reflux-induced cricopharyngeal dysphagia. Five-year review. *J Thorac Cardiovasc Surg.* 1989;98:428–433.
9. Williams RB, Ali GN, Hunt DR, et al. Cricopharyngeal myotomy does not increase the risk of esophagopharyngeal acid regurgitation. *Am J Gastroenterol.* 1999;94: 3448–3454.
10. Migliore M1, Payne HR, Jeyasingham K. Pharyngo-oesophageal dysphagia: surgery based on clinical and manometric data. *Eur J Cardiothorac Surg.* 1996;10(5): 365–371.
11. Sanei-Moghaddam A1, Kumar S, Jani P, Brierley C. Cricopharyngeal myotomy for cricopharyngeus stricture in an inclusion body myositis patient with hiatus hernia: a learning experience. *BMJ Case Rep.* 2013;2013.
12. Alfonsi E, Merlo IM, Ponzio M, Montomoli C, Tassorelli C, Biancardi C, Lozza A, Martignoni E. An electrophysiological approach to the diagnosis of neurogenic dysphagia: implications for botulinum toxin treatment. *J Neurol Neurosurg Psychiatry.* 2010;81(1):54–60.
13. Baredes S, Shah CS, Kaufman R. *Am J Otolaryngol.* The frequency of cricopharyngeal dysfunction on videofluoroscopic swallowing studies in patients with dysphagia. 1997;18(3):185–189.
14. Frederick MG, Ott DJ, Grishaw EK, Gelfand DW, Chen MY. Functional abnormalities of the pharynx: a prospective analysis of radiographic abnormalities relative to age and symptoms. *AJR Am J Roentgenol.* 1996;166(2):353–357.
15. Allen JE. Cricopharyngeal function or dysfunction: what's the deal? *Curr Opin Otolaryngol Head Neck Surg.* 2016;24(6):494–499.
16. Tokashiki R, Funato N, Suzuki M. Globus sensation and increased upper esophageal sphincter pressure with distal esophageal acid perfusion. *Eur Arch Otorhinolaryngol.* 2010;267(5):737–741.
17. Chavez YH, Ciarleglio MM, Clarke JO, Nandwani M, Stein E, Roland BC. Upper esophageal sphincter abnormalities: frequent finding on high-resolution esophageal manometry and associated with poorer treatment response in achalasia. *J Clin Gastroenterol.* 2015;49(1):17–23.
18. Wauters L, Van Oudenhove L, Selleslagh M, et al. Balloon dilation of the esophagogastric junction affects lower and upper esophageal sphincter function in achalasia. *Neurogastroenterol Motil.* 2014;26(1):69–76.
19. Yao S, Linghu E. Peroral endoscopic myotomy can improve esophageal motility in patients with achalasia from a large sample self-control research (66 patients). *PLoS One.* 2015;10(5):e0125942.
20. Ren Y, Tang X, Chen F, et al. Myotomy of distal esophagus influences proximal esophageal contraction and upper esophageal sphincter relaxation in patients with achalasia after peroral endoscopic myotomy. *J Neurogastroenterol Motil.* 2016;22(1):78–85.
21. Alkan Z, Demir A, Yigit O, et al. Cricopharyngeal muscle electromyography findings in patients with gastroesophageal reflux disease. *Otolaryngol Head Neck Surg.* 2012;147(2):295–301.

22. Celik M, Alkan Z, Ercan I, Ertasoglu H, Alkm C, Erdem L, Turgut S, Ertekin C. Cricopharyngeal muscle electromyography in laryngopharyngeal reflux. *Laryngoscope.* 2005;115(1):138–142.

23. Ashman A, Dale OT, Baldwin DL. Management of isolated cricopharyngeal dysfunction: systematic review. *J Laryngol Otol.* 2016;130(7):611–615.

24. Schrey A, Airas L, Jokela M, Pulkkinen J. Botulinum toxin alleviates dysphagia of patients with inclusion body myositis. *J Neurol Sci.* 2017;380:142–147.

25. Sharma SD, Kumar G, Eweiss A, Chatrath P, Kaddour H. Endoscopic-guided injection of botulinum toxin into the cricopharyngeus muscle: our experience. *J Laryngol Otol.* 2015;129(10):990–995.

26. Kocdor P, Siegel ER, Tulunay-Ugur OE. Cricopharyngeal dysfunction: a systematic review comparing outcomes of dilatation, botulinum toxin injection, and myotomy. *Laryngoscope.* 2016;126(1):135–141.

CHAPTER 55

Systemic Sclerosis/CREST Syndrome and Swallow Dysfunction

Silvia G. Marinone-Lares and Jacqueline Allen

Silvia G. Marinone-Lares and Jacqueline Allen

INTRODUCTION

Systemic conditions, particularly those resulting in vasculitis or connective tissue disorders, may present with or include swallow dysfunction in the range of symptoms that affect patients. These include autoimmune conditions such as granulomatosis with polyangiitis, rheumatoid arthritis, systemic lupus erythematosus, polymyositis, and systemic sclerosis.[1]

Systemic sclerosis (SSc) is an autoimmune disease that affects the microvasculature and connective tissue, causing progressive fibrosis of the skin and visceral organs.[1,2] SSc can be classified as *diffuse cutaneous disease* when skin thickening is seen proximal to the knees and elbows, *limited cutaneous disease* when skin thickening is distal to the knees and elbows, and *overlap syndrome* when features of other connective tissue diseases are present.[3]

This group of sclerosing skin disorders is well known to affect the gastrointestinal tract (GIT), with the overwhelming majority (>90%) of patients reporting GIT symptoms.[4] The esophagus is the most commonly affected subsite of the GIT.[2,4,5] In these cases, dysfunctional deglutition may occur with attendant secondary problems, including weight loss, respiratory complaints, and choking. The treatment of these disorders is evolving with both medical and surgical therapy offering benefit.

DEFINITION

SSc is a group of autoimmune disorders characterized by abnormal small blood vessels and progressive fibrotic changes in the dermis and connective tissue. It is classified as diffuse cutaneous disease, limited cutaneous disease, and overlap syndrome.[3] CREST syndrome is a variant of limited cutaneous disease, with the acronym "CREST" representing Calcinosis, Raynaud's phenomenon, Esophageal dysfunction, Sclerodactyly, and Telangiectasia. SSc has multi-organ effects that may include esophageal dysmotility. SSc occurs most often in women aged 40 to 65 years (M:F, 2:8).[5]

PATHOPHYSIOLOGY OF SWALLOWING DYSFUNCTION IN SSC

The pathogenesis of SSc is not fully understood, but there is some evidence that has led to the description of four stages of progression that are thought to lead to GIT dysfunction: microvasculopathy, neural dysfunction, smooth muscle atrophy, and, finally, fibrosis.[6,7] Symptoms present during the neural stage, at which point patients describe dysphagia, gastroesophageal reflux disease (GERD), and abdominal distension. Prokinetic drugs may reverse the functional abnormalities at this early stage. When smooth muscle atrophy develops, there is only partial response to drugs, and when fibrosis ensues, drugs are no longer useful.[6,7] The specific cause of the first stage of microvasculopathy is yet unknown. Once initiated, endothelial abnormalities result in an inflammatory response with the release of numerous cytokines, chemokines, and polypeptide growth factors that recruit fibroblasts and other cells that differentiate into myofibroblasts, eventually causing fibrosis of the musculature of the GIT.[4,5]

587

It is thought that episodes of vasoconstriction and reperfusion result in tissue ischemia and stimulate reparative processes. A fibrogenic process ensues with replacement of connective tissue elements with fibrosis.[5]

The vasculopathy described above in conjunction with immune dysfunction as evidenced by the presence of auto-antibodies are believed to be the main pathogenic drivers of GIT dysfunction in SSc.[4,5]

CASE PRESENTATION

A 71-year-old woman was referred for evaluation of dysphagia and globus sensation present for a decade but progressing over the past 5 months. Additional complaints of regurgitation of food, coughing and vomiting after meals, eructation, and mucus in the throat were reported. Mild solid food dysphagia, early satiety, and reflux symptoms with bitter flavor in the oral cavity were also present. Acid reflux symptoms had been medicated with proton pump inhibitors with some response for heartburn symptoms but no assistance with swallowing. Liquids were not problematic, and no weight loss was described. Mild dysphonia was reported but she was not concerned about this. She is a non-smoker and her current medications include omeprazole, aspirin, hydroxyurea, diltiazem, and venlafaxine.

INITIAL ASSESSMENT

History

Initial evaluation includes a comprehensive inquiry of symptoms, most importantly dysphagia, odynophagia, weight loss, dysphonia, and breathing issues. Patient-reported symptom instruments such as the Eating Assessment Tool (EAT-10) and the Voice Handicap Index (VHI-10) can be useful to track symptoms over time. Characteristics of dysphagia (solids, liquids, pills, multiple), onset, and sequelae (weight loss, malnutrition, pneumonia) should be evaluated. Reports of chest infection, pneumonia, food bolus impaction, and reflux symptoms reflect severe swallow dysfunction. Cough and mucus production may also be relevant.

Further history regarding medical and surgical comorbidities, previous surgery or radiation treatments, exposure to tobacco and alcohol, and family history of relevant disorders should be obtained. Current medications, allergies, and family history are helpful.

Examination

Initial examination includes assessment of vocal quality, secretions, and volitional cough. Lower cranial nerve (CN V–XII) examination is undertaken by assessing facial and masticatory muscle function and sensation, palate and tongue function, and shoulder elevation. During this exam mucosal appearance, hydration, jaw mobility, and dental quality can also be evaluated. The neck should be inspected for scars and masses, including lymphadenopathy.

Endoscopy

Endoscopic visualization of the laryngopharynx is vital and can be combined with administration of food and fluid through a functional endoscopic evaluation of swallowing (FEES). This provides information regarding pharyngolaryngeal sensation, motor function, secretion presence, pharyngeal strength (through the validated pharyngeal squeeze maneuver), regurgitation on hard phonation, and penetration or aspiration if present. Esophageal endoscopy, performed in-office (transnasal esophagoscopy [TNE]) or under sedation as an esophagogastroduodenoscopy (EGD) is helpful to assess mucosal integrity, gastroesophageal junction structure, hiatus hernia, and the presence of strictures and other pathologies such as Barrett's esophagus.

Additional Testing

Fluoroscopic evaluation of swallowing in the form of a videofluoroscopic swallow study (VFSS) provides additional crucial information. Quantitative displacement and timing measures can be gathered and airway violation demonstrated. Furthermore, if the bolus is followed distally, then esophageal evaluation is also possible. Delay in esophageal transit of bolus, redirection, stasis, strictures and rings, or herniae can be identified (particularly if a barium tablet of 13 mm diameter is also given to swallow). SSc often affects esophageal smooth muscle with dysmotility a common finding. Pharyngoesophageal manometry (preferably high resolution) will also provide quantitative swallowing metrics, and there are clearly defined parameters that are diagnostic for primary esophageal motility disorders as set out by the Chicago classification.[8] Low esophageal body pressures and hypotonic lower esophageal sphincter (LES) with incomplete bolus transfer are hallmarks of SSc.[1,9,10] Around 70% of SSc patients demonstrate esophageal symptoms thought to be due to smooth muscle atrophy, fibrosis, and incoordination.[1,10,11] Raja et al report HRM findings in 31 SSc patients, with 89% demonstrating dysmotility, 63% hypotonic LES, and 84% with positive pH-metry criteria. Those with worse gastroesophageal reflux parameters (eg, higher DeMeester score and total acid times) also demonstrated significant lung disease but did not necessarily report typical reflux symptoms such as heartburn and regurgitation.[9]

Blood work may also be performed primarily looking for positive anti-centromere (15–43%), anti-topoisomerase I (21–34%), anti-RNA polymerase III (5%), or anti-ribonucleoprotein (5%) antibodies.[11]

SCENARIO 1

History is as above; however, the patient also reports a diagnosis of CREST syndrome under the care of a rheumatologist. The patient's examination shows no mass lesions but a perceptually diplophonic voice. In-office TNE reveals mild pooling of secretions within the pyriform apices, normal laryngeal mobility function but left-sided atrophy and weak glottal closure, poor distal esophageal contractility, and a hiatus hernia (Figure 55–1). Her VHI-10 is 17 and EAT-10 is 18.

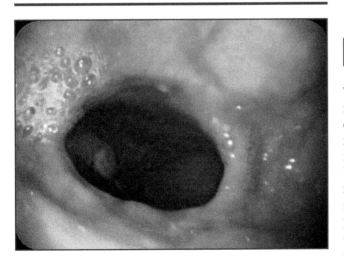

Figure 55–1. Endoscopic image demonstrating peptic stricture, grade B esophagitis, hiatus hernia containing refluxate.

VFSS confirmed poor esophageal motility with a hiatal hernia, bolus stasis and oscillation, and moderate gastroesophageal escape.

Diagnosis

Esophageal dysmotility with concomitant gastroesophageal reflux secondary to CREST syndrome

Investigations

As reported, the VFSS reveals poor esophageal transit of bolus, redirection of bolus, and a hiatus hernia (also identified by TNE).

Management

The patient is counseled regarding eating strategies, including texture management (alternating solids and liquids), use of lubrication, body position during meals (upright during meals and for a further 90 minutes), and during sleep (head of the bed elevated by 30°). She is recommended a trial of prokinetic medication (domperidone 10 mg three times a day) and post-prandial alginate. Review is planned for 8 weeks time with repeat VFSS in 12 months (unless symptoms deteriorate).

SCENARIO 2

The patient's examination shows marked pooling of foamy saliva in the hypopharynx, with penetration episodes and reduced pharyngeal clearance, but fully mobile vocal folds. TNE reveals glottal insufficiency, fluid in the lower esophagus, frank reflux through the LES, grade B esophagitis, peptic stricture, hiatal hernia, and mild gastritis (Figure 55–2). Fingers demonstrate shiny tight skin with flexion of the distal interphalangeal joints. Multiple telangiectasia are identified on facial and limb skin. Her blood work is positive for anti-centromere antibodies and a VFSS demonstrates profound esophageal dysmotility and stasis. EAT-10 score is 26.

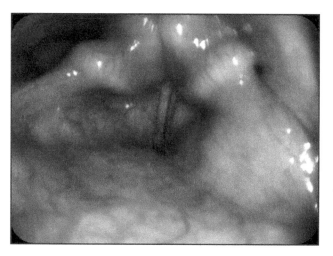

Figure 55–2. Endoscopic image of the larynx, demonstrating left vocal fold atrophy and left false vocal fold compensatory hyperadduction.

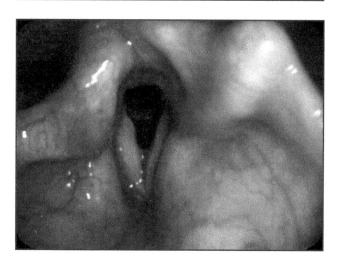

Figure 55–3. Endoscopic image of the glottis demonstrating left vocal fold atrophy with endolaryngeal mucus and inter-arytenoid edema.

Diagnosis

CREST syndrome variant of limited cutaneous systemic sclerosis and esophageal dysmotility.

Management

The patient is referred back to her rheumatologist for further systemic management of CREST syndrome with scleroderma. The patient is started on methotrexate with improvement in symptoms. Speech language therapy is involved with a tailored swallow strengthening plan, behavioral eating strategies, and body positioning. Trial of prokinetic domperidone is undertaken with only a limited response. High-resolution manometry is performed (Figure 55–3). This demonstrates severely weakened esophageal body pressures and hypotonic LES. She is scheduled for a microlaryngoscopy and bilateral vocal fold injection augmentation with balloon dilation of the peptic stricture and biopsies of the esophagus.

DIFFERENTIAL DIAGNOSIS

Systemic sclerosis may mimic several conditions, including primary esophageal motility disorders, gastroesophageal reflux disease, dyspepsia, neurodegenerative conditions (Parkinson's disease, amyotrophic lateral sclerosis, or stroke), and other autoimmune disorders (systemic lupus erythematosus, granulomatosis with polyangiitis, dermatomyositis). Diagnosis typically revolves around the combination of symptoms and blood work. Women are affected more often than men (M:F, 2:8).[1,5,12] Characteristic HRM or VFSS findings can be suggestive of SSc and associated peripheral limb and digit deformities should prompt referral to a rheumatologist for evaluation.

PITFALLS

It may be difficult to establish a firm diagnosis early in the disease course as symptoms can emerge gradually and can often be attributed to alternate diagnoses. A high index of suspicion and willingness to revisit the diagnosis of autoimmune systemic conditions causing dysphagia complaints is valuable. As these disorders affect a range of systems, it is important that they are managed in a multidisciplinary team environment. Dysphagia is a symptom, not a diagnosis, and causative factors should be sought to account for the observed changes in deglutition. This should include structural and functional esophageal evaluations to reduce the rate of false-negative evaluations.

DISCUSSION

Given that esophageal involvement is almost universal in those with SSc, complaints of swallow dysfunction and dyspepsia/reflux-type symptoms (regurgitation, bilious taste in mouth, eructation, or heartburn) may be the earliest presenting symptoms. Although GERD is far more common than SSc, the diagnosis of SSc requires consideration particularly in women between 30 and 50 years old, or those with dermatologic manifestations. Early diagnosis is important in that the condition may affect multiple organs, and systemic treatment can be effective in reducing disease burden. Clear diagnosis requires the combination of symptoms, fluoroscopic or preferentially manometric signs and metrics, alongside blood work indicating abnormal antibodies to certain cellular components. GERD coexists in SSc in up to 30% of patients (population incidence) and reports of Barrett's esophagus in as many as 37% of SSc patients.[5]

Manometry

Manometric evaluation of systemic sclerosis patients has been incorporated into the diagnostic paradigm, as it allows the distinction between the generalized disorder of SSc and the less common localized form sometimes known as morphea.[13] Further, it also distinguishes SSc from GERD or other primary esophageal motility disorders that may present with similar symptom complexes. HRM provides clear information about sphincter competence, typically revealing a hypotensive LES.[1,5,9,13] The combination of distal aperistalsis with a hypotensive LES has been termed scleroderma esophagus.[5] There is little reported on whether pharyngeal parameters are affected in SSc and, as HRM is now being applied to the pharynx and upper esophageal sphincter (UES), this information will likely emerge in the near future.[14,15]

Patient-Reported Tools

UCLA Scleroderma Clinical Trials Consortium Gastrointestinal Scale (UCLA SCTC GIT 2.0) is a multi-item symptoms scale measuring GIT complaint in SSc patients. It consists of 34 items that evaluate activity and severity of GIT involvement on seven subscales: reflux, distention/bloating, diarrhea, fecal soilage, constipation, emotional well-being, and social functioning. It is a useful marker of symptom severity and health-related quality of life. It is scored from 0 to 3 and distinguishes symptoms very mild/mild to severe/very severe. Validated in 2009, it may be used both in clinical practice and for research purposes.[16] Further, reflux and overall UCLA SCTC GIT 2.0 scores have been shown to have moderate to strong inverse correlation, with distal esophageal amplitude and resting LES pressure detected by HRM in a group of 40 patients in a recent study, suggesting that the UCLA SCTC GIT 2.0 may be a useful, non-invasive screening tool for this group of patients.[17]

The Scleroderma Assessment Questionnaire (SAQ) has also been validated to assess symptom severity and changes over time in these patients. It evaluates symptoms of vascular, respiratory, GIT, and musculoskeletal dysfunction.[18]

Other validated patient-reported tools for SSc patients are available on the website of the European League Against Rheumatism (EULAR); however, the UCLA SCTC GIT 2.0 and the SAQ are the only ones that evaluate GIT function.[19]

Multisystem Involvement

Generalized SSc requires a multidisciplinary team management approach which includes rheumatology, speech language therapy, gastroenterology, otolaryngology, pulmonology, and physiotherapy services. Supportive care, behavioral strategies, counseling, and education are important. Over time, repeated endoscopic evaluations may be needed to assess gut integrity in light of the incongruity of symptoms with esophageal damage.

Medical Therapy

A diet with food of soft consistency and small bolus sizes is easier to manage for those with reduced mouth opening secondary to fibrosis of the facial and perioral skin. Similarly, general lifestyle measures to reduce reflux are recommended. These include weight loss, avoiding large meals, maintaining an upright position for 90 minutes following meals, avoiding alcohol and tobacco, and elevating the head of the bed by 30°.

Patients with secondary Sjogren's syndrome are recommended to have meticulous oral hygiene, preferably with early consultation by an oral health specialist.

Artificial saliva and cholinergic drugs such as pilocarpine may be of benefit for dry mouth.[4]

If simple lifestyle therapy is ineffective, then pharmacotherapy may be required. In 2017, EULAR published recommendations for the treatment of SSc. These include the immunomodulatory drugs methotrexate and cyclophosphamide to treat skin and lung disease, as well as a number of drugs for treatment of Raynaud's phenomenon, digital ulcers, pulmonary arterial hypertension, scleroderma renal crisis, and SSc-related GIT disease.[20] Other immunomodulatory drugs that have shown promise in the treatment of SSc are rituximab, tocilizumab, and tumor necrosis factor antagonists, but as of yet there is insufficient evidence to support their use.[20]

Use of high dose corticosteroid can be effective for many autoimmune diseases but carries the risks attendant with long-term steroid use. Steroids are not first-line treatment for systemic sclerosis, and further caution in their use for SSc is advised, as they may be associated with scleroderma renal crisis.[20] Proton pump inhibitors (PPIs) are recommended for management of reflux and to aid in the prevention of esophageal ulcers and strictures. Prokinetics are also recommended despite a lack of strong evidence for their use. These include cisapride, erythromycin, metoclopramide, and domperidone.[4,5,20] Prokinetics have a potential cardiac side effect profile and should be used with caution, in particular cisapride, as there have been reports of cardiac arrhythmias (due to prolonged Q-T syndrome) related to its use.[20] A recent paper has described improved symptom control and manometrically increased LES pressures after 4 weeks of buspirone 20 mg daily.[20] This 5-hydroxytryptamine 1A receptor agonist was well tolerated and reduced heartburn and regurgitation symptoms significantly while increasing LES pressure and mildly increasing esophageal body pressures.[5] Further studies are required to ascertain buspirone's place in treatment.

Occasionally, patients report resolution of dysphagia solely with treatment directed at SSc,[21] but most patients require treatment for reflux disease and dysmotility. The management of these patients should be coordinated by an experienced rheumatologist.

LES Treatment

There are several surgical procedures available to address incompetent LES: Nissen or Toupet fundoplication, radiofrequency energy application (Stretta™), or even a circlet of magnets (Linx™ device). The problem in SSc is that the weakened esophageal body pressures cannot overcome increased pressure at the LES, and therefore these procedures may result in symptomatic deterioration. In fact, a recent manometric study in 8 SSc patients and 13 control subjects suggested that the SSc patients increased their LES barrier function (increased LES pressure during forced inspiration) spontaneously compared with normal adults, indicating a possible training or compensatory effect. There are few additional studies that discuss surgical outcomes in patients with SSc who have undergone anti-reflux surgery, and the results are controversial due to the concerns described above.[5,22,23] Esophageal strictures are often treated surgically with balloon or bougie dilation[4,7]; however, there is a paucity of literature reporting outcomes of this procedure in patients with SSc.

SUMMARY

Systemic sclerosis and its variant CREST syndrome are rare connective tissue disorders that profoundly affect swallowing and may present first with impairment of deglutition to otolaryngologists. A high index of suspicion is crucial in identifying these conditions, with early intervention and referral to a rheumatologist beneficial for symptom control and possibly delay in disease progression highlighting the importance of multidisciplinary cooperation. Frequent reassessment is prudent given the evolving nature of the disorders. Systematic assessment of outcomes related to interventions, prospective record keeping, and use of measurable functional outcomes is critical.

REFERENCES

1. Amos J, Baron A, Rubin AD. Autoimmune swallowing disorders. *Curr Opin Otolaryngol Head Neck Surg.* 2016;24 (6):483–488. doi:10.1097/MOO.0000000000000312
2. Paravina M, Stanojević M, Spalević L, Ljubisavljević D, Zlatanović Z, Popović D. CREST syndrome—a limited form of systemic scleroderma: a case report and literature review. *Serbian J Dermatol Venereol.* 2015;7(3):97–114. doi:10.1515/sjdv-2015-0009
3. Domsic R, Fasanella K, Bielefeldt K. Gastrointestinal manifestations of systemic sclerosis. *Dig Dis Sci.* 2008;53 (5):1163–1174. doi:10.1007/s10620-007-0018-8
4. Kumar S, Singh J, Rattan S, DiMarino AJ, Cohen S, Jimenez SA. Review article: pathogenesis and clinical man-

ifestations of gastrointestinal involvement in systemic sclerosis. *Aliment Pharmacol Ther.* 2017;45(7):883–898. doi:10.1111/apt.13963

5. Denaxas K, Ladas SD, Karamanolis GP. Evaluation and management of esophageal manifestation in systemic sclerosis. *Ann Gastroenterol,* 2018;31:165–170.

6. Sjogren RW. Gastrointestinal features of scleroderma. *Curr Opin Rheumatol.* 1996;8(6):569–575. doi:10.1097/00002281-199611000-00012

7. Gyger G, Baron M. Systemic sclerosis: gastrointestinal disease and its management. *Rheum Dis Clin North Am.* 2015;41(3):459–473. doi:10.1016/j.rdc.2015.04.007

8. Kahrilas PJ, Bredenoord AJ, Fox M, et al. The Chicago Classification of esophageal motility disorders, v3.0. *Neurogastroenterol Motil.* 2015;27(2):160–174. doi:10.1111/nmo.12477

9. Raja J, Ng CT, Sujau I, Cin KF, Sockalingam S. High-resolution oesophageal manometry and 24-hour impedance-pH study in systemic sclerosis patients: association with clinical features, symptoms and severity. *Clin Exp Rheumatol.* 2016;34:115–121.

10. Fynne L, Liao D, Aksglæde K, et al. Esophagogastric junction in systemic sclerosis: a study with the functional lumen imaging probe. *Neurogastroenterol Motil.* 2017;29(8). doi:10.1111/nmo.13073

11. Desbois AC, Cacoub P. Systemic sclerosis: an update in 2016. *Autoimmun Rev.* 2016;15(5):417–426. doi:10.1016/j.autrev.2016.01.007

12. Ji J, Sundquist J, Sundquist K. Gender-specific incidence of autoimmune diseases from national registers. *J Autoimmun.* 2016;69:102–106. doi:10.1016/j.jaut.2016.03.003

13. Arif T, Masood Q, Singh J, Hassan I. Assessment of esophageal involvement in systemic sclerosis and morphea (localized scleroderma) by clinical, endoscopic, manometric and pH metric features: a prospective comparative hospital-based study. *BMC Gastroenterol.* 2015;15(1). doi:10.1186/s12876-015-0241-2

14. Hila A, Castell JA, Castell DO. Pharyngeal and upper esophageal sphincter manometry in the evaluation of dysphagia. *J Clin Gastroenterol.* 2001;33(5):355–361. doi:10.1097/00004836-200111000-00003

15. Pinna BR, Herbella FAM, de Biase N, Vaiano TCG, Patti MG. High-resolution manometry evaluation of pressures at the pharyngo-upper esophageal area in patients with oropharyngeal dysphagia due to vagal paralysis. *Dysphagia.* 2017;32(5):657–662. doi:10.1007/s00455-017-9811-5

16. Khanna D, Hays RD, Maranian P, et al. Reliability and validity of the University of California, Los Angeles Scleroderma Clinical Trial Consortium gastrointestinal tract instrument. *Arthritis Care Res.* 2009;61(9):1257–1263. doi:10.1002/art.24730

17. Abozaid HSM, Imam HMK, Abdelaziz MM, EL-Hammady DH, Fathi NA, Furst DE. High-resolution manometry compared with the University of California, Los Angeles Scleroderma Clinical Trials Consortium GIT 2.0 in Systemic Sclerosis. *Semin Arthritis Rheum.* 2017;47(3):403–408. doi:10.1016/j.semarthrit.2017.05.005

18. Ostojic P, Damjanov N. Indices of the Scleroderma Assessment Questionnaire (SAQ) can be used to demonstrate change in patients with systemic sclerosis over time. *Jt Bone Spine.* 2008;75(3):286–290. doi:10.1016/j.jbspin.2007.06.014

19. Ingegnoli F, Carmona L, Castrejon I. Systematic review of systemic sclerosis-specific instruments for the EULAR outcome measures library: an evolutional database model of validated patient-reported outcomes. *Semin Arthritis Rheum.* 2017;46(5):609–614. doi:https://doi.org/10.1016/j.semarthrit.2016.10.002

20. Kowal-Bielecka O, Fransen J, Avouac J, et al. Update of EULAR recommendations for the treatment of systemic sclerosis. *Ann Rheum Dis.* 2017;76(8):1327–1339. doi:10.1136/annrheumdis-2016-209909

21. Rajapakse C. Pharyngoesophageal dysphagia: an under recognised, potentially fatal, but very treatable feature of systemic sclerosis. *Intern Med J.* 2016;46(11):1340–1344. doi:10.1111/imj.13243

22. Thompson JS, Langenfeld SJ, Hewlett A, et al. Surgical treatment of gastrointestinal motility disorders. *Curr Probl Surg.* 2016;53(11):503–549. doi:10.1067/j.cpsurg.2016.08.006

23. Ebert EC. Esophageal disease in progressive systemic sclerosis. *Curr Treat Options Gastroenterol.* 2008;11(1-2):157–169. doi:10.1007/s11938-008-0008-8

Index

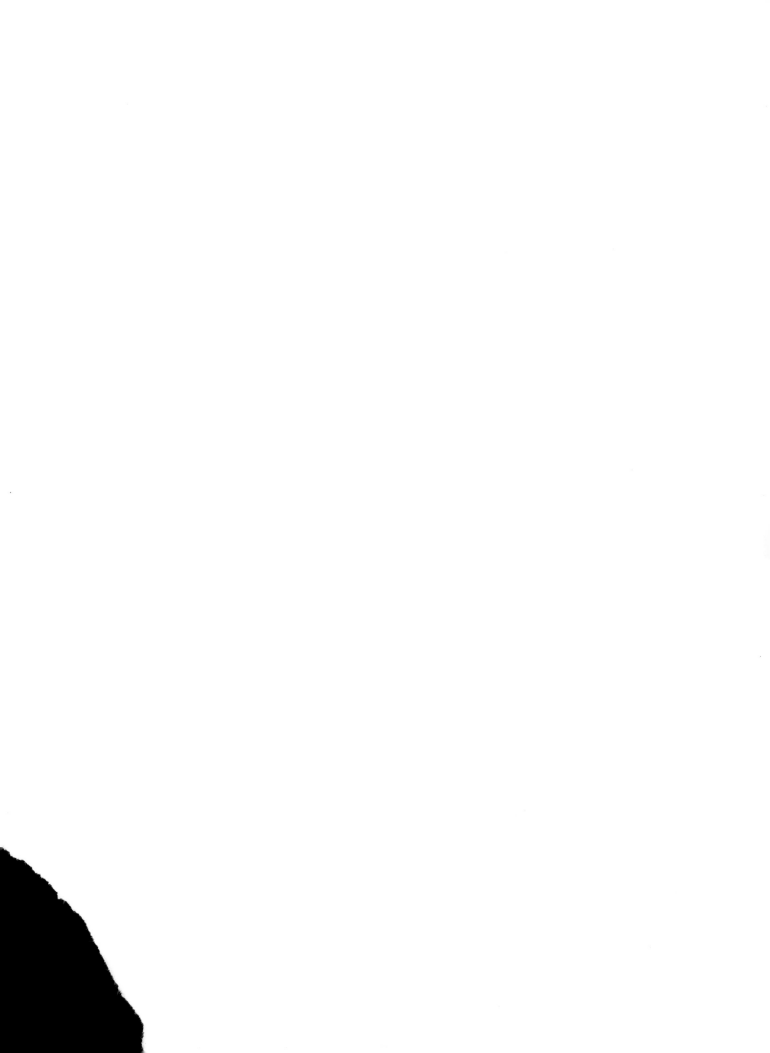